Clinical Handbook of Insulin Resistance

Clinical Handbook of
Insulin Resistance

Editor: Jessica Morris

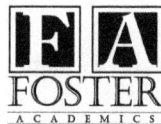

FA FOSTER
ACADEMICS

www.fosteracademics.com

www.fosteracademics.com

FA
FOSTER
ACADEMICS

Cataloging-in-Publication Data

Clinical handbook of insulin resistance / edited by Jessica Morris.
    p. cm.
Includes bibliographical references and index.
ISBN 978-1-63242-954-4
1. Insulin resistance. 2. Insulin antibodies. 3. Diabetes--Complications. 4. Diabetes clinics. I. Morris, Jessica.
RC662.4 .C55 2020
61646--dc23

Foster Academics,
118-35 Queens Blvd., Suite 400,
Forest Hills, NY 11375, USA

ISBN 978-1-63242-954-4 (Hardback)

Contents

Preface

The hormone insulin, which is produced by the beta cells of the pancreatic islets, regulates carbohydrate, fat and protein metabolism. When glucose generated due to the digestion of carbohydrate is released into the bloodstream, insulin is produced by the body. Under conditions of normal insulin reactivity, glucose is absorbed by the cells. When cells have an inhibited response to this hormone, a pathological condition known as insulin resistance occurs. Under this, excess blood sugar is not absorbed by the cells and results in symptoms such as polyphagia, polydipsia and polyuria. This is believed to occur due to a high intake of carbohydrates, mainly fructose. The diagnosis of insulin resistance is generally done by evaluating fasting insulin levels, glucose tolerance testing, hyperinsulinemic euglycemic clamp and modified insulin suppression test. Often a low carbohydrate diet and fasting helps in reversing insulin resistance. This book unravels the recent studies related to insulin resistance. It provides significant information of this condition to help develop a good understanding of its diagnosis and management. This book includes contributions of experts and scientists which will provide innovative insights into this metabolic condition.

This book has been the outcome of endless efforts put in by authors and researchers on various issues and topics within the field. The book is a comprehensive collection of significant researches that are addressed in a variety of chapters. It will surely enhance the knowledge of the field among readers across the globe.

It gives us an immense pleasure to thank our researchers and authors for their efforts to submit their piece of writing before the deadlines. Finally in the end, I would like to thank my family and colleagues who have been a great source of inspiration and support.

Editor

Common Genetic Variation in the Human *CTF1* Locus, Encoding Cardiotrophin-1, Determines Insulin Sensitivity

Stefan Z. Lutz[1,2,3]**, Olga Franck**[1]**, Anja Böhm**[1,2,3]**, Jürgen Machann**[2,3,4]**, Fritz Schick**[2,3,4]**, Fausto Machicao**[2,3]**, Andreas Fritsche**[1,2,3,5]**, Hans-Ulrich Häring**[1,2,3]*****, Harald Staiger**[1,2,3]

1 Department of Internal Medicine, Division of Endocrinology, Diabetology, Vascular Disease, Nephrology and Clinical Chemistry, University of Tübingen, Tübingen, Germany, 2 Institute for Diabetes Research and Metabolic Diseases of the Helmholtz Centre Munich at the University of Tübingen, Tübingen, Germany, 3 German Centre for Diabetes Research (DZD), Tübingen, Germany, 4 Department of Diagnostic and Interventional Radiology, Section on Experimental Radiology, Eberhard Karls University Tübingen, Tübingen, Germany, 5 Department of Internal Medicine, Division of Nutritional and Preventive Medicine, University of Tübingen, Tübingen, Germany

Abstract

Aims/Hypothesis: Recently, cardiotrophin-1, a member of the interleukin-6 family of cytokines was described to protect beta-cells from apoptosis, to improve glucose-stimulated insulin secretion and insulin resistance, and to prevent streptozotocin-induced diabetes in mice. Here, we studied whether common single nucleotide polymorphisms (SNPs) in the *CTF1* locus, encoding cardiotrophin-1, influence insulin secretion and insulin sensitivity in humans.

Methods: We genotyped 1,771 German subjects for three *CTF1* tagging SNPs (rs1046276, rs1458201, and rs8046707). The subjects were metabolically characterized by an oral glucose tolerance test. Subgroups underwent magnetic resonance (MR) imaging/spectroscopy and hyperinsulinaemic-euglycaemic clamps.

Results: After appropriate adjustment, the minor allele of *CTF1* SNP rs8046707 was significantly associated with decreased *in vivo* measures of insulin sensitivity. The other tested SNPs were not associated with OGTT-derived sensitivity parameters, nor did the three tested SNPs show any association with OGTT-derived parameters of insulin release. In the MR subgroup, SNP rs8046707 was nominally associated with lower visceral adipose tissue. Furthermore, the SNP rs1458201 showed a nominal association with increased VLDL levels.

Conclusions: In conclusion, this study, even though preliminary and awaiting further confirmation by independent replication, provides first evidence that common genetic variation in *CTF1* could contribute to insulin sensitivity in humans. Our SNP data indicate an insulin-desensitizing effect of cardiotrophin-1 and underline that cardiotrophin-1 represents an interesting target to influence insulin sensitivity.

Editor: Juergen Eckel, GDC, Germany

Funding: The study was supported in part by a grant (01GI0925) from the German Federal Ministry of Education and Research (BMBF) to the German Centre for Diabetes Research (DZD e.V.). The funders had no role in study design, data collection and analysis, decision to publish, or preparation of the manuscript. Furthermore, we acknowledge the support by the Deutsche Forschungsgemeinschaft and the Open Access Publishing Fund of the University of Tübingen.

Competing Interests: The authors have declared that no competing interests exist.

* Email: hans-ulrich.haering@med.uni-tuebingen.de

Introduction

Diabetes, which is characterized by chronic hyperglycaemia, occurs either by developing insulin resistance and/or by beta-cell failure. Possible trigger for both are cytokines, which may be produced by the liver (hepatokines), skeletal muscle (myokines), or adipose tissue (adipokines). Beyond a large number of cytokines which have been shown to be involved as mediators in cellular insulin resistance and beta-cell failure often under inflammatory conditions, other cytokines are reported to exert beneficial effects with regard to improved glucose tolerance and insulin sensitivity [1–3].

Cardiotrophin-1 (CT-1) is a member of the interleukin-6 (IL-6) family of cytokines with a molecular mass of 21.5 kDa, which interacts with the glycoprotein 130 (gp130)/leukaemia inhibitory factor receptor (LIFR) heterodimer [4]. CT-1 was originally isolated from cardiac tissue and first described by its ability to protect cardiomyocytes from apoptosis but also to induce cardiac hypertrophy [5].

In several previous *in vitro* and mouse studies, CT-1 was shown to exert an important role in glucose and lipid metabolism. CT-1 knockout mice display mature-onset obesity, insulin resistance, and hypercholesterolemia. Moreover, recombinant CT-1 treatment corrected insulin resistance and reduced adiposity in ob/ob and high-fat diet (HFD) receiving mice, pointing to a key regulatory role of CT-1 in glucose and lipid metabolism [6]. Beside regenerative and anti-apoptotic functions in several tissues, e.g. motoneurons and hepatocytes [7,8], in a recent study, CT-1 was reported to protect beta cells from apoptosis and to enhance glucose-stimulated insulin secretion, and additionally, to prevent streptozotocin-induced diabetes in a mouse model [9].

Some members of the IL-6 family like ciliary neurotrophic factor (CNTF) have been shown to improve insulin resistance and glucose tolerance by activating skeletal muscle AMPK [10].

Moreover, in a recent study, CT-1 was also referred to stimulate the oxidative metabolism through phosphorylation and activation of AMPK [6]. Thus, CT-1 is involved in AMPK signalling and represents a conceivable trigger for a cytokine-mediated improvement of insulin sensitivity and/or beta-cell survival and function.

These mouse and in vitro studies point to an important involvement of CT-1 in improving insulin secretion and insulin sensitivity. For this reason, and because of its high expression in tissues that play a pivotal role in the pathogenesis of type 2 diabetes like beta-cells, skeletal muscle and liver [6,8,9], the CT-1 gene (CTF1) would be a promising candidate to associate with diabetes, insulin secretion and insulin sensitivity. Thus, we asked whether genetic variation within or near CTF1 has an impact on insulin secretion and insulin sensitivity in humans. To this end, we assessed in 1,771 German individuals at increased risk for type 2 diabetes, recruited from the Tübingen family (TÜF) study for type 2 diabetes, whether common single nucleotide polymorphisms (SNPs) with minor allele frequencies (MAFs) ≥ 0.05 tagging the human CTF1 locus associate with prediabetic traits. Our data support a robust association of the CTF1 SNP rs8046707 with insulin sensitivity in humans.

Materials and Methods

Ethics statement

The protocol of the study adhered to the Declaration of Helsinki and was approved by the local ethics board (Ethics Committee of the Medical Faculty of the Eberhard Karls University Tübingen). From all participants, informed written consent to the study was obtained.

Subjects

An overall study group of 1,771 White European individuals from Southern Germany was recruited from the ongoing Tübingen Family study for type 2 diabetes (TÜF). This study group currently encompasses more than 2,700 participants at increased risk for type 2 diabetes (i.e., diagnosis of impaired fasting glycaemia, obesity, family history of type 2 diabetes, and/or previous gestational diabetes) [11]. All participants underwent the standard procedures of the protocol: assessment of medical history, routine blood analyses, alcohol and smoking status, physical examination, and oral glucose tolerance tests (OGTTs). The subjects were not on medication known to affect glucose tolerance, insulin sensitivity, or insulin secretion. 41 subjects were on lipid-lowering drugs (37 on statins, one on fibrates, two on ezetrol, and one on a combination of statins, fibrates, and ezetrol). From the overall study group, a subgroup of 312 subjects agreed to undergo magnetic resonance (MR) imaging and spectroscopy and another subgroup of 443 subjects a hyperinsulinaemic-euglycaemic clamp procedure. The clinical characteristics of the overall study group, the MR and the clamp subgroups are presented in Table 1.

OGTT

A standard 75-g OGTT was performed after a 10 h-overnight fast. For the determination of plasma glucose, insulin, C-peptide, and free fatty acid (FFA) concentrations, venous blood samples were taken at time-points 0, 30, 60, 90, and 120 min [11].

Hyperinsulinaemic-euglycaemic clamp

In subjects who agreed to undergo the hyperinsulinaemic-euglycaemic clamp, the clamp procedure was started after the 10-h overnight fast. The subjects received a primed infusion of insulin $(40 \text{ mU}^*\text{m}^{-2}*\text{min}^{-1})$ for 120 min, and glucose infusion was started to clamp the plasma glucose concentration at 5.5 mmol/

L. For the measurement of plasma glucose, venous blood samples were drawn in 5-min intervals. Plasma insulin levels were determined at baseline and in the steady state of the clamp [11].

Measurements of body fat content and body fat distribution

Waist circumference was measured in the upright position at the midpoint between the lateral iliac crest and the lowest rib (in cm). Body mass index (BMI) was determined as weight divided by height squared (kg/m²). In addition, the percentage of body fat was measured by bioelectrical impedance (BIA-101, RJL systems, Detroit, MI, USA). Total and visceral adipose tissue (TAT, VAT) contents were determined by whole-body MR imaging (% of body weight) [12]. The intrahepatic lipid content was determined by localized STEAM ¹H-MR spectroscopy, as described earlier (% of signal) [13].

Laboratory measurements

Plasma glucose was measured using a bedside glucose analyzer (glucose oxidase method, Yellow Springs Instruments, Yellow Springs, OH, USA) (mmol/L). Plasma insulin and C-peptide concentrations were measured by commercial chemiluminescence assays for ADVIA Centaur (Siemens Medical Solutions, Fernwald, Germany) (both pmol/L). Total-, high-density lipoprotein (HDL)-, and low-density lipoprotein (LDL)-cholesterol, and triglycerides were measured using the ADVIA 1800 clinical chemical analyzer. FFA concentrations were determined with an enzymatic method (WAKO Chemicals, Neuss, Germany).

Selection of tagging SNPs

Based on publicly available phase III data of the International HapMap Project derived from Utah residents with Central European ancestry (release #28 August 2010, http://hapmap.ncbi.nlm.nih.gov/index.html.en), we screened in silico the complete CTF1 gene spanning 6.953 kb (3 exons, 2 introns) on human chromosome 16p11.2 as well as 3 and 5 kb of its 5'- and 3'-flanking regions, respectively (Figure 1). Within this genomic locus, four informative SNPs with MAFs ≥ 0.05 (according to HapMap) were present: rs1046276 (C/T), rs1458201 (C/T), rs8046707 (G/A), and rs11649653 (C/G). The HapMap linkage disequilibrium (r^2) data of these four common SNPs are schematically presented in Figure 1. Except SNP rs1046276, that is located in the 3'-untranslated region of exon 3, all SNPs reside in the 3'-flanking region of the gene. Since rs11649653 and rs8046707 were in complete linkage ($r^2 = 1.0$) according to HapMap, only SNPs rs8046707, rs1046276, and rs1458201 were genotyped and further analyzed.

Genotyping

In the TÜF study, DNA was isolated from the whole blood using a commercial DNA isolation kit (NucleoSpin, Macherey & Nagel, Düren, Germany). The three CTF1 tagging SNPs were genotyped using the Sequenom mass ARRAY system with iPLEX software (Sequenom, Hamburg, Germany). The genotyping success rates were $\geq 99.8\%$. The Sequenom and TaqMan assays were validated by bidirectional sequencing in 50 randomly selected subjects, and both methods gave 100% identical results.

Calculations

HOMA-IR was calculated as: $c(\text{glucose}[\text{mmol/L}])_0 * c(\text{insulin}[\text{mU/L}])_0$, c = concentration [14]. The insulin sensitivity index derived from the OGTT (ISI OGTT) was calculated as formerly reported: $10,000/\{c(\text{glucose}[\text{mmol/L}])_0 * c(\text{insulin}[\text{pmol/L}])_0 *$

Table 1. Clinical characteristics of the study groups.

	Overall study group	MR subgroup	ISI clamp subgroup
Sample size (N)	1,771	312	443
Women/men (%)	66.3/33.7	60.6/39.4	54.2/45.8
Age (y)	40±13	46±12	40±12
BMI (kg/m^2)	29.9±8.9	29.9±5.1	27.4±5.6
Body fat (%)	28.6±9.7	32.7±8.7	28.6±9.7
Waist circumference (cm)	95.5±18.6	97.3±13.4	92.5±15.0
Fasting glucose (mmol/L)	5.15±0.53	5.26±0.50	5.02±0.54
Glucose 120 min OGTT (mmol/L)	6.36±1.61	6.93±1.57	6.22±1.70
Fasting insulin (pmol/L)	69.7±57.4	64.6±42.7	53.6±38.8
HOMA-IR (*10^{-6} mol*U*L^{-2})	2.73±2.41	2.55±1.82	2.05±1.65
ISI OGTT (*10^{15} L^2*mol^{-2})	15.2±10.4	12.4±6.8	18.1±11.5
ISI Clamp (10^{*6} L*kg^{-1}*min^{-1})	–	–	0.085±0.054
HOMA-B (U*mol^{-1})	144.5±119.3	126.8±80.8	124.9±102.1
AUC$_{Ins\ 0-30}$/AUC$_{Glc0-30}$ OGTT (*10^{-9})	45.0±32.7	42.9±27.7	37.3±24.2
AUC$_{C-Peptid\ 0-120}$/AUC$_{Glc\ 0-120}$ OGTT (*10^{-9})	318.7±103.3	307.1±90.9	310.7±97.7
Fasting FFA (µmol/L)	585.2±247.6	656.3±267.3	577.6±257.6
AUC$_{FFA}$ (µmol/l)	480.9±214.4	526.6±186.6	452.0±197.7
Fasting triglycerides (mg/dL)[a]	119.0±78.2	124.4±98.5	114.4±88.6
Total cholesterol (mg/dL)[a]	192±37	194±36	191±36
LDL-cholesterol (mg/dL)[a]	118±33	122±30	118±31
HDL-cholesterol (mg/dL)[a]	54±14	52±13	56±15
Body fat (%)	32.8±12.1	32.7±8.7	28.6±9.7
Total adipose tissue (% BW)	–	30.2±9.0	–
Visceral adipose tissue (% BW)	–	3.32±1.71	–
Intrahepatic lipids (%)	–	5.97±6.51	–

Data are given as counts, percentages, or means ±SD. AUC - area under the curve; BMI - body mass index; BW - body weight; Glc - glucose; HOMA-IR - homeostasis model assessment of insulin resistance; Ins - insulin; ISI - insulin sensitivity index; MR - magnetic resonance; OGTT - oral glucose tolerance test; FFA - free fatty acid.
[a]Available in 1,628 participants of the overall study group.

$c(glucose[mmol/L])_{mean}*c(insulin[pmol/L])mean\}^{1/2}$ [15]. The insulin sensitivity index derived from the hyperinsulinaemic-euglycaemic clamp (ISI clamp) was determined as glucose infusion rate to maintain euglycaemia during the last 20 min of the clamp (steady state) ($\mu mol*kg^{-1}*min^{-1}$) divided by the steady-state insulin concentration (pmol/L). HOMA-B was calculated as: $\{20* \quad c(insulin[mU/L])_0\}/\{c(glucose[mmol/L])_0-3.5\}$. The OGTT-derived insulin release was calculated by $AUC_{Ins\ 0-30}$/$AUC_{Glc\ 0-30}$ and $AUC_{C-Pep\ 0-120}$/$AUC_{Glc\ 0-120}$, Ins = insulin (pmol/L), C-Pep = C-peptide (pmol/L), Glc = glucose (mmol/L). $AUC_{Ins\ 0-30}$/$AUC_{Glc\ 0-30}$ was calculated as: $\{c(insulin)_0+c(insulin)_{30}\}/\{c(glucose)_0+c(glucose)_{30}$. $AUC_{C-Pep\ 0-120}$/$AUC_{Glc\ 0-120}$ was calculated by the trapezoid method: $½\{½c(C-peptide)_0+ c(C-peptide)_{30}+c(C-peptide)_{60}+c(C-peptide)_{90}+½c(C-peptide)_{120}\}/½\{½c(glucose)_0+c(glucose)_{30}+ c(glucose)_{60}+c(glucose)_{90}+ ½c(glucose)_{120}\}$. Both $AUC_{Ins\ 0-30}$/$AUC_{Glc\ 0-30}$ and $AUC_{C-Pep\ 0-120}$/$AUC_{Glc\ 0-120}$ were found to be superior to fasting state or OGTT-derived parameters for genetically determined beta-cell failure [16].

Statistical analyses

Hardy-Weinberg equilibrium was tested by χ^2 test. Linkage disequilibrium data (r^2) between the SNPs were obtained with MIDAS 1.0 (http://www.genes.org.uk/software/midas). All con-

tinuous variables not normally distributed were $\log_e$-transformed prior to regression analysis. Multiple linear regression analysis was performed using the least-squares method with the trait of interest (measure of body fat content/distribution, glycaemia, insulin secretion, insulin sensitivity, or plasma lipid) as dependent variable, the SNP genotype (in the additive inheritance model) as independent variable, and gender, age, BMI, and insulin sensitivity as confounding variables where applicable. Based on the three non-linked SNPs tested, a p-value <0.0170 was considered statistically significant according to Bonferroni correction for multiple comparisons ($\alpha_{corrected} = 1-0.95^{1/N}$ with N = number of null hypotheses). We did not correct for the tested traits of interest since these were not considered as independent. The analyses were performed with the statistical software package JMP 8.0 (SAS Institute, Cary, NC, USA). In the dominant inheritance model, our overall study cohort was sufficiently powered ($\alpha<0.05$; $1-\beta\geq 0.8$) to detect effect sizes ≥ 0.13 (Cohen's d). Power calculations were performed using G*power 3.0 software available at http://www.psycho.uni-duesseldorf.de/aap/projects/gpower/.

Results

Clinical characteristics of the study groups

The overall population derived from the TÜF study consisted of 1,771 relatively young (median age 40 y) non-diabetic White

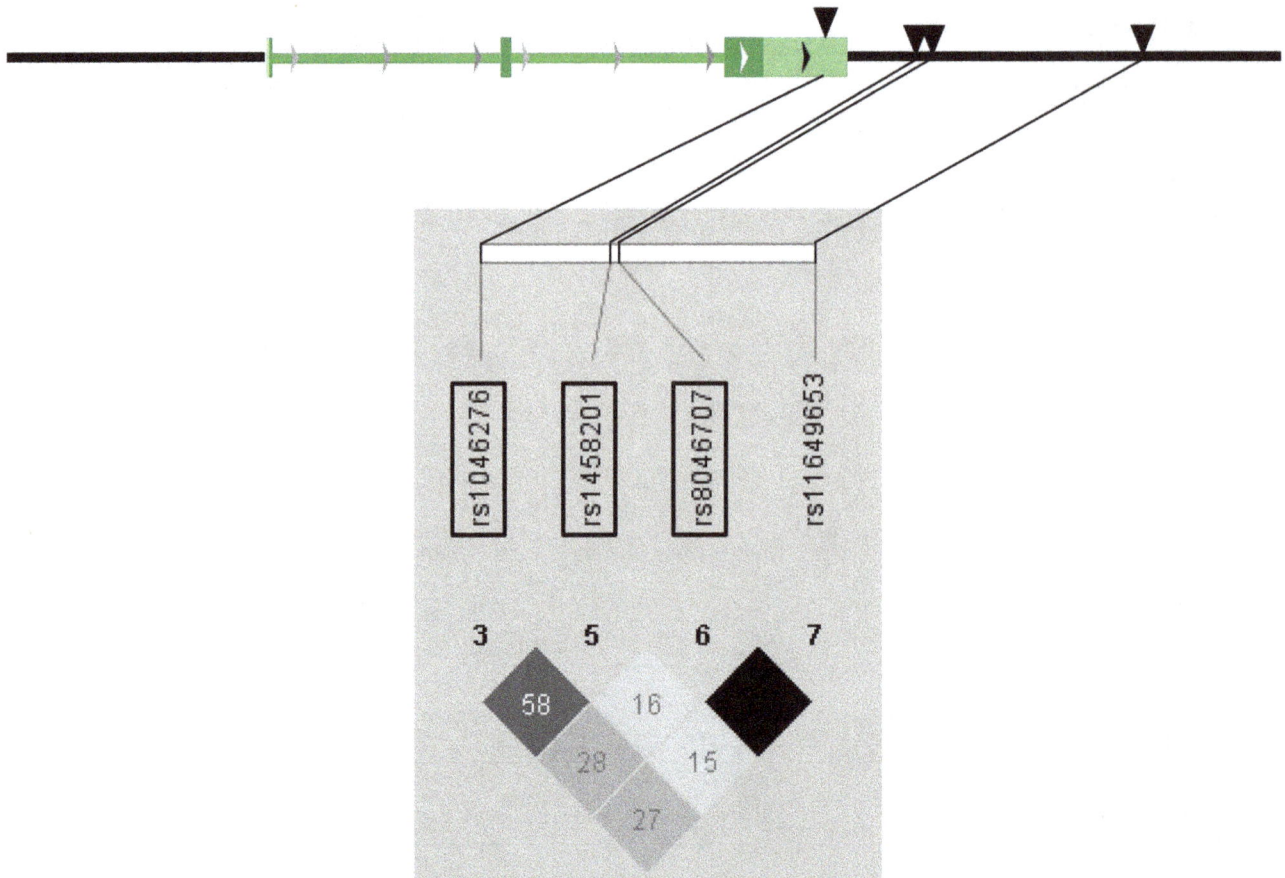

Figure 1. Genomic region of human chromosome 16p11.2 harbouring the *CTF1* gene and HapMap linkage disequilibrium (r²) data of common (MAF≥0.05) informative SNPs within this region. The *CTF1* gene consists of three exons and two introns and spans 6.953 kb from nucleotide 30,815,429 to nucleotide 30,822,381 (HapMap coordinates). The analyzed region additionally included 3 kb of the 5'-flanking region and 5 kb of the 3'-flanking region. The genotyped SNPs are highlighted by black frames. In the diamonds below the SNPs, r² values are given (black diamonds: r² = 1.0).

European subjects with a median BMI of 29.9 kg/m². Two thirds were women, one third men. The majority (~71%) of the subjects were normal glucose tolerant (NGT), ~29% were prediabetic: 11.2% had isolated impaired fasting glycaemia (IFG), 9.6% isolated impaired glucose tolerance (IGT), and 8.2% both IFG and IGT. The clinical characteristics of the overall population, MR and ISI clamp subgroups were largely comparable and given in Table 1. Though, the ISI clamp subgroup was somewhat more insulin-sensitive.

Genotyping of *CTF1* tagging SNPs

The 1,771 study participants were genotyped for the SNPs rs1046276, rs1458201, and rs8046707 covering all common genetic variation in the *CTF1* gene locus with MAF ≥0.05 (Figure 1). All SNPs were in Hardy-Weinberg equilibrium (p≥0.1 all). The observed MAFs were 0.25 (rs1458201), 0.36 (rs1046276), and 0.41 (rs8046707) and were comparable to those provided by HapMap for the CEU population (0.21, 0.33, and 0.40, respectively). As expected from the HapMap data (Figure 1), the observed genetic linkage between the three SNPs was modest with r² = 0.60 for the linkage between rs1046276 and rs1458201, r² = 0.38 between rs1046276 and rs8046707, and r² = 0.23 between rs1458201 and rs8046707.

Genetic associations of *CTF1* with body fat content and body fat distribution

After adjustment for gender and age, none of the three tagging SNPs showed significant association (p>0.1) with parameters of body fat content (BMI, bioelectrical impedance-derived percentage of body fat, MR imaging-derived TAT) or body fat distribution (waist circumference, MR imaging-derived VAT, MR spectroscopy-derived intrahepatic lipids). After identical adjustment, the minor A-allele of SNP rs8046707 was nominally associated with reduced VAT (Table S1, p = 0.044).

Genetic associations of *CTF1* with insulin sensitivity and glycaemia

We then asked whether *CTF1* SNPs are associated with insulin sensitivity and/or glycaemia. After adjustment for gender, age and BMI, the minor A-allele of SNP rs8046707 was significantly associated with increased HOMA-IR (p = 0.013) and decreased ISI OGTT (p = 0.008) revealing an insulin-desensitizing effect of this allele (Figure 2 and Table 2). The SNP revealed effect sizes of 4.6% on HOMA-IR and -5.1% on ISI OGTT per allele. None of the other tested SNPs showed associations with insulin sensitivity and/or glycaemia (p>0.1).

A

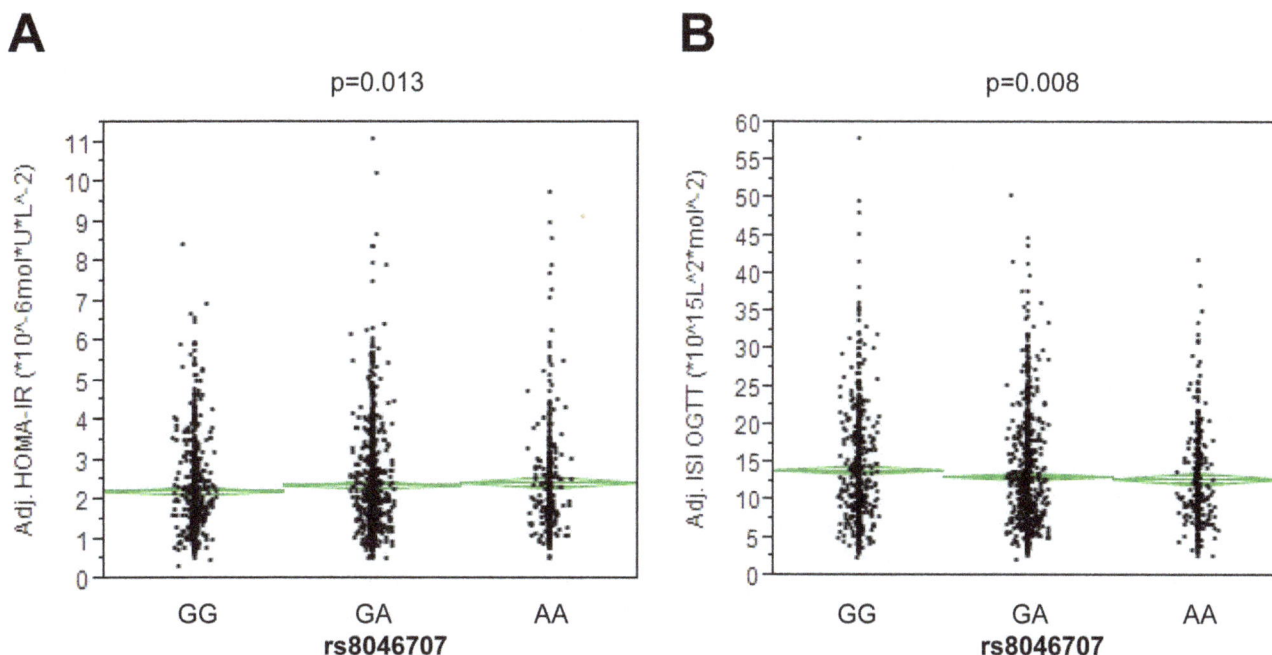

B

Figure 2. Association of SNP rs8046707 with HOMA-IR (A) and ISI OGTT (B). Data were adjusted for gender, age, and BMI. Diamonds represents means ± SE. HOMA-IR – homeostasis model assessment of insulin resistance; ISI OGTT – oral glucose tolerance test-derived insulin sensitivity index. SNP – single nucleotide polymorphism.

Genetic associations of *CTF1* with insulin release

After adjustment of gender, age, BMI and ISI OGTT, none of the tagging SNPs was significantly or nominally associated with OGTT-derived parameters of insulin release (p>0.3) as given in Table S2.

Genetic associations of *CTF1* with indices of lipid metabolism

From 1,628 subjects of the overall group, quantitative measurements of triglycerides (TG), total-, LDL-, and HDL-cholesterol were available. The number of the subjects receiving lipid-lowering drugs is denoted in the Materials and Methods section. An additional adjustment for the drug classes by introducing appropriate dummy variables in the regression models was carried out. In our study, the minor T-allele of SNP rs1458201 was nominally associated with increased VLDL levels (p = 0.024) (Table S3).

Interrogation of MAGIC data for replication

We screened the MAGIC data from 37,037 non-diabetic subjects of European descent (HOMA-IR dataset) to replicate the effects of SNP rs8046707 on HOMA-IR [17]. However, SNP rs8046707 was not depicted on the arrays used by MAGIC. Therefore, we looked for proxies for SNP rs8046707 to investigate whether they show associations with fasting insulin and HOMA-IR. Using SNAP (http://www.broadinstitute.org/mpg/snap/ldsearch.php), we found two proxies, rs11649653 ($r^2 = 0.967$) and rs4889603 ($r^2 = 0.870$). They showed no significant association with fasting insulin (p = 0.262 and p = 0.285, respectively) or HOMA-IR (p = 0.171 and p = 0.196, respectively). Two other proxies, rs12917722 and rs11640961, were not depicted on the arrays.

Discussion

Up to now, several different studies tried to highlight the role of CT-1 with regard to metabolic disorders *in vitro* as well as *in vivo*, both in murine models and in humans. Among a variety of metabolic and cytoprotective activities reported so far, CT-1 has been shown to play an important protective role in beta-cell viability and to improve glucose-stimulated insulin secretion, and moreover, to prevent streptozotocin-induced diabetes in mice [9]. In addition, recombinant CT-1 treatment corrected insulin resistance and reduced adiposity in ob/ob and high-fat diet receiving mice, pointing to a key regulatory role of CT-1 in insulin sensitivity and lipid metabolism [6].

In this study, we report a significant insulin-desensitizing effect of the minor A-allele of *CTF1* SNP rs8046707. After adjustment for gender, age and BMI, the minor A-allele of SNP rs8046707 was significantly associated with increased HOMA-IR and reduced ISI OGTT. However, we could not confirm these results in the ISI clamp subgroup, as there was no association either of the SNP rs8046707 or of the other two analyzed common variants with hyperinsulinaemic-euglycaemic clamp-derived insulin sensitivity parameters. One possible reason for this discrepancy may be due to the limited sample size of this subgroup. Of interest, the ISI clamp subgroup showed somewhat higher insulin sensitivity compared to the overall group, so that a possible selection bias can not be excluded. We hypothesize that the more insulin sensitive subgroup possess protective compensatory mechanisms to counteract the adverse effects of the minor A-allele of *CTF1* SNP rs8046707, while the more insulin resistant overall group may lack these compensatory mechanisms. Otherwise, ISI clamp-derived parameters mainly reflect skeletal muscle specific insulin sensitivity, whereas elevated HOMA-IR is commonly due to hepatic insulin resistance. Hence, the isolated detection of reduced insulin sensitivity by HOMA-IR and ISI OGTT, without corresponding alterations in ISI clamp-derived indices, could reflect a selective

Table 2. Associations between CTF1 SNPs and glycaemia and insulin sensitivity.

	Genotype	N overall	Fasting glc (mmol/L)	120 min glc OGTT (mmol/L)	AUC glc (mmol/L)	Fasting ins (pmol/L)	HOMA-IR ($*10^{-6}$ mol$*$U$*$L^{-2})	ISI, OGTT ($*10^{15}$ L^{2*}mol^{-2})	N subgroup	ISI clamp (10^{-6} L$*$kg$^{-1}*$min^{-1})
rs1046276	CC	732	5.16±0.54	6.34±1.64	14.88±3.21	70.73±57.91	2.79±2.45	14.82±10.19	182	0.087±0.057
	CT	794	5.14±0.52	6.39±1.60	14.76±3.05	69.33±57.33	2.71±2.37	15.24±10.52	185	0.083±0.052
	TT	245	5.11±0.56	6.35±1.57	14.70±3.01	68.05±56.29	2.67±2.40	15.86±10.87	76	0.085±0.051
P_{add}	-	-	0.325	0.502	0.555	0.325	0.104	0.11	-	0.392
rs1458201	CC	988	5.16±0.54	6.36±1.65	14.85±3.19	69.75±56.69	2.75±2.40	15.01±10.25	240	0.084±0.054
	CT	666	5.12±0.51	6.34±1.56	14.67±3.01	69.76±58.39	2.71±2.37	15.36±10.74	171	0.085±0.052
	TT	117	5.18±0.58	6.55±1.58	15.11±3.01	69.39±58.26	2.79±2.65	15.25±10.19	32	0.088±0.060
P_{add}	-	-	0.459	0.371	0.989	0.459	0.453	0.464	-	0.875
rs8046707	GG	624	5.13±0.56	6.34±1.60	14.67±3.09	68.43±56.85	2.68±2.40	15.72±10.75	171	0.083±0.049
	GA	858	5.16±0.50	6.43±1.62	14.87±3.02	70.93±57.76	2.78±2.40	14.76±10.39	189	0.086±0.058
	AA	289	5.15±0.59	6.21±1.61	14.86±3.44	68.98±57.64	2.71±2.45	15.10±9.80	83	0.085±0.053
P_{add}	-	-	0.347	0.945	0.122	0.347	**0.013***	**0.008***	-	0.414

Data represents means ± SD. Prior to statistical analysis, glucose concentrations and insulin sensitivity measures were adjusted for gender, age and BMI. Nominal associations marked by bold fonts. AUC - area under the curve; glc - glucose; HOMA-IR - homeostasis model assessment of insulin resistance; ins - insulin; ISI - insulin sensitivity index; OGTT - oral glucose tolerance test.

hepatic insulin resistance in minor A-allele carriers of SNP rs8046707. Thus, both in the overall study group and the ISI clamp subgroup neither fasting glucose nor fasting insulin were associated with *CTF1* variations. It would be interesting to carry out further replications of our results in larger comparably phenotyped study populations.

Our finding that the *CTF1* SNP rs8046707 determines insulin sensitivity, appears in good agreement with previous *in vitro* and *in vivo* mouse studies, reporting on CT-1 mediated enhanced insulin signaling in muscle and adipocyte and an amelioration of insulin resistance in obese mice after chronic administration of CT-1 [6]. Asrih et al. reported a concentration-dependent dual effect of CT-1 on insulin-stimulated glucose transport in cardiomyocytes, with stimulated glucose transport at high concentrations CT-1 (10 nM) and inhibited glucose transport at low concentrations (1 nM), also pointing to an involvement of CT-1 in insulin sensitivity [18]. The first finding at low CT-1 concentrations was proposed to be due to a reduction of GLUT-4 expression and, concomitantly, reduced insulin signaling due to enhanced SOCS-3 expression, whereas this inhibitory mechanism seemed to be overridden at high CT-1 concentrations.

Several members of the IL-6 family like ciliary neurotrophic factor (CNTF) have been shown to improve insulin resistance and glucose tolerance by activating skeletal muscle AMPK [10] and further, in a recent study, CT-1 itself was also found to stimulate the oxidative metabolism through phosphorylation and activation of AMPK [6]. Interestingly, an insulin-independent effect of CT-1 on glucose uptake is likely, based on the study mentioned before, showing an AMPK activation through calmodulin-dependent kinase II after exposure to high concentrations of CT-1 [18], but also on the study reported by Chopra et al. demonstrating AMPK to phosphorylate the insulin receptor independently of insulin [19]. Hence, CT-1 is involved in AMPK signalling and, in agreement with our data, it may represent a conceivable trigger for a cytokine-mediated improvement of insulin sensitivity.

On the other hand, several previous *in vitro* and *in vivo* reports demonstrate also an involvement of CT-1 in insulin sensitivity, though, a deleterious effect of CT-1 on the development of insulin resistance [20]. Moreover, some studies point to a positive correlation between upregulation of CT-1 and impaired fasting glucose (IFG), hyperglycemia, newly diagnosed DM or obesity [21–23]. As already mentioned, CT-1 may exert opposite effects in insulin stimulated glucose uptake depending on the CT-1 concentration [18]. As previously discussed [24], based on mouse studies, elevated CT-1 plasma levels in obesity may represent a potential protective way to antagonize the deleterious metabolic dysregulations. For the moment, it is unclear whether CT-1 exerts similar biochemical features in humans and in mice, and this could be a possible explanation for the different results regarding insulin sensitivity between the mentioned studies above.

Surprisingly, our findings with regard to insulin release do not support the previous mouse study results of Jiménez-Gonzales, who reported CT-1 to protect beta cells from apoptosis and to enhance glucose-stimulated insulin release [9]. In our study, we didnt find an impact of the three investigated *CTF1* SNPs on insulin secretion. One possible explanation might be a smaller impact of *CTF1* polymorphisms in humans on CT-1 plasma levels compared to the used CT-1 concentrations in the *in vitro* experiments. In addition, perhaps more relevantly, a germline knockout mouse with potentially massive genetic variation may display a diverse phenotype than humans with expectedly weaker alterations due to common variations in the *CTF1* gene.

Beside significant associations with insulin sensitivity markers, we also found a nominal association between reduced VAT and

SNP rs8046707 (p = 0.044). Up to now, several groups reported an impact of CT-1 on obesity. In a previous study, recombinant CT-1 reversed obesity, due to reduction of fat stores and remodeling of white adipose tissue, insulin resistance and DM in *ob/ob* and high-fat diet fed mice, related to an increase in energy expenditure and decreased food intake [6]. However, because of the weak nominal association, without achieving significance after Bonferroni correction, and moreover, because of the controversy, that the minor A-allele of SNP rs8046707, which associates with significantly reduced insulin sensitivity in our study, was concomitantly nominally associated with decreased VAT, we think that this result may represent a chance finding due to the limited number of subjects included in the MR subgroup needing further replication in larger study populations.

Although CT-1 was reported to be upregulated in human and murine steatotic livers and, chronic CT-1 treatment to reverse hepatic steatosis in obese mice after AMPK activation [25], we could not detect any involvement of the three SNPs in intrahepatic lipid content. Finally, in our study, SNP rs1458201 showed a nominal association with increased VLDL levels. With regard to the small study population used for this measurement, this result should be replicated in a similarly well characterized study population.

A limitation of the study could be the comparatively small number of subjects included in the ISI clamp subgroup, for which reason we probably could not confirm the significant HOMA-IR- and ISI OGTT-associations with SNP rs8046707, as found in the overall study group. Furthermore, only relatively young (median age 40 y) White European subjects were included in this study, so that the impact of *CTF1* SNPs on insulin sensitivity and other related metabolic traits in elderly or other ethnical groups is not assessable based on this study. In addition, due to the limited number of participants of the TÜF study, only common variants with MAFs ≥0.05 were analyzed, so that additional rare SNPs with direct effect on CT-1 may exist. Finally, we could not replicate our results in the MAGIC dataset (using two closely linked SNPs as proxies), which may have several reasons. First, the HOMA-IR data from the 37,037 non-diabetic subjects were not adjusted for BMI, as compared to our data. Second, the MAGIC dataset is a result of meta-analyses of 21 genome-wide association studies, with a considerable heterogeneity, e.g., with respect to age of the participants.

In conclusion, the present study indicates that the *CTF1* gene, encoding the cytokine cardiotrophin-1, could be involved in the control of insulin sensitivity in humans. This cytokine therefore represents a promising target to influence insulin resistant states in diabetes.

Supporting Information

Table S1 Associations between CTF1 SNPs and parameters of body fat content/distribution. Data represents means±SD. Prior to statistical analysis, all measures were adjusted for gender and age. Nominal associations marked by bold fonts. BMI - body mass index; Waist - waist circumference; TAT - total adipose tissue; VAT - visceral adipose tissue; IHL - intrahepatic lipids.

Table S2 Associations between CTF1 SNPs and insulin secretion. Data represents means±SD. Prior to statistical analysis, indices of insulin secretion were adjusted for gender, age, BMI and ISI OGTT. AUC - area under the curve; Glc - glucose; Ins - insulin; HOMA-B - homeostasis model assessment of beta-cell function; ISI - insulin sensitivity index; OGTT - oral glucose tolerance test.

Table S3 Associations between CTF1 SNPs and indices of lipid metabolism. Data represents means±SD. Prior to statistical analysis, indices of lipid metabolism were adjusted for gender, age, BMI and lipid-lowering medication. AUC - area under the curve; TG, triglyceride; Chol, cholesterol; LDL, low-density lipoprotein; HDL, high-density lipoprotein; VLDL, very low-density lipoprotein.

Acknowledgments

We thank all study participants for their cooperation. We gratefully acknowledge the excellent technical assistance of Alke Guirguis, and Roman-Georg Werner.

Author Contributions

Conceived and designed the experiments: AF HS FM FS HUH. Performed the experiments: AB JM FM. Analyzed the data: SZL OF HS. Wrote the paper: SZL.

References

1. Febbraio MA (2007) gp130 receptor ligands as potential therapeutic targets for obesity. J Clin Invest 117: 841–849.
2. Stefan N, Haring HU (2013) The role of hepatokines in metabolism. Nat Rev Endocrinol 9: 144–152.
3. Weigert C, Hennige AM, Brodbeck K, Haring HU, Schleicher ED (2005) Interleukin-6 acts as insulin sensitizer on glycogen synthesis in human skeletal muscle cells by phosphorylation of Ser473 of Akt. Am J Physiol Endocrinol Metab 289: E251–E257.
4. Pennica D, Shaw KJ, Swanson TA, Moore MW, Shelton DL, et al. (1995) Cardiotrophin-1. Biological activities and binding to the leukemia inhibitory factor receptor/gp130 signaling complex. J Biol Chem 270: 10915–10922.
5. Pennica D, King KL, Shaw KJ, Luis E, Rullamas J, et al. (1995) Expression cloning of cardiotrophin 1, a cytokine that induces cardiac myocyte hypertrophy. Proc Natl Acad Sci U S A 92: 1142–1146.
6. Moreno-Aliaga MJ, Perez-Echarri N, Marcos-Gomez B, Larequi E, Gil-Bea FJ, et al. (2011) Cardiotrophin-1 is a key regulator of glucose and lipid metabolism. Cell Metab 14: 242–253.
7. Mitsumoto H, Klinkosz B, Pioro EP, Tsuzaka K, Ishiyama T, et al. (2001) Effects of cardiotrophin-1 (CT-1) in a mouse motor neuron disease. Muscle Nerve 24: 769–777.
8. Bustos M, Beraza N, Lasarte JJ, Baixeras E, Alzuguren P, et al. (2003) Protection against liver damage by cardiotrophin-1: a hepatocyte survival factor up-regulated in the regenerating liver in rats. Gastroenterology 125: 192–201.

9. Jimenez-Gonzalez M, Jaques F, Rodriguez S, Porciuncula A, Principe RM, et al. (2013) Cardiotrophin 1 protects beta cells from apoptosis and prevents streptozotocin-induced diabetes in a mouse model. Diabetologia 56: 838–846.
10. Watt MJ, Dzamko N, Thomas WG, Rose-John S, Ernst M, et al. (2006) CNTF reverses obesity-induced insulin resistance by activating skeletal muscle AMPK. Nat Med 12: 541–548.
11. Stefan N, Machicao F, Staiger H, Machann J, Schick F, et al. (2005) Polymorphisms in the gene encoding adiponectin receptor 1 are associated with insulin resistance and high liver fat. Diabetologia 48: 2282–2291.
12. Machann J, Thamer C, Schnoedt B, Haap M, Haring HU, et al. (2005) Standardized assessment of whole body adipose tissue topography by MRI. J Magn Reson Imaging 21: 455–462.
13. Machann J, Thamer C, Schnoedt B, Stefan N, Haring HU, et al. (2006) Hepatic lipid accumulation in healthy subjects: a comparative study using spectral fat-selective MRI and volume-localized 1H-MR spectroscopy. Magn Reson Med 55: 913–917.
14. Matthews DR, Hosker JP, Rudenski AS, Naylor BA, Treacher DF, et al. (1985) Homeostasis model assessment: insulin resistance and beta-cell function from fasting plasma glucose and insulin concentrations in man. Diabetologia 28: 412–419.
15. Matsuda M, DeFronzo RA (1999) Insulin sensitivity indices obtained from oral glucose tolerance testing: comparison with the euglycemic insulin clamp. Diabetes Care 22: 1462–1470.
16. Herzberg-Schafer SA, Staiger H, Heni M, Ketterer C, Guthoff M, et al. (2010) Evaluation of fasting state-/oral glucose tolerance test-derived measures of

insulin release for the detection of genetically impaired beta-cell function. PLoS One 5: e14194.

17. Dupuis J, Langenberg C, Prokopenko I, Saxena R, Soranzo N, et al.(2010) New genetic loci implicated in fasting glucose homeostasis and their impact on type 2 diabetes risk. Nat Genet 42: 105–116.

18. Asrih M, Gardier S, Papageorgiou I, Montessuit C (2013) Dual effect of the heart-targeting cytokine cardiotrophin-1 on glucose transport in cardiomyocytes. J Mol Cell Cardiol 56: 106–115.

19. Chopra I, Li HF, Wang H, Webster KA (2012) Phosphorylation of the insulin receptor by AMP-activated protein kinase (AMPK) promotes ligand-independent activation of the insulin signalling pathway in rodent muscle. Diabetologia 55: 783–794.

20. Zvonic S, Hogan JC, Arbour-Reily P, Mynatt RL, Stephens JM (2004) Effects of cardiotrophin on adipocytes. J Biol Chem 279: 47572–47579.

21. Natal C, Fortuno MA, Restituto P, Bazan A, Colina I, et al. (2008) Cardiotrophin-1 is expressed in adipose tissue and upregulated in the metabolic syndrome. Am J Physiol Endocrinol Metab 294: E52–E60.

22. Hung HC, Lu FH, Ou HY, Wu HT, Wu JS, et al. (2013) Increased cardiotrophin-1 in subjects with impaired glucose tolerance and newly diagnosed diabetes. Int J Cardiol 169: e33–e34.

23. Malavazos AE, Ermetici F, Morricone L, Delnevo A, Coman C, et al. (2008) Association of increased plasma cardiotrophin-1 with left ventricular mass indexes in normotensive morbid obesity. Hypertension 51: e8–e9.

24. Moreno-Aliaga MJ, Romero-Lozano MA, Castano D, Prieto J, Bustos M (2012) Role of cardiotrophin-1 in obesity and insulin resistance. Adipocyte 1: 112–115.

25. Castano D, Larequi E, Belza I, Astudillo AM, Martinez-Anso E, et al. (2014) Cardiotrophin-1 eliminates hepatic steatosis in obese mice by mechanisms involving AMPK activation. J Hepatol 60(5): 1017–1025.

2

Up-Regulation of MicroRNA-190b Plays a Role for Decreased IGF-1 that Induces Insulin Resistance in Human Hepatocellular Carcinoma

Tzu-Min Hung[1,2], Cheng-Maw Ho[1,3], Yen-Chun Liu[1,2], Jia-Ling Lee[1], Yow-Rong Liao[1], Yao-Ming Wu[1], Ming-Chih Ho[1], Chien-Hung Chen[4], Hong-Shiee Lai[1], Po-Huang Lee[1,5]*

1 Department of Surgery, National Taiwan University Hospital and National Taiwan University College of Medicine, Taipei, Taiwan, 2 Department of Medical Research, E-DA Hospital, Kaohsiung, Taiwan, 3 Graduate Institute of Clinical Medicine, College of Medicine, National Taiwan University, Taipei, Taiwan, 4 Department of Internal Medicine, National Taiwan University Hospital and National Taiwan University College of Medicine, Taipei, Taiwan, 5 Department of Surgery, E-DA Hospital, Kaohsiung, Taiwan

Abstract

Background & Aims: Insulin-like growth factor, (IGF)-1, is produced mainly by the liver and plays important roles in promoting growth and regulating metabolism. Previous study reported that development of hepatocellular carcinoma (HCC) was accompanied by a significant reduction in serum IGF-1 levels. Here, we hypothesized that dysregulation of microRNAs (miRNA) in HCC can modulate IGF-1 expression post-transcriptionally.

Methods: The miRNAs expression profiles in a dataset of 29 HCC patients were examined using illumina BeadArray. Specific miRNA (miR)-190b, which was significantly up-regulated in HCC tumor tissues when compared with paired non-tumor tissues, was among those predicted to interact with 3′-untranslated region (UTR) of *IGF-1*. In order to explore the regulatory effects of miR-190b on IGF-1 expression, luciferase reporter assay, quantitative real-time PCR, western blotting and immunofluorecence analysis were performed in HCC cells.

Results: Overexpression of miR-190b in Huh7 cells attenuated the expression of IGF-1, whereas inhibition of miR-190b resulted in up-regulation of IGF-1. Restoration of IGF-1 expression reversed miR-190b-mediated impaired insulin signaling in Huh7 cells, supporting that IGF-1 was a direct and functional target of miR-190b. Additionally, low serum IGF-1 level was associated with insulin resistance and poor overall survival in HCC patients.

Conclusions: Increased expression of miR-190 may cause decreased IGF-1 in HCC development. Insulin resistance appears to be a part of the physiopathologic significance of decreased IGF-1 levels in HCC progression. This study provides a novel miRNA-mediated regulatory mechanism for controlling IGF-1 expression in HCC and elucidates the biological relevance of this interaction in HCC.

Editor: Dong-Yan Jin, University of Hong Kong, Hong Kong

Funding: This work was supported in part by research grants NSC-99-2314-B-002-068-MY2, NSC-101-2314-B -650-005 and NSC-102-2314-B-650-007-MY3 from the National Science Council. The funders had no role in study design, data collection and analysis, decision to publish, or preparation of the manuscript.

Competing Interests: The authors have declared that no competing interests exist.

* E-mail: pohuang1115@ntu.edu.tw

Introduction

IGF-1 is a potent mitogenic factor that exerts anti-apoptotic effects on many cell systems. Experimental and epidemiologic evidence indicate that the IGF axis plays an important role in carcinogenesis [1,2]. High serum IGF-1 levels are associated with an increased risk for prostate, breast, colon, and lung cancers [2]. As a circulating peptide hormone, IGF-1 is also an important factor in regulating metabolism. IGF-1 has structural homology with insulin and exerts insulin-like effects on glucose and lipid metabolism [3]. Cross-sectional studies suggest that IGF-1 levels may be reduced in insulin resistance and type 2 diabetes [4]. Altered IGF-1 levels have also been implicated in cardiovascular disease, with compelling data suggesting that reduced IGF-1 levels are associated with increased cardiovascular risk [5,6]. In animal models, mice become insulin resistant when liver synthesis of IGF-1 is deleted [7,8], and IGF-1 administration corrects this insulin resistance [8].

Since alterations of IGF levels have been implicated in the pathogenesis of several diseases, understanding the mechanisms controlling IGF-1 expression are of great interest. Post-transcriptional regulatory mechanisms, some of which involve microRNAs (miRNAs), have been reported to influence IGF-1 expression [9]. Among neoplasm with activated IGF signaling, some miRNAs acted as tumor suppressors to inhibit the expression of IGF-1 receptor (IGF-1R), such as miR-145, and miR-99a in breast cancer and HCC, respectively [10,11]. Additionally, miR-29 acts as an antifibrogenic mediator by interfering with profibrogenic cell communication via IGF-1 [12]. Furthermore, miR-1 and miR-206 have been shown to target the 3′-untranslated region (3′-UTR) of IGF-I mRNA and reduce IGF-1 expression; miR-1 levels increased in rat cardiomyoctes during glucose-induced apoptosis and antagonized the anti-apoptotic action of IGF-1 [13,14]. IGF-I was downregulated by miR-320 in myocardial microvascular endothelial cells of type 2 diabetic rats. Expression of miR-320 was up-regulated in the diabetic rat model, impairing angiogenesis by repressing IGF-I expression [15].

Unlike the positive correlation between IGF-1 levels and other cancers, a reduced serum level of IGF-1 has been documented in hepatocellular carcinoma (HCC) [16,17]. In patients with hepatitis C virus–related cirrhosis, HCC development was accompanied by significant reduction in serum IGF-1 levels [18]. Serum IGF-1 levels were significantly decreased in HCC patients compared to healthy subjects [19]. Since most serum IGF-1 originates in the liver, destruction of the liver parenchyma would reduces serum IGF-1 levels [20]. However, in HCC, upstream regulators that may lead to this decrease are not well defined. Furthermore, the physiopathological significance of decreased IGF-1 levels in the progression of HCC remains unclear. In the present study, we hypothesized that dysregulation of miRNAs in HCC may modulate IGF-1 expression post-transcriptionally. In addition, we demonstrated that IGF-1 plays a role in insulin resistance other than the expected reduction in its own levels in HCC.

Materials and Methods

Ethics Statement

This study was approved by the Research Ethics Committee of the National Taiwan University Hospital, Taipei, Taiwan. Written informed consent was obtained from all included subjects. Another cohort of 29 HCC patients, which tissues were used to conduct the gene expression analysis, was registered at ClinicalTrials.gov (NCT01247506) as described in our previous study [21].

Subjects

This study collected preoperative serum samples from 102 HCC patients who underwent curative resection between January 2004 and December 2005 at National Taiwan University Hospital and were followed until December 2011. Patients' clinical and pathological data were retrieved from medical records. Deaths of enrolled patients were confirmed using the mortality data bank of Taiwan Cancer Registry. Two control groups were included. Serum from healthy subjects was obtained from living liver donors at the same hospital. A second "viral hepatitis" group included chronic hepatitis B virus or hepatitis C virus patients without HCC.

Enzyme-linked Immunosorbent Assay (ELISA)

Serum IGF-1 levels of all subjects were measured using a commercial enzyme-linked immunosorbent assay (ELISA) kit (R&D Systems, Minneapolis, MN, USA). Basal serum insulin was measured using a commercially available insulin ELISA kit (Mercodia, Uppsala, Sweden). ELISA assays were performed according to the manufacturer's instructions. The index of insulin resistance (IR) was calculated using the homeostasis model of assessment (HOMA) formula: fasting plasma glucose (mg/dL) × fasting serum insulin (mU/L)/405.

Isolation of Total RNA, miRNA Microarray and Quantitative Real-time PCR Analysis of miRNA and mRNA

Total RNA from human HCC samples and cancer cell lines were extracted using Trizol reagent (Invitrogen, Carlsbad, CA, USA). 29 HCC tumor tissues (T) and their paired nontumor tissues (NT) were selected for microRNA profiling. Total RNA was analyzed by illumina BeadArray (human v2 miRNA panel)

according to the manufacturer's instructions. miRNAs with false discovery rate (FDR) <0.05 using paired t-test and T/NT ratio > 2 or <0.5 were identified as differentially expressed genes. For miRNA analyses by quantitative real-time polymerase chain reaction (qRT-PCR), 100 ng of total RNA was reverse-transcribed using the TaqMan miRNA Reverse Transcription Kit (Applied Biosystems, Carlsbad, CA, USA). The expression levels of mature miR-190b and control RNU6B were determined by qRT-PCR with the TaqMan Universal PCR Master Mix in StepOne Real-time PCR System (Applied Biosystems). TaqMan probes from Applied Biosystems were used to assess the expression of miR-190b (ID 002263) and RNU6B (ID 001093). For mRNA expression detection, one microgram total RNA was reverse-transcribed using random hexamer and MMLV reverse transcriptase (Fermentas, Glen Burnie, MD, USA). qRT-PCR was subsequently performed using TaqMan Gene Expression Assays (Applied Biosystems). The assay ID numbers of the validated genes are as follows: Hs01555481 for IGF-1 and Hs99999905 for GAPDH. miRNA and mRNA transcript levels were normalized to RNU6B and GAPDH mRNA levels (ΔCT), respectively.

Expression Plasmids

The EGFP-tagged pEZX-MR04 vectors expressing precursor miR-190b and scrambled sequences [named pre-miR-190b and pre-negative control (NC)], the mCherry-tagged pEZX-AM01 vectors expressing the miR-190b inhibitor and scrambled sequences (named anti-miR-190b and anti-NC), as well as luciferase vectors (pEZX-MT01) containing IGF-1 3′UTRs, were obtained from GeneCopoeia, Rockville MD. Human TrueClone IGF-1 plasmid was purchased from OriGene Technologies (Rockville, MD). The cloning expression vector is pCMV6-XL.

Luciferase Reporter Assay

HEK293T cells ($1*10^5$) were seeded in 24-well plates the day before transfection. Luciferase vectors and precursor control or precursor-miR-190b or inhibitor control or inhibitor miR-190b were co-transfected into cells using TurboFect reagent (Fermentas, Glen Burnie, MD, USA) following the manufacturer's protocol. Forty-eight hours post-transfection, cell extracts was assayed for luciferase activity using the Luc-Pair miR luciferase assay kit (Genecoepia, Rockville, MD). Relative luciferase activities were expressed as luminescence units normalized to Renilla luciferase activity.

miRNA Transfection and Establishment of Stable Cell Clones

The human HCC cell lines, Huh7 and HepG2, were maintained at 37°C with 5% CO2 in Dulbecco's modified Eagle's medium (Invitrogen, Carlsbad, CA) supplemented with 10% heat-inactivated fetal bovine serum and 100 U of penicillin and 100 µg of streptomycin/ml. Stable cell clones were established by transfecting plasmids (as described above) into Huh7 cells using TurboFect reagent. Stable cell clones were generated with 2 µg/ml and maintained in culture with 1 µg/ml of puromycin (Invitrogen, Carlsbad, CA, USA). These subclones were named Huh7-Pre-NC-1, Huh7-Pre-miR190b-3, Huh7-Pre-miR190b-6, Huh7-Anti-NC-1, Huh7-Anti-miR190b-2 and Huh7-Anti-miR190b-5.

Western Blotting

Whole cell lysate was subjected to 12.5% sodium dodecyl sulfate (SDS)–polyacrylamide electrophoresis gel, transferred to polyvinylidene difluoride membrane, blotted with rabbit polyclonal IGF-

1 antibody (Santa Cruz Biotechnology, Santa Cruz, CA, USA) and followed by the secondary antibody. The enhanced chemi-luminescence detection system was used to detect the immuno-complex. Antibodies directed against IRS1, FOXO1, GSK3β, and phosphor-specific antibodies directed against p-IRS1 (Ser612 or 318), p-FOXO1 (Ser256) and p-GSK3β (Ser9) were supplied by Cell Signaling Technology (Danvers, MA, USA). Anti-β-actin antibody was purchased from Novus (Littleton, CO, USA).

Immunofluorescence

Cells were plated onto glass cover slips and fixed in 4% (vol/vol) paraformaldehyde/phosphate-buffered saline (PBS). They were subsequently permeabilized in PBS containing 0.5% (vol/vol) Triton X-100 for 15 min and were blocked in PBS containing 5% (wt/vol) bovine serum albumin for an hour. Cells were labeled with rabbit anti-IGF-1 or anti-FOXO1 antibody, followed by AF-488-conjugated goat anti-rabbit immunoglobulin G (Molecular Probes, Carlsbad, CA). Nucleus was stained with Hoechst 33258. Photographs were taken using a fluorescence microscope (Axio Imager A1, ZEISS).

Glucose Production Assay

Glucose production was measured using a commercial kit (Glucose Colorimetric Assay Kit II, BioVision, Milpitas,CA). Briefly, Huh7 stable cells were washed with PBS and incubated with glucose production buffer consisting of glucose-free Dulbec-co's modified Eagle's medium (Invitrogen, Carlsbad, CA, USA), without phenol red, supplemented with a gluconeogenic substrate (2 mM sodium pyruvate and 20 mM sodium lactate). After incubation for 4 hours, the medium was collected, and the total glucose concentration was measured.

Statistical Analysis

All statistical analyses were performed using SPSS 16.0 statistical software package (SPSS, Chicago, IL, USA). Data were presented as mean ± SD. Data were analyzed using the Wilcoxon signed rank test for comparison of paired data, the One-way ANOVA for more than two groups and the Student's t-test for unpaired comparison. Pearson correlations were used to deter-mine correlation coefficients. Kaplan-Meier method was used for survival analysis, and log-rank test was used to compare differences. $P < 0.05$ was considered statistically significant.

Results

Circulating and Hepatic Levels of IGF-1 were Decreased in Patients with HCC

The circulating levels of IGF-1 were analyzed in the cohort of 102 HCC patients. When compared to patients with viral hepatitis and healthy subjects, serum IGF-1 levels were significantly decreased in patients with HCC (Table 1). Besides, HCC and viral hepatitis groups showed significantly higher levels of AST, ALT and bilirubin than those of healthy controls (Table 1), which supported that destruction of the liver parenchyma reduced serum IGF-1 levels. However, compared to the viral hepatitis group, the HCC group showed no significant differences in AST levels ($P = 1.000$) and even had significantly lower levels of ALT ($P = 0.022$) and bilirubin ($P = 0.019$). Liver damage alone seems not to explain the greater decreases in IGF-1 levels of HCC patients compared with those of the viral hepatitis group.

The levels of hepatic IGF-1 were analyzed in a further cohort of 29 HCC patients from whom tumor and adjacent non-tumor tissues were collected. As shown in Figure 1A, using qRT-PCR demonstrated that IGF-1 expression was downregulated >2-fold in 90% (26/29) of tumor tissues examined. The relative expression of IGF-1 was significantly lower in tumor tissues as compared to paired non-tumor tissues ($P < 0.001$; Figure 1A). This result raises a possibility that tumor-specific factors might also contribute to the decline of IGF-1 in HCC.

Identification of miRNA that Targets IGF-1

Determination of miRNA expression profiles of 29 HCC tumor tissues and their paired non-tumor tissues identified 16 miRNAs that were significantly and differentially expressed between HCC tumor tissues and their paired non-tumor tissues, including 8 up-regulated and 8 down-regulated (Table S1). Since miRNAs act as negative regulators, up-regulated miRNAs resulted in down-regulated target mRNAs, 8 up-regulated miRs were chosen for further in silico analysis. Using TargetScan Human V5.1 predic-tion, 5 miRNAs that potentially bind to the 3′ UTR of IGF-1 mRNA were selected (Figure 1B). To validate the reliability of the microarray test, miR-190b, one of the most statistically significant miR, was selected for qRT-PCR examination. The expression of miR-190b was significantly up-regulated in 66% (19/29) of HCC samples compared with the paired nontumor tissues (Figure 1C). Next, we correlated the expression of IGF-1 to that of miR-190b in the 29 HCC tumor tissues and identified a marginally reverse correlation ($P = 0.057$; Figure 1D), implying that miR-190b dysregulation might be associated with the decline of IGF-1.

IGF-1 is a Direct Target of miR-190b

Analysis of the 3′UTR sequence of IGF-1 using TargetScan revealed two possible binding sites for miR-190b at positions 844–850 and 1752–1758 (Figure 2A). To determine whether miR-190b affects IGF-1 expression through these putative elements, a luciferase reporter construct carrying these elements was em-ployed. Precursor miR-190b transfection significantly decreased luciferase activities whereas its inhibitor transfection increased them (Figure 2B). Inclusion of the IGF-1 3′ UTR into a luciferase reporter construct reduced luciferase activity compared to a reporter lacking IGF-1 3′ UTR (Figure 2C), suggesting that this 3′UTR of IGF-1 was inhibited by the endogenous expression of miRs. Overexpression of miR-190b led to further reduction of luciferase activity when the reporter construct contained IGF-1 3′UTR (Figure 2C). Two reporter constructs were generated carrying mutations for each predicted miR-190b binding site. As shown in Figure 2C, the suppressive effect of miR-190b was significantly reversed on mutation of binding site 2 (7mer-m8), whereas no significant changes were noted on mutation of binding site 1 (7mer-A1). Taken together, these results revealed that IGF-1 is a direct target of miR-190b.

The Regulatory Effects of miR-190b on IGF-1 Expression

To learn whether miR-190b can affect endogenous IGF-1 protein levels, we established Huh7 stable cells that constitutively express precursor negative control, precursor miR-190b, inhibitor negative control or miR-190b inhibitor. Results of qRT-PCR confirmed that clones expressing precursor miR-190b exhibited greatly increased miR-190b expression when compared to negative controls (Figure 3A, left). However, the principle of our inhibitor is to de-repress microRNA targets [22], so the transfected inhibitors would not alter the amount of endogenous miR-190b (Figure 3A, right). Next, when exploring the corresponding IGF-1 protein levels in these stable clones, western blotting showed dose-dependent reduced expression of IGF-1 in Huh7 stable cells expressing precursor miR-190b (Figure 3B, left). Conversely,

Table 1. Demographic data and clinical features of healthy control, viral hepatitis and hepatocellular carcinoma groups.

Variable mean ± SD	Healthy control[1] (n = 38)	Viral hepatitis[2] (n = 50)	HCC[3] (n = 102)	P vale (1 vs.2)	P vale (1 vs.3)	P vale (2 vs.3)
Sex (Male/Female)	19/19	30/20	77/25			
Age (years)	33.6±11	56.4±4.2	58.1±11.6	<0.001	<0.001	0.970
Serum IGF-1 level (ng/mL)	106.3±46.7	70.0±29.1	46.4±13.9	<0.001	<0.001	<0.001
AST (U/L)	17.8±5.6	61.4±49.2	58.3±40.6	<0.001	<0.001	1.000
ALT (U/L)	16.5±10.3	96.3±112.2	63.6±52.5	<0.001	<0.01	0.022
Bilirubin (mg/dL)	0.7±0.3	1.1±0.4	0.9±0.4	<0.001	<0.05	0.019

The significance of the difference between the three groups was tested first using an analysis of variance (ANOVA); then, if proven significant, the Bonferroni test was used to assess the individual differences between each pair of groups.
n = number of subjects.
AST, aspartate aminotransferase; ALT, alanine aminotransferase.

increased expression of IGF-1 was observed in stable cells expressing miR-190b inhibitor (Figure 3B, right).

Expression of IGF-1 proteins was also verified by immunofluorescence. Among the miR-190b stable cells, analysis of two representative subclones, namely Huh7-Pre-miR190b-6 and

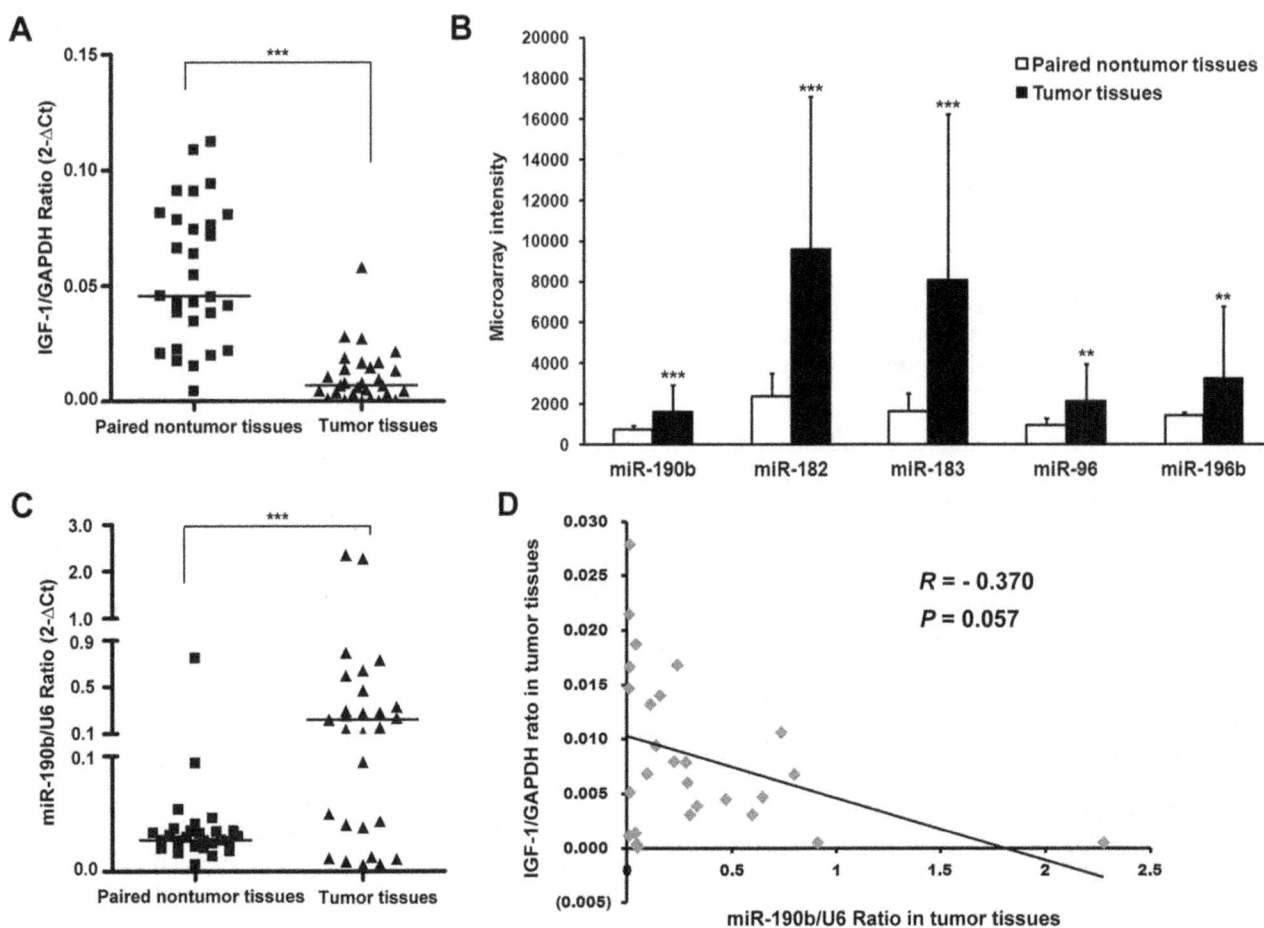

Figure 1. Identification of miRNA that targets IGF-1. (A) qRT-PCR analysis showing that IGF-1 expression levels were significantly down-regulated in HCC tumor tissues as compared with paired nontumor tissues. The horizontal line indicates the median. The expression level of IGF-1 was normalized by GAPDH. (B) An integrative analysis of miRNA BeadArray with TargetScan predictions defined 5 miRNAs that are up-regulated in HCC tumor tissues and could potentially bind to the 3′-UTR of IGF-1 mRNA. (C) qRT-PCR analysis of miR-190b expression in HCC tumor and nontumor tissues. The horizontal line indicates the median. The expression level of miR-190b was normalized by U6. (D) Correlation between expression levels of IGF-1 and miR-190b of tumor tissues in 29 HCC patients. Linear regression coefficients and statistical significance are indicated. ***$P<0.001$; **$P<0.01$.

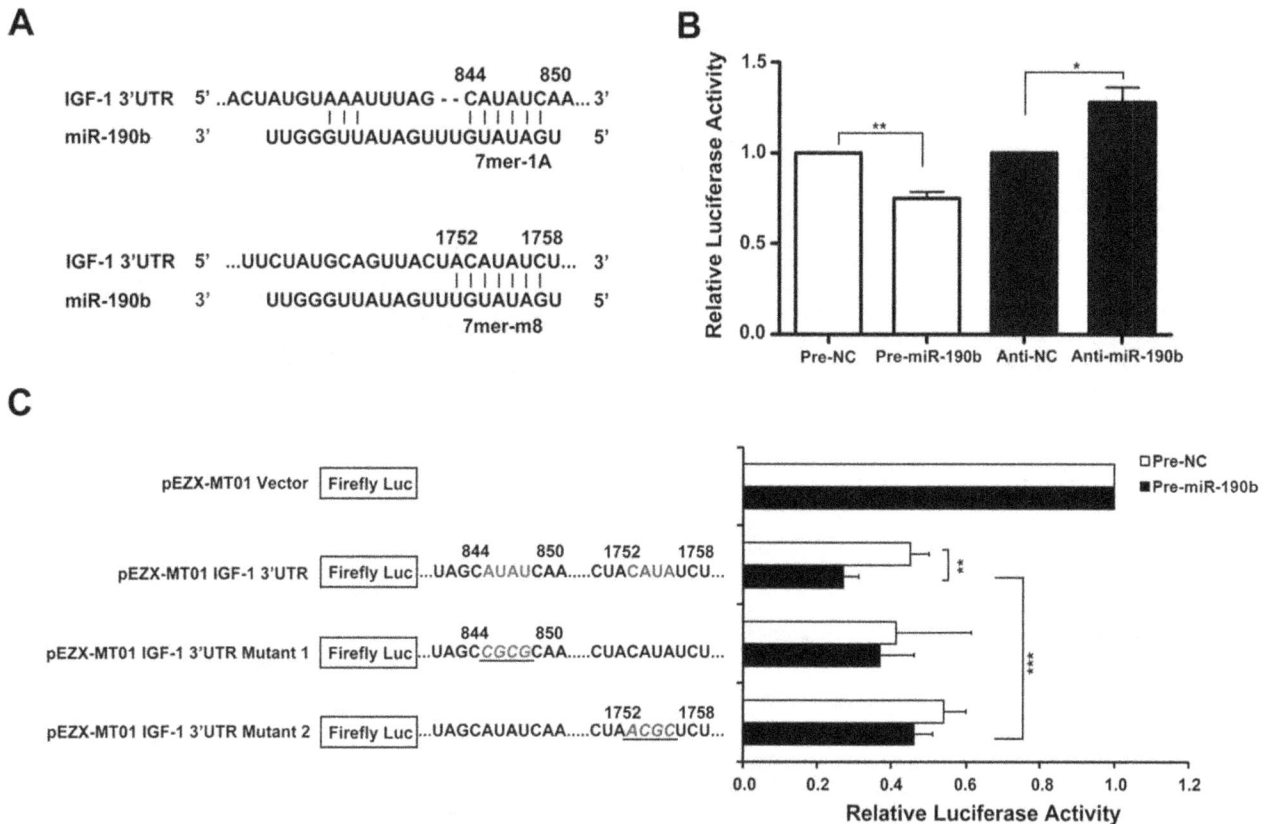

Figure 2. IGF-1 was a direct target of miR-190b. (A) Base pairing complement suggests two putative miR-190b binding positions at 844–850 and 1752–1758 of the IGF-1 3′UTR. (B) The effect of precursor miR-190b or miR-190b inhibitor on pEZX-IGF-1 3′UTR luciferase activity. Luciferase assays were done on HEK293 T cells. Significant differences were compared to each negative control (NC). (C) HEK293T cells were transiently transfected with pre-miR-190b or pre-NC vector together with the pEZX-MT01 empty vector, a modified pEZX-MT01 vector containing wild-type IGF-1 3′UTR, or two mutant IGF-1 3′UTR carrying mutations for each putative miR-190b binding site. Luciferase activity of pEZX-MT01 empty plasmid was set to 1. ***, $P<0.001$; **, $P<0.01$; *, $P<0.05$.

Huh7-Anti-miR190b-5, revealed an attenuated IGF-1 signal in Huh7-Pre-miR190b-6 cells and a moderately elevated IGF-1 signal in Huh7-Anti-miR190b-5 (Figure 3C). Because inhibition of expression by miRNA may also be mediated by mRNA degradation, we examined whether IGF-1 mRNA levels might be affected by miR-190b; consistent overexpression of miR-190b decreased IGF-1 mRNA levels, whereas inhibition of miR-190b increased the levels (Figure 3D), indicating that miR-190b might act to destabilize or degrade IGF-1 mRNA transcripts. To further confirm this, we analyzed the turnover of IGF-1 mRNA in miR-190b overexpressed and control cells. IGF-1 mRNA stability was determined by qRT-PCR after treatment with actinomycin D to inhibit de novo RNA synthesis. As shown in Figure S1, overexpression of miR-190b resulted in a significant decrease in IGF-1 mRNA levels after 6 hr with actinomycin D, on the contrary, IGF-1 mRNA was stable in control cells.

Transient transfection was also performed to clarify that IGF-1 repression was not due to clonal effects of miR-190b stable cells. Analysis of IGF-1 expression confirmed decreased IGF-1 protein levels in cells transfected with precursor miR-190b as compared to precursor controls (Figure S2-A and B). Conversely, IGF-1 expression in cells transfected with miR-190b inhibitor was increased when compared to inhibitor controls (Figure S2-A and B). Immunofluorescence analysis was used to further confirm the relationship between miR-190b and IGF-1. Representative staining is shown in Figure S2-C and D. IGF-1 expression was suppressed in cells transfected with precursor miR-190b (Figure S2-D, indicated by arrows). Cells transfected with empty vector showed no change in IGF-1 expression (Figure S2-C). Collectively, these results indicate that *IGF-1* gene expression is directly and post-transcriptionally suppressed by miR-190b.

Because the endogenous levels of miR-190b were marginally expressed in Huh7 cells, the other cell was used to conduct the loss-of-function analysis of miR-190b again. We transfected the miR-190b inhibitors into HepG2 cells, which have a relatively higher basal levels of miR-190b and lower levels of IGF-1 compared to those of Huh7 cells (Figure 3E). We expected that our miRNAs inhibitor should function more by entrapping than by degradation of the target mature miRNA. But qRT-PCR showed a modest decrease in miR-190b after transfection of the miR-190b inhibitor (Figure 3F) [22]. Furthermore, inhibition of miR-190b in HepG2 cells led to a clear increase of IGF-1 expression both in the mRNA (Figure 3G) and protein levels (Figure 3H). Taken together, these data further confirm that miR-190b can regulate IGF-1 expression.

Low IGF-1 is Associated with Insulin Resistance and Poor Prognosis in Patients with HCC

To clarify the clinical significance of decreased IGF-1 levels in HCC, we determined whether serum IGF-1 levels correlated with prognosis. The median serum IGF-1 level of these 102 HCC patients was 44.8 ng/mL. On the basis of serum IGF-1 levels, we

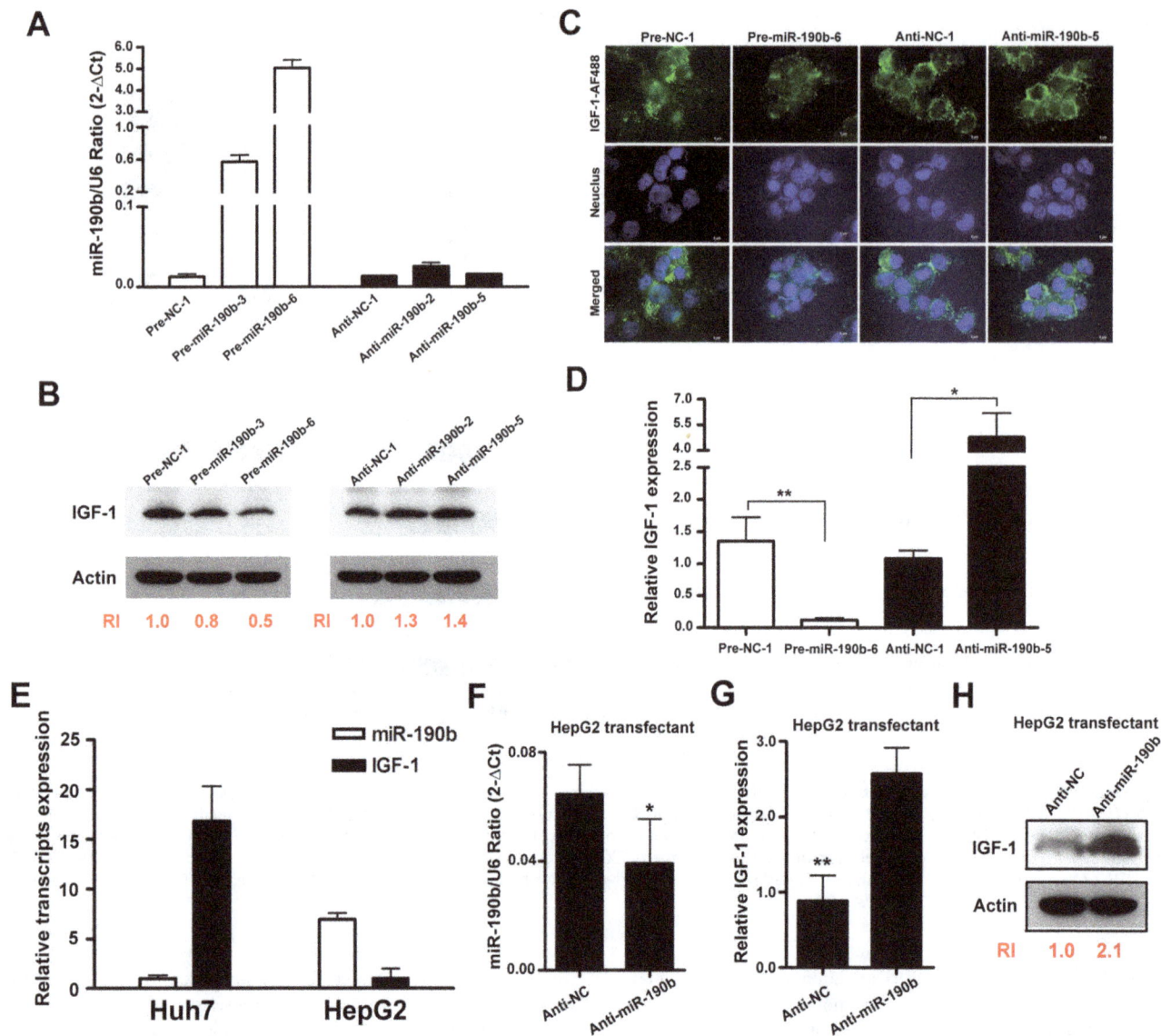

Figure 3. The regulatory effects of miR-190b on IGF-1 expression. (A) qRT-PCR assay verified the relative miR-190b expression in Huh7 stable cells clones. (B&C) Overexpression of miR-190b attenuated IGF-1 protein expression, and blocking miR-190b moderately increased IGF-1 protein expression. These results were assayed by western blotting (B) and immunofluorescence staining (C), respectively. (D) IGF-1 mRNA was detected by qRT-PCR in stable cells expressing precursor miR-190b or inhibitor miR-190b. Relative expression of IGF-1 compared to negative control (NC) was calculated using the $2^{-\Delta\Delta CT}$ methods. (E) The endogenous transcript levels of miR-190b and IGF-1 were dertermined by qRT-PCR in Huh7 and HepG2 cells. (F&G) qRT-PCR analysis of miR-190b (F) and IGF-1 (G) in HepG2 cells transfected with anti-NC or anti-miR-190b vectors. (H) Western blotting of IGF-1 in HepG2 cells transfected with anti-NC or anti-miR-190b vectors. Relative intensity (RI) shown was calculated by normalization of the intensities of IGF-1 from the internal controls. **, $P<0.01$ and *, $P<0.05$ as compared to each of the negative control cells.

divided the whole study group into low (<44.8 ng/mL) and high serum IGF-1 (>44.8 ng/mL) level groups. Kaplan-Meier curves showed a significant association between low serum IGF-1 levels and poor overall survival (Figure 4A). However, the intergroup difference in the recurrence-free survival of patients was not statistically significant (Figure 4B). Further, the relationship between serum IGF-1 levels and clinicopathological features was examined. A significant inverse association was found between IGF-1 and insulin levels (Figure 4C), as well as between IGF-1 levels and insulin resistance index (HOMA-IR) (Figure 4D). However, there were no significant correlations between serum IGF-1 levels and tumor characteristics among HCC patients (Table S2). Taken together, these results suggest that low serum

IGF-1 level is associated with insulin resistance and poor overall survival in HCC patients.

Over-expression of miR-190b Contributes to Hepatic Insulin Resistance through Down-regulation of IGF-1 Expression

As a potential regulator of IGF-1, we reasoned that expression of miR-190b might be involved in insulin resistance. To address this issue, we investigated the phosphorylation status of insulin signaling mediators by western blotting in the presence of miR-190b overexpression. The down-regulation of IGF-1 in Huh7-Pre-miR190b-6 cells was confirmed again in Figure 5A. Overexpression of miR-190b increased hepatic expression and insulin-

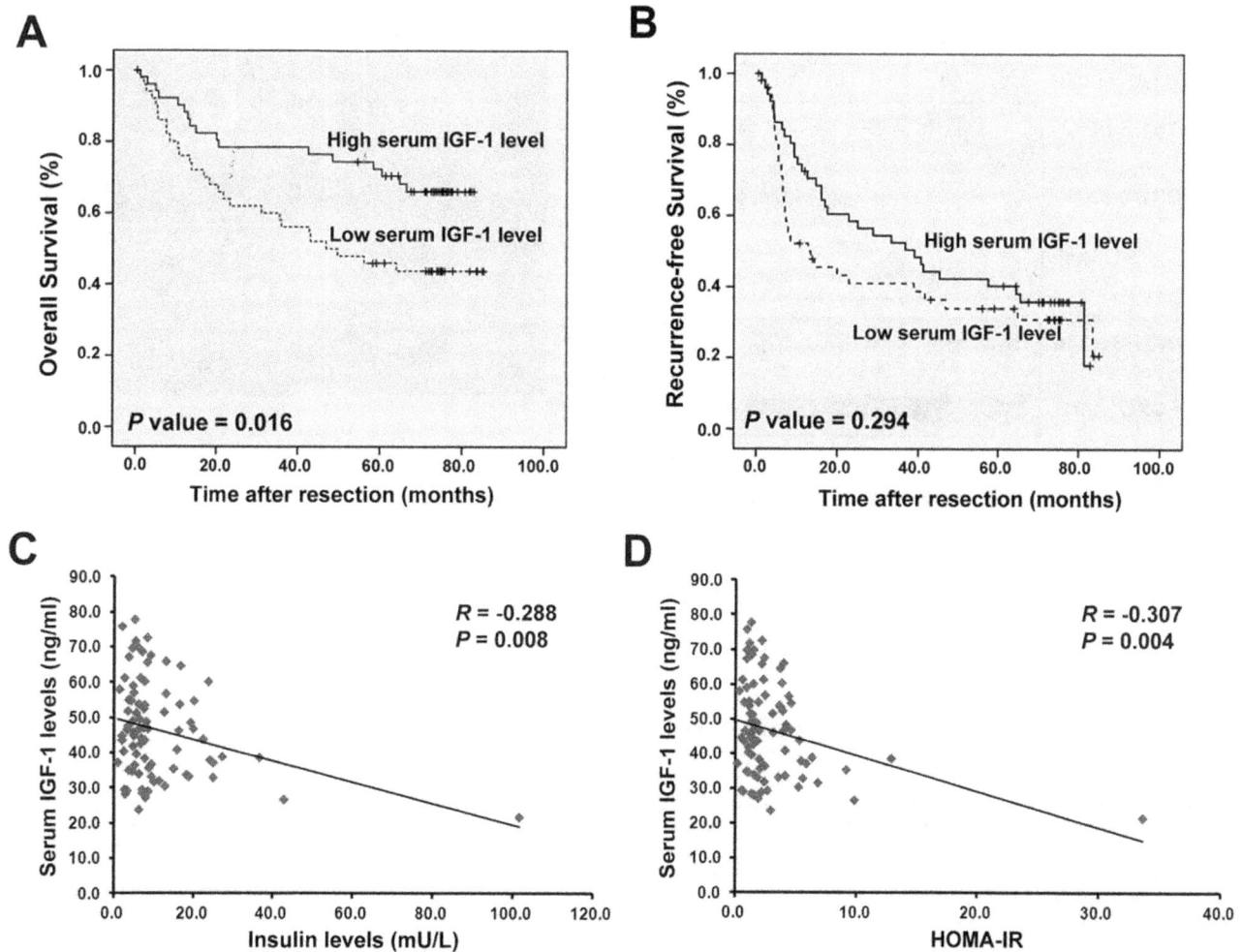

Figure 4. Low IGF-1 is associated with insulin resistance and poor prognosis in HCC patients. (A, B) Kaplan-Meier curves for overall survival (A) and recurrence-free survival (B) in patients with HCC after curative resection. Compared with patients with high IGF-1 levels, patients with low IGF-1 levels exhibited significantly shorter overall survival but no significant difference in recurrence-free survival. Statistical significance was calculated using the log-rank test. (C, D) Correlations of insulin levels (C) and homeostasis model assessment of insulin resistance (HOMA-IR) (D) with serum IGF-1 levels in HCC patients. Linear regression coefficients and statistical significance are indicated.

stimulated phosphorylation of IRS1 (insulin receptor substrate-1) at Ser612 and Ser318 (Figure 5A), verifying impairment of insulin signaling [23]. Phosphorylation of forkhead box class O1 (FOXO1) and glycogen synthase kinase 3β (GSK3β), two downstream effectors of insulin action [24], revealed that overexpression of miR-190b critically decreased FOXO1 and GSK3β phosphorylation at Ser256 and Ser9, respectively (Figure 5A). In addition, upon treatment of insulin, miR-190b overexpression resulted in the diminished ability of insulin to phosphorylate GSK3β. Abnormalities in the signaling pathway, including IRS1, FOXO1 and GSK3β, marked the main characteristics of insulin resistance in Huh7-Pre-miR190b-6 cells.

The phosphorylated form of FOXO1, a transcription factor controlling gene expression of gluconeogenesis, is exported from the nucleus and thereby loses its transcriptional function [25]. Measurement of FOXO1 translocation and glucose production revealed that the majority of FOXO1 accumulated in the nucleus upon miR-190b overexpression, whereas in control cells, FOXO1 was distributed in both nucleus and cytoplasm (Figure 5B). Cells that overexpressed miR-190b produced greater amounts of glucose than did control cells (Figure 5C). Taken together, these results indicate the critical role of miR-190b in impairing insulin signaling and promoting hepatic gluconeogenesis in HCC cells.

Restoration of IGF-1 Inhibits miR-190b-mediated Insulin Resistance

We next asked whether the insulin-resistance effects of miR-190b in HCC cells was attributed to its suppressive effect on IGF-1 expression. Transfection of Huh7-Pre-miR190b-6 cells with IGF-1 cDNA in a dose-dependent manner revealed that 20 microgram cDNA expresses comparable IGF-1 levels as control cells. A faster migrating band in IGF-1-overexpressing lysates may be IGF-1 isoform protein (Figure 6A).

Consistent with previously observed (Figure 5A), Huh7-Pre-miR190b-6 cells exhibited a significantly increased level of IRS1-Ser612&318 and decreased level of FOXO1-Ser256 and GSK3β-Ser9 when compared with control cells (Figure 6B). Restoring IGF-1 levels via cDNA transfection reversed the altered phophorylation status of Huh7-Pre-miR190b-6 cells to the similar level as control cells (Figure 6B). IGF-1 has been functionally validated as a *bona fide* target of miR-190b. In conclusion, the involvement of

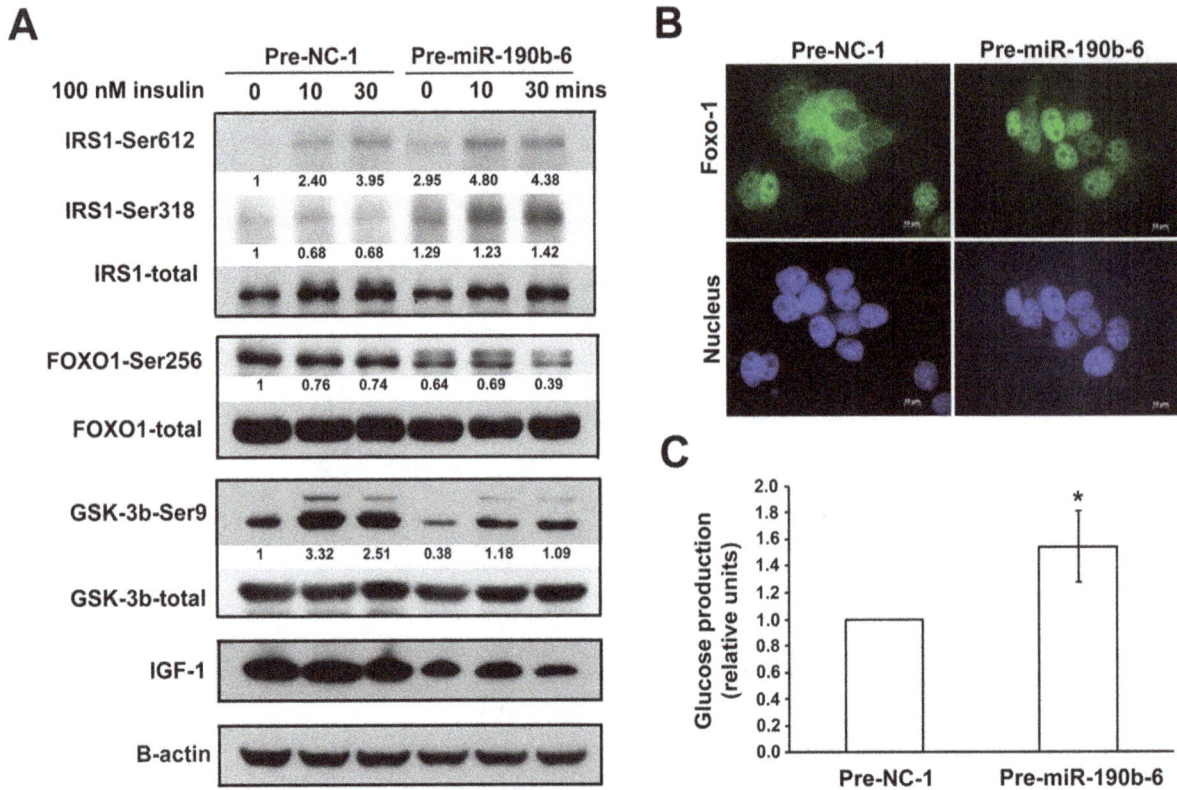

Figure 5. Over-expression of miR-190b in HCC cells leads to insulin resistance through down-regulation of IGF-1 expression. (A) Representative western blotting and quantification of expression and insulin-stimulated phosphorylation of IRS1, FOXO1 and GSK3β in Huh7 stable cells expressing precursor negative control (NC) or miR-190b. Cells were starved for 24 hours and then treated with 100 nM insulin for 10 and 30 minutes. Band intensity and ratio of phospho-form/total proteins were calculated by Image J. (B) immunofluorescence staining showing the subcellular localization of FOXO1 in Huh7 stable cells. (C) Extracellular glucose production in Huh7 stable cells was measured as described in Materials and Methods (*$P < 0.05$).

insulin resistance in response to IGF-1 deficiency was further substantiated by this *in vitro* evidence.

Discussion

Since the decline of IGF-1 in HCC is not well understood, this study investigated whether dysregulation of a specific miRNA may modulate IGF-1 reduction, and if so, what the biological consequences may be. Results of this study have shown that HCC significantly increases expression of miR-190b, which targets to IGF-1 3′UTR directly, resulting in impaired insulin signaling and gluconeogenesis. These findings suggest a novel mechanism for the development of insulin resistance in HCC by providing the first evidence that miR-190b mediates the repression of IGF-1 expression.

Most circulating IGF-1 is produced by the liver and production is regulated by growth hormone (GH) [20]. IGF-1 deficiency in HCC is thought to result primarily from the reduced synthetic capacity of hepatic mass. Alternatively, it might be the result of reduced GH stimulation because GH receptor expression in hepatoma tissue is also low [26]. However, some studies report that reduction of IGF-1 among HCC patients is greater than that attributed to liver damage alone. Mazziotti et al. found that IGF-1 levels decreased independently from the progression of cirrhosis from Child Grade A to Child Grade B [18]. After controlling for the degree of liver damage, as assessed by prothrombin time and serum albumin level, Stuver et al. reported that reduction of

serum IGF-1 levels in HCC patients appeared to be largely independent of liver damage [16]. Results of the present study have consistently shown that the gradually decreased IGF-1 levels among healthy subjects, viral hepatitis patients and HCC patients were partially independent of AST, ALT and total bilirubin levels. The idea that tumor-specific factors also contribute to the decline of IGF-1 in HCC was supported by evidence that overexpressed miR-190b in HCC tumor tissues regulated IGF-1 expression. Along the same line, some tumor cytokines, including Interleukin-1 beta, tumor necrosis factor-alpha and interleukin-6, were found to be elevated in HCC patients [27], have been reported to block IGF-1 production in the liver [28,29].

IGF-1 gene is heavily epigenetically regulated. A study of intrauterine growth restriction (IUGR) in rats found that the modest extent of IGF-1 promoter DNA hypermethylation appears to dampen IGF-1 expression in the IUGR liver [30]. Another study of traumatic brain injury in rats demonstrated that increased hippocampal IGF-1B mRNA is associated with DNA methylation and/or histone modifications at the promoter site 1 or exon 5 regions [31]. Furthermore, it becomes increasingly clear that HCC initiation and promotion can occur by way of epigenetic mechanisms [32]. Therefore, effects of epigenetic modification on the down-regulation of IGF-1 expression in HCC might be worth future research.

The production levels of many metabolic factors, including insulin and IGF-1, are critically controlled at the post-transcriptional level. Post-transcriptional regulations that alter the stability

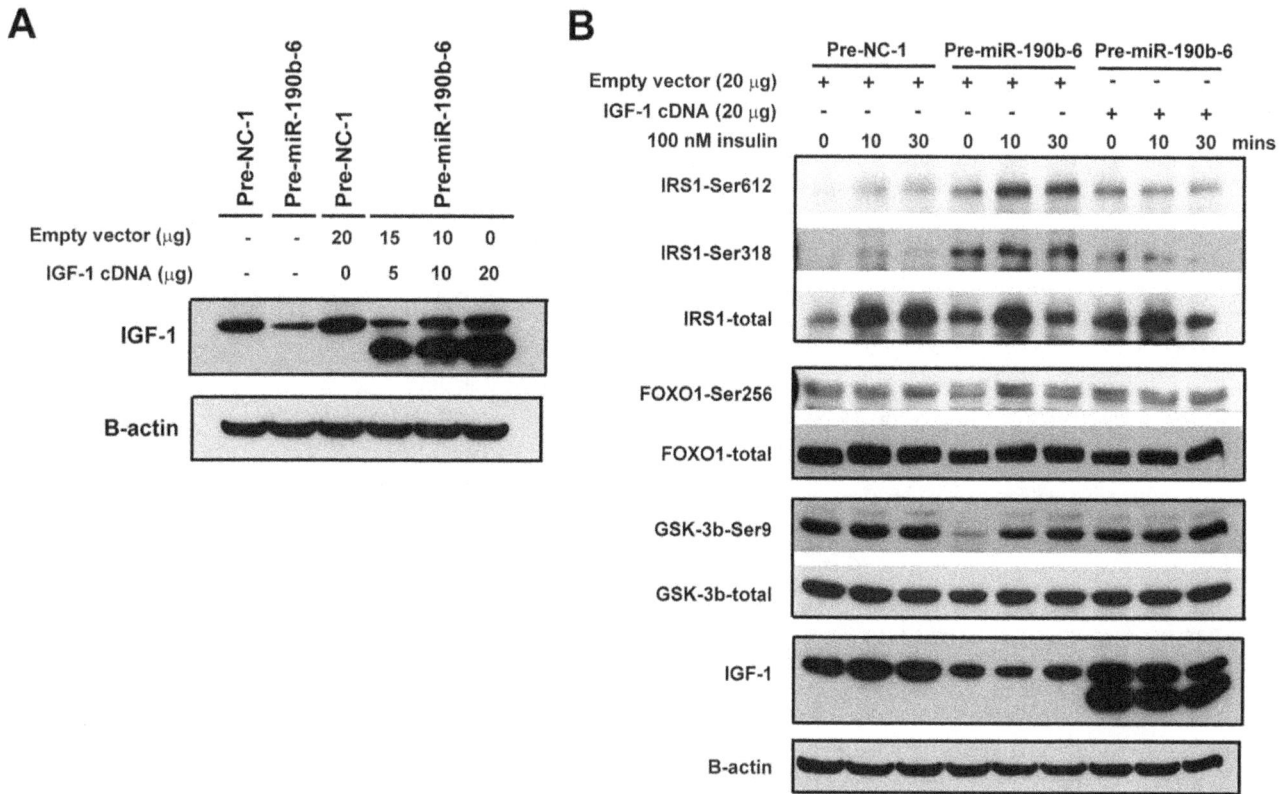

Figure 6. Restoration of IGF-1 inhibited miR-190b-mediated insulin resistance. (A) Western blotting of IGF-1 expression in Huh7-Pre-NC-1 cells or Huh7-Pre-miR190b-6 cells transfected with IGF-1 expression vector in different amounts. (B) Western blotting of expression and insulin-stimulated phosphorylation of IRS1, FOXO1 and GSK3β in Huh7-Pre-NC-1 cells transfected with empty vector, and Huh7-Pre-miR190b-6 cells transfected with empty vector or IGF-1 expression vector. β-actin was used as an internal control.

and translation of encoding mRNA allow the cell to respond effectively to stimuli such as altered glucose levels [9,33]. The liver is the principal organ that regulates glucose homeostasis because of its capacity to consume and produce glucose [34]. The liver's central role in glucose homeostasis offers a clue to the hypothesis that reduction of IGF-1 in HCC is due to miRNA-mediated post-transcriptional regulation. Our finding that miR-190b has a regulatory role for IGF-1 expression in human HCC supports this hypothesis. Dysregulated miRNAs, which was identified by our experimental observations and those of other studies [13–15], indicate that defects in post-transcriptional regulation contribute to the pathogenesis of metabolic disorders at multiple levels, including impaired insulin signaling, gluconeogenesis, glucose-induced apoptosis and impaired angiogenesis.

The effect of IGF-1 on tumor formation in humans is demonstrated by the finding that patients with acromegaly with elevated serum IGF-1 levels exhibit increased risk of colon and thyroid cancer [35]. This increased level of IGF-1 is in keeping with its known mitogenic and anti-apoptotic effects. However, contrary to IGF-1 levels in other cancers, IGF-1 levels are decreased in HCC and the underlying mechanisms are difficult to explain based on the proliferative effect of IGF-1. We consistently found no significant correlations between serum IGF-1 levels and tumor characteristics among HCC patients (Table S2). Further, this study showed that serum IGF-1 levels can predict overall survival of HCC patients, but not recurrence-free survival (Figure 4A and B). Accordingly, we propose that the association of low serum IGF-1 levels with poor prognosis in HCC may be attributable to mechanisms beyond development of tumor itself.

In contrast to its negative effects on growth and proliferation, reduced IGF-1 signaling has been reported to positively correlated insulin resistance [3,4]. Recently, many evidence points to a link between insulin resistance and cancer [36,37]. In patients with chronic hepatitis C, HCC subjects have a higher insulin resistance index than those with chronic hepatitis [38]. Moreover, prognosis is worse in HCC patients with glucose intolerance or increased fasting serum insulin level [39,40]. In accordance with these lines of evidence, low serum IGF-1 levels were associated with insulin resistance and poor prognosis in our HCC patients. Besides, we showed that the impaired insulin signaling caused by overexpression of miR-190b in HCC cells can partly reverse by restoring IGF-1 expression. These data indicated decreased expression of IGF-1 have a role in the development of HCC-associated insulin resistance. For the first time, this study demonstrated that insulin resistance appears to be part of the physiopathologic significance of decreased IGF-1 levels in HCC progression.

Recently, an association between IGF-1 and HCC patient outcome had been reported in the literature [41,42]. Shao et al. reported that high pretreatment IGF-1 level were associated with better survival and disease control rate of patients who received antiangiogenic therapy for advanced HCC [41]. Because of the lack of a control group not receiving therapy, it was uncertain that the better survival outcomes of high IGF-1 group resulted from better tumor prognosis or better therapeutic efficacy, or both. Kaseb et al. reported that low plasma IGF-1 levels correlated with poor overall survival in the other HCC patient cohort with heterogeneous disease status and treatment [42]. The main difference between our and the previous studies is that all patients in this study received curative resection, which resulted in a more homogeneous patient population. Moreover, after resection of HCC, none of the patients had received adjuvant therapy. Thus, we can conclude that the better survival outcomes of patients with high preoperative serum IGF-1 were derived from better tumor prognosis. In this study, we were able to substantiate earlier observations and extended our investigations to determine the biological role of IGF-1 in HCC.

As miR-190b was indentified between HCC tissues and their paired non-tumor tissues, we wondered whether miR-190b has potential effects on the characteristics of HCC. We checked the relationship of miR-190b with overall survival and found that high miR-190b levels could infer a poorer overall survival prospect of HCC patients (Figure S3-A). However, the intergroup difference was not statistically significant, which may be beset with small sample-size (n = 29). Further, the relationship between miR-190b levels and clinicopathological features was examined. However, there were no significant correlations between miR-190b levels and tumor characteristics among HCC patients (Table S3). Additional studies with large sample sizes are required to confirm these results.

Besides HCC, up-regulation of miR-190b has been reported in miRNA profile studies of other cancers such as rectal cancer and lung cancer [43,44]. However, in none of these reports has the biological consequences of miR-190b dysregulation in human cancers been characterized further. We examined whether the miR-190b overexpression would affect the cancer biology. The WST-1 assay demonstrated a modest, but significant, decrease in cell viability upon miR-190b overexpression (Figure S3-B). In general, slowly proliferating cells are far more resistant to chemotherapeutic drug treatment [45]. Therefore, an *in vitro* chemosensitivity assay was then performed. We observed that the overexpression of miR-190b increased resistance to 5-Fluorouracil (Figure S3-C). These results are in line with a previous report showing the up-regulation of miR-190b in rectal tumors of non-reponders to chemoradiotherapy [43]. Next, we evaluated the apoptosis potential of miR-190b by caspase 3/7 activity assay. As shown in Figure S3-D, increased expression of miR-190b inhibited cell apoptosis in HCC cells. Given that IGF-1 is the main anti-apoptoic factor, we supposed that additional mechanisms induced by miR-190b were involved in this anti-apoptosis ability, independently of IGF-1 inhibition. Our present study substantiates the notion that a single miRNA could pleiotropically regulate several oncogenic targets.

In summary, the present study not only uncovered that post-transcriptional regulation is responsible for the decline of IGF-1,

but also elucidated the mechanisms by which IGF-1 affects the clinical course of HCC patients. The therapeutic strategy that supplementation of IGF-1 to improve metabolic control after curative resection for HCC may be worth further study. Furthermore, the findings that the dysregulation of miR-190b had effects on drug resistance and anti-apoptosis indicate that miR-190b could be a therapeutic target of HCC.

Supporting Information

Figure S1   miR-190b repressed IGF-1 mRNA stability.

Figure S2   miR-190b regulated IGF-1 protein expression. Huh7 cells were transiently transfected with pre-NC, pre-miR-190b, anti-NC or anti-miR-190b vectors.

Figure S3   miR-190b overexpression was correlated with prognosis in HCC patients and regulated cell viability, chemosensitivity and apoptosis in HCC cells.

Table S1   List of 16 significantly dysregulated micro-RNAs in human hepatocelluar carcinoma (HCC) (miRNA beadarray data).

Table S2   Comparison of tumor characteristics between low and high serum insulin-like growth factor (IGF)-1 levels in patients with hepatocellular carcinoma.

Table S3   Comparison of tumor characteristics between low and high miR-190b levels in patients with hepato-cellular carcinoma.

Acknowledgments

We are grateful to Lih-Hwa Hwang (National Yang-Ming University) for providing the HEK293T cell line and Chia-Hung Chou (National Taiwan University Hospital) for providing the Huh7 cell line.

Author Contributions

Conceived and designed the experiments: TMH CMH PHL. Performed the experiments: TMH YCL JLL. Analyzed the data: TMH CMH YCL YRL. Contributed reagents/materials/analysis tools: YMW MCH CHC HSL. Wrote the paper: TMH PHL.

References

1. Pollak MN, Schernhammer ES, Hankinson SE (2004) Insulin-like growth factors and neoplasia. Nat Rev Cancer 4: 505–518.
2. Renehan AG, Zwahlen M, Minder C, O'Dwyer ST, Shalet SM, et al. (2004) Insulin-like growth factor (IGF)-I, IGF binding protein-3, and cancer risk: systematic review and meta-regression analysis. Lancet 363: 1346–1353.
3. Ohlsson C, Mohan S, Sjogren K, Tivesten A, Isgaard J, et al. (2009) The Role of Liver-Derived Insulin-Like Growth Factor-I. Endocr Rev 30: 494–535.
4. Rajpathak SN, Gunter MJ, Wylie-Rosett J, Ho GYF, Kaplan RC, et al. (2009) The role of insulin-like growth factor-I and its binding proteins in glucose homeostasis and type 2 diabetes. Diabetes Metab Res Rev 25: 3–12.
5. Abbas A, Grant PJ, Kearney MT (2008) Role of IGF-1 in glucose regulation and cardiovascular disease. Expert Rev Cardiovasc Ther 6: 1135–1149.
6. Juul A, Scheike T, Davidsen M, Gyllenborg J, Jorgensen T (2002) Low serum insulin-like growth factor I is associated with increased risk of ischemic heart disease - A population-based case-control study. Circulation 106: 939–944.
7. Yu R, Yakar S, Liu YL, Lu YR, LeRoith D, et al. (2003) Liver-specific IGF-I gene deficient mice exhibit accelerated diabetes in response to streptozotocin, associated with early onset of insulin resistance. Mol Cell Endocrinol 204: 31–42.
8. Yakar S, Liu JL, Fernandez AM, Wu YP, Schally AV, et al. (2001) Liver-specific igf-1 gene deletion leads to muscle insulin insensitivity. Diabetes 50: 1110–1118.
9. Lee EK, Gorospe M (2010) Minireview: posttranscriptional regulation of the insulin and insulin-like growth factor systems. Endocrinology 151: 1403–1408.
10. Kim SJ, Oh JS, Shin JY, Lee KD, Sung KW, et al. (2011) Development of microRNA-145 for therapeutic application in breast cancer. J Control Release 155: 427–434.
11. Li D, Liu X, Lin L, Hou J, Li N, et al. (2011) MicroRNA-99a inhibits hepatocellular carcinoma growth and correlates with prognosis of patients with hepatocellular carcinoma. J Biol Chem 286: 36677–36685.
12. Kwiecinski M, Elfimova N, Noetel A, Tox U, Steffen HM, et al. (2012) Expression of platelet-derived growth factor-C and insulin-like growth factor I in hepatic stellate cells is inhibited by miR-29. Lab Invest 92: 978–987.
13. Yu XY, Song YH, Geng YJ, Lin QX, Shan ZX, et al. (2008) Glucose induces apoptosis of cardiomyocytes via microRNA-1 and IGF-1. Biochem Biophys Res Commun 376: 548–552.
14. Shan ZX, Lin QX, Fu YH, Deng CY, Zhou ZL, et al. (2009) Upregulated expression of miR-1/miR-206 in a rat model of myocardial infarction. Biochem Biophys Res Commun 381: 597–601.
15. Wang XH, Qian RZ, Zhang W, Chen SF, Jin HM, et al. (2009) MicroRNA-320 expression in myocardial microvascular endothelial cells and its relationship with insulin-like growth factor-1 in type 2 diabetic rats. Clin Exp Pharmacol Physiol

36: 181–188.

16. Stuver SO, Kuper H, Tzonou A, Lagiou P, Spanos E, et al. (2000) Insulin-like growth factor 1 in hepatocellular carcinoma and metastatic liver cancer in men. Int J Cancer 87: 118–121.

17. Rehem RN, El-Shikh WM (2011) Serum IGF-1, IGF-2 and IGFBP-3 as Parameters in the Assessment of Liver Dysfunction in Patients with Hepatic Cirrhosis and in the Diagnosis of Hepatocellular Carcinoma. Hepatogastroenterology 58: 949–954.

18. Mazziotti G, Sorvillo F, Morisco F, Carbone A, Rotondi M, et al. (2002) Serum insulin-like growth factor I evaluation as a useful tool for predicting the risk of developing hepatocellular carcinoma in patients with hepatitis C virus-related cirrhosis - A prospective study. Cancer 95: 2539–2545.

19. Su WW, Lee KT, Yeh YT, Soon MS, Wang CL, et al. (2010) Association of Circulating Insulin-Like Growth Factor 1 With Hepatocellular Carcinoma: One Cross-Sectional Correlation Study. J Clin Lab Anal 24: 195–200.

20. Bonefeld K, Moller S (2011) Insulin-like growth factor-I and the liver. Liver Int 31: 911–919.

21. Hung TM, Hu RH, Ho CM, Chiu YL, Lee JL, et al. (2011) Downregulation of alpha-fetoprotein expression by LHX4: a critical role in hepatocarcinogenesis. Carcinogenesis 32: 1815–1823.

22. Haraguchi T, Ozaki Y, Iba H (2009) Vectors expressing efficient RNA decoys achieve the long-term suppression of specific microRNA activity in mammalian cells. Nucleic Acids Res 37: e43.

23. Boura-Halfon S, Zick Y (2009) Phosphorylation of IRS proteins, insulin action, and insulin resistance. Am J Physiol Endocrinol Metab 296: E581–591.

24. Cohen P (2006) The twentieth century struggle to decipher insulin signalling. Nat Rev Mol Cell Biol 7: 867–873.

25. Tikhanovich I, Cox J, Weinman SA (2013) Forkhead box class O transcription factors in liver function and disease. J Gastroenterol Hepatol 28 Suppl 1: 125–131.

26. Su TS, Liu WY, Han SH, Jansen M, Yang-Fen TL, et al. (1989) Transcripts of the insulin-like growth factors I and II in human hepatoma. Cancer Res 49: 1773–1777.

27. Budhu A, Wang XW (2006) The role of cytokines in hepatocellular carcinoma. J Leukoc Biol 80: 1197–1213.

28. Thissen JP, Verniers J (1997) Inhibition by interleukin-1 beta and tumor necrosis factor-alpha of the insulin-like growth factor I messenger ribonucleic acid response to growth hormone in rat hepatocyte primary culture. Endocrinology 138: 1078–1084.

29. DeBenedetti F, Alonzi T, Moretta A, Lazzaro D, Costa P, et al. (1997) Interleukin 6 causes growth impairment in transgenic mice through a decrease in insulin-like growth factor-I - A model for stunted growth in children with chronic inflammation. J Clin Invest 99: 643–650.

30. Fu Q, Yu X, Callaway CW, Lane RH, McKnight RA (2009) Epigenetics: intrauterine growth retardation (IUGR) modifies the histone code along the rat hepatic IGF-1 gene. FASEB J 23: 2438–2449.

31. Schober ME, Ke XR, Xing BH, Block BP, Requena DF, et al. (2012) Traumatic brain injury increased IGF-1B mRNA and altered IGF-1 exon 5 and promoter region epigenetic characteristics in the rat pup hippocampus. J Neurotrauma 29: 2075–2085.

32. Sceusi EL, Loose DS, Wray CJ (2011) Clinical implications of DNA methylation in hepatocellular carcinoma. HPB (Oxford) 13: 369–376.

33. Adeli K (2011) Translational control mechanisms in metabolic regulation: critical role of RNA binding proteins, microRNAs, and cytoplasmic RNA granules. Am J Physiol Endocrinol Metab 301: E1051–1064.

34. Raddatz D, Ramadori G (2007) Carbohydrate metabolism and the liver: actual aspects from physiology and disease. Z Gastroenterol 45: 51–62.

35. Loeper S, Ezzat S (2008) Acromegaly: re-thinking the cancer risk. Rev Endocr Metab Disord 9: 41–58.

36. Tsugane S, Inoue M (2010) Insulin resistance and cancer: epidemiological evidence. Cancer Sci 101: 1073–1079.

37. Kawaguchi T, Taniguchi E, Itou M, Sakata M, Sumie S, et al. (2011) Insulin resistance and chronic liver disease. World J Hepatol 3: 99–107.

38. Hung CH, Wang JH, Hu TH, Chen CH, Chang KC, et al. (2010) Insulin resistance is associated with hepatocellular carcinoma in chronic hepatitis C infection. World J Gastroentero 16: 2265–2271.

39. Sumie S, Kawaguchi T, Komuta M, Kuromatsu R, Itano S, et al. (2007) Significance of glucose intolerance and SHIP2 expression in hepatocellular carcinoma patients with HCV infection. Oncol Rep 18: 545–552.

40. Miuma S, Ichikawa T, Taura N, Shibata H, Takeshita S, et al. (2009) The level of fasting serum insulin, but not adiponectin, is associated with the prognosis of early stage hepatocellular carcinoma. Oncol Rep 22: 1415–1424.

41. Shao YY, Huang CC, Lin SD, Hsu CH, Cheng AL (2012) Serum insulin-like growth factor-1 levels predict outcomes of patients with advanced hepatocellular carcinoma receiving antiangiogenic therapy. Clin Cancer Res 18: 3992–3997.

42. Kaseb AO, Morris JS, Hassan MM, Siddiqui AM, Lin E, et al. (2011) Clinical and prognostic implications of plasma insulin-Like growth factor-1 and vascular endothelial growth factor in patients with hepatocellular carcinoma. J Clin Oncol 29: 3892–3899.

43. Svoboda M, Sana J, Fabian P, Kocakova I, Gombosova J, et al. (2012) MicroRNA expression profile associated with response to neoadjuvant chemoradiotherapy in locally advanced rectal cancer patients. Radiat Oncol 7: 195.

44. Patnaik SK, Yendamuri S, Kannisto E, Kucharczuk JC, Singhal S, et al. (2012) MicroRNA expression profiles of whole blood in lung adenocarcinoma. PLoS One 7: e46045.

45. Boni V, Bitarte N, Cristobal I, Zarate R, Rodriguez J, et al. (2010) miR-192/miR-215 influence 5-Fluorouracil resistance through cell cycle-mediated mechanisms complementary to its post-transcriptional thymidilate synthase regulation. Mol Cancer Ther 9: 2265–2275.

3

Jejunal Proteins Secreted by *db/db* Mice or Insulin-Resistant Humans Impair the Insulin Signaling and Determine Insulin Resistance

Serenella Salinari[1]**, Cyrille Debard**[2]**, Alessandro Bertuzzi**[3]**, Christine Durand**[2]**, Paul Zimmet**[4]**, Hubert Vidal**[2]**, Geltrude Mingrone**[5]*

1 Department of Computer and System Science, University of Rome "Sapienza", Rome, Italy, 2 Lyon 1 University, CarMeN Laboratory, INSERM U1060, Oullins, France, 3 Institute of Systems Analysis and Computer Science, National Research Council, Rome, Italy, 4 Baker IDI Heart and Diabetes Institute, Melbourne, Victoria, Australia, 5 Department of Internal Medicine, Catholic University, School of Medicine, Rome, Italy

Abstract

Background: Two recent studies demonstrated that bariatric surgery induced remission of type 2 diabetes very soon after surgery and far too early to be attributed to weight loss. In this study, we sought to explore the mechanism/s of this phenomenon by testing the effects of proteins from the duodenum-jejunum conditioned-medium (CM) of *db/db* or Swiss mice on glucose uptake *in vivo* in Swiss mice and *in vitro* in both Swiss mice soleus and L6 cells. We studied the effect of sera and CM proteins from insulin resistant (IR) and insulin-sensitive subjects on insulin signaling in human myoblasts.

Methodology/Principal Findings: *db/db* proteins induced massive IR either *in vivo* or *in vitro*, while Swiss proteins did not. In L6 cells, only *db/db* proteins produced a noticeable increase in basal ^{473}Ser-Akt phosphorylation, lack of GSK3β inhibition and a reduced basal ^{389}Thr-p70-S6K1 phosphorylation. Human IR serum markedly increased basal ^{473}Ser-Akt phosphorylation in a dose-dependent manner. Human CM IR proteins increased by about twofold both basal and insulin-stimulated ^{473}Ser-Akt. Basal ^{9}Ser-GSK3β phosphorylation was increased by IR subjects serum with a smaller potentiating effect of insulin.

Conclusions: These findings show that jejunal proteins either from *db/db* mice or from insulin resistant subjects impair muscle insulin signaling, thus inducing insulin resistance.

Editor: Massimo Federici, University of Tor Vergata, Italy

Funding: Financed by the Catholic University. The funders had no role in study design, data collection and analysis, decision to publish, or preparation of the manuscript.

Competing Interests: The authors have declared that no competing interests exist.

* E-mail: gmingrone@rm.unicatt.it

Introduction

Type 2 diabetes (T2D) is a heterogeneous disorder usually associated with insulin resistance and hyperinsulinemia leading to impaired glucose tolerance or frank diabetes as pancreatic insulin response declines [1].

Typically, obesity promotes insulin resistance with a compensatory increase in insulin production via increased β-cell mass [2,3]. In obese T2D subjects, a prompt diabetes remission is observed after bariatric surgery [4,5] and insulin sensitivity is restored [4,6] along with the normalization of the first phase of insulin secretion [7]. Bariatric operations reroute food through the upper small intestine, possibly reducing the production of putative factor/s inducing insulin resistance and whose secretion is stimulated by nutrients. The mechanisms of T2D remission have been investigated in experimental animals. These suggest a pivotal role of the small intestine [8]. The bypass of duodenum and jejunum in Goto-Kakizaki (GK) rats, an animal model of non-obese T2D, was shown to control diabetes directly and not as a secondary effect of weight loss [9]. That food intake reduction is

not implicated in the amelioration of glucose disposal was then demonstrated by the observation that GK rats which had undergone duodenal-jejunal bypass had a markedly better oral glucose tolerance compared to pair-fed sham-operated rats [9]. Duodenal-jejunal bypass surgery in rats normalized glucose disposal in streptozotocin-induced diabetes as well as in insulin deficient autoimmune type 1 diabetes [10].

Obese, diabetic C57BL/Ks *db/db* mice are an extensively studied genetic model of obesity and type 2 diabetes [11]. These animals show characteristics similar to human T2D including obesity and severe insulin resistance [12]. Brozinick et al. [13] have reported that despite the marked *in vivo* insulin resistance observed for the normal-glucose tolerant *db/db* mice during hyperinsulinemic clamps, their muscles are completely insulin responsive *in vitro*. On the basis of these findings, they suggested the presence of a humoral factor impairing the insulin action *in vivo* [13].

To test the hypothesis that the small intestine of *db/db* mice produces factors/hormones inducing insulin resistance, proteins enriched from the conditioned medium (CM) of *db/db* and Swiss duodenum-jejunum or of insulin resistant and insulin sensitive subjects were obtained. Their molecular cutoff was chosen in a range between 10 and 100 kDa, on the basis of a series of previous experiments. The biological activity of mouse CM proteins was assessed both *in vivo* in Swiss mice which underwent an intra-peritoneal insulin tolerance test, and *in vitro* in Swiss skeletal muscle tissue as well as in L6 cell cultures to measure insulin-mediated glucose uptake and insulin signaling. Furthermore, the effect on insulin signaling of serum or CM proteins from jejunum specimens obtained during abdominal surgery in insulin resistant and insulin sensitive human subjects was studied in human myotubes.

Materials and Methods

Experimental Animals

Animals. One-hundred fifty-eight (108M and 50F) Swiss mice 12–14 weeks old were from in-house breeding colonies. Eighty-one C57BL/6 (*db/db*) mice (31M and 50F) 12–14 weeks old were from Charles River Laboratories (Calco, Italy).

The protocol was approved by the Catholic University Animal Experimentation Ethics Committee in accordance with European guidelines for the use of animals.

Intestinal protein secretion. In order to enhance the secretion of intestinal factor/s inducing insulin resistance, fed mice were sacrificed by intraperitoneal injection with pentobarbital (12 mg/mouse, ip, Nembutal, Abbott Laboratories, Abbott Park, IL). Everted duodenum-jejunum sacs [14] were washed with saline and incubated in oxygenated (O_2:CO_2, 95:5, v/v) Krebs-Henseleit solution (37°C, pH 7.4) for 1 h to isolate proteins secreted into the medium. Conditioned medium was lyophilized and stored at -80°C for protein purification.

Protein purification. Lyophilized powders were re-suspended in bidistilled water ($\sim$10 mg/ml) and ultra-filtered through a hydrophilic 100 kDa cutoff membrane (Centripep, Amicon, Beverly) at 4°C. The fraction containing compounds <100 kDa was passed through a Centripep with membrane cutoff of 10 kDa. The material retained by the filter was removed with a pipette and dried.

Protein concentrations were determined with bicinchoninic acid (Pierce, Rockford, IL, USA), using bovine serum albumin as a concentration standard.

Intraperitoneal Insulin Tolerance Test (IPITT). 1 IU Actrapid insulin/kg bodyweight was injected into the peritoneum of Swiss mice after 16 h of fasting. Swiss mice were injected intravenously with saline (control) or proteins secreted from small intestine of *db/db* or Swiss mice 20 min before the IPITT. $t=0$ is the starting time of intraperitoneal insulin injection. Blood samples were drawn from the orbital sinus and blood glucose measured by Accu-Chek blood glucose meter (Roche Diagnostics, Basel, Switzerland) at 0, 15, 30, 45, 60, and 90 min. Serum insulin was analyzed by radioimmunoassay (Linco Research, St. Charles, MO).

IPITT data were analyzed by adapting the minimal model [15], which is currently used to assess insulin sensitivity (S_I, $min^{-1} \cdot pM^{-1}$) and glucose effectiveness (S_G, min^{-1}) from intravenous or oral glucose tolerance-tests and has been validated in mice [16]. Minimal model equations were written in the following form

$$\dot{G} = -(S_G + S_I Z)\,G + S_G G_b, \quad G(0) = G_b \tag{1}$$

$$\dot{Z} = p(-Z + I - I_b), \quad Z(0) = 0 \tag{2}$$

where the overdot means d/dt, G is glucose concentration (basal value, G_b), I insulin concentration (basal value, I_b), Z a variable related to the insulin action, and p a rate constant (min^{-1}) governing Z kinetics.

Insulin data, linearly interpolated, were assigned to $I - I_b$ in Eq. (2), and the model parameters S_G, S_I, G_b and p were estimated by fitting glucose concentration data. Direct estimation of the population parameters was obtained by the NONMEM method [17].

Glucose transport in soleus muscle. Experiments were performed as reported elsewhere [18]. Briefly, Swiss soleus muscle was incubated for 20 min (glucose 5 mM, insulin 60 nM) in the absence (control) or in the presence of 10 μg/ml and 20 μg/ml of either db/db or Swiss CM proteins.

L6 cell culture. Skeletal L6 myoblasts were grown to 70–80% confluence in DMEM as described elsewhere [19,20]. Cells were serum deprived for 2 h (glucose 25 mM) before treatment with various concentrations of insulin for 5 min. The rate of 2-DG uptake versus insulin concentration in L6 myoblasts was measured in the absence (control) or presence of 30 μg/ml Swiss or db/db CM.

2-deoxyglucose uptake data were fitted with a function of the insulin concentration, I :

$$R(I) = R_b + \Delta R \frac{I}{K_{0.5} + I} \tag{3}$$

where R_b ($pmol \cdot min^{-1} \cdot well^{-1}$) is the rate of glucose uptake at zero insulin concentration, ΔR ($pmol \cdot min^{-1} \cdot well^{-1}$) is the maximal insulin-stimulated increase in the rate of uptake, and $K_{0.5}$ (nM) is the insulin concentration that yields the half-maximal increase.

Western blot analysis. L6 cells were harvested and lysed in ice-cold lysis buffer as previously described [21]. Akt phosphorylations were detected using anti-phospho-Ser[473] and anti-phospho-Thr[308] antibodies. For the characterization of the other signaling pathways in L6 cells, we used anti-[9]Ser-GSK3β and anti-[389]Thr-p70 S6K1. More details are given in the Supporting Information (Appendix S1).

Humans

Demographic data. Seven obese and 3 normal weight subjects were enrolled. The study protocol was approved by the ethics committee of the Catholic University, School of Medicine, Rome, Italy. All the subjects signed two written informed consents, one prior to the study and the other before surgery.

The seven IR subjects had an mean age of 41.7±4.6 years and a body mass index (BMI) of 43.24±1.91 kg/m². The three normal weight subjects were 41.0±3.6 (mean ± s.d.) years old with a BMI of 22.28±1.85 kg/m².

Insulin sensitivity assessment. Insulin sensitivity was assessed by the euglycemic hyperinsulinemic clamp [22]. Insulin sensitivity was determined during the last 40 min of the clamp by computing the whole-body glucose uptake (M, $μmol \cdot min^{-1} \cdot kg_{bw}^{-1}$) during the steady-state euglycemic hyperinsulinemia.

Surgery. The obese, insulin resistant subjects underwent Roux-en-Y gastric bypass after an overnight fast. Specimens of the jejunum of circa 500 mg were obtained during the operation and immediately placed in the oxygenated incubation medium. After an overnight fast, the three insulin sensitive subjects underwent elective small bowel resection for stenosis of the terminal ileum in inactive Crohn's disease, taking care during the operation to obtain the jejunal specimens (ca. 500 mg) at a distance of at least 15 cm from the diseased portion of the small intestine.

Human skeletal muscle cell culture and Western blot analysis. Human myoblasts were plated on 6-well plates coated with collagen I and grown in Ham's F10 medium supplemented with 2% FCS, 2% Ultroser G, and 1% antibiotics. Differentiation was induced in DMEM (1 g/l glucose) without serum and polynucleated myotubes were obtained after 4 days [23]. Myotubes were treated for 15 min with serum from IR patients or with conditioned medium proteins (25 µg/ml) from IR or insulin sensitive patients in the presence or absence of 100 nM of human recombinant insulin.

The western blot conditions are described in the Supporting Information (Appendix S1).

Statistical analysis. Data are presented as mean ± s.d. unless otherwise indicated. ANOVA test for repeated measurements followed by Tukey-test was used for intergroup comparisons. Two-sided $P<0.05$ was significant.

Results

Experimental Animal Data

Intraperitoneal insulin tolerance test. The effect on insulin sensitivity of saline (control) and CM proteins from *db/db* or Swiss mice injected in Swiss mice was evaluated by the intraperitoneal insulin test (IPITT) and minimal model analysis (Fig. 1, A and B). Amounts of proteins injected were 15 or 150 µg, which corresponded to circulating levels of 2.1 or, respectively, 21 µg/ml assuming that the distribution volume of these proteins equals that of glucose (7.1 ml, see [16]). The overall profile of glucose concentration was significantly increased in animals injected with either 15 or 150 µg proteins from *db/db* mice, compared with animals injected with saline (Fig. 1A), strongly suggesting that *db/db* proteins induce insulin resistance in control Swiss mice. In contrast, glucose concentration profiles in mice injected with Swiss proteins did not differ from those of controls (Fig. 1B). The estimates of minimal model parameters (Eqs. (1)-(2) in Methods) demonstrate that the insulin sensitivity, S_I, that accounts for cumulative insulin action in liver and peripheral tissues, was significantly decreased in mice injected with *db/db* proteins (ca. 40% with both 15 and 150 µg) (Table 1). The glucose effectiveness, S_G, representing the capacity of glucose to regulate its own disposal, was also significantly reduced in the presence of *db/db* proteins. By contrast, the parameters from mice treated with Swiss proteins did not differ significantly from those of controls.

Glucose uptake in soleus muscle. To test the effect of CM proteins on glucose uptake in muscle, 2-deoxyglucose transport in response to a constant insulin concentration of 60 nM was measured *in vitro* in the isolated soleus muscle of Swiss mice (Fig. 1C). Glucose transport – equal in control to 2.48±0.44 (mean ± s.d.) µmol of 2-deoxyglucose (2-DG) per ml intracellular water over 20 min – was reduced by 39.5% when muscle samples were exposed to 10 µg/ml of *db/db* proteins and 49.7% when exposed to 20 µg/ml. By contrast, in the presence of the same concentrations of Swiss proteins, the rate of glucose transport underwent a smaller, not significant reduction.

Glucose uptake in L6 cells. The effects of the exposure to proteins from *db/db* mice on the insulin-stimulated glucose uptake in L6 myoblasts (Fig. 1D) were consistent with those observed during the IPITT and the glucose transport experiments in the isolated soleus muscle. After preincubation with 30 µg/ml *db/db* proteins, the 2-DG rate of uptake, expressed as pmol·min^{-1}.''' well^{-1}, was significantly reduced with respect to control at all insulin concentrations from 1 nM to 10 µM. In contrast, the response to insulin under the exposure to the same concentration

of Swiss proteins was not statistically different from that observed in response to saline.

Table 2 reports the parameters R_b, ΔR, and $K_{0.5}$ of Eq. (3) in Methods, estimated by fitting the glucose uptake data. The ratio $\Delta R/R_b$ was close to the unity in all cases because, as also shown by the raw data, the maximal 2-DG uptake was about twofold the basal uptake either in control or in the presence of the intestinal proteins. However, the insulin-independent rate of uptake, R_b, which is possibly related to the activity of GLUT1, was found to be largely decreased only in cells exposed to *db/db* proteins.

A measure of the sensitivity to insulin of glucose uptake was obtained by computing from Eq. (3) the derivative of the rate of uptake R with respect to I at $I=0$, which gives $(dR/dI)|_{I=0} = \Delta R/K_{0.5}$. The values of this ratio (µl·min^{-1}·well^{-1}) were 7.1±1.8 in control, 4.1±1.8 in the presence of Swiss proteins and 2.3±0.3 in the presence of *db/db* proteins, respectively, showing that insulin sensitivity was significantly decreased ($P<0.0002$) in the L6 cells exposed to *db/db* proteins.

We found that the average reduction in glucose uptake (37.2%) by the L6 cells in the presence of *db/db* proteins at 60 nM insulin concentration as computed by Eq. (3) was in the same order of the decrease found in the isolated soleus muscle.

Effects of mice CM proteins on insulin signaling in L6 cells. CM proteins at a concentration of 25 µg/ml increased ^{473}Ser Akt phosphorylation in the absence of insulin, with a tendency toward a stronger effect of medium prepared from *db/db* than from Swiss mice (Fig. 2A). This effect was very rapid, already observed after 5 min of incubation, and approached saturation at 15–30 min (Fig. 2C). Insulin was still able to increase ^{473}Ser Akt phosphorylation in the presence of CM proteins from *db/db* mice, but the amplitude of the maximal increase over basal was markedly reduced (Fig. 2A). Accordingly, the sigmoidal profile of the dose-response curve of insulin action on ^{473}Ser Akt phosphorylation was lost in the presence of *db/db* proteins (Fig. 2B). Rapamycin, a classical inhibitor of mammalian target of Rapamycin complex 1 (mTORC1), did not counteract the effect of CM proteins from *db/db* mice on ^{473}Ser Akt phosphorylation, while the global mTOR inhibitor PP242 completely abolished this phosphorylation, particularly in cells incubated with *db/db* CM proteins (Fig. 2D). This result suggests that CM proteins probably increased ^{473}Ser Akt phosphorylation in muscle cells through stimulation of mTORC2 complex.

Insulin stimulated ^{308}Thr Akt phosphorylation had a tendency toward a decrease ($P=0.08$) in the presence of *db/db* but not Swiss CM proteins (Fig. S1A), indicating that *db/db* CM proteins tend to inhibit phosphoinositide-dependent kinase 1 (PDK1) activity. Accordingly, the dose-response curve of insulin action on ^{308}Thr Akt phosphorylation was reduced in the presence of *db/db* proteins (Fig. S1B).

To further confirm the implication of mTOR signaling in the effect of CM proteins, we measured the phosphorylation of S6Kinase in L6 cells. In control conditions, both Rapamycin and PP242 abolished the basal ^{389}Thr phosphorylation of p70 S6K1 (Fig. 3A), consistent with the role of mTORC1 in mediating ^{389}Thr phosphorylation in its downstream substrate S6K1. Interestingly, *db/db* CM proteins in the absence of inhibitors reduced by about 50% ($P<0.05$) the basal ^{389}Thr phosphorylation of p70 S6K1 (Fig. 3A). Addition of the mTOR inhibitors further suppressed the phosphorylation of S6K1 in the presence of the *db/db* CM, suggesting that CM proteins could negatively control mTORC1 activity (Fig. 3A) while concomitantly activating mTORC2 (Fig. 2D).

Glycogen synthase kinase 3 (GSK3) is a well-known downstream substrate of Akt. In human muscle cells, insulin stimulates

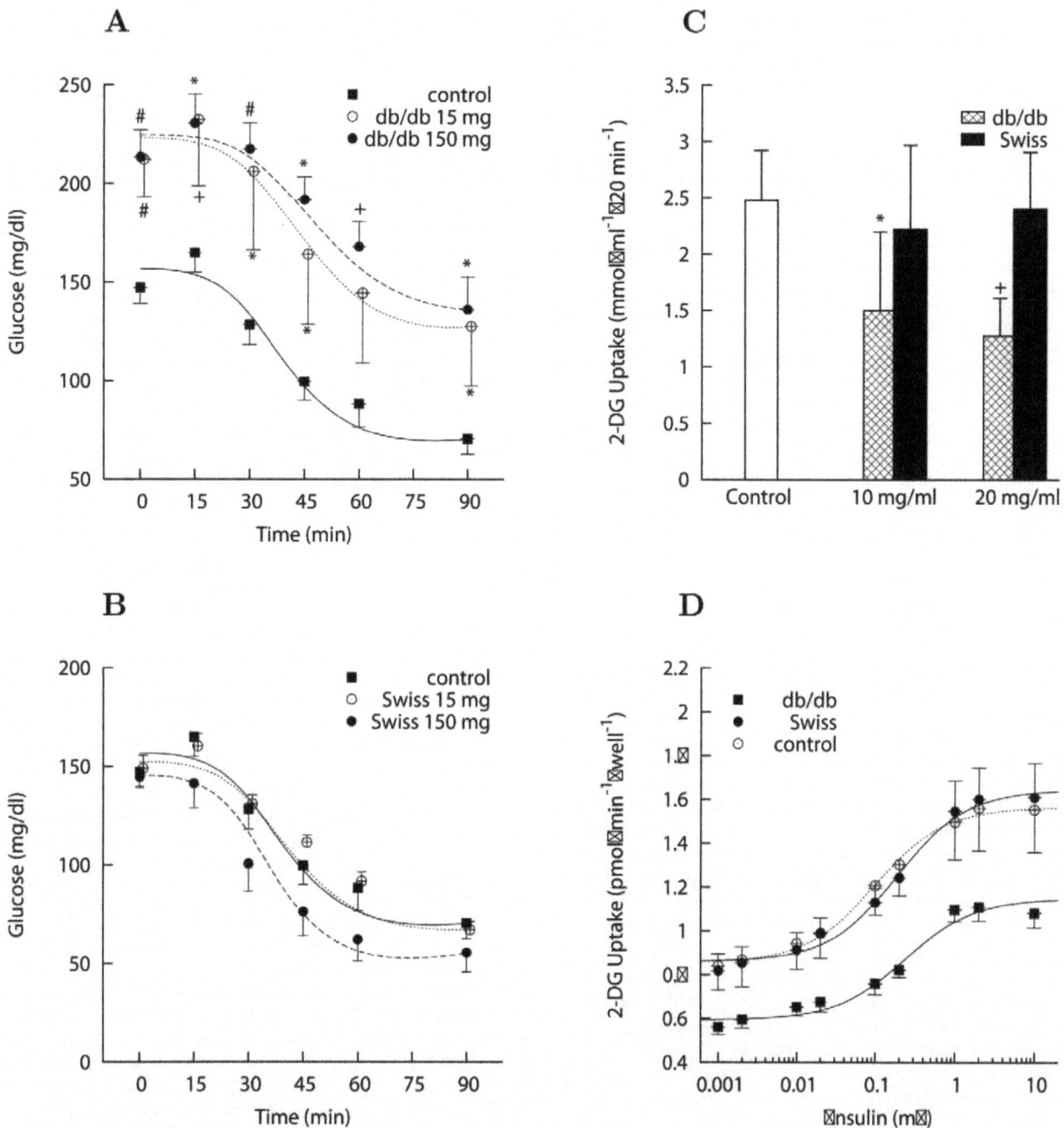

Figure 1. Intraperitoneal insulin tolerance test on Swiss mice and effect of *db/db* and Swiss conditioned medium (CM) proteins on the *in vitro* glucose uptake. *Panel A*: Glucose concentration profiles during the IPITT in controls ($n = 23$) and mice injected with 15 ($n = 10$) or 150 μg ($n = 11$) of *db/db* CM proteins. Values are mean ± s.e.m. *$P < 0.05$, +$P < 0.01$, and #$P < 0.001$, *db/db* 15 or 150 μg vs. control. The lines are the fitting curves obtained by the model of Eqs. (1)-(2) in Methods with the parameter values reported in Table 1. *Panel B*: Glucose concentration profiles during the IPITT (mean ± s.e.m.) in controls ($n = 23$) and mice injected with 15 ($n = 11$) or 150 μg ($n = 7$) of Swiss CM proteins. *Panel C*: Transport of 2-deoxyglucose (2-DG) in isolated soleus muscle. Values are mean ± s.d. of $n = 7$ determinations of 2-DG uptake expressed as μmol per ml intracellular water per 20 min. *$P < 0.02$, *db/db* 10 μg/ml CM proteins vs. control; +$P < 0.0005$, *db/db* 20 μg/ml CM proteins vs. control. *Panel D*: Rate of 2-DG uptake versus insulin concentration in L6 myoblasts. Insulin mediated glucose uptake was determined in cells exposed to 30 μg/ml of *db/db* or Swiss CM proteins vs. control. Data points are mean ± s.d. of $n = 7$ determinations for each insulin concentration expressed as pmol per min per well. $P < 0.0001$ for 2-DG uptake reduction with *db/db* CM proteins vs. control and Swiss CM at all insulin concentrations. Fitting curves are given by Eq. 3 in Methods with the parameter values reported in Table 2.

GSK3β phosphorylation on the [9]Ser residue, leading to inhibition of its activity [24]. In L6 cells, incubation with *db/db* CM proteins led to a marked inhibition of insulin-stimulated increase of [9]Ser GSK3β phosphorylation (Fig. 3B). Furthermore, lower molecular

weight bands appeared on the blot, suggesting proteolysis of the phosphorylated form of GSK3β especially upon *db/db* CM protein treatment (Fig. 3B). Actually, a rapid proteolysis of [9]Ser phosphorylated GSK3β was observed, readily after 5 min

Table 1. Estimates of parameters (mean $\pm$ s.d. over the population) of Eqs. (1)-(2) used to fit IPITT data.

CM proteins	Control n = 23	Swiss 15 μg n = 11	Swiss 150 μg n = 7	db/db 15 μg n = 10	db/db 150 μg n = 11
S_G (min^{-1}) $\times 10^2$	2.61±0.43	2.95±1.04	2.15±1.63	2.20±0.34	1.01±0.75[#*°]
S_I (min$^{-1}\cdot$pM^{-1}) $\times 10^5$	8.45±1.95	8.73±4.55	9.51±3.50	4.50±1.52[×]	5.42±1.22[&°]
G_b (mg$\cdot$dl^{-1})	156.9±38.6	152.2±21.6	145.4±12.7	223.0±59.9[+]	224.5±46.0[+]
p (min^{-1}) $\times 10^2$	1.77±1.22	1.47±0.40	2.32±1.56	3.01±1.32	2.93±1.43

[#]$P < 0.001$, db/db 150 μg vs. control and Swiss 15 μg;
[+]$P < 0.005$, db/db 15 or 150 μg vs. Swiss 15 or 150 μg;
$P < 0.005$, db/db 15 μg vs. control;
[×]$P < 0.01$, db/db 15 μg vs. Swiss 15 and 150 μg;
[*]$P < 0.05$, db/db 15 vs. db/db 150 μg;
[°]$P < 0.05$, db/db 150 μg vs. Swiss 150 μg;
[&]$P < 0.05$, db/db 150 μg vs. control and Swiss 15 μg.

incubation, in the presence of db/db CM, and this effect was fully reversible on 15 min washout with fresh culture medium (Fig. 3C). Finally, mTOR inhibitors had no effect on the proteolysis of phosphorylated GSK3β induced by the db/db CM proteins, either in the presence or absence of insulin (Fig. 3D).

Human Data

Euglycemic-hyperinsulinemic clamp. The insulin mediated glucose disposal (M) in the IR subjects was much lower than in Crohn's patients. The M value of the former group was 16.4 ± 2.8 μmol·min^{-1}·kg$_{bw}^{-1}$ with a steady state plasma insulin concentration of 460.3 ± 89.7 pmol/l, whereas in the in Crohn's patients the M value was 47.4 ± 3.6 μmol·min^{-1}·kg$_{bw}^{-1}$ with a plasma insulin concentration at the steady state of 420.0 ± 26.2 pmol/l.

Effects of human serum and CM proteins on insulin signaling in human myotubes. To assess whether the findings in L6 cells are replicated in humans, Akt and GSK3β phosphorylation was measured in human myotubes treated with serum or CM proteins from insulin sensitive and insulin resistant subjects. Incubation of human myotubes with 5, 10 or 20% serum from IR subjects induced a rapid (15 min) and dose dependent increase of basal (no insulin) ^{473}Ser Akt phosphorylation, which attained a level comparable with that induced by 100 nM insulin (Fig. 4A). Similarly, serum induced ^{9}Ser GSK3β phosphorylation with levels comparable with that of insulin (Fig. 4B). By contrast, no significant changes were obtained with sera from insulin sensitive subjects (data not shown).

Table 2. Estimates of parameters (estimate $\pm$ s.d. of the estimate) of Eq. (3) used to fit the rate of deoxyglucose uptake in L6 cells.

Secreted proteins	Control	Swiss	db/db
R_b (pmol·min^{-1}·well^{-1})	0.855±0.112	0.847±0.077	0.593±0.033[*&]
ΔR (pmol·min^{-1}·well^{-1})	0.713±0.130	0.782±0.150	0.555±0.055 [#]
$K_{0.5}$ (nM)	100.7±34.7	190.8±120.2	240.5±52.1[+]

[*]$P < 0.00005$, db/db vs. control;
[+]$P < 0.02$, db/db vs. control;
[&]$P < 0.00005$, db/db vs. Swiss;
[#]$P < 0.01$, db/db vs. Swiss.

The intestinal CM proteins from insulin resistant subjects almost doubled the basal level of ^{473}Ser Akt phosphorylation with respect to insulin sensitive controls, but also its insulin stimulated level was markedly increased (Fig. 5A). The degree of insulin sensitivity (M in μmol·min^{-1}·kg$_{bw}^{-1}$ normalized by the steady state insulin, I, in pM) measured by the euglycemic clamp inversely correlated with the relative amount of ^{473}Ser Akt during insulin stimulation. The linear regression equation is: M/I = 0.128 − 0.018 ^{473}Ser Akt ($R^2 = 0.613$, $P = 0.007$).

Basal ^{9}Ser GSK3β phosphorylation had a tendency to increase in the presence of CM proteins from IR subjects compared with insulin sensitive subjects, while the differential increase of phosphorylation under insulin stimulation was pretty low (Fig. 5B).

Discussion

Two recent studies demonstrated that bariatric surgery induced remission of T2D and significant improvement in metabolic control of the diabetes over and above medical therapy [5,25]. The improvement in glycemia occurs very soon after the surgery and far too early to be attributed to weight loss. In this study, we sought to explore the mechanism/s of this phenomenon. Jejunal conditioned medium proteins from both diabetic, insulin resistant animals and insulin resistant humans impaired insulin signaling in skeletal muscle cell cultures. A similar effect was obtained with the human serum from insulin resistant subjects, suggesting that circulating (and thus by definition endocrine) factors are inducing insulin resistance.

An in vivo and in vitro state of insulin resistance was reproduced in the presence of proteins secreted by the duodenal-jejunal mucosa of db/db mice. Contrary to the conditioned medium proteins from Swiss mice, those secreted by the db/db mice small intestine induced insulin resistance when injected in normal Swiss mice or when added to the incubation medium of skeletal muscle preparations in vitro. Also the experiments with the L6 cells were congruent, as shown by ~65% and ~30% reduction of insulin-dependent ($\Delta R/K_{0.5}$) and insulin-independent (R_b) glucose uptake in the presence of db/db proteins, respectively. Notably, Swiss mice proteins failed to decrease glucose uptake either in vivo or in vitro.

Our study demonstrates that the molecular mechanism through which proteins secreted by the duodenal-jejunal mucosa of db/db mice induce insulin resistance could be mediated by interference with intracellular signaling pathways. We found that db/db proteins robustly induced the phosphorylation of the Akt ^{473}serine residue at zero insulin, leading to a prompt saturation of the insulin dose-response curve. Moreover, db/db CM proteins tended

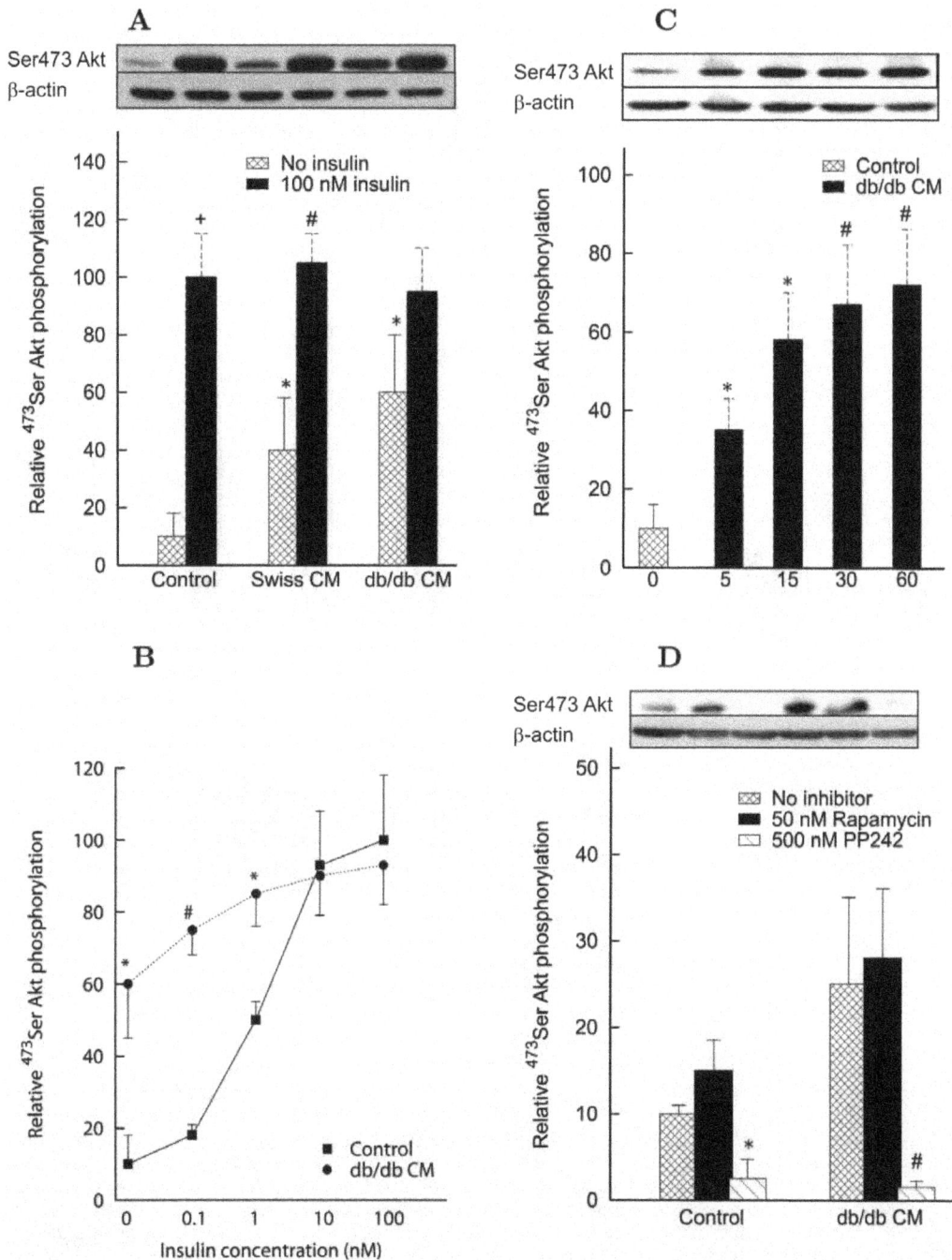

Figure 2. Effect of conditioned medium (CM) on ^{473}Ser Akt phosphorylation in differentiated L6 myotubes. Each bar is the mean of experiments in triplicate with 3 to 5 different preparations of CM. Data are normalized by β-actin amount and expressed as fold change versus control condition (control at 100 nM insulin set at 100). Data are mean ± s.d. *Panel A*: 15 min incubation of L6 myotubes with 25 μg/ml of CM proteins increased ^{473}Ser Akt phosphorylation level in the absence of insulin, with an effect that tended to be stronger of medium prepared from *db/db* (*$P<0.05$ vs. control) than from Swiss mice. The stimulatory effect of 100 nM insulin in control (+$P<0.01$ vs. no insulin) was preserved in the presence of Swiss CM (#$P<0.05$) but did not reach significance in the presence of *db/db* CM. *Panel B*: Dose-response profile of insulin action on ^{473}Ser Akt phosphorylation vs. insulin concentration (nM) in logarithmic scale after 15 min co-incubation in the absence (squares) or presence (circles) of 25 μg/ ml *db/db* CM proteins (#$P<0.01$ and *$P<0.05$ vs. control). *Panel C*: Basal (no insulin) ^{473}Ser Akt phosphorylation determined after different incubation times with 25 μg/ml *db/db* CM proteins. An increased ^{473}Ser Akt phosphorylation was already observed after 5 min of incubation and approached saturation at 15–30 min (*$P<0.05$ and #$P<0.01$ vs. control). *Panel D*: Effect of mTORC inhibitors on basal ^{473}Ser Akt phosphorylation. L6 myotubes were treated with Rapamycin or PP242 for 1 hour before 15 min incubation with 25 μg/ml CM proteins. The stimulatory effect of *db/db* proteins was inhibited by PP242 in both control (*$P<0.05$ vs. no inhibitor) and *db/db* CM treated cells (#$P<0.01$ vs. no inhibitor).

A

B

C

D

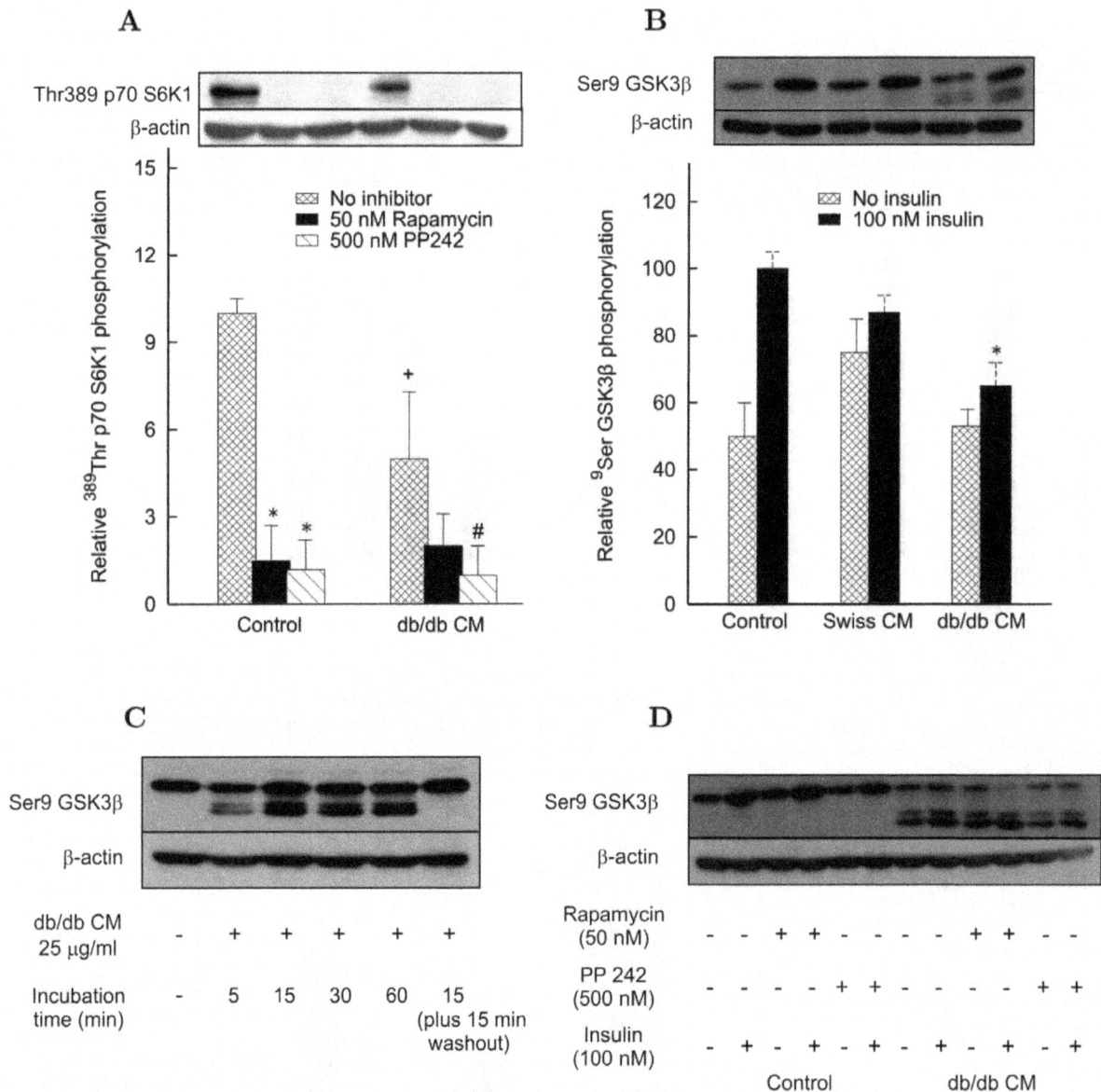

Figure 3. Effect of conditioned medium (CM) on p70 S6kinase and GSK3β phosphorylation in differentiated L6 myotubes. Each bar is the mean of experiments in triplicate with 3 to 5 different preparations of CM. Data are normalized by β-actin amount and expressed as fold change versus control condition (no insulin nor CM) set at 10. Data are mean ± s.d. *Panel A*: ^{389}Thr p70 S6K1 phosphorylation. L6 myotubes were treated with Rapamycin or PP242 for 1 hour before 15 min incubation with 25 μg/ml of *db/db* CM. *db/db* CM proteins inhibited the basal ^{389}Thr p70 S6K1 phosphorylation ($^{+}P<0.05$ vs. control no inhibitors). PP242 further reduced the phosphorylation level in both control ($^{*}P<0.01$, Rapamycin and PP242 vs. no inhibitor) and *db/db* CM ($^{#}P<0.05$ vs. no inhibitor). *Panel B*: ^{9}Ser GSK3β phosphorylation after 15 min co-incubation with 25 μg/ml CM with or without insulin. *db/db* CM proteins inhibited the insulin-stimulated increase of ^{9}Ser GSK3β phosphorylation ($^{*}P<0.05$ vs. insulin-induced phosphorylation in control set at 100). Lower molecular weight bands in the blot suggest proteolysis of phosphorylated form of GSK3β upon *db/db* CM treatment. *Panel C*: Time course of the effect of 25 μg/ml *db/db* CM on ^{9}Ser GSK3β phosphorylation and proteolysis. The *db/db*-derived conditioned medium did not significantly affect basal phosphorylation of GSK3β on ^{9}Ser, while it induced a rapid degradation of GSK3β, measurable since 5 min of incubation. After 15 min of pretreatment with *db/db* CM, a washout for 15 min with medium replacement was able to fully correct the alterations induced by the *db/db* CM. *Panel D*: Pretreatment of L6 myotubes with Rapamycin or PP242 for 1 hour before incubation with 25 μg/ml CM from *db/db* for 15 min in the absence or presence of 100 nM insulin. mTOR inhibitors had no effect on proteolysis of phosphorylated GSK3β induced by *db/db* CM proteins either in the presence or absence of insulin.

to reduce the insulin-induced phosphorylation of Akt on ^{308}Thr residue. Thus, 100 nM insulin treated L6 cells in the presence of *db/db* CM exhibited maximal Akt phosphorylation at ^{473}Ser residue but about 50% phosphorylation at ^{308}Thr residue, so full Akt activation could not be attained, consistent with the observed reduction of 2DG uptake in the soleus muscle and L6 cells. CM

db/db also determined a marked proteolysis of GSK3β phosphorylated form and inhibited the basal activation of the p70 S6kinase.

Interestingly, when compared with insulin sensitive individuals, both serum and intestinal CM proteins from insulin resistant subjects determined a higher basal ^{473}Ser Akt and ^{9}Ser GSK3β phosphorylation in human myotubes. A tendency toward an increased basal phosphorylation of ^{9}Ser GSK3β was also observed

A

B

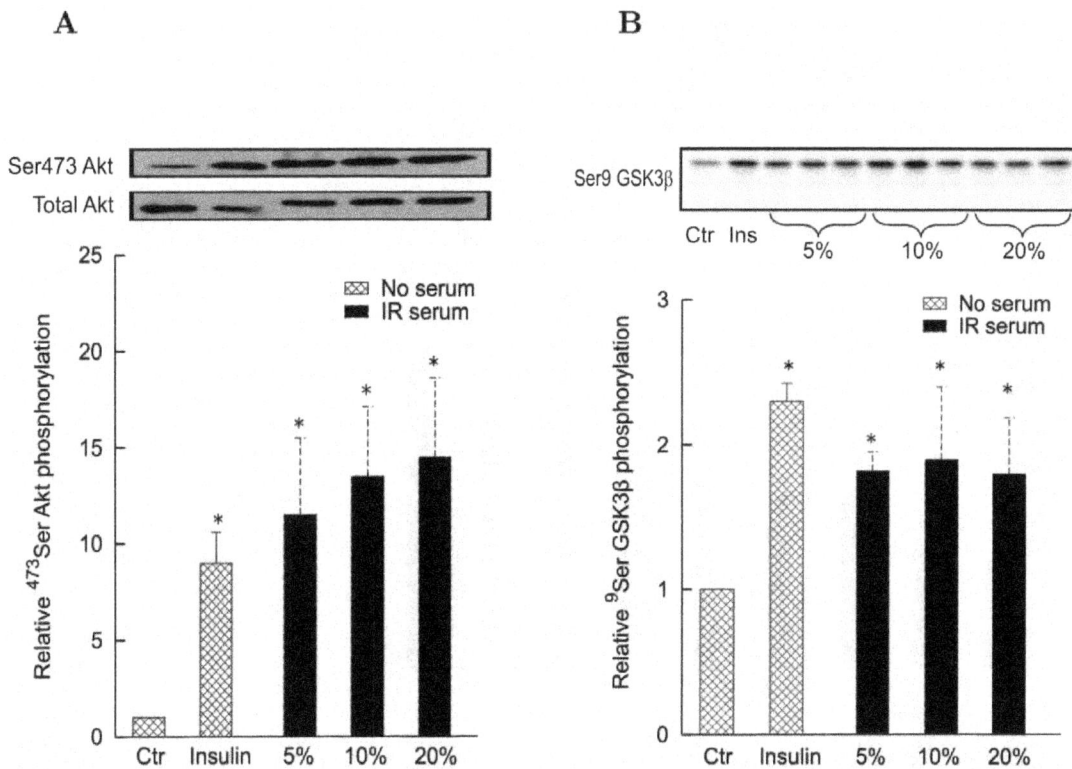

Figure 4. Effect of serum from IR subjects (15 min) on Akt and GSK3β phosphorylation in differentiated human myotubes. Each bar is the mean of the results with sera from 7 IR subjects. Experiments were performed in triplicate for each individual. Ctr denotes controls. *Panel A*: Basal [473]Ser Akt phosphorylation in the presence of 100 nM insulin or of different serum concentrations (5%, 10% and 20%) from IR subjects. Blots are representative western blots of [9]Ser Akt phosphorylation and total Akt amounts. Data (mean ± s.d.) are expressed as fold change versus control condition (no insulin nor serum) set at 1 (*$P<0.05$ vs. control). *Panel B*: Basal [9]Ser GSK3β phosphorylation in the presence of 100 nM insulin or of different serum concentrations (5%, 10% and 20%) from IR subjects. The blot is a representative western blots of [9]Ser GSK3β phosphorylation. Data (mean ± s.d.) are expressed as fold change versus control condition (no insulin nor serum) set at 1 (*$P<0.05$ vs. control).

in the presence of CM from insulin sensitive subjects. Furthermore, the incremental [9]Ser GSK3β phosphorylation over basal in the presence of insulin was reduced in IR subjects. Overall, these data suggest that serum and conditioned medium contain factor/s, which are likely in a larger amount in the insulin resistant than in insulin sensitive subjects, that induce insulin resistance. We observe that we could not compare insulin resistant with healthy control subjects because it is near impossible to obtain sufficient duodenal/jejunal mucosa during endoscopy to provide sufficient intestinal secreted proteins for testing in human myoblasts. Our controls were in an inactive phase of their disease with stenosis of the ileum which required elective surgery. We cannot exclude a certain degree of general inflammation, and thus they could not be considered as healthy subjects. However these patients were still insulin sensitive according to a previous observation [26] and as assessed by the euglycemic clamp.

The Akt phosphorylation of [473]Ser residue is a target of the mTOR complex 2 [27], while the Akt phosphorylation at [308]Thr is operated by PDK1, this last step being essential for the full Akt catalytic activity [28,29]. Fraenkel et al. [30] showed that, in the fasting state, basal [473]Ser Akt phosphorylation was higher in the skeletal muscle of diabetic than in normoglycemic *Psammomys obesus* (*P. obesus*), while there was a net reduction of the stimulation by insulin in agreement with the high insulin resistance state of these diabetic animals. Furthermore, it was found that Akt directly mediates Ser/Thr phosphorylation of the insulin receptor substrate 1 (IRS-1), resulting in a negative feedback loop that

reduces insulin action [31]. Interestingly, this effect was inhibited by Rapamycin [31].

Akt phosphorylates [9]Ser in GSK3β with subsequent inhibition of the enzymatic function of GSK [32]. It was recently demonstrated that GSK activity can also be regulated by calpain-induced proteolysis of its N terminus, which gives way to a short-lived constitutively active form of the enzyme [33]. Our data suggest that similar mechanisms could occur in the presence of small intestine *db/db* CM. If the products of GSK3β degradation induced by *db/db* CM proteins are active, they might contribute to enhance the recognition of GSK substrates. In addition to the well-known effect on glycogen synthase activity [34,35], GSK3 has been implicated in the phosphorylation of the IRS-1 on serine residues with a consequent impairment of insulin signaling [36,37]. Furthermore, GSK3 overexpression was found in peripheral tissues in a variety of diabetic animals and also in humans [38–42]. It has also been shown that Rapamycin markedly decreased GSK3 phosphorylation in muscle of normoglycemic and diabetic *P. obesus*, indicating increased GSK3β activity [30], while diabetes was reversed in obese diabetic mice treated with GSK3 inhibitors [43,44].

The mammalian target of rapamycin (mTOR) exists in two forms, mTORC1 and mTORC2. mTORC1 regulates protein synthesis by S6K1 and the eukaryotic initiation factor 4E-binding protein 1 at ribosomal level [45], while mTORC2 phosphorylates Akt at [473]Ser. Rapamycin is an mTORC1 inhibitor, which acts specifically on S6K1, whereas the ATP-competitive inhibitor

A

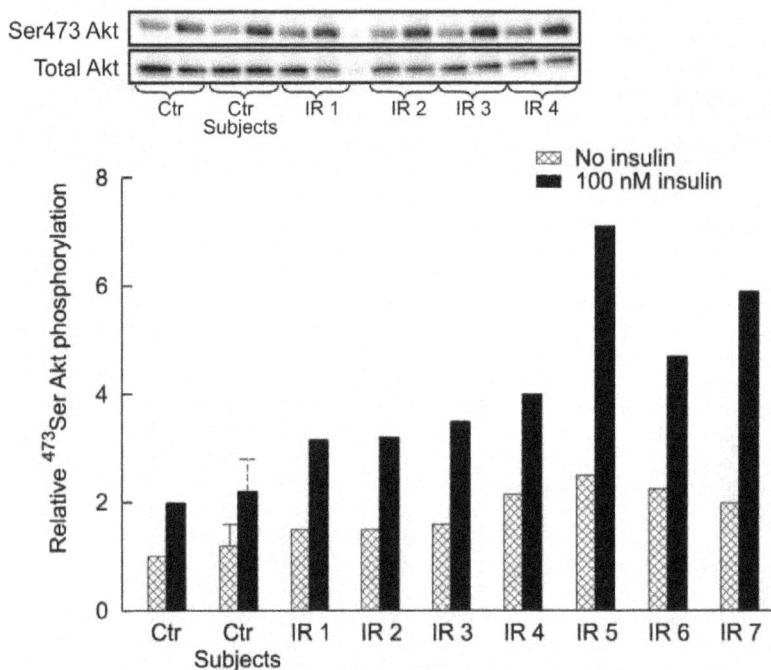

B

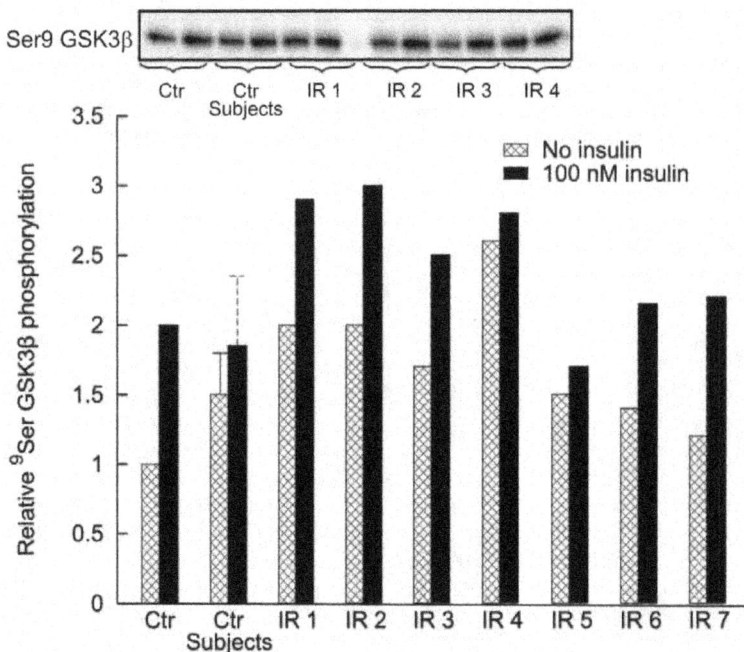

Figure 5. Effect of conditioned medium (CM) from insulin sensitive subjects and IR subjects on Akt and GSK3β phosphorylation in differentiated human myotubes. Control denotes phosphorylation in the absence of CM, with phosphorylation level in the absence of insulin set at 1. Data are reported as mean ± s.d. for control subjects (Crohn's patients denoted as control subjects), while individual values are reported for each IR subject. Each bar is the mean of experiments in triplicate. *Panel A*: 15 min incubation of human myotubes from insulin sensitive subjects with 25 μg/ml of CM proteins increased ^{473}Ser Akt phosphorylation level in the absence of insulin, with a stronger effect of medium prepared from IR subjects than from insulin sensitive subjects ($P<0.05$ vs. control subjects). The stimulatory effect of 100 nM insulin in control was increased in the presence of CM from IR subjects ($P<0.01$ vs. control subjects). Blots are representative western blots of ^{473}Ser Akt phosphorylation and total Akt amounts. *Panel B*: 15 min incubation of human myotubes from insulin sensitive subjects with 25 μg/ml of CM proteins increased ^{9}Ser GSK3β phosphorylation level in the absence of insulin, with a stronger effect of medium prepared from IR subjects than from insulin sensitive subjects ($P<0.05$ vs. control subjects). The incremental stimulatory effect of 100 nM insulin over basal was reduced mainly in the presence of CM from IR subjects. Blot is a representative western blot of ^{9}Ser GSK3β phosphorylation.

PP242 completely blocks both mTORCs [46]. We found that the effect of *db/db* CM proteins on Akt [473]Ser phosphorylation was fully prevented by PP242, but not by Rapamycin, indicating a preferential role of mTORC2 in the response to CM proteins in L6 cells. Furthermore, inhibition of p70S6K1 phosphorylation suggested a negative modulation of mTORC1 inhibitors.

Taken together, these results support a possible mechanism of action of the *db/db* or IR subjects CM on insulin signaling and action in skeletal muscle cells by which proteins produced by small intestine could act via activation of mTORC2 while inhibiting mTORC1. Activation of mTORC2 may be regulated by activation of TSC1/TSC2 complex, which directly binds to mTORC2 while inhibiting Rheb and thus mTORC1 [47]. So, the increased [473]Ser Akt phosphorylation is accompanied by decrease in basal (no insulin) p70 S6K1 [389]Thr phosphorylation. Accordingly, Rapamycin and PP242 inhibit p70 S6K1 [389]Thr phosphorylation (as also observed in the absence of *db/db* CM). This is accompanied by the lack of inhibition of GSK3 due to the proteolysis of its phosphorylated form, and may in turn lead to the phosphorylation of IRS-1 on serine/threonine residues that determines inhibition of insulin signaling by reducing IRS-1 tyrosine phosphorylation with consequent insulin resistance [48] (Fig. 6).

Our finding that *db/db* CM promotes Akt [473]Ser phosphorylation in L6 cells, likely via mTORC2 or TSC activation and Akt recruitment to plasma membrane, may provide a new insight on the upstream regulation of mTORC2 [49]. Finally, the reversibility of CM proteins action after washout suggests that these proteins may act through the activation of a membrane receptor. We conclude that, although some difference in the effect of mice and human CM proteins on the insulin signaling does exist, the

mechanism of action, as summarized in Figure 6, likely involves the mTOR pathway.

The strength of the present study is the demonstration that the small intestine of insulin resistant humans and mice secrete a protein factor/s inducing insulin resistance by impairing the insulin signaling.

The limitations of our investigation are that insulin sensitivity in mice was assessed by the IPITT instead of a more sophisticated euglycemic hyperinsulinemic clamp and that the insulin signaling pathway was studied in two different cellular lines, the L6 cells to test the proteins secreted by the mice intestine and human myoblasts to test the proteins secreted by the human intestine. Concerning the first point we note that the steady state conditions of plasma concentration, required by the clamp, could not be assured for the jejunal proteins, whose kinetics is not known. Moreover, the minimal model analysis also provides the estimate of the glucose effectiveness that has been found decreased after the *in vivo* injection of *db/db* proteins.

As for the second point, it is well accepted that insulin action is comparable in L6 cells and primary muscle cells. Because the use of human primary muscle cells requires biopsies and time-consuming expansion and differentiation, we restricted the use of these cells to the study of the human secreted proteins. Actually, we found similar results by using the secreted proteins from *db/db* mice and insulin resistant humans, although the proteolytic degradation of phopsphorylated GSK3, observed in the rodent study, was not present in the human study.

Ideally, the best model to investigate the role of the small intestine in inducing insulin resistance would be that of studying the same insulin resistant subjects and animals before and after bariatric surgery, in particular the bilio-pancreatic diversion that

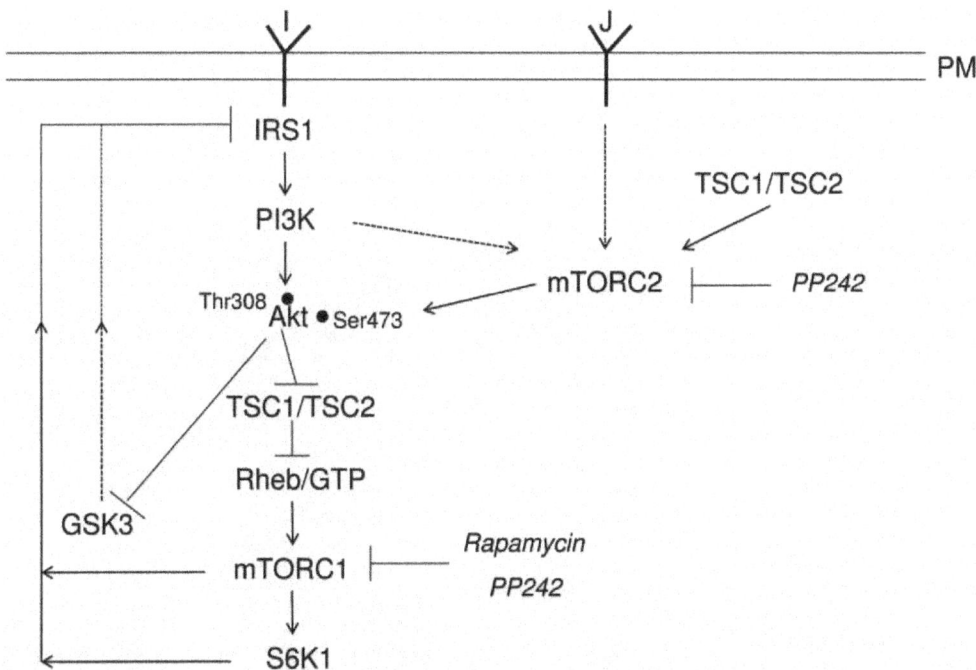

Figure 6. Interaction between IRS1−PI3K−Akt signaling pathway and mTOR. Upon insulin binding insulin receptor activates, through insulin receptor substrate 1 (IRS1), phosphatidylinositol-3-kinase (PI3K), which results in Akt phosphorylation at [308]Thr residue via Phosphatidylinositol 4,5-bisphosphate (PIP2) to Phosphatidylinositol 3,4,5-bisphosphate (PIP3) conversion followed by Akt and PDK1 recruitment to plasma membrane (not shown). A factor J present in duodenal-jejunal conditioned medium activates, possibly via the tuberous sclerosis complex TSC1-TSC2, the mammlian target of rapamycin complex 2 (mTORC2). mTORC2 also appears to be regulated by the PI3K pathway and phosphorylates Akt at [473]Ser residue. Through TSC1-TSC2 and the GTPase Rheb, Akt activates mTORC1 and its direct substrate S6K1. Akt also inhibits GSK3. S6K1, mTORC1 and GSK3 phosphorylate serine residues on IRS1, thus attenuating insulin signalling. Hypothetical signalling is denoted by dotted lines.

was proven to allow diabetes remission through the normalization of insulin resistance [4–7]. After this operation as well as after Roux-en-Y gastric bypass, however, the biliary limb is excluded from food transit and it is no further explorable endoscopically to obtain mucosal biopsies. To harmonize the experimental design in humans and animals, we have thus chosen to demonstrate that the duodenum/jejunum of insulin resistant humans and mice secrete hormone/s inducing insulin resistance.

The natural evolution our study will be the isolation and identification of the IR hormone/s secreted by the duodenum-jejunum tracts. Their future identification might permit the development of new pharmacological agents for the treatment of type 2 diabetes. Insulin resistance is, in fact, a characteristic feature of type 2 diabetes and plays a central role in the pathogenesis of this disease although the presence of a concomitant β-cell failure is necessary. It is worldwide recognized that the skeletal muscle insulin resistance develops decades before β-cell failure [50]. The clinical implications of our study are related to the mechanisms of action of the jejunal hormone/s inducing IR which can explain the immediate metabolic and longer term effects of bariatric surgery in inducing the remission of type 2 diabetes [50].

Supporting Information

Figure S1   Effect of conditioned medium (CM) on ^{308}**Thr Akt phosphorylation in differentiated L6 myotubes.** *Panel A*: Effect of 25 μg/ml CM proteins on ^{308}Thr Akt phosphorylation in differentiated L6 myotubes in the absence or presence of 100 nM insulin. Each bar is the mean of triplicate experiments with 4 different preparations of control and *db/db* CM and 1 preparation of Swiss CM. Data are normalized by β-actin amount and expressed as fold change versus control condition (control at 100 nM insulin set at 100). Data are mean ± s.d. $^{\#}P = 0.08$ vs. insulin stimulated ^{308}Thr Akt phosphorylation in control. *Panel B*: Dose-response profile of insulin action on ^{308}Thr Akt phosphorylation versus insulin concentration (nM) in logarithmic scale after 15 min co-incubation in the absence (squares) or presence (circles) of 25 μg/ml *db/db* CM proteins ($^{*}P<0.05$ and $^{\#}P = 0.08$ vs. control).

Appendix S1   L6 cells western blot analysis. Human skeletal muscle cell culture western blot analysis.

Acknowledgments

We would like to thank Mrs. Anna Caprodossi for her precious technical assistance and commitment to this specific study.

Author Contributions

Conceived and designed the experiments: GM SS AB HV. Performed the experiments: C. Debard C. Durand HV. Analyzed the data: SS AB. Contributed reagents/materials/analysis tools: HV GM. Wrote the paper: GM SS AB HV PZ.

References

1. DeFronzo RA (2004) Pathogenesis of type 2 diabetes mellitus. Med Clin N Am 88: 787–835.
2. Kasuga M (2006) Insulin resistance and pancreatic β cell failure. J Clin Invest 116: 1756–1760.
3. Prentki M, Nolan CJ (2006) Islet β cell failure in type 2 diabetes. J Clin Invest 116: 1802–1812.
4. Guidone C, Manco M, Valera Mora E, Iaconelli A, Gniuli D, et al. (2006) Mechanisms of recovery from type 2 diabetes after malabsorptive bariatric surgery. Diabetes 55: 2025–2031.
5. Mingrone G, Panunzi S, De Gaetano A, Guidone C, Iaconelli A, et al. (2012) Bariatric surgery vs. conventional medical therapy for type 2 diabetes. New Engl J Med 336: 1577–1585.
6. Mari A, Manco M, Guidone C, Nanni G, Castagneto M, et al. (2006) Restoration of normal glucose tolerance in severely obese patients after bilio-pancreatic diversion: role of insulin sensitivity and beta cell function. Diabetologia 49: 2136–2143.
7. Salinari S, Bertuzzi A, Asnaghi S, Guidone C, Manco M, et al. (2009) First-phase insulin secretion restoration and differential response to glucose load depending on the route of administration in type 2 diabetic subjects after bariatric surgery. Diabetes Care 32: 375–380.
8. Rubino F, Marescaux J (2004) Effect of duodenal-jejunal exclusion in a non-obese animal model of type 2 diabetes: a new perspective for an old disease. Ann Surg 239: 1–11.
9. Rubino F, Forgione A, Cummings DE, Vix M, Gnuli D, et al. (2006) The mechanism of diabetes control after gastrointestinal bypass surgery reveals a role of the proximal small intestine in the pathophysiology of type 2 diabetes. Ann Surg 244: 741–749.
10. Breen DM, Rasmussen BA, Kokorovic A, Wang R, Cheung GW, et al. (2012) Jejunal nutrient sensing is required for duodenal-jejunal bypass surgery to rapidly lower glucose concentrations in uncontrolled diabetes. Nature Med 18: 950–955.
11. Hummel KP, Dickie MM, Coleman DL (1966) Diabetes, a new mutation in the mouse. Science 153: 1127–1128.
12. Kodama H, Fujita M, Yamaguchi I (1994) Development of hyperglycaemia and insulin resistance in conscious genetically diabetic (C57BL/KsJ-db/db) mice. Diabetologia 37: 739–744.
13. Brozinick JT Jr., McCoid SC, Reynolds TH, Nardone NA, Hargrove DM, et al. (2001) GLUT4 over-expression in db/db mice dose-dependently ameliorates diabetes but is not a lifelong cure. Diabetes 50: 593–600.
14. Russell MS, Bailey J, Duffy SJ, Vogels CM, Broderick TL, et al. (2006) Gut transport of a molybdenum/ascorbic acid complex. Drugs R D 7: 111–117.
15. Bergman RN, Ider YZ, Bowden CR, Cobelli C (1979) Quantitative estimation of insulin sensitivity. Am J Physiol 236: E667–E677.
16. Pacini G, Thomaseth K, Ahrén B (2001) Contribution to glucose tolerance of insulin-independent vs. insulin-dependent mechanisms in mice. Am J Physiol Endocrinol Metab 281: E693–E703.
17. Sheiner LB, Beal SL (1980) Evaluation of methods for estimating population pharmacokinetics parameters. I. Michaelis-Menten model: routine clinical pharmacokinetic data. J Pharmacokinet Biopharm 8: 553–571.
18. Burcelin R, Crivelli V, Dacosta A, Roy-Tirelli A, Thorens B (2002) Heterogeneous metabolic adaptation of C57BL/6J mice to high-fat diet. Am J Physiol Endocrinol Metab 282: E834–E842.
19. Ueyama A, Yaworsky KL, Wang Q, Ebina Y, Klip A (1999) GLUT-4myc ectopic expression in L6 myoblasts generates a GLUT-4-specific pool conferring insulin sensitivity. Am J Physiol Endocrinol Metab 277: E572–E578.
20. Koivisto UM, Martinez-Valdez H, Bilan PJ, Burdett E, Ramlal P, et al. (1991) Differential regulation of the GLUT-1 and GLUT-4 glucose transport systems by glucose and insulin in L6 muscle cells in culture. J Biol Chem 266: 2615–2621.
21. Cozzone D, Fröjdö S, Disse E, Debard C, Laville M, et al. (2008) Isoform-specific defects of insulin stimulation of Akt/protein kinase B (PKB) in skeletal muscle cells from type 2 diabetic patients. Diabetologia 51: 512–521.
22. DeFronzo RA, Tobin JD, Andres R (1979) Glucose clamp technique: a method for quantifying insulin secretion and resistance. Am J Physiol 237: E214–E223.
23. Bouzakri K, Roques M, Gual P, Espinosa S, Guebre-Egziabher F, et al. (2003) Reduced activation of phosphatidylinositol-3 kinase and increased serine 636 phosphorylation of insulin receptor substrate-1 in primary culture of skeletal muscle cells from patients with type 2 diabetes. Diabetes 52: 1319–1325.
24. Montori-Grau M, Guitart M, Lerin C, Andreu AL, Newgard CB, et al. (2007) Expression and glycogenic effect of glycogen-targeting protein phosphatase I regulatory subunit GL in cultured human muscle. Biochem J 405: 107–113.
25. Schauer PR, Kashyap SR, Wolski K, Brethauer SA, Kirwan JP, et al. (2012) Bariatric surgery versus intensive medical therapy in obese patients with diabetes. N Engl J Med 366: 1567–1576.
26. Capristo E, Mingrone G, Addolorato G, Greco AV, Gasbarrini G (1998) Metabolic features of inflammatory bowel disease in a remission phase of the disease activity. J Intern Med 243: 339–347.
27. Sarbassov DD, Ali SM, Sabatini D M (2005) Growing roles for the mTOR pathway. Curr Opin Cell Biol 17: 596–603.
28. Alessi DR, James SR, Downes CP, Holmes AB, Gaffney PR, et al. (1997) Characterization of a 3-phosphoinositide-dependent protein kinase which phosphorylates and activates protein kinase Balpha. Curr Biol 7: 261–269.
29. Stephens L, Anderson K, Stokoe D, Erdjument-Bromage H, Painter GF, et al. (1998) Protein kinase B kinases that mediate phosphatidylinositol 3,4,5-trisphosphate-dependent activation of protein kinase B. Science 279: 710–714.

30. Fraenkel M, Ketzinel-Gilad M, Ariav Y, Pappo O, Karaca M, et al. (2008) mTOR inhibition by rapamycin prevents beta-cell adaptation to hyperglycemia and exacerbates the metabolic state in type 2 diabetes. Diabetes 57: 945–957.

31. Li J, DeFea K, Roth RA (1999) Modulation of insulin receptor substrate-1 tyrosine phosphorylation by an Akt/phosphatidylinositol 3-kinase pathway. J Biol Chem 274: 9351–9356.

32. Frame S, Cohen P (2001) GSK3 takes centre stage more than 20 years after its discovery. Biochem J 359: 1–16.

33. Goñi-Oliver P, Lucas JJ, Avila J, Hernandez F (2007) N-terminal cleavage of GSK-3 by calpain. A new form of GSK-3 regulation. J Biol Chem 282: 22406–22413.

34. Cross DAE, Alessi DR, Cohen P, Andjelkovich M, Hemmings BA (1995) Inhibition of glycogen synthase kinase-3 by insulin mediated by protein kinase B. Nature 378: 785–789.

35. McManus EJ, Sakamoto K, Armit LJ, Ronaldson L, Shapiro N, et al. (2005) Role that phosphorylation of GSK3 plays in insulin and Wnt signalling defined by knockin analysis. EMBO J 24: 1571–1583.

36. Eldar-Finkelman H, Krebs EG (1997) Phosphorylation of insulin receptor substrate 1 by glycogen synthase kinase 3 impairs insulin action. Proc Natl Acad Sci U S A 94: 9660–9664.

37. Liberman Z, Eldar-Finkelman H (2005) Serine 332 phosphorylation of insulin receptor substrate-1 by glycogen synthase kinase-3 attenuates insulin signaling. J Biol Chem 280: 4422–4428.

38. Wang QM, Fiol CJ, DePaoli RAA, Roach PJ (1994) Glycogen synthase kinase-3 beta is a dual specificity kinase differentially regulated by tyrosine and serine/ threonine phosphorylation. J Biol Chem 269: 14566–14574.

39. Eldar-Finkelman H, Schreyer SA, Shinohara MM, LeBoeuf RC, Krebs EG (1999) Increased glycogen synthase kinase-3 activity in diabetes- and obesity-prone C57BL/6J mice. Diabetes 48: 1662–1666.

40. Dokken BB, Sloniger JA, Henriksen EJ (2005) Acute selective glycogen synthase kinase-3 inhibition enhances insulin signaling in pre-diabetic insulin-resistant rat skeletal muscle. Am J Physiol Endocrinol Metab 288: E1188–E1194.

41. Wente SR, Villalba M, Schramm VL, Rosen OM (1990) Mn2(+)-binding properties of a recombinant protein-tyrosine kinase derived from the human insulin receptor. Proc Natl Acad Sci U S A 87: 2805–2809.

42. Ciaraldi TP, Nikoulina SE, Bandukwala SA, Carter L, Henry RR (2007) Role of glycogen synthase kinase-3 alpha in insulin action in cultured human skeletal muscle cells. Endocrinology 148: 4393–4399.

43. Ring DB, Johnson KW, Henriksen EJ, Nuss JM, Goff D, et al. (2003) Selective glycogen synthase kinase 3 inhibitors potentiate insulin activation of glucose transport and utilization in vitro and in vivo. Diabetes 52: 588–595.

44. Mora A, Sakamoto K, McManus EJ, Alessi DR. (2005) Role of the PDK1-PKB-GSK3 pathway in regulating glycogen synthase and glucose uptake in the heart. FEBS Lett 579: 3632–3638.

45. Hay N, Sonenberg N. (2004) Upstream and downstream of mTOR. Genes Dev 18: 1926–1945.

46. Feldman ME, Apsel B, Uotila A, Loewith R, Knight ZA, et al. (2009) Active-site inhibitors of mTOR target rapamycin-resistant outputs of mTORC1 and mTORC2. PLoS Biol 7(2): e38.

47. Huang J, Dibble CC, Matsuzaki M, Manning BD (2008) The TSC1-TSC2 complex is required for proper activation of mTOR complex 2. Mol Cell Biol 28: 4104–4115.

48. Huang J, Manning BD (2009) A complex interplay between Akt, TSC2 and the two mTOR complexes. Biochem Soc Trans 37: 217–222.

49. Cybulski N, Hall MN (2009) TOR complex 2: a signaling pathway of its own. Trends Biochem Sci 34: 620–627.

50. Dixon JB, le Roux CW, Rubino F, Zimmet P (2012) Bariatric surgery for type 2 diabetes. Lancet 379: 2300–2311.

4

Higher Fetal Insulin Resistance in Chinese Pregnant Women with Gestational Diabetes Mellitus and Correlation with Maternal Insulin Resistance

Qiuwei Wang, Ruiping Huang, Bin Yu, Fang Cao, Huiyan Wang, Ming Zhang, Xinhong Wang, Bin Zhang, Hong Zhou, Ziqiang Zhu*

Changzhou Women and Children Health Hospital Affiliated to Nanjing Medical University, Changzhou, Jiangsu Province, China

Abstract

Objective: The aim of this study was to determine the effect of gestational diabetes mellitus (GDM) on fetal insulin resistance or β-cell function in Chinese pregnant women with GDM.

Measurements: Maternal fasting blood and venous cord blood samples (reflecting fetal condition) were collected in 65 well-controlled Chinese GDM mothers (only given dietary intervention) and 83 control subjects. The insulin, glucose and proinsulin concentrations of both maternal and cord blood samples were measured, and the homeostasis model assessment of insulin resistance (HOMA-IR) and the proinsulin-to-insulin ratios (an indicator of fetal β-cell function) were calculated in maternal and cord blood respectively.

Results: Both maternal and fetal levels of insulin, proinsulin and HOMA-IR but not proinsulin-to-insulin ratios were significantly higher in the GDM group than in the control group (maternal insulin, 24.8 vs. 15.4 μU/mL, $P = 0.004$, proinsulin, 23.3 vs. 16.2 pmol/L, $P = 0.005$, and HOMA-IR, 5.5 vs. 3.5, $P = 0.041$, respectively; fetal: insulin, 15.1 vs. 7.9 μU/mL, $P < 0.001$, proinsulin, 25.8 vs. 15.1 pmol/L, $P = 0.015$, and HOMA-IR, 2.8 vs. 1.4, $P = 0.017$, respectively). Fetal HOMA-IR but not proinsulin-to-insulin ratios was significantly correlated to maternal HOMA-IR ($r = 0.307$, $P = 0.019$), in the pregnant women with GDM.

Conclusions: Fetal insulin resistance was higher in Chinese pregnant women with GDM than control subjects, and correlated with maternal insulin resistance.

Editor: Victor Sanchez-Margalet, Virgen Macarena University Hospital, School of Medicine, Spain

Funding: This study was supported by funding from the Changzhou Health Bureau (No. ZD201013) and Changzhou Women and Children Health Hospital affiliated to Nanjing Medical University supported this study. The funders had no role in study design, data collection and analysis, decision to publish, or preparation of the manuscript.

Competing Interests: The authors have declared that no competing interests exist.

* E-mail: answercn@163.com

Introduction

The rapid and significant increase in the incidence of metabolic syndrome and type II diabetes has become a worldwide concern in both developed and developing countries [1,2]. There are strong evidential supports for the "fetal origins" hypothesis, which connects adult metabolic syndrome to adverse intrauterine conditions and related disproportionate fetal growth [3–5], especially in the type II diabetes [6–14].

A great deal of research has revealed the pivotal role of insulin resistance and β-cell function in the development of type II diabetes in adults. Offspring of mothers with insulin resistance (e.g. GDM or obese mothers) are far more likely to develop metabolic syndrome and type II diabetes [9, 10, and 15]. However, only a few latest studies focused on the effect of GDM on fetal levels of insulin resistance or β-cell function in pregnant women with GDM. In 2009, it was firstly reported that fetuses of obese mothers (who had insulin resistance) developed insulin resistance in utero [16]. Furthermore, in 2010, another study reported that oral glucose tolerance test (OGTT) blood glucose concentrations were strongly negatively associated with decreased fetal insulin sensitivity in pregnant women with GDM [17]. Similarly, our study was to determine the effect of GDM on fetal insulin resistance or β-cell function in Chinese pregnant women with GDM. Such related research may be help to find a potential effective intervention during pregnancy to halt the increasing epidemic of metabolic syndromes and type II diabetes.

Subjects and Methods

Ethics Statement

This study was approved by Changzhou Health Bureau and the ethics committee of Changzhou Women and Children Health Hospital affiliated to Nanjing Medical University (No. ZD201013). The written informed consent was obtained from each subject in this manuscript.

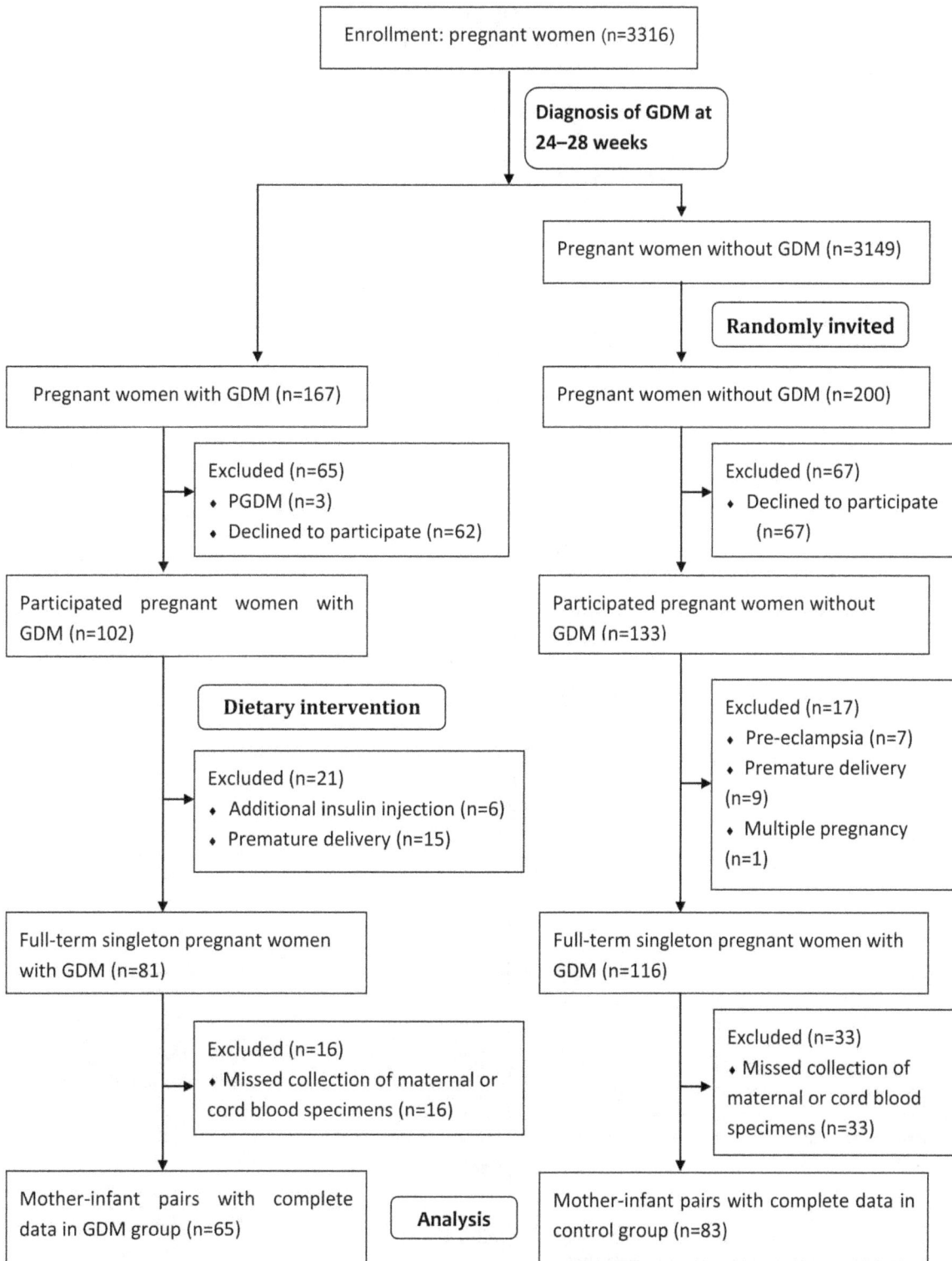

Figure 1. Flow diagram. GDM, gestational diabetes mellitus; PGDM, pregestational diabetes mellitus.

Study Subjects

This was a prospective maternal-fetal case-controlled cohort study. Pregnant women were recruited from Changzhou Women and Children Health Hospital affiliated to Nanjing Medical University from March 2010 to June 2011, as shown in figure 1.

167 GDM and 3149 control subjects were included as candidates in this study, on the basis of a diagnosis of GDM at 24–28 weeks of gestation. 200 subjects were randomly invited in the control group. 62 GDM and 67 control subjects declined to participate this study, and 3 pregnant women with pregestational

diabetes mellitus was not invited in the GDM group. 102 GDM and 133 control subjects participated in this study. The pregnant women with GDM were well managed by dietary intervention and blood glucose monitoring for achieving euglycemia. Dietary intervention included low-carbohydrate and low-fat diets intake, as well as optimizing of dietary fatty acid composition. In the GDM group, 21 were excluded as 6 for additional insulin injection, and 15 for premature delivery. In the control group, 17 were excluded, as 7 for pre-eclampsia, 9 for premature delivery, and 1 for a multiple pregnancy. 16 GDM and 33 control subjects were excluded, as we missed collection of their maternal blood or cord blood specimens. 65 GDM and 83 control mother-infant pairs (total 75.1% of eligible participants) constituted our final study cohort, with complete data on all studied biomarkers in maternal and cord blood specimens. There were no significant differences in maternal characteristics between patients included versus those excluded in this study.

Diagnosis of GDM was established by a 75-g oral glucose tolerance test (OGTT) at 24–28 weeks of gestation. GDM was diagnosed if the woman had two or more of the three plasma glucose values exceeding the following cutoffs: fasting, 5.3 mmol/L; 1 hour, 10.0 mmol/L; or 2 hour, 8.6 mmol/L (American Diabetes Association criteria) (18). There was no abnormal labor (e.g., prolonged labor or precipitate delivery) in every subject with or without GDM in this study. Every woman had been fasting since the beginning of the active phase in the first stage of labor. Exclusion criteria were: 1) a multiple pregnancy; 2) gestational age <37 weeks; 3) maternal age <18 or >45 years; 4) illicit drug use; 5) severe preexisting illnesses including pregestational diabetes mellitus, chronic hypertension, renal failure, pre-eclampsia, active or chronic liver diseases, epilepsy, serious pulmonary disease, serious hematological disorders, cancer, heart disease, or other life-threatening conditions; and 6) known fetal congenital anomalies or chromosomal abnormalities.

Data and Blood Sample Collection

Maternal prepregnancy weight was obtained by face-to-face interview. Maternal weight close to delivery and height were measured in the hospital, and maternal body mass index (BMI) and weight gain were calculated. Neonatal birth weight and length were measured within one hour after delivery. Body mass index (BMI) and ponderal index (PI) were calculated: BMI = [weight (kilograms)/height $(m)^2$], and PI = [birth weight (grams)/length (centimeters)^3] ×100. Maternal fasting blood samples were collected about 1–3 days before delivery, at 37–41 weeks. Venous cord blood samples were obtained by syringe from the double-clamped venous cord immediately after delivery. Serum was separated by centrifugation and kept frozen in multiple aliquots at −80°C until analysis. Hemoglobin A1c levels were measured during the late pregnancy in the GDM group.

Metabolic Parameters Assays

Glucose levels were assessed using Hitachi 7180 automated analyzer (Wako Diagnostics, Japan). Hemoglobin A1c levels were estimated using VARIANT II automated analyser (Bio-Rad, laboratories, Inc.). Insulin levels were measured using the electrochemistry immunoassay (ECL) method, with a COBAS e601 automated analyser (Roche Diagnostics, Germany). Pro-insulin levels were determined by ELISA (R&D Systems, America), with an intra-assay CV of 5.6% and an inter-assay CV of 8.3%. The insulin resistance indexes were calculated according to the homeostasis model assessment of insulin resistance (HOMA-IR): (fasting serum insulin [microunits per milliliter] × fasting glucose [millimoles per liter])/22.5 [19].

Statistical Analysis

Results were expressed as means ± SEM. Log transformation was applied for variables with skewed data distribution (insulin, proinsulin, HOMA-IR, and proinsulin-to-insulin ratio) in all statistical analysis. Differences between groups were examined with the Student's t-test, and adjusted for potential confounders (maternal age, prepregnancy weight, and prepregnancy BMI), using univariate ANOVA analysis. The correlation analysis was tested with Pearson's correlation analysis, and adjusted for potential confounders (maternal age and prepregnancy BMI), using partial correlations. All statistical analysis were performed with the software package SPSS version 17.0 (SPSS Inc., Chicago, IL, USA). A P-value <0.05 was considered statistically significant.

Results

Maternal and Pregnancy Characteristics

Maternal and fetal characteristics of total 148 Chinese pregnant women with or without GDM were shown in Table 1. The fetal condition was reflected by cord blood metabolic parameters. The pregnant women with GDM were slightly older, and had a higher prepregnancy weight and BMI than the control subjects. Maternal height, weight gain and Caesarean section rate did not differ between the two groups. Hemoglobin A1c level of GDM mothers was 5.29±0.06%, and in the mormal interval ranges. Neonatal birth weight, length and ponderal index were higher in the GDM group than the control group, although neonates in two groups were born at the similar gestational weeks.

Differences in Metabolic Parameters between the GDM and Control Groups

Both maternal and fetal levels of insulin, proinsulin and HOMA-IR were significantly higher in the GDM groups than the control subjects. Those differences were still significant, after adjustment for potential confounders (maternal age, prepregnancy weight and prepregnancy BMI) (Table 2). There're no significant

Table 1. Maternal and fetal characteristics of pregnant women with or without GDM.

	Control	GDM	P value
Subjects (n)	83	65	
Maternal Age (years)	28.06±0.37	29.68±0.48	0.009
Maternal height (m)	161.25±0.48	161.05±0.53	NS
Prepregnancy weight (kg)	53.43±0.79	57.27±1.10	0.005
Prepregnancy BMI (kg/m²)	20.52±0.27	22.01±0.39	0.002
Maternal weight gain (kg)	13.62±0.34	14.76±0.66	NS
Gestational age (weeks)	39.02±0.13	38.78±0.11	NS
Caesarean section (% (n))	47.7% (31)	38.6% (32)	NS
Female sex, % (n)	52.3%(24)	50.6%(33)	NS
Birth weight (g)	3343±40	3581±58	0.001
Birth length (cm)	49.36±0.14	49.87±0.16	0.023
Ponderal index (g/cm³)	2.76±0.03	2.86±0.03	0.013

Data was expressed as means ± SEM.
[a]log-transformed skewed data were used for statistical comparisons.
[b]Maternal and fetal serum parameters were adjusted for maternal age, prepregnancy weight and prepregnancy BMI.
NS, not significant.

Table 2. Maternal and fetal metabolic parameters of pregnant women with or without GDM.

	Control	GDM	P value	Adjusted P value[b]
Maternal				
Fasting glucose (mmol/L)	4.69±0.07	4.73±0.11	NS	NS
Insulin (μU/mL)[a]	15.38±1.19	24.79±1.70	<0.001	0.004
Proinsulin (pmol/L)[a]	16.17±1.84	23.30±2.05	0.005	0.005
HOMA-IR[a]	3.48±0.32	5.46±0.48	0.002	0.041
Proinsulin/insulin ratio (pmol/mU)[a]	1.36±0.21	1.28±0.13	NS	NS
Fetal				
Glucose (mmol/L)	3.89±0.05	4.08±0.08	NS	NS
Insulin (μU/mL)[a]	7.91±0.64	15.08±1.52	<0.001	<0.001
Proinsulin (pmol/L)[a]	15.07±1.23	25.82±2.92	0.017	0.015
HOMA-IR[a]	1.38±0.12	2.80±0.35	<0.001	0.017
Proinsulin/insulin ratio (pmol/mU)[a]	2.83±0.31	2.66±0.35	NS	NS

Data was expressed as means ± SEM.
[a]log-transformed skewed data were used for statistical comparisons.
[b]Maternal and fetal serum parameters were adjusted for maternal age, prepregnancy weight and prepregnancy BMI.
NS, not significant.

differences in maternal or fetal levels of glucose and proinsulin-to-insulin ratios between the GDM and control groups (Table 2).

Correlations between Fetal HOMA-IR and Maternal Metabolic Parameters

In the GDM group, fetal HOMA-IR was significantly correlated with maternal insulin, fasting glucose, HOMA-IR and proinsulin-to-insulin ratios (Table 2). Fetal proinsulin-to-insulin ratios were not significantly correlated with maternal HOMA-IR. After adjustment for maternal age and prepregnancy BMI, fetal HOMA-IR was significantly correlating with maternal HOMA-IR or insulin (adjusted, r = 0.307, P = 0.019, and r = 0.261, P = 0.047, respectively) (Table 3). Similar correlations were observed in all the subjects with or without GDM (adjusted, r = 0.424, P = 0.008, and r = 0.415, P = 0.007, respectively). In the GDM group, neonatal ponderal index was significantly correlated with maternal or fetal HOMA-IR and insulin (Table 4). Those correlations remained significant after adjustment for maternal age and prepregnancy BMI (Table 4).

Table 3. Correlations between fetal HOMA-IR and metabolic parameters in pregnant women with GDM.

	Fetal HOMA-IR[a]			
	r	P	r[b] (Adjusted)	P[b] (Adjusted)
Maternal				
HOMA-IR[a]	0.421	<0.001	0.307	0.019
Proinsulin/insulin (pmol/mU)[a]	−0.297	0.016	0.008	0.950
Insulin (μU/mL)[a]	0.378	0.002	0.261	0.047
Fasting glucose (mmol/L)	0.316	0.010	0.257	0.052

[a]log-transformed skewed data were used for statistical analysis.
[b]Partial correlations were adjusted for maternal age and prepregnancy BMI.

Table 4. Correlations between neonatal ponderal index and maternal or fetal metabolic parameters in pregnant women with GDM.

	Neonatal ponderal index (g/cm³)			
	r	P	r[b] (Adjusted)	P[b] (Adjusted)
Maternal HOMA-IR[a]	0.290	0.012	0.259	0.036
Maternal insulin (μU/mL)[a]	0.270	0.020	0.262	0.033
Fetal HOMA-IR[a]	0.471	<0.001	0.490	<0.001
Fetal insulin (μU/mL)[a]	0.510	<0.001	0.521	<0.001

[a]log-transformed skewed data were used for statistical analysis.
[b]Partial correlations were adjusted for maternal age and prepregnancy BMI.

Discussion

Several studies on GDM have reported on the metabolic abnormalities of GDM mothers. Quite a few focused on maternal-fetal metabolic mechanisms in pregnant women with GDM.

This study tried to determine the effect of GDM on fetal insulin resistance or β-cell function in Chinese pregnant women with GDM. Our study reported i) fetal insulin resistance but not proinsulin-to-insulin ratios was significantly higher in Chinese pregnant women with GDM than control subjects, ii) fetal insulin resistance was correlated with maternal insulin resistance,iii) neonatal ponderal index was correlated with maternal or fetal insulin and insulin resistance.

In this study, we reported significantly higher levels of insulin, proinsulin and HOMA-IR, in Chinese pregnant women with GDM than control subjects, within 1–3 days before delivery, after adjustment for potential confounders. Similarly, we also reported significantly higher levels of insulin, proinsulin and HOMA-IR, in fetuses of Chinese pregnant women with GDM than control subjects, after adjustment for potential confounders. Such data clearly show a more highly insulin-resistant condition in fetuses of Chinese pregnant women with GDM than control subjects. Similar with this study of Chinese pregnant women, higher levels of insulin, proinsulin and HOMA-IR in fetuses of pregnant women with GDM were also reported in other different races and countries [17, 20, and 21].

However, even though both fetal levels of insulin and proinsulin levels were higher in GDM group, there're no significant differences in fetal proinsulin-to-insulin ratios between the GDM and control groups. Such data agree with related fetal studies [17], and show no observably impaired β-cell function, in fetuses of GDM mothers than control subjects.

Several studies have focused on the effect of fetal growth on insulin resistance in infants, children, adolescents or adults [22–24]. While only a few latest data is available about the effects of maternal metabolic parameters on fetal insulin resistance. It was reported that there's a strong positive correlation ($r = 0.35$) between maternal insulin resistance of obese mothers and fetal insulin resistance [16]. Similarly, it was reported that there's a negative association between maternal OGTT blood glucose levels in mothers with GDM and fetal insulin sensitivity ($r = -0.31$) [17]. In accord with such data, this study reported that maternal insulin resistance significantly correlated with fetal insulin resistance in Chinese pregnant women with GDM ($r = 0.307$). As maternal insulin can not cross the placenta, GDM may thus affect fetal metabolic condition (such as insulin resistance) by maternal-fetal metabolic and/or epigenetic mechanisms. For example, a latest study from Salomón C et al. reported GDM reduces adenosine transport in human placental microvascular endothelium, by an effect of insulin [25]. Further research increasing that understanding may facilitate the development of potential effective interventions

during GDM pregnancy, for breaking the mother-baby metabolic programming cycle.

As expected, neonatal ponderal index was significantly correlated with fetal levels of HOMA-IR and insulin in this study. We also reported significant correlations between neonatal ponderal index and maternal levels of HOMA-IR and insulin. In view of the associations of HOMA-IR or insulin levels between mothers and fetuses presented above, it was suggested that increased fetal insulin may play an important role in the GDM effect on increased neonatal fat mass.

The prevalence of GDM and macrosomia increased rapidly in Asia, especially in China. In view of Asian traditional custom of striving to ingest nutrition in gestation, this problem would become more and more seriously in future. It was suggested that glucose control may have attenuated the impact of GDM on fetal overgrowth in Chinese women in this study. Furthermore, our data presented higher fetal insulin resistance in Chinese pregnant women with GDM. As fetuses of a more highly insulin-resistant condition are more likely to develop metabolic syndromes and type II diabetes, this finding would be help to understand the mechanism in development and prevention of mother-baby diabetic cycle.

In summary, this study reported a higher fetal insulin resisitance in well-controlled Chinese pregnant women with GDM, which was correlated with maternal insulin resistance. Our findings demonstrate the effect of GDM on higher fetal insulin resistance, which may be help to present an opportunity for potential effective intervention during pregnancy on prevention of metabolic syndrome and type II diabetes.

Author Contributions

Conceived and designed the experiments: ZZ QW RH BY FC. Performed the experiments: ZZ QW RH BY FC MZ HW XW BZ HZ. Analyzed the data: ZZ RH BY FC. Contributed reagents/materials/analysis tools: HW XW BZ. Wrote the paper: ZZ QW RH BY FC.

References

1. Prasad H, Ryan DA, Celzo MF, Stapleton D (2012) Metabolic syndrome: definition and therapeutic implications. Postgrad Med 124: 21–30.
2. Eberle C, Merki E, Yamashita T, Johnson S, Armando AM, et al. (2012) Rising diabetes prevalence among urban-dwelling black South Africans. PLoS One 7: e45361.
3. Barker DJ, Hales CN, Fall CH, Osmond C, Phipps K, et al. (1993) Type 2 (non-insulin-dependent) diabetes mellitus, hypertension and hyperlipidaemia (syndrome X): relation to reduced fetal growth. Diabetologia 36: 62–67.
4. Hales CN, Barker DJ (1992) Type 2 (non-insulin-dependent) diabetes mellitus: the thrifty phenotype hypothesis. Diabetologia 35: 595–601.
5. Knowler WC, Pettitt DJ, Savage PJ, Bennett PH (1981) Diabetes incidence in Pima indians: contributions of obesity and parental diabetes. Am J Epidemiol 113: 144–156.
6. Dabelea D, Crume T (2011) Maternal environment and the transgenerational cycle of obesity and diabetes. Diabetes 60: 1849–1855.
7. Meas T (2010) Fetal origins of insulin resistance and the metabolic syndrome: a key role for adipose tissue? Diabetes Metab 36: 11–20.
8. Symonds ME, Sebert SP, Hyatt MA, Budge H (2009) Nutritional programming of the metabolic syndrome. Nat Rev Endocrinol 5: 604–610.
9. Dabelea D, Hanson RL, Lindsay RS, Pettitt DJ, Imperatore G, et al. (2000) Intrauterine exposure to diabetes conveys risks for type 2 diabetes and obesity: a study of discordant sibships. Diabetes 49: 2208–2211.
10. Krishnaveni GV, Veena SR, Hill JC, Kehoe S, Karat SC, et al. (2010) Intrauterine exposure to maternal diabetes is associated with higher adiposity and insulin resistance and clustering of cardiovascular risk markers in Indian children. Diabetes Care 33: 402–404.
11. Langer O, Yogev Y, Xenakis EM, Brustman L (2005) Overweight and obese in gestational diabetes: the impact on pregnancy outcome. Am J Obstet Gynecol 192: 1768–1776.
12. Schaefer-Graf UM, Kjos SL, Kilavuz O, Plagemann A, Brauer M, et al. (2003) Determinants of fetal growth at different periods of pregnancies complicated by gestational diabetes mellitus or impaired glucose tolerance. Diabetes Care 26: 193–198.
13. Misra VK, Trudeau S, Perni U (2011) Maternal serum lipids during pregnancy and infant birth weight: the influence of prepregnancy BMI. Obesity 19: 1476–1481.
14. Schaefer-Graf UM, Graf K, Kulbacka I, Kjos SL, Dudenhausen J, et al. (2008) Maternal lipids as strong determinants of fetal environment and growth in pregnancies with gestational diabetes mellitus. Diabetes Care 31: 1858–1863.
15. Dabelea D (2007) The predisposition to obesity and diabetes in offspring of diabetic mothers. Diabetes Care (Suppl. 1): S169–S174.
16. Catalano PM, Presley L, Minium J, Hauguel-de Mouzon S (2009) Fetuses of obese mothers develop insulin resistance in utero. Diabetes Care 32: 1076–1080.
17. Luo ZC, Delvin E, Fraser WD, Audibert F, Deal CI, et al. (2010) Maternal glucose tolerance in pregnancy affects fetal insulin sensitivity. Diabetes Care 33: 2055–2061.
18. American Diabetes Association (2003) Gestational diabetes mellitus. Diabetes Care (Suppl. 1): S103–S105.
19. Matthews DR, Hosker JP, Rudenski AS, Naylor BA, Treacher DF, et al. (1985) Homeostasis model assessment: insulin resistance and beta-cell function from fasting plasma glucose and insulin concentrations in man. Diabetologia 28: 412–419.
20. Ortega-Senovilla H, Schaefer-Graf U, Meitzner K, Abou-Dakn M, Graf K, et al. (2011) Gestational diabetes mellitus causes changes in the concentrations of adipocyte fatty acid-binding protein and other adipocytokines in cord blood. Diabetes Care 34: 2061–2066.
21. Schaefer-Graf UM, Meitzner K, Ortega-Senovilla H, Graf K, Vetter K, et al. (2011) Differences in the implications of maternal lipids on fetal metabolism and growth between gestational diabetes mellitus and control pregnancies. Diabet Med 28: 1053–1059.
22. Vielwerth SE, Jensen RB, Larsen T, Holst KK, Molgaard C, et al. (2008) The effect of birthweight upon insulin resistance and associated cardiovascular risk factors in adolescence is not explained by fetal growth velocity in the third trimester as measured by repeated ultrasound fetometry. Diabetologia 51: 1483–1492.

23. Fabricius-Bjerre S, Jensen RB, Faerch K, Larsen T, Molgaard C, et al. (2011) Impact of birth weight and early infant weight gain on insulin resistance and associated cardiovascular risk factors in adolescence. PLoS One 6: e20595.

24. Ortega FB, Ruiz JR, Hurtig-Wennlof A, Meirhaeghe A, Gonzalez-Gross M, et al. (2011) Physical activity attenuates the effect of low birth weight on insulin resistance in adolescents: findings from two observational studies. Diabetes 60: 2295–2299.

25. Salomón C, Westermeier F, Puebla C, Arroyo P, Guzmán-Gutiérrez E, et al. (2012) Gestational diabetes reduces adenosine transport in human placental microvascular endothelium, an effect reversed by insulin. PLoS One 7: e40578.

5

Common Genetic Variation in the Human *FNDC5* Locus, Encoding the Novel Muscle-Derived 'Browning' Factor Irisin, Determines Insulin Sensitivity

Harald Staiger[1,2,3], Anja Böhm[1,3,4], Mika Scheler[3,4], Lucia Berti[3,4], Jürgen Machann[2,3,5], Fritz Schick[2,3,5], Fausto Machicao[2,3], Andreas Fritsche[1,2,3,6], Norbert Stefan[1,2,3], Cora Weigert[1,2,3], Anna Krook[7], Hans-Ulrich Häring[1,2,3,4]*, Martin Hrabě de Angelis[3,4,8]*

1 Department of Internal Medicine, Division of Endocrinology, Diabetology, Angiology, Nephrology and Clinical Chemistry, Eberhard Karls University Tübingen, Tübingen, Germany, 2 Institute for Diabetes Research and Metabolic Diseases of the Helmholtz Centre Munich at the University of Tübingen, Tübingen, Germany, 3 German Centre for Diabetes Research (DZD), Neuherberg, Germany, 4 Institute of Experimental Genetics, Helmholtz Centre Munich, German Research Centre for Environmental Health, Neuherberg, Germany, 5 Department of Diagnostic and Interventional Radiology, Section on Experimental Radiology, Eberhard Karls University Tübingen, Tübingen, Germany, 6 Department of Internal Medicine, Division of Nutritional and Preventive Medicine, Eberhard Karls University Tübingen, Tübingen, Germany, 7 Department of Physiology and Pharmacology, Karolinska Institute, Stockholm, Sweden, 8 Chair for Experimental Genetics, Technical University Munich, Freising, Germany

Abstract

Aims/hypothesis: Recently, the novel myokine irisin was described to drive adipose tissue 'browning', to increase energy expenditure, and to improve obesity and insulin resistance in high fat-fed mice. Here, we assessed whether common single nucleotide polymorphisms (SNPs) in the *FNDC5* locus, encoding the irisin precursor, contribute to human prediabetic phenotypes (overweight, glucose intolerance, insulin resistance, impaired insulin release).

Methods: A population of 1,976 individuals was characterized by oral glucose tolerance tests and genotyped for *FNDC5* tagging SNPs. Subgroups underwent hyperinsulinaemic-euglycaemic clamps, magnetic resonance imaging/spectroscopy, and intravenous glucose tolerance tests. From 37 young and 14 elderly participants recruited in two different centres, muscle biopsies were obtained for the preparation of human myotube cultures.

Results: After appropriate adjustment and Bonferroni correction for the number of tested variants, SNPs rs16835198 and rs726344 were associated with *in vivo* measures of insulin sensitivity. Via interrogation of publicly available data from the Meta-Analyses of Glucose and Insulin-related traits Consortium, rs726344's effect on insulin sensitivity was replicated. Moreover, novel data from human myotubes revealed a negative association between *FNDC5* expression and appropriately adjusted *in vivo* measures of insulin sensitivity in young donors. This finding was replicated in myotubes from elderly men.

Conclusions/interpretation: This study provides evidence that the *FNDC5* gene, encoding the novel myokine irisin, determines insulin sensitivity in humans. Our gene expression data point to an unexpected insulin-desensitizing effect of irisin.

Editor: Yong-Gang Yao, Kunming Institute of Zoology, Chinese Academy of Sciences, China

Funding: The study was supported in part by a grant (01GI0925) from the German Federal Ministry of Education and Research (BMBF) to the German Centre for Diabetes Research (DZD e.V.). Norbert Stefan is supported by a Heisenberg professorship from the Deutsche Forschungsgemeinschaft (STE 1096/3-1), Anna Krook by the Swedish Research Council. The funders had no role in study design, data collection and analysis, decision to publish, or preparation of the manuscript.

Competing Interests: The authors have declared that no competing interests exist.

* E-mail: hans-ulrich.haering@med.uni-tuebingen.de (H-UH); hrabe@helmholtz-muenchen.de (MHdA)

Introduction

The importance of adipose tissue-derived hormones, collectively termed adipokines, for the regulation of glucose, lipid, and energy metabolism was convincingly shown, and it appears by now very plausible that dysregulated adipokine secretion significantly contributes to the pathogenesis of human metabolic diseases (i.e., obesity, atherosclerosis, type 2 diabetes) [1]. More recently, it was recognized that skeletal muscle and liver are also able to secrete, e.g., upon metabolic or physical stress, substantial amounts of metabolically active hormones, in analogy termed myokines and hepatokines, respectively [2–5]. Pathophysiological roles of in-

dividual myokines, such as interleukin-6 [6], and hepatokines, such as sex hormone-binding globulin and fetuin-A [7–9], in the development of human metabolic diseases are currently emerging.

A novel intriguing myokine, termed irisin, was very recently described by Boström et al. [10]. Irisin is released upon cleavage of the plasma membrane protein fibronectin type III domain-containing protein 5 (FNDC5). Expression of its gene was shown to be driven by muscle-specific transgenic overexpression of the exercise-responsive transcriptional co-activator peroxisome proliferator-activated receptor (PPAR)-γ co-activator-1α (PGC-1α) and, more physiologically, by three weeks of free wheel running in mice and by ten weeks of supervised endurance exercise training in humans [10]. After FNDC5 cleavage by a still unknown protease, irisin is released from muscle cells, enters the circulation, and is detectable in murine and human plasma [10]. Irisin treatment of differentiating primary murine preadipocytes induced, in a PPAR-α-dependent manner, the expression of brown fat genes (including *Ucp1*) [10], pointing to trans-determination and/or trans-differentiation of white adipose precursor cells [11]. This finding is in keeping with the observation of subcutaneous white adipose tissue 'browning' in PGC-1α-transgenic mice due to an increase in brown adipocyte number [10]. Finally, adenoviral *Fndc5* over-expression in mice increased energy expenditure (probably via enhanced thermogenesis) and improved obesity and insulin resistance induced by high-fat feeding [10].

Whether irisin or the *FNDC5* gene, encoding its membrane-resident protein precursor (MIM ID *611906), is involved in human metabolic disease is currently unknown. Therefore, we assessed in 1,976 German individuals at increased risk for type 2 diabetes whether common single nucleotide polymorphisms (SNPs; with minor allele frequencies [MAFs] ≥0.05) in the human *FNDC5* locus contribute to the prediabetic phenotypes overweight, glucose intolerance, insulin resistance, or impaired insulin release. In addition, we examined whether *in vitro FNDC5* gene expression in human myotubes reflects prediabetes-related metabolic *in vivo* traits of the donors.

Materials and Methods

Ethics statement. The study adhered to the Declaration of Helsinki, and its protocol was approved by the local ethics boards (Ethics Committees of the Eberhard Karls University Tübingen and the Karolinska Institute Stockholm). From all participants, informed written consent to the study was obtained.

Subjects. An overall study group of 1,976 White European individuals from Southern Germany was recruited from the ongoing Tübingen Family study for type 2 diabetes (TÜF) that currently encompasses more than 2,300 participants at increased risk for type 2 diabetes (i.e., non-diabetic individuals with family history of type 2 diabetes and/or diagnosis of impaired fasting glycaemia [12]. All subjects underwent the standard procedures of the protocol: assessment of medical history, smoking status, and alcohol consumption habits, physical examination, routine blood tests, and OGTTs. Selection of the overall study group was based on (i) the absence of newly diagnosed diabetes and (ii) the availability of complete phenotypic data sets. The participants were not taking any medication known to affect glucose tolerance, insulin sensitivity, or insulin secretion. From the overall study group, a subgroup of 486 subjects voluntarily agreed to undergo a hyperinsulinaemic-euglycaemic clamp procedure, a subgroup thereof (N = 360) additionally underwent MRI and magnetic resonance spectroscopy (MRS), and another subgroup (N = 305) IVGTTs. The clinical characteristics of the overall study group and the clamp, MRI/MRS, and IVGTT subgroups are presented in Table 1.

OGTT. After a 10-h overnight fast, a standard 75-g OGTT was performed, and venous blood samples were drawn at time-points 0, 30, 60, 90, and 120 min for the determination of plasma glucose, insulin, and C-peptide concentrations [12].

IVGTT and hyperinsulinaemic-euglycaemic clamp. In those individuals who agreed to undergo both the IVGTT and the hyperinsulinaemic-euglycaemic clamp, the IVGTT was performed prior to the clamp after a 10-h overnight fast, as described by the Botnia protocol [13]. For the IVGTT, glucose (0.3 g/kg body weight) was given, and blood samples for the measurement of

plasma glucose and insulin were obtained at time-points 0, 2, 4, 6, 8, 10, 20, 30, 40, 50, and 60 min [12]. For the hyperinsulinaemic-euglycaemic clamp, subjects received a primed infusion of insulin ($40 \text{ mU*m}^{-2}\text{*min}^{-1}$) for 120 min, and glucose infusion was started to clamp the plasma glucose concentration at 5.5 mmol/L. Blood samples for the measurement of plasma glucose were obtained at 5-min intervals, plasma insulin levels were measured at baseline and in the steady state of the clamp [12]. In subjects who agreed to undergo the hyperinsulinaemic-euglycaemic clamp only, the clamp procedure was started after the 10-h overnight fast.

Measurements of body fat content and body fat distribution. Waist circumference (in cm) was measured in the upright position at the midpoint between the lateral iliac crest and the lowest rib. BMI was calculated as weight divided by height squared (kg/m^2). The percentage of body fat was measured by bioelectrical impedance (BIA-101, RJL systems, Detroit, MI, USA). In addition, total and visceral fat contents (in % of body weight) were determined by whole-body MRI, as described earlier [14]. The intrahepatic lipid content (in % of signal) was determined by localized STEAM ^{1}H-MRS, as formerly reported in detail [15].

Laboratory measurements. Plasma glucose (in mmol/L) was determined using a bedside glucose analyzer (glucose oxidase method, Yellow Springs Instruments, Yellow Springs, OH, USA). Plasma insulin and C-peptide concentrations (in pmol/L both) were measured by commercial chemiluminescence assays for ADVIA Centaur (Siemens Medical Solutions, Fernwald, Germany) according to the manufacturer's instructions.

Calculations. HOMA-IR was calculated as {c(glucose[mmol/L])$_0$*c(insulin[mU/L])$_0$}/22.5 with c = concentration [16]. Therefore, HOMA-IR and fasting insulin concentrations are closely correlated (p<0.0001). The insulin sensitivity index derived from the OGTT (ISI OGTT) was estimated as proposed earlier [17]: 10,000/{c(glucose[mmol/L])$_0$*c(insulin[pmol/L])$_0$*c(glucose[mmol/L])$_{mean}$*c(insulin[pmol/L])$_{mean}$}$^{1/2}$. The insulin sensitivity index derived from the hyperinsulinaemic-euglycaemic clamp (ISI clamp) was calculated as glucose infusion rate necessary to maintain euglycaemia during the last 20 min (steady state) of the clamp (in $\mu\text{mol*kg}^{-1}\text{*min}^{-1}$) divided by the steady-state insulin concentration (in pmol/L). OGTT-derived insulin release was estimated by AUC$_{\text{Ins } 0-30}$/AUC$_{\text{Glc } 0-30}$ and AUC$_{\text{C-Pep } 0-120}$/AUC$_{\text{Glc } 0-120}$ with Ins = insulin (in pmol/L), C-Pep = C-peptide (in pmol/L), and Glc = glucose (in mmol/L). AUC$_{\text{Ins } 0-30}$/AUC$_{\text{Glc } 0-30}$ was calculated as {c(insulin)$_0$+c(insulin)$_{30}$}/{c(glucose)$_0$+c(glucose)$_{30}$}. AUC$_{\text{C-Pep } 0-120}$/AUC$_{\text{Glc } 0-120}$ was calculated by the trapezoid method as ½{½c(C-peptide)$_0$+c(C-peptide)$_{30}$+c(C-peptide)$_{60}$+c(C-peptide)$_{90}$+½c(C-peptide)$_{120}$}/½{½c(glucose)$_0$+c(glucose)$_{30}$+c(glucose)$_{60}$+c(glucose)$_{90}$+½c(glucose)$_{120}$}. Both indices were recently shown to be superior to several fasting state−/OGTT-derived indices for the detection of genetically determined β-cell failure [18]. Acute insulin response (AIR) from the IVGTT was calculated according to the trapezoid method as ½{½c(insulin)$_0$+c(insulin)$_2$+c(insulin)$_4$+c(insulin)$_6$+c(insulin)$_8$+½c(insulin)$_{10}$}.

Selection of tagging SNPs. Based on publicly available phase III data of the International HapMap Project derived from the Central European (CEU) population (release #28 August 2010, http://hapmap.ncbi.nlm.nih.gov/index.html.en), we screened *in silico* a genomic area on human chromosome 1p35.1 encompassing the complete *FNDC5* gene (8.47 kb, 6 exons, 5 introns) as well as 5 and 3 kb of its 5'- and 3'-flanking regions, respectively (Figure 1). The *FNDC5* locus is flanked ~16 kb upstream by the *HPCA* gene and ~3.5 kb downstream by the *S100PBP* gene, but no high-linkage-disequilibrium blocks within the screened *FNDC5* locus region were found to overlap with these

Table 1. Clinical characteristics of the study groups.

	Overall study group	Clamp subgroup	MRI/MRS subgroup	IVGTT subgroup	Myotube donors TÜ	Myotube donors ST
Sample size (N)	1,976	486	360	305	37	14
Women/men (%)	66.1/33.9	54.1/45.9	61.9/38.1	58.0/42.0	48.6/51.4	0/100
NGT/IFG/IGT/IFG&IGT/DIA (%)	70.4/11.3/9.8/8.5/0	75.7/7.4/10.1/6.8/0	63.1/12.2/13.6/11.1/0	65.9/10.5/14.1/9.5/0	91.9/0/5.4/0/2.7	57.1/0/0/0/42.9
Age (y)	40±13	40±12	45±12	45±11	28±7	62±4
BMI (kg/m^2)	30.2±9.3	27.5±5.8	30.0±5.3	29.5±5.7	23.9±5.0	28.0±2.1
Body fat (%)	32.7±12.1	28.6±9.7	33.0±8.9	32.2±8.8	22.4±8.0	–
Waist circumference (cm)	96±19	93±15	97±14	97±15	82±11	–
Total adipose tissue (% BW)	–	–	30.5±9.1	–	–	–
Visceral adipose tissue (% BW)	–	–	3.33±1.74	–	–	–
Intrahepatic lipids (%)	–	–	5.88±6.43	–	–	–
Fasting glucose (mmol/L)	5.14±0.55	5.01±0.55	5.24±0.51	5.18±0.50	4.85±0.53	6.27±1.24
Glucose 120 min OGTT (mmol/L)	6.36±1.65	6.21±1.74	6.92±1.58	6.81±1.66	5.68±1.96	–
AUC$_{Ins\ 0-30}$/AUC$_{Glc\ 0-30}$ OGTT (*10^{-9})	45.6±34.2	37.4±24.2	42.1±27.1	41.5±26.2	27.1±13.0	–
AUC$_{C-Pep\ 0-120}$/AUC$_{Glc\ 0-120}$ OGTT (*10^{-9})	322±106	311±97	307±89	309±95	288±72	–
AIR IVGTT (pmol/L)	–	–	–	936±633	–	–
Fasting insulin (pmol/L)	71.3±61.0	53.7±39.1	63.8±42.4	61.6±42.2	45.2±26.1	67.8±37.1
HOMA-IR (*10^{-6} mol*U*L^{-2})	2.80±2.60	2.05±1.66	2.51±1.79	2.41±1.82	1.66±1.11	3.00±1.53
ISI OGTT (*10^{15} L^2*mol^{-2})	15.1±10.4	18.0±11.4	12.6±6.9	13.6±7.7	23.3±11.3	–
ISI Clamp (*10^6 L*kg^{-1}*min^{-1})	–	0.084±0.055	–	–	0.112±0.062*	–

Data are given as counts, percentages, or means ±SD. AIR – acute insulin response; AUC – area under the curve; BMI – body mass index; BW – body weight; C-Pep – C-peptide; DIA – diabetes; Glc – glucose; HOMA-IR – homeostasis model assessment of insulin resistance; IFG – impaired fasting glycaemia; IGT – impaired glucose tolerance; Ins – insulin; ISI – insulin sensitivity index; IVGTT – intravenous glucose tolerance test; MRI – magnetic resonance imaging; MRS – magnetic resonance spectroscopy; NGT – normal glucose tolerance; OGTT – oral glucose tolerance test; ST – Stockholm; TÜ – Tübingen; *data available from 27 subjects.

neighbouring genes, based on HapMap r^2-data (Figure S1). Within the *FNDC5* locus, twelve HapMap SNPs were present and in Hardy-Weinberg equilibrium (HapMap data). Among these, eleven SNPs showed MAFs ≥0.05 (HapMap data), and one SNP, i.e., rs1284368, was rare (MAF = 0.004). As our study population is too small to assess rare variants with sufficient statistical power, we focussed on the common SNPs. Among the eleven common SNPs, only seven were genotyped in ≥50% of the HapMap individuals (HapMap CEU population: 46 family trios) and, thus, provide reliable data. All of these seven SNPs are located in non-coding regions of the locus. Their HapMap linkage disequilibrium (r^2) data are schematically presented in Figure 1. Among these SNPs, four SNPs were selected as tagging SNPs covering all the other common SNPs within the locus with an r^2 >0.8 (100% coverage) based on Tagger analysis using Haploview software (http://www.broadinstitute.org/scientific-community/science/programs/medical-and-population-genetics/haploview/haploview). As highlighted in Figure 1, the four tagging SNPs were rs16835198 (G/T) in the 3′-flanking region, rs3480 (A/G) in exon 6 (3′-untranslated region), rs726344 (G/A) in intron 5, and rs1746661 (G/T) in intron 2.

Genotyping. DNA was isolated from whole blood using a commercial DNA isolation kit (NucleoSpin, Macherey & Nagel, Düren, Germany). The four *FNDC5* tagging SNPs were genotyped using the Sequenom massARRAY system with iPLEX software (Sequenom, Hamburg, Germany). The genotyping success rates were ≥99.7%. The Sequenom results were validated by bi-

directional sequencing in 50 randomly selected subjects, and both methods gave 100% identical results (r = 1.00).

Human myotube culture. Thirty-seven mostly young study participants (including two subjects with impaired glucose tolerance and one newly diagnosed treatment-naive diabetic patient) recruited in Tübingen and 14 elderly men (including 6 diabetic patients not under insulin treatment) recruited in Stockholm voluntarily agreed to undergo percutaneous needle biopsy of the vastus lateralis muscle (clinical characteristics of the donors presented in Table 1). From satellite cells that were obtained from the biopsies via collagenase digestion, primary human skeletal muscle cells were grown as formerly described in detail [19]. Basal gene expression was assessed in first-pass cells after growth to 80–90% confluence and five days of differentiation to myotubes [19]. The medium in which the myotubes were kept until cell lysis contained 2% fetal calf serum and 1 mg/L glucose.

Quantitative PCR (qPCR). Myotubes were washed and harvested by trypsinization. RNA was isolated with RNeasy columns (Qiagen, Hilden, Germany). Total RNA treated with RNase-free DNase I was transcribed into cDNA using AMV reverse transcriptase and the First Strand cDNA kit from Roche Diagnostics (Mannheim, Germany). QPCR was performed in duplicates with fluorescence-labelled probes from Roche Universal ProbeLibrary on a LightCycler^{TM} (Roche Diagnostics, Mannheim, Germany). Primers were purchased from TIB MOLBIOL (Berlin, Germany). Primer sequences and PCR conditions are available upon request. All quantitative mRNA data were

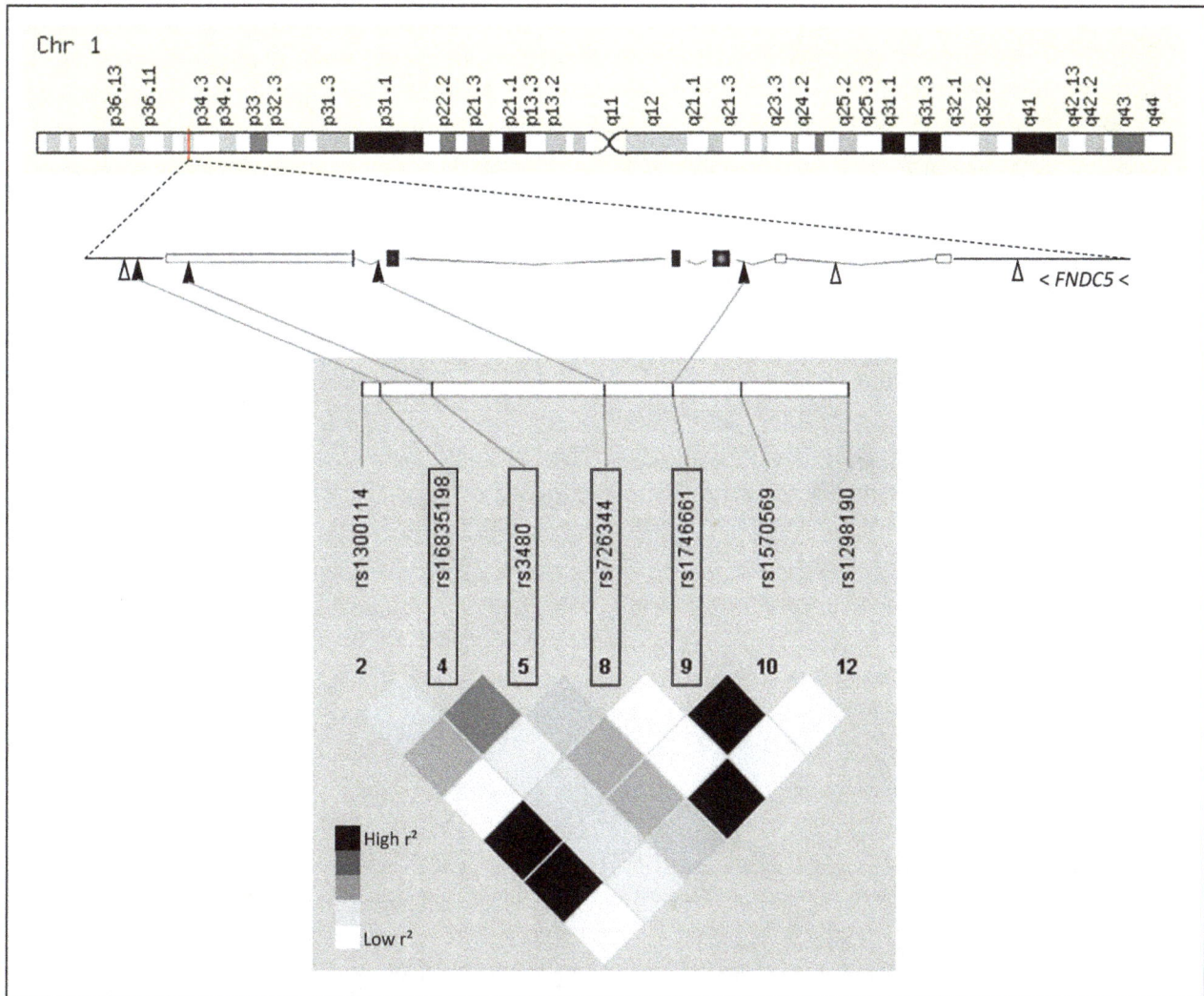

Figure 1. *FNDC5* **gene locus on human chromosome 1p35.1 and tagging SNPs.** The *FNDC5* gene consists of 6 exons and 5 introns and spans 8.47 kb from nucleotide position 33,100,464 to nucleotide position 33,108,934. The analyzed region additionally included 5 kb of the 5'-flanking region and 3 kb of the 3'-flanking region. This genomic region did not overlap with other known gene loci. The locations of the seven common (minor allele frequencies ≥0.05) SNPs in the region and the four tagging SNPs (highlighted by boxes) are indicated by white and black triangles, respectively. HapMap CEU-derived linkage disequilibrium data (r^2-values) are presented as shaded diamonds (white – $r^2 = 0.0$; black – $r^2 = 1.0$; grey – in between). CEU – Central Europeans; SNP – single nucleotide polymorphism.

normalized to the housekeeping gene *RPS13* using the ΔC_t method.

Statistical analyses. Hardy-Weinberg equilibrium was tested using χ^2 test (one degree of freedom). Linkage disequilibrium (D', r^2) between the tagging SNPs was analysed using MIDAS 1.0 freeware (http://www.genes.org.uk/software/midas, [20]). Continuous variables with non-normal distribution were log$_e$-transformed prior to linear regression analysis. Multiple linear regression analysis was performed using the least-squares method. In the regression models, the trait of interest (measure of body fat content/distribution, glycaemia, insulin sensitivity, or insulin release) was chosen as outcome variable, the SNP genotype (in the additive inheritance model) as independent variable, and gender, age, body fat content/BMI as possible confounding variables. Based on screening four non-linked tagging SNPs in parallel, a p-value <0.0127 was considered statistically significant according to Bonferroni correction for multiple comparisons. We did not correct for the tested metabolic traits since these were far

from being independent. In all subsequent analyses addressing exclusively the effects of SNPs rs16835198 and rs726344 on insulin sensitivity in more detail, a p-value <0.0253 was considered statistically significant. We did this because we assumed that the chance to get a statistical chance finding in a hypothesis-driven replication effort in the absence of multiple testing is extremely low. For all these analyses, the statistical software package JMP 10.0 (SAS Institute, Cary, NC, USA) was used. The effects of SNPs rs726344 and rs16835198 on insulin sensitivity in our TÜF-derived overall study group and in the Meta-Analyses of Glucose and Insulin-related traits Consortium (MAGIC) was studied by inverse variance weighted meta-analysis using MetaXL freeware (http://www.epigear.com/index_files/metaxl.html). Our study was sufficiently powered (1-β≥0.8) to detect effect sizes between 6.2% (rs3480) and 10% (rs726344) on ISI OGTT (two-sided type 1 error rate <0.05). Power calculations were performed using Quanto 1.2.4 freeware (http://hydra.usc.edu/gxe). For gene expression studies, t-tests, simple and multiple linear regression analyses were applied wherever appropriate, and the significance threshold was set to p≤0.05.

Results

Clinical characteristics of the study groups. The overall study group (N = 1,976) consisted of relatively young (median age –39 y) and moderately overweight (median BMI –27.6 kg/m²) non-diabetic individuals with a proportion of 66% being female and a proportion of 34% being male. The majority (~70%) of the subjects were normal glucose tolerant (NGT), ~30% were prediabetic: 11.3% had isolated impaired fasting glycaemia (IFG), 9.8% isolated impaired glucose tolerance (IGT), and 8.5% both IFG and IGT. The clinical characteristics of the study participants are presented in Table 1. The clinical characteristics of the clamp, MRI/MRS, and IVGTT subgroups were largely comparable (Table 1).

Genotyping of *FNDC5* tagging SNPs. The 1,976 study participants were genotyped for the four tagging SNPs rs16835198, rs3480, rs726344, and rs1746661 covering all other common variants in the *FNDC5* gene locus with MAFs ≥0.05 (Figure 1). The genotyping success rates were ≥99.7%, and three tagging SNPs obeyed the Hardy-Weinberg equilibrium (p≥0.2, Table 2). SNP rs1746661 significantly deviated from Hardy-Weinberg equilibrium (p = 0.0292, Table 2). Since no genotyping errors could be detected, we included this SNP in our analyses. The MAFs observed in our overall study group ranged from 0.10 to 0.42 and were close to those reported for the HapMap CEU population (Table S1). Based on r² data, the observed genetic linkage between the tagging SNPs was low or moderate (r² range – 0.03–0.50, Table S2).

Genetic associations of *FNDC5* with body fat content and body fat distribution. After adjustment for gender and age, none of the four tagging SNPs showed significant or nominal association (p≥0.1, Table S3) with parameters of body fat content (BMI, bioelectrical impedance-derived percentage of body fat, MRI-derived total adipose tissue mass) or body fat distribution (waist circumference, MRI-derived visceral adipose tissue mass, MRS-derived intrahepatic lipids).

Genetic associations of *FNDC5* with insulin release. After adjustment for gender, age, bioelectrical impedance-derived percentage of body fat, and ISI OGTT, none of the tagging SNPs was significantly or nominally associated with OGTT-derived parameters of insulin release (p≥0.6) or with IVGTT-derived AIR (p≥0.5) as given in Table S4.

Genetic associations of *FNDC5* with insulin sensitivity and glycaemia. After adjustment for gender, age, and percentage of body fat, the major G-allele of SNP rs16835198 was significantly associated with elevated fasting insulin concentrations (p = 0.0118) and reduced ISI OGTT (p = 0.0126) and nominally associated with increased HOMA-IR (p = 0.0179) revealing an additive insulin-desensitizing effect of this allele (raw data shown in Table S5, adjusted data shown in Figure 2A and B, statistics shown in Table 2). After identical adjustment, the minor A-allele of SNP rs726344 was significantly associated with increased HOMA-IR (p = 0.0073) and reduced ISI OGTT (p = 0.0074) and nominally associated with increased fasting insulin concentrations (p = 0.0131) demonstrating an additive insulin-desensitizing effect of this allele (raw data shown in Table S5, adjusted data shown in Figure 2C and D, statistics shown in Table 2). Furthermore, the insulin-desensitizing allele of rs726344 was nominally associated with increased fasting glucose concentrations (p = 0.0281, Table 2, raw data shown in Table S5). None of the other tested SNPs showed associations with insulin sensitivity and/or glycaemia. To

Table 2. Association of *FNDC5* SNPs rs16835198, rs3480, rs726344, and rs1746661 with glycaemia and insulin sensitivity (statistics).

SNP	Genotype	N Overall study group	HWE	Fasting glucose (mmol/L)	Glucose 120 min OGTT (mmol/L)	Fasting insulin (pmol/L)	HOMA-IR (*10⁻⁶ mol*U*L⁻²)	ISI OGTT (*10¹⁵ L²*mol⁻²)	N Clamp subgroup	ISI Clamp (*10⁶ L*kg⁻¹*min⁻¹)
rs16835198	GG/GT/TT	844/892/238	p=0.9	β=-0.0003 p=1.0	β=0.0005 p=1.0	**β=-0.0457 p=0.0118#**	β=-0.0459 p=0.0179	**β=0.0480 p=0.0126#**	209/221/55	β=0.0081 p=0.8
rs3480	AA/AG/GG	689/928/355	p=0.2	β=0.0012 p=0.7	β=0.0007 p=0.9	β=0.0281 p=0.1	β=0.0294 p=0.1	β=-0.0286 p=0.1	159/240/86	β=0.0022 p=0.9
rs726344	GG/GA/AA	1,590/359/22	p=0.7	**β=0.0111 p=0.0281**	β=0.0071 p=0.6	**β=0.0708 p=0.0131**	**β=0.0817 p=0.0073#**	**β=-0.0809 p=0.0074#**	381/94/9	β=0.0778 p=0.1
rs1746661	GG/GT/TT	1,240/627/105	p=0.0292	β=-0.0010 p=0.8	β=0.0050 p=0.6	β=0.0243 p=0.2	β=0.0237 p=0.3	β=-0.0094 p=0.7	304/151/30	β=-0.0361 p=0.3

Prior to statistical analysis, all parameters were adjusted for gender, age, and bioelectrical impedance-derived percentage of body fat. Nominal associations are marked by bold fonts; #significant after Bonferroni correction (p<0.0127). HOMA-IR – homeostasis model assessment of insulin resistance; HWE – Hardy-Weinberg equilibrium; ISI – insulin sensitivity index; OGTT – oral glucose tolerance test; SNP – single nucleotide polymorphism.

test whether the effects of SNP rs16835198 were mediated by the weakly linked SNP rs726344 ($r^2 = 0.061$, Table 2) and vice versa, we performed conditional analyses. After adjustment of SNP rs16835198 for gender, age, percentage of body fat and SNP rs726344, the associations of SNP rs16835198 with fasting insulin concentrations and ISI OGTT were still nominal (p = 0.0424 and p = 0.0496, respectively), whereas its association with HOMA-IR was no longer nominal (p = 0.07). The associations of SNP rs726344 with fasting glucose concentrations, fasting insulin concentrations, HOMA-IR, and ISI OGTT were still nominal after additional adjustment for SNP rs16835198 (p = 0.0252, p = 0.0497, p = 0.0275, and p = 0.0298, respectively) pointing to independent effects of both SNPs and weaker effects of SNP rs16835198. Furthermore, both SNPs provided divergent results in NGT vs. prediabetic (sum of IFG, IGT, and IFG+IGT) subjects: the effect of SNP rs16835198 on insulin sensitivity (as assessed by fasting insulin concentrations, HOMA-IR, and ISI OGTT) was present in NGT ($\beta \geq 0.0492$, $p \leq 0.0216$), but not in prediabetic ($\beta \leq 0.0216$, $p \geq 0.5$), subjects, whereas the effect of SNP rs726344 emerges in prediabetic ($\beta \geq 0.0875$, $p \leq 0.09$), but not in NGT ($\beta \leq 0.0490$, $p \geq 0.1$), subjects. The effect of SNP rs726344 on fasting glucose concentrations was detectable in prediabetic subjects only ($\beta = 0.0210$, p = 0.0131; NGT subjects: $\beta = 0.0029$, p = 0.6).

Interrogation of MAGIC data for replication. To replicate the effects of SNPs rs16835198 and rs726344 on fasting insulin concentrations and HOMA-IR, we screened the publicly available MAGIC data from 38,238 (fasting insulin dataset) and 37,037 (HOMA-IR dataset) subjects (http://www.magicinvestigators.org/downloads, [21]) and found a concordant and significant association of the A-allele of SNP rs726344 with elevated fasting insulin concentrations (p = 0.01669) and a nonsignificant trend for association with increased HOMA-IR (p = 0.08). SNP rs16835198 was not associated with either parameter in MAGIC ($p \geq 0.7$). To further corroborate the effect of SNP rs726344 on insulin sensitivity, we meta-analysed the effects on fasting insulin and HOMA-IR reported for this SNP's A-allele in MAGIC and the effects of the A-allele derived from comparably performed multiple linear regression models in our overall study group. In the meta-analysis, the effect sizes of the A-allele were shifted to higher (and more significant) values compared to those reported by MAGIC (fasting insulin −0.018 vs. 0.015, p = 0.0002; HOMA-IR −0.015 vs. 0.012, p = 0.0015), as depicted in Figure 3. As expected from the MAGIC data alone, meta-analysis did not reveal significant effects of SNP rs16835198 on insulin sensitivity (Figure S2).

Association of human myotube FNDC5 expression with insulin sensitivity. To further address the role of FNDC5/irisin in humans, we quantified FNDC5 mRNA expression in myotubes derived from 37 mostly young participants (Table 1) of the overall study group. This gene's basal expression levels were not influenced by donors' gender, age, or percentage of body fat ($p \geq 0.3$, Figure S3). Then, we addressed whether we can replicate, in human myotubes, the close association between PGC-1α and FNDC5 that was observed in mice upon muscle-specific transgenic PGC-1α overexpression [10]. As depicted in Figure 4A, the basal *PPARGC1A* (encoding PGC-1α) and *FNDC5* mRNA contents of human myotubes were closely associated (r = 0.60, $p = 8.6 \times 10^{-5}$). Based on our SNP data, we finally asked whether myotube *FNDC5* expression is associated with *in vivo* insulin sensitivity of the donors. In contrast to the findings in mice, i.e., insulin sensitization of high fat-fed mice upon adenoviral *Fndc5* overexpression [10], basal *FNDC5* expression in human myotubes was positively associated with fasting insulin concentrations (p = 0.0366, Figure 4B) and

HOMA-IR (p = 0.0204, Figure 4C), negatively associated with ISI OGTT (p = 0.0149, Figure 4D), and positively associated with 2-h glucose concentrations (p = 0.0500, Figure 4E) after adjustment of the metabolic trait for gender, age, and percentage of body fat. Even though there was a weak trend for association of the insulin-desensitizing minor A-allele of *FNDC5* SNP rs726344 with higher *FNDC5* mRNA contents (p = 0.19), this SNP's MAF was too low to allow a reliable evaluation (only four heterozygous and no homozygous carriers of the minor allele were present among the myotube donors).

Replication of the *in vitro* results. To this end, we determined *FNDC5* expression in human myotubes from 14 elderly men (8 normal glucose tolerant subjects, 6 diabetic patients; Table 1) recruited at the Karolinska Institute in Stockholm. Importantly, none of the diabetic patients was under insulin treatment. From these donors, only age, BMI, and fasting glucose and insulin concentrations were available. Again, the basal *FNDC5* expression levels were not influenced by donors' age or BMI ($p \geq 0.5$). After adjustment for BMI, basal *FNDC5* expression was positively associated with fasting insulin levels (p = 0.0326, Figure 4F) and showed a trend towards positive association with HOMA-IR (p = 0.06). In further support of our data, a recent report by Timmons et al. also provided a trend for positive association between *FNDC5* expression in freshly isolated skeletal muscle biopsies (without isolation and culture of myocytes) from 118 diabetes medication-free subjects and donors' fasting insulin levels (r = 0.2, not significant [22]).

Discussion

In this study, we report a significant and replicated insulin-desensitizing effect of the minor A-allele of *FNDC5* SNP rs726344 (adjusted effect size on HOMA-IR in our study population − +9.5% per A-allele). Since this SNP and the only HapMap SNP reported to be in high linkage with it, i.e., rs1298190 ($r^2 = 0.96$, Figure 1), are both intronic, the molecular mechanisms how these SNPs affect insulin sensitivity remain obscure. Unfortunately, we were not able to reliably study this SNP's impact on *FNDC5* expression in our myotube donors due to the SNP's low MAF (= 0.10).

The replicated finding that *FNDC5* expression is inversely associated with the donors' insulin sensitivity appears conflicting with the mouse data from Boström et al. who reported reduced insulin resistance in high fat-fed mice upon adenoviral *Fndc5* overexpression via ('browning'-mediated) elevated energy expenditure and attenuated weight gain [10]. The reasons for this discrepancy may be diverse. Even though it was recently convincingly demonstrated that functional brown adipose tissue exists in adult humans [23–26], it is currently unclear whether 'browning', i.e., trans-determination and/or trans-differentiation of human white adipose precursor cells into brown adipocytes occurs in humans *in vivo*, as was shown in mice [10,27–29]. Moreover, it is completely unknown whether the FNDC5-derived myokine irisin exerts similar biological functions in mice and humans, and mice and humans may differ, e.g., in the regulation of FNDC5's post-translational processing (glycosylation, protease-stimulated cleavage) and/or in the regulation of cellular irisin release. Interestingly and in very good agreement with our results, a positive association between irisin plasma levels and fasting insulin levels, as a rough estimate of insulin resistance, was very recently demonstrated by Stengel et al. [30]. Moreover, Timmons et al. [22] could not establish irisin as an exercise factor in humans, but this was shown by Boström et al. in mice. Thus, irisin's role in humans is far from being understood, and there are

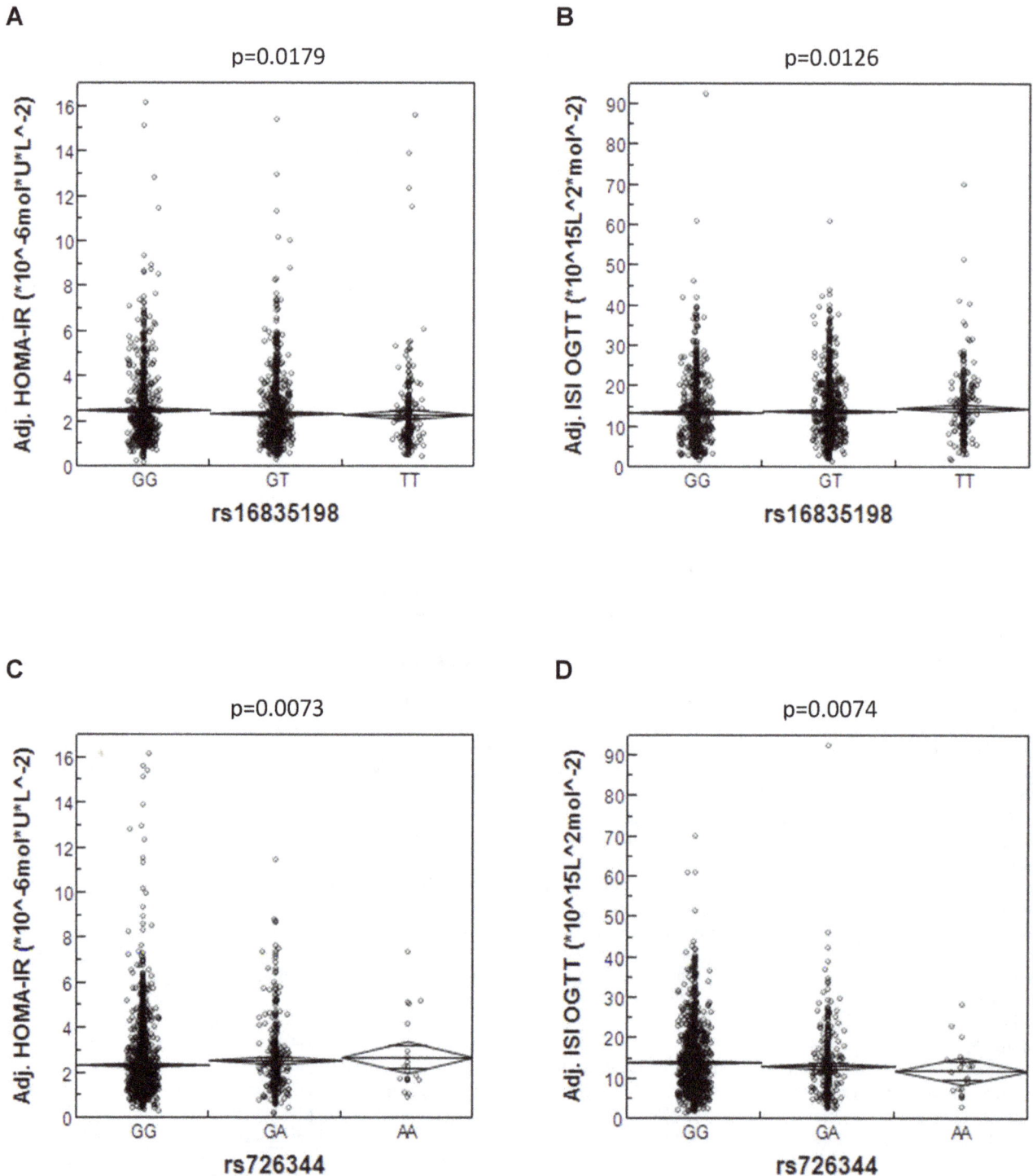

Figure 2. Association of *FNDC5* SNPs rs16835198 and rs726344 with insulin sensitivity. HOMA-IR (A and C) and ISI OGTT (B and D) data were adjusted for gender, age, and bioelectrical impedance-derived percentage of body fat. Diamonds represent means ±SE. HOMA-IR – homeostasis model assessment of insulin resistance; ISI OGTT – oral glucose tolerance test-derived insulin sensitivity index; SNP – single nucleotide polymorphism.

several lines of evidence for species-specific differences between mice and humans.

Our translational data showing an association between myotube *FNDC5* expression and insulin sensitivity of the donors imply that *FNDC5* expression in vivo is maintained during muscle biopsy, isolation of stellate cells, and in vitro differen-

tiation to myotubes. Since we observed similar associations between *ANGPTL4*, *PDK4*, *SCD*, and *ADIPOR1* expression in human myotubes and in vivo traits of the donors earlier [3,31–33], we suggest that the expression of a series of genes is indeed stable, and this may have genetic and/or epigenetic reasons.

A

Adj. fasting insulin (pmol/L, log)

	Effect size (log) [95% CI]	% Weight	N
TÜF	0.063 [0.012, 0.114]	5.8	1,947
MAGIC	0.015 [0.002, 0.028]	94.2	38,238
Overall	0.018 [0.006, 0.030]	100.0	40,185

Q=3.26, p=0.07, I²=69%

Effect size (pmol/L, log)

B

Adj. HOMA-IR (*10⁻⁶mol*U*L⁻², log)

	Effect size (log) [95% CI]	% Weight	N
TÜF	0.074 [0.020, 0.128]	5.5	1,947
MAGIC	0.012 [-0.001, 0.025]	94.5	37,037
Overall	0.015 [0.003, 0.028]	100.0	38,984

Q=4.84, p=0.03, I²=79%

Effect size (*10⁻⁶mol*U*L⁻², log)

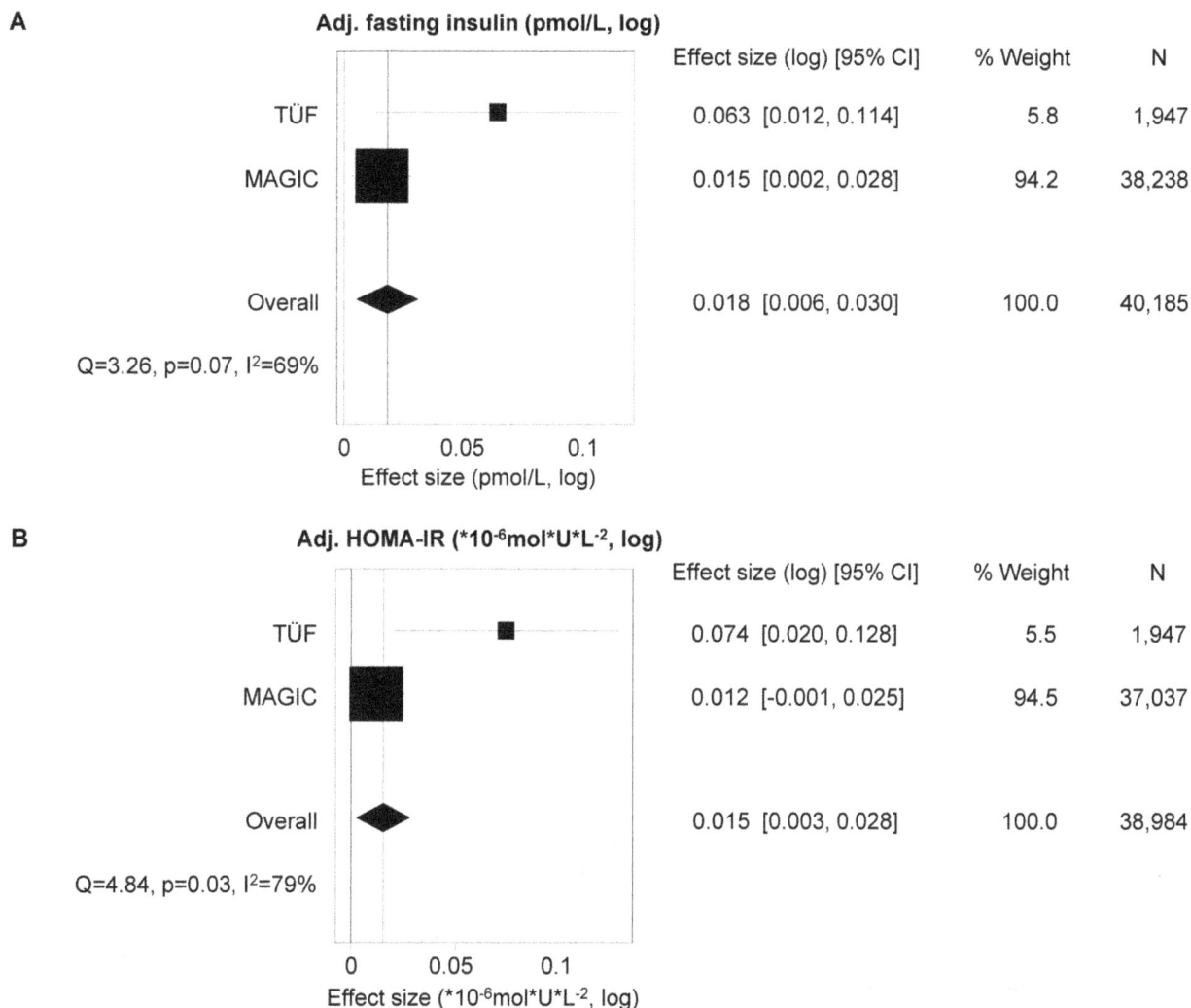

Figure 3. Meta-analysis of the effect of *FNDC5* SNP rs726344 on insulin sensitivity in TÜF and MAGIC. The effects of the minor A-allele of SNP rs726344 on fasting insulin (A) and HOMA-IR (B), as derived from multiple linear regression analysis with gender, age, and BMI as confounding variables, were subjected to inverse variance weighted meta-analysis. Effect sizes, 95% confidence intervals, weights, sample sizes, and heterogeneity data are given. HOMA-IR – homeostasis model assessment of insulin resistance; MAGIC – Meta-Analyses of Glucose and Insulin-related traits Consortium; SNP – single nucleotide polymorphism; TÜF – overall study group derived from the Tübingen Family study for type 2 diabetes.

Notably, we identified a second *FNDC5* SNP, i.e., rs16835198, with markedly weaker, but significant, effects on parameters of insulin sensitivity (adjusted effect size on HOMA-IR in our study population –4.7% per major G-allele). This SNP is located in the 3'-flanking region of the gene and was in rather low linkage with SNP rs726344 ($r^2 = 0.061$). Furthermore, both SNPs exerted independent effects on insulin sensitivity and revealed divergent effects on insulin sensitivity in NGT vs. prediabetic subjects. The latter finding, however, has to be interpreted with caution due to the limited sample sizes of the subgroups (NGT subjects: N = 1,392; prediabetic subjects: N = 584), but could point to SNP-specific genotype-glycaemia interactions. This clearly needs deeper examination in larger study populations. In contrast to rs726344, this SNP's major allele revealed an insulin-desensitizing effect. This difference could be, for instance, explained by transcription rate-attenuating versus -enhancing effects of these two rather independent nucleotide exchanges. To assess whether the SNPs indeed affect the transcription rate and transcription factor binding sites in enhancer/silencer elements, further functional studies are needed.

Notably, both SNPs rs726344 and rs16835198 revealed smaller effect sizes on fasting insulin and HOMA-IR in MAGIC as compared to TÜF and the effect of SNP rs16835198 was no longer significant in MAGIC. One explanation for this observation may be the greater heterogeneity of MAGIC genome-wide association studies, e.g., in measured insulin values. In our experience, the method of insulin measurement is one of the most critical points whenever insulin data have to be compared between different studies.

An intriguing finding of our study is the lack of association of *FNDC5* SNPs rs726344 and rs16835198 with hyperinsulinaemic-euglycaemic clamp-derived insulin sensitivity. This may reflect the limited statistical power of the substantially smaller clamp subgroup. On the other hand, this could also be due to organ-specific insulin-desensitizing effects of irisin that are better detected by fasting- and OGTT-derived measures of insulin sensitivity. In this regard, it has been suggested that HOMA-IR and the OGTT-derived insulin sensitivity index used in this study are proxies reflecting, to a large part, hepatic insulin sensitivity, whereas

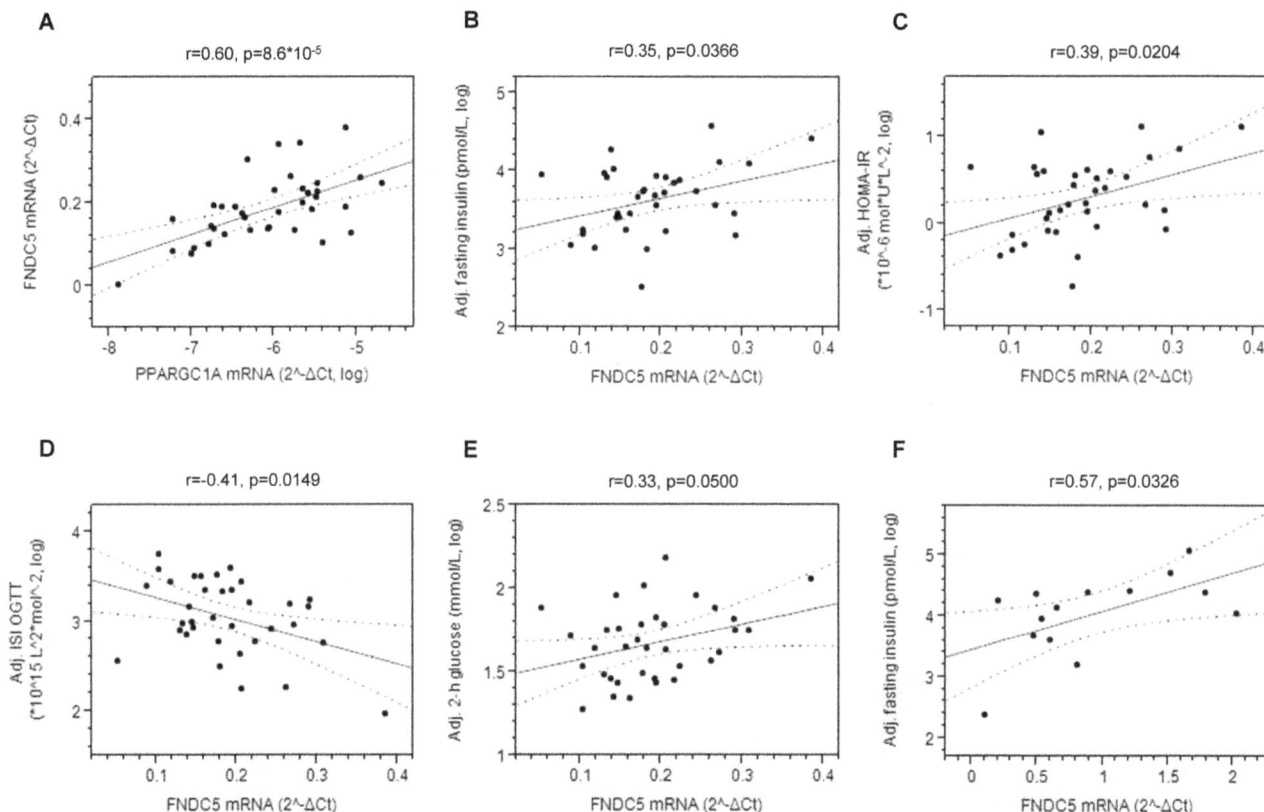

Figure 4. Association of human myotube *FNDC5* mRNA expression with *PPARGC1A* mRNA expression *in vitro* and donors' insulin sensitivity *in vivo*. The association between human myotube *FNDC5* and *PPARGC1A* mRNA contents (A) was assessed using simple linear regression analysis. The association between human myotube *FNDC5* mRNA expression and fasting insulin levels (B), HOMA-IR (C), ISI OGTT (D), and 2-h plasma glucose levels (E) of 37 young healthy donors recruited in Tübingen and with fasting insulin levels (F) of 14 elderly men recruited in Stockholm was tested by multiple linear regression analysis with gender, age, and bioelectrical impedance-derived percentage of body fat (Tübingen volunteers) or with BMI (Stockholm volunteers) as confounding variables (leverage plots shown). Dotted lines indicate the 95% confidence interval of the regression. HOMA-IR – homeostasis model assessment of insulin resistance.

hyperinsulinaemic-euglycaemic clamp-derived insulin sensitivity indices measure whole-body insulin sensitivity [34,35]. Clearly, this issue needs further investigation, e.g., by measurement of organ-specific insulin sensitivity via tracer methods [36].

A limitation of the study could be that we applied Bonferroni correction of the significance threshold for the four non-linked tagging SNPs only. We did not perform additional correction for the four prediabetic phenotypes tested, i.e., overweight, glucose intolerance, insulin resistance, and impaired insulin release, since these traits are far from being independent, and testing highly dependent traits is well known to result in actual error rates far below the adjusted error rates. A more rigorous correction, at the costs of an increasing number of statistical type II errors, would have rendered most of our significant results nominal. The fact that we identified two non-linked SNPs within the same locus – and not just a single one – both with effects on insulin sensitivity, but not on body adiposity or insulin secretion, further argues against mere chance findings.

In conclusion, this study provides evidence that the *FNDC5* gene, encoding the novel myokine irisin, influences insulin sensitivity in humans. Our gene expression data revealed an unexpected and currently inexplicable insulin-desensitizing effect of irisin. Based on this finding, it would now be interesting to study this gene's impact on type 2 diabetes risk.

Supporting Information

Figure S1   Linkage disequilibrium structure of the 200-kb genomic region surrounding the *FNDC5* gene. Genes (with exon-intron structure) are written in red colour. *FNDC5* is marked by yellow shading. HapMap CEU-derived linkage disequilibrium data (r^2-values) are presented as shaded diamonds (white – $r^2 = 0.0$; black – $r^2 = 1.0$; grey – in between). CEU – Central Europeans.

Figure S2   Meta-analysis of the effect of *FNDC5* SNP rs16835198 on insulin sensitivity in TÜF and MAGIC. The effects of the major G-allele of SNP rs16835198 on fasting insulin (A) and HOMA-IR (B), as derived from multiple linear regression analysis with gender, age, and BMI as confounding variables, were subjected to inverse variance weighted meta-analysis. Effect sizes, 95% confidence intervals, weights, sample sizes, and heterogeneity data are given. HOMA-IR – homeostasis model assessment of insulin resistance; MAGIC – Meta-Analyses of Glucose and Insulin-related traits Consortium; SNP – single nucleotide polymorphism; TÜF – overall study group derived from the Tübingen Family study for type 2 diabetes.

Figure S3   Association of human myotube *FNDC5* mRNA expression with donors' gender, age, and body fat

content. The association between human myotube *FNDC5* mRNA contents and donors' gender (A) was assessed by Student's t-test. The association between human myotube *FNDC5* mRNA expression and donors' age (B) and body fat content (C) was tested by multiple linear regression analysis. Dotted lines indicate the 95% confidence interval of the regression.

Table S1 Minor allele frequencies of *FNDC5* tagging SNPs. CEU – Central Eurpeans; SNP – single nucleotide polymorphism.

Table S2 Linkage disequilibrium between *FNDC5* tagging SNPs. Data represent linkage disequilibrium data: D' values are given below empty cell, r^2 values above empty cells. CEU – Central Europeans; SNP – single nucleotide polymorphism.

Table S3 Association of *FNDC5* SNPs rs16835198, rs3480, rs726344, and rs1746661 with body fat content and body fat distribution. Data are shown as unadjusted raw data (means ±SD). Prior to statistical analysis, all parameters were adjusted for gender and age. BMI – body mass index; BW – body weight; MRI – magnetic resonance imaging; MRS – magnetic resonance spectroscopy; SNP – single nucleotide polymorphism.

Table S4 Association of *FNDC5* SNPs rs16835198, rs3480, rs726344, and rs1746661 with insulin release. Data are shown as unadjusted raw data (means ±SD). Prior to statistical analysis, all parameters were adjusted for gender, age,

percentage of body fat, and OGTT-derived insulin sensitivity. AIR – acute insulin response; AUC – area under the curve; C-Pep – C-peptide; Glc – glucose; Ins – insulin; IVGTT – intravenous glucose tolerance test; OGTT – oral glucose tolerance test; SNP – single nucleotide polymorphism.

Table S5 Association of *FNDC5* SNPs rs16835198, rs3480, rs726344, and rs1746661 with glycaemia and insulin sensitivity (raw data). Data are shown as unadjusted raw data (means ±SD). HOMA-IR – homeostasis model assessment of insulin resistance; ISI – insulin sensitivity index; OGTT – oral glucose tolerance test; SNP – single nucleotide polymorphism.

Acknowledgments

We thank all study participants for their cooperation. We gratefully acknowledge the excellent technical assistance of Anna Bury, Alke Guirguis, Carina Haas, Roman-Georg Werner, and Eva Palmer. Data on glycaemic traits have been contributed by MAGIC investigators and have been downloaded from www.magicinvestigators.org.

Author Contributions

Reviewed and edited the manuscript, FS AF NS AK HUH MHA. Conceived and designed the experiments: HS AB MS LB CW FS AF NS AK HUH MHdA. Performed the experiments: HS JM FM AK. Analyzed the data: HS JM FM. Contributed reagents/materials/analysis tools: AF NS HUH MHdA. Wrote the paper: HS.

References

1. Maury E, Brichard SM (2010) Adipokine dysregulation, adipose tissue inflammation and metabolic syndrome. Mol Cell Endocrinol 314: 1–16.
2. Febbraio MA, Pedersen BK (2005) Contraction-induced myokine production and release: is skeletal muscle an endocrine organ? Exerc Sport Sci Rev 33: 114–119.
3. Staiger H, Haas C, Machann J, Werner R, Weisser M et al. (2009) Muscle-derived angiopoietin-like protein 4 is induced by fatty acids via peroxisome proliferator-activated receptor (PPAR)-delta and is of metabolic relevance in humans. Diabetes 58: 579–589.
4. Hansen J, Brandt C, Nielsen AR, Hojman P, Whitham M et al. (2011) Exercise induces a marked increase in plasma follistatin: evidence that follistatin is a contraction-induced hepatokine. Endocrinology 152: 164–171.
5. Dutchak PA, Katafuchi T, Bookout AL, Choi JH, Yu RT et al. (2012) Fibroblast growth factor-21 regulates PPARgamma activity and the antidiabetic actions of thiazolidinediones. Cell 148: 556–567.
6. Pedersen BK (2006) The anti-inflammatory effect of exercise: its role in diabetes and cardiovascular disease control. Essays Biochem 42: 105–117.
7. Peter A, Kantartzis K, Machann J, Schick F, Staiger H et al. (2010) Relationships of circulating sex hormone-binding globulin with metabolic traits in humans. Diabetes 59: 3167–3173.
8. Weikert C, Stefan N, Schulze MB, Pischon T, Berger K et al. (2008) Plasma fetuin-a levels and the risk of myocardial infarction and ischemic stroke. Circulation 118: 2555–2562.
9. Stefan N, Fritsche A, Weikert C, Boeing H, Joost HG et al. (2008) Plasma fetuin-A levels and the risk of type 2 diabetes. Diabetes 57: 2762–2767.
10. Bostrom P, Wu J, Jedrychowski MP, Korde A, Ye L et al. (2012) A PGC1-alpha-dependent myokine that drives brown-fat-like development of white fat and thermogenesis. Nature 481: 463–468.
11. Barbatelli G, Murano I, Madsen L, Hao Q, Jimenez M et al. (2010) The emergence of cold-induced brown adipocytes in mouse white fat depots is determined predominantly by white to brown adipocyte transdifferentiation. Am J Physiol Endocrinol Metab 298: E1244–E1253.
12. Stefan N, Machicao F, Staiger H, Machann J, Schick F et al. (2005) Polymorphisms in the gene encoding adiponectin receptor 1 are associated with insulin resistance and high liver fat. Diabetologia 48: 2282–2291.
13. Tripathy D, Wessman Y, Gullstrom M, Tuomi T, Group L (2003) Importance of obtaining independent measures of insulin secretion and insulin sensitivity during the same test: results with the Botnia clamp. Diabetes Care 26: 1395–1401.
14. Machann J, Thamer C, Schnoedt B, Haap M, Haring HU et al. (2005) Standardized assessment of whole body adipose tissue topography by MRI. J Magn Reson Imaging 21: 455–462.
15. Thamer C, Machann J, Haap M, Stefan N, Heller E et al. (2004) Intrahepatic lipids are predicted by visceral adipose tissue mass in healthy subjects. Diabetes Care 27: 2726–2729.
16. Matthews DR, Hosker JP, Rudenski AS, Naylor BA, Treacher DF et al. (1985) Homeostasis model assessment: insulin resistance and beta-cell function from fasting plasma glucose and insulin concentrations in man. Diabetologia 28: 412–419.
17. Matsuda M, DeFronzo RA (1999) Insulin sensitivity indices obtained from oral glucose tolerance testing: comparison with the euglycemic insulin clamp. Diabetes Care 22: 1462–1470.
18. Herzberg-Schafer SA, Staiger H, Heni M, Ketterer C, Guthoff M et al. (2010) Evaluation of fasting state−/oral glucose tolerance test-derived measures of insulin release for the detection of genetically impaired beta-cell function. PLoS One 5: e14194.
19. Krutzfeldt J, Kausch C, Volk A, Klein HH, Rett K et al. (2000) Insulin signaling and action in cultured skeletal muscle cells from lean healthy humans with high and low insulin sensitivity. Diabetes 49: 992–998.
20. Gaunt TR, Rodriguez S, Zapata C, Day IN (2006) MIDAS: software for analysis and visualisation of interallelic disequilibrium between multiallelic markers. BMC Bioinformatics 7: 227.
21. Dupuis J, Langenberg C, Prokopenko I, Saxena R, Soranzo N et al. (2010) New genetic loci implicated in fasting glucose homeostasis and their impact on type 2 diabetes risk. Nat Genet 42: 105–116.
22. Timmons JA, Baar K, Davidsen PK, Atherton PJ (2012) Is irisin a human exercise gene? Nature 488: E9–10.
23. Cypess AM, Lehman S, Williams G, Tal I, Rodman D et al. (2009) Identification and importance of brown adipose tissue in adult humans. N Engl J Med 360: 1509–1517.
24. Marken Lichtenbelt WD, Vanhommerig JW, Smulders NM, Drossaerts JM, Kemerink GJ et al. (2009) Cold-activated brown adipose tissue in healthy men. N Engl J Med 360: 1500–1508.
25. Stefan N, Pfannenberg C, Haring HU (2009) The importance of brown adipose tissue. N Engl J Med 361: 416–417.
26. Nedergaard J, Cannon B (2010) The changed metabolic world with human brown adipose tissue: therapeutic visions. Cell Metab 11: 268–272.
27. Cao L, Choi EY, Liu X, Martin A, Wang C et al. (2011) White to brown fat phenotypic switch induced by genetic and environmental activation of a hypothalamic-adipocyte axis. Cell Metab 14: 324–338.
28. Vitali A, Murano I, Zingaretti MC, Frontini A, Ricquier D et al. (2012) The adipose organ of obesity-prone C57BL/6J mice is composed of mixed white and brown adipocytes. J Lipid Res 53: 619–629.
29. Fisher FM, Kleiner S, Douris N, Fox EC, Mepani RJ et al. (2012) FGF21

regulates PGC-1alpha and browning of white adipose tissues in adaptive thermogenesis. Genes Dev 26: 271–281.

30. Stengel A, Hofmann T, Goebel-Stengel M, Elbelt U, Kobelt P et al. (2012) Circulating levels of irisin in patients with anorexia nervosa and different stages of obesity - Correlation with body mass index. Peptides 39C: 125–130.

31. Ordelheide AM, Heni M, Thamer C, Machicao F, Fritsche A et al. (2011) In vitro responsiveness of human muscle cell peroxisome proliferator-activated receptor delta reflects donors' insulin sensitivity in vivo. Eur J Clin Invest 41: 1323–1329.

32. Peter A, Weigert C, Staiger H, Machicao F, Schick F et al. (2009) Individual stearoyl-coa desaturase 1 expression modulates endoplasmic reticulum stress and inflammation in human myotubes and is associated with skeletal muscle lipid storage and insulin sensitivity in vivo. Diabetes 58: 1757–1765.

33. Staiger H, Kaltenbach S, Staiger K, Stefan N, Fritsche A et al. (2004) Expression of adiponectin receptor mRNA in human skeletal muscle cells is related to in vivo parameters of glucose and lipid metabolism. Diabetes 53: 2195–2201.

34. Tripathy D, Almgren P, Tuomi T, Groop L (2004) Contribution of insulin-stimulated glucose uptake and basal hepatic insulin sensitivity to surrogate measures of insulin sensitivity. Diabetes Care 27: 2204–2210.

35. Muniyappa R, Lee S, Chen H, Quon MJ (2008) Current approaches for assessing insulin sensitivity and resistance in vivo: advantages, limitations, and appropriate usage. Am J Physiol Endocrinol Metab 294: E15–E26.

36. Choukem SP, Gautier JF (2008) How to measure hepatic insulin resistance? Diabetes Metab 34: 664–673.

6

Relationship between Insulin Resistance and Coronary Artery Calcium in Young Men and Women

Ki-Chul Sung[1]*, Jin-Ho Choi[2], Hyeon-Cheol Gwon[2], Seung-Hyuk Choi[2], Bum-Soo Kim[1], Hyon Joo Kwag[3], Sun H. Kim[4]

1 Division of Cardiology, Department of Medicine, Kangbuk Samsung Hospital, Sungkyunkwan University School of Medicine, Seoul, Republic of Korea, 2 Division of Cardiology, Cardiac and Vascular Center, Department of Medicine, Samsung Medical Center, Sungkyunkwan University School of Medicine, Seoul, Republic of Korea, 3 Department of Radiology, Kangbuk Samsung Hospital Sungkyunkwan, University School of Medicine, Seoul, Republic of Korea, 4 Division of Endocrinology, Department of Medicine, Stanford University School of Medicine, Stanford, California, United States of America

Abstract

Background: The gender disparity in cardiovascular disease (CVD) risk is greatest between young men and women. However, the causes of that are not fully understood. The objective of this study was to evaluate the relationship between insulin resistance and the presence of coronary artery calcium (CAC) to identify risk factors that may predispose young men and women to CVD.

Methodology/Principal Findings: Insulin resistance and CVD risk factors were examined in 8682 Korean men and 1829 women aged 30–45 years old. Insulin resistance was estimated using the homeostasis model assessment of insulin resistance (HOMA-IR), and CAC was measured using computed tomography. Women were less likely to be insulin resistant (upper quartile of HOMA-IR, 18% vs. 27%, $p<0.001$) and had a lower prevalence of CAC (1.6% vs. 6.4%, $p<0.001$). Even when equally insulin resistant men and women were compared, women continued to have lower prevalence of CAC (3.1% vs. 7.2%, $p=0.004$) and a more favorable CVD risk profile. Finally, after adjustment for traditional CVD risk factors, insulin resistance remained an independent predictor of CAC only in men ($p=0.03$).

Conclusions/Significance: Young women have a lower risk for CVD and a lower CAC prevalence compared with men. This favorable CVD risk profile in women appears to occur regardless of insulin sensitivity. Unlike men, insulin resistance was not a predictor of CAC in women in this cohort. Therefore, insulin resistance has less impact on CVD risk and CAC in young women compared with men, and insulin resistance alone does not explain the gender disparity in CVD risk that is observed at an early age.

Editor: Alexander G. Obukhov, Indiana University School of Medicine, United States of America

Funding: This work was partially supported by a Samsung Biomedical Research Institute grant [SBRI C-B1-114-1]. S.H.K. is funded by a NIH Career Development Award [K23 MH079114]. The funders had no role in study design, data collection and analysis, decision to publish, or preparation of the manuscript.

Competing Interests: The authors have declared that no competing interests exist.

* E-mail: kcmd.sung@samsung.com

Introduction

Women have a lower risk for cardiovascular disease (CVD) than men of equal age [1,2]. This disparity in CVD risk narrows with aging [1,3] and the presence of diabetes [4,5,6]. Both aging and diabetes are associated with increased prevalence of insulin resistance and insulin-resistance related CVD risk factors, including dysglycemia, dyslipidemia, and hypertension [7,8]. These risk factors are present less commonly in young women compared with similarly aged men, despite the increased adiposity that is observed in women [9]. Therefore, one simple explanation for the gender disparity in CVD risk factors has been that young women are more insulin sensitive than young men [10,11]. Another explanation could be that, for a given level of insulin resistance, young women may have fewer CVD risk factors.

To examine these two possibilities, we evaluated the relationship between insulin sensitivity and CVD risk factors, including presence of coronary artery calcium (CAC), in 8682 Korean men and 1829 women aged 30–45 years old. To the best of our knowledge, this study contains the largest population of young adults characterized by measurements of CAC and other CVD risk factors. In addition, this is the first study to evaluate the role of insulin resistance in modulating gender disparities in CAC in young adults.

Methods

Subjects

The study population consisted of patients aged 30–45 years old who participated in a comprehensive health examination in 2010 at Kangbuk Samsung Hospital, College of Medicine, Sungkyunkwan University. Initially, 10596 individuals were identified who met the age criterion. Individuals were excluded for the following reasons: missing weight (n = 10), unclear diabetes status (n = 47), unclear coronary disease history (n = 2), and reported history of coronary artery disease (n = 26). After exclusion, 8682 men and 1829 women were included.

The study was approved by the institutional review board at Kangbuk Samsung Hospital. Informed consent requirement was waived because personal identifying information was not accessed.

Data Collection

The health examination included a medical history, physical examination, fasting blood samples and an imaging study for assessment of CAC. Trained clinical staff measured weight, height and blood pressure. Body mass index (BMI) was calculated by dividing weight (kilogram) by height (meters) squared.

Patients also completed self-administered questionnaires related to their medical and social histories. Individuals were asked to designate their highest level of education. They were classified as having higher education if they had completed 16 or more years of school. Smoking status was reported as never, past, or current. For the current study, only current smoking status was considered. Hypertension was diagnosed if individuals met one of the following criteria: systolic blood pressure ≥ 140 or diastolic blood pressure ≥ 90 mmHg [12], history of hypertension, or use of anti-hypertensive medications. Diabetes was diagnosed when individuals had a fasting glucose concentration ≥ 126 mg/dL [13], a prior history of diabetes, or treatment with anti-diabetic medications. Type of diabetes was not differentiated in this study.

Blood samples were collected after an overnight fast. Fasting plasma glucose and lipid profile were measured using Bayer Reagent Packs on an automated chemistry analyzer (Advia 1650 Autoanalyzer; Bayer Diagnostics, Leverkusen, Germany). Insulin concentration was measured with the electrochemiluminescence immunoassay (Roche Diagnostics, Mannheim, Germany) with a repeatability and precision coefficient of variation of 0.8–1.5% and 2.4–4.9%, respectively. High-sensitivity C-reactive protein levels were measured using a nephelometric assay (BNII nephelometer, Dade Behring, Deerfield, IL). The limit of measurement was 1.67 nmol/L with a sample dilution of 1:20.

To measure CAC, a 64-slice multidetector computed tomography scanner (Lightspeed VCT XTe-64 slice; GE Healthcare, Milwaukee,WI) was used. A standard scanning protocol was employed: 32×0.625-mm section collimation, 400-msec rotation time, 120-kV tube voltage, and 31 mAS (310 mA*0.1 sec) tube current under electrocardiographic-gated dose modulation. The Agatston scoring method was used to quantify CAC [14]. CAC scores were positively skewed with 95% having zero value. Therefore, coronary calcification was defined as the presence of any calcium (CAC>0).

Calculations

The homeostasis model assessment of insulin resistance (HOMA-IR) was calculated using fasting plasma glucose and insulin concentration: [fasting glucose (mmol/L) X fasting insulin (mU/L)/22.5] [15]. Framingham risk score was also calculated using gender-specific equations [16].

Statistical Analysis

Continuous variables were expressed as mean $\pm$ SD or median [interquartile range] if not normally distributed. Continuous variables were compared using the independent t-test. Nonparametric variables were log-transformed prior to analyses. Categorical variables were expressed as percentage and compared using the chi-squared test.

To better understand the role of insulin resistance on gender differences in CVD risk, men and women were classified based on HOMA-IR as insulin sensitive (lowest quartile of HOMA-IR) or insulin resistant (highest quartile of HOMA-IR). Individuals with diabetes were separately evaluated, as previous studies have shown differential CVD risk in individuals with diabetes compared with those without diabetes. Differential CVD risk was especially apparent in women [5,6]. CVD risk factors and CAC>0 were then compared between men and women matched for insulin sensitivity or diabetes status. Crude and adjusted logistic regression analyses also were used to determine the association between CAC>0 and insulin resistance or diabetes. Covariates in the model included traditional risk factors for CVD: age, current smoking status (yes, no), hypertension (yes, no), low density lipoprotein cholesterol (LDL-C) and high density lipoprotein cholesterol (HDL-C) concentration. In a secondary model, BMI was also included as a covariate in addition to the traditional CVD risk factors. $P \leq 0.05$ was considered significant. All statistical analysis was conducted using SPSS (version 16 for Windows; SPSS, Chicago, IL).

Results

Characteristics of the young men and women are shown in Table 1. Despite similar age, most CVD risk factors were more favorable in women. Women also had a lower HOMA-IR and a lower prevalence of diabetes. Given the more favorable CVD risk profile, women had a lower Framingham risk score and a lower prevalence of CAC.

To better understand the role of insulin resistance and diabetes on gender differences, we compared CVD risk factors between men and women with similar states of insulin sensitivity, insulin resistance or overt diabetes (Table 2). Beginning with the insulin sensitive group, more women qualified as being insulin sensitive compared with men (33% vs. 23%, p<0.001). Despite having similar age and HOMA-IR in insulin-sensitive men and women, women had a more favorable CVD risk profile, with the exception of HgA1c, which was slightly higher in women despite having a lower fasting glucose.

In the insulin resistant group, the HOMA-IR was more than three times higher than that in the insulin sensitive group. There were more men than women (27% vs.18%, p<0.001) in the insulin resistant group, but HOMA-IR was similar in men and women. In both men and women, values of CVD risk factors were worse in the insulin resistant group compared with the insulin sensitive group. However, within the insulin resistant group, women again maintained a more favorable CVD risk profile.

The prevalence of diabetes was low in this young cohort. Men and women with diabetes were more similar in age, BMI, and glucose indices compared with men and women in the other groups, although men had a higher prevalence of diabetes compared with women (3.8% vs. 2%, p<0.001). Despite being more comparable in demographic and metabolic variables, women still had significantly lower blood pressure and triglyceride concentration and higher HDL-C concentration than men. As a result, Framingham risk score was also significantly lower in women compared with men.

Figure 1 shows the prevalence of CAC stratified by insulin resistance and diabetes status in men and women. Regardless of the category, the proportion of individuals with CAC was greater in men than women. Nonetheless, in both men and women, the proportion with CAC increased significantly in insulin resistant individuals compared with insulin sensitive individuals. For men, there was a 1.5 fold increase in prevalence of CAC in insulin resistant individuals compared with insulin sensitive individuals (p = 0.001); for women, there was a 2.6 fold increase in prevalence of CAC in insulin resistant individuals compared with insulin sensitive individuals, but this difference did not reach statistical significance (p = 0.07).

Table 1. Characteristics of the study population by gender.

	Men (n = 8682)	Women (n = 1829)	p Value
Age, years	38.8±4.2	38.9±4.1	0.19
BMI, kg/m²	25.0±3.0	22.4±3.4	<0.001
Higher education, no. (%)	6685 (80%)	1106 (62%)	<0.001
Current smoker, no. (%)	2595 (30%)	23 (1%)	<0.001
Diabetes, no. (%)	332 (3.8%)	37 (2%)	<0.001
Blood pressure, mmHg			
Systolic blood pressure	119±11	108±12	<0.001
Diastolic blood pressure	76±9	68±9	<0.001
Lipids, mmol/L			
LDL-C	3.3±0.8	2.9±0.8	<0.001
HDL-C	1.3±0.3	1.6±0.4	<0.001
Triglyceride	1.4	0.9	<0.001
	[1.0,2.0]	[0.7,1.2]	
Glucose, mmol/L	5.3±0.8	5.1±0.7	<0.001
Hemoglobin A1c, %	5.67±0.53	5.64±0.43	0.02
Insulin, pmol/L	38	33	<0.001
	[25,54]	[22,47]	
HOMA-IR	1.26	1.05	<0.001
	[0.83, 1.88]	[0.70, 1.54]	
High-sensitivity C-reactive protein,	5.7	3.8	<0.001
nmol/L	[2.9,10.5]	[2.9,7.6]	
Framingham 10 year risk, %	4	1	<0.001
	[3,6]	[1,2]	
CAC>0, no. %	553 (6.4%)	29 (1.6%)	<0.001
CAC>100, no. %	56 (0.6%)	2 (0.1%)	0.003

Data are mean ± SD or median [interquartile range] unless otherwise noted. LDL-C, low density lipoprotein cholesterol; HDL-C, high density lipoprotein cholesterol; CAC, coronary artery calcium.

For men, the proportion with CAC was highest in those with diabetes. As high as 18% of the men with diabetes had detectable CAC, which was 3.8 fold greater than men classified as insulin sensitive without diabetes (p<0.001). In contrast, for women, the proportion of those with diabetes with CAC was not statistically different from those who were insulin sensitive or insulin resistant with CAC (p≥0.39).

Table 3 shows the association between CAC and insulin resistance and diabetes. For men, HOMA-IR and diabetes were significantly associated with the presence of CAC, even when adjusted for traditional CVD risk factors. When this association was further adjusted for BMI, HOMA-IR and the presence of diabetes remained significantly associated with CAC. For women, insulin resistance, defined as being in the upper quartile of HOMA-IR, was significantly associated with CAC. However, this association was no longer significant when adjusted for CVD risk factors. For women, diabetes was not significantly associated with CAC.

Discussion

Although both young men and women are at low risk for CVD [17], we found a clear gender disparity in risk for CVD in our cohort. Overall, young women had a better CVD risk profile and lower CAC compared with men. Women were also more likely to be insulin sensitive which might have explained the gender disparity in CVD risk. On the other hand, even when matched for level of insulin resistance, young women maintained a lower CVD risk profile and prevalence of CAC. Therefore, women had a better CVD risk profile independent of insulin sensitivity.

To the best of our knowledge, our study contains the largest cohort of young adults (aged 45 and less) characterized by measurement of CAC. In previous studies of young adults with CAC, the population sample has ranged from 630 to 3043 individuals [3,18,19,20]. In those studies, the prevalence of CAC has ranged from 11–31% in men and 4–10% in women, with men having 2–4 times greater prevalence of CAC compared with women [3,18,19,20]. Similarly, we show here that men have approximately a four-fold increase in CAC compared with women. The lower overall prevalence of CAC in our study may reflect differences in race [21,22] and age.

Our study is also unique because it evaluates the role of insulin resistance in mediating the gender disparity in CAC in young adults. Previous studies have suggested that women without diabetes may be more insulin sensitive compared with men [10,23,24], which could drive the development of CAC and CVD over time. However, those studies included individuals with wider age ranges than the current study and did not match men and women based on insulin resistance. In our study, when men and women were specifically matched for level of insulin resistance, women continued to have a more favorable CVD risk profile and

Table 2. Cardiovascular risk factors in young men and women by insulin resistance and diabetes status.

	No Diabetes						Diabetes		
	Insulin Sensitive			Insulin Resistant			–		
	(HOMA-IR <0.79)			(HOMA-IR ≥1.76)					
	Men	Women	p	Men	Women	p	Men	Women	p
	(n = 1950)	(n = 585)	Value	(n = 2213)	(n = 323)	Value	(n = 332)	(n = 37)	Value
HOMA-IR	0.6	0.6	0.09	2.3	2.3	0.96	2.6	2.9	0.82
	[0.4,0.7]	[0.4,0.7]		[2.0,2.9]	[2.0,2.9]		[1.6, 3.9]	[1.4,3.9]	
Age, years	38.9±4.2	38.8±4.3	0.49	38.5±4.1	39.5±3.9	<0.001	41.4±2.7	41.2±3.4	0.61
BMI, kg/m²	23.1±2.4	21.0±2.4	<0.001	27.0±3.0	25.3±4.2	<0.001	26.6±3.3	25.7±5.1	0.16
Higher education, no. (%)	1499	376	<0.001	1676	166	<0.001	225	16	0.003
	(79%)	(66%)		(79%)	(53%)		(69%)	(43%)	
Current smoker, no. (%)	587	10	<0.001	682	5	<0.001	135	0	<0.001
	(30%)	(2%)		(31%)	(2%)		(41%)	(0%)	
Blood pressure, mmHg									
Systolic blood pressure	115±11	105±11	<0.001	122±12	113±12	<0.001	122±13	113±12	<0.001
Diastolic blood pressure	73±8	66±8	<0.001	78±9	71±9	<0.001	78±9	72±8	<0.001
Lipids, mmol/L									
LDL-C	3.2±0.8	2.8±0.8	<0.001	3.4±0.8	3.2±0.8	<0.001	3.2±1.0	3.3±0.9	0.58
HDL-C	1.5±0.3	1.7±0.3	<0.001	1.2±0.2	1.4±0.3	<0.001	1.2±0.3	1.4±0.3	<0.001
Triglyceride	1.0	0.7	<0.001	1.9	1.3	<0.001	1.9	1.6	0.002
	[0.7,1.3]	[0.6,0.9]		[1.4, 2.6]	[1.0,1.8]		[1.3,2.8]	[0.9,2.4]	
Glucose, mmol/L	4.9±0.4	4.7±0.4	<0.001	5.5±0.5	5.4±0.5	<0.001	8.0±2.4	7.9±2.8	0.83
Insulin, pmol/L	18	18	0.35	67	68	0.43	54	60	0.66
	[14,21]	[14,22]		[58,82]	[59,84]		[35,79]	[31,72]	
HgA1c, %	5.5±0.2	5.6±0.3	0.01	5.7±0.3	5.7±0.3	0.12	7.4±1.6	7.3±1.7	0.87
Hs-CRP, nmol/L	3.8	2.9	<0.001	7.6	6.7	0.008	8.6	7.6	0.39
	[2.9,8.6]	[2.9,4.8]		[4.8,14.3]	[3.8, 12]		[4.8,17]	[3.8,14]	
Framingham 10 year risk	3	1	<0.001	5	1	<0.001	7	4	<0.001
(%)	[1,6]	[1,1]		[1,8]	[1,1]		[6,11]	[3,6]	

Data are mean ± SD or median [interquartile range] unless otherwise noted. LDL-C, low density lipoprotein cholesterol; HDL-C, high density lipoprotein cholesterol.

lower CAC compared with men, suggesting that insulin resistance does not solely mediate the risk difference between young women and men.

Insulin resistance was also not an independent predictor of CAC in women as it is in men. In older cohorts, studies have shown that insulin resistance has a significant impact on CAC in both men and women [25,26]. In our study, insulin resistance was not a significant predictor of CAC when adjusted for other CVD risk factors. This finding may relate to the low prevalence of CAC in women in this cohort; a greater number of women may be required to observe a measurable effect of insulin resistance on CAC. Our results also suggest that the immediate clinical impact of insulin resistance may be minimal in young women given their low overall risk. As seen in Table 2, CVD risk factors were extremely favorable in women classified as being insulin sensitive. Although the absolute values of CVD risk factors worsened in women with insulin resistance, they remained normal according to accepted criteria for CVD risk [27]. For example, the median triglyceride concentration in insulin resistant women was 1.3 mmol/L, which is almost twice the value of the triglyceride concentration in insulin sensitive women (0.7 mmol/L). However, a triglyceride concentration of 1.3 mmol/L does not meet the cut-

point for CVD risk of 1.7 mmol/L [27]. In comparison, insulin resistant men also had a near doubling of triglyceride concentration compared with insulin sensitive men. However, in contrast to women, insulin resistant men had a median triglyceride concentration of 1.9 which is above the risk cut-point. Therefore, although insulin resistance was associated with a less favorable CVD risk profile in both women and men, the incremental impact of insulin resistance on CVD risk factors and thus CAC was lower in young women compared with men due to the lower baseline risk in women.

The lack of impact of diabetes status on CAC in women deserves mention. In older cohorts, diabetes has been suggested to increase CAC prevalence and progression in both men and women [28,29]. The impact of diabetes on atherosclerotic risk is not isolated to individuals with type 2 diabetes and has been observed in women with type 1 diabetes [30]. Therefore, factors beyond insulin resistance may account for the higher CVD risk in individuals with diabetes. In our study, men with diabetes had a significant 3.8-fold increase in CAC prevalence compared with insulin sensitive men without diabetes. In contrast, women with diabetes had a 2.5-fold increase in CAC prevalence, but this was not statistically significant. The lack of a statistical effect may relate

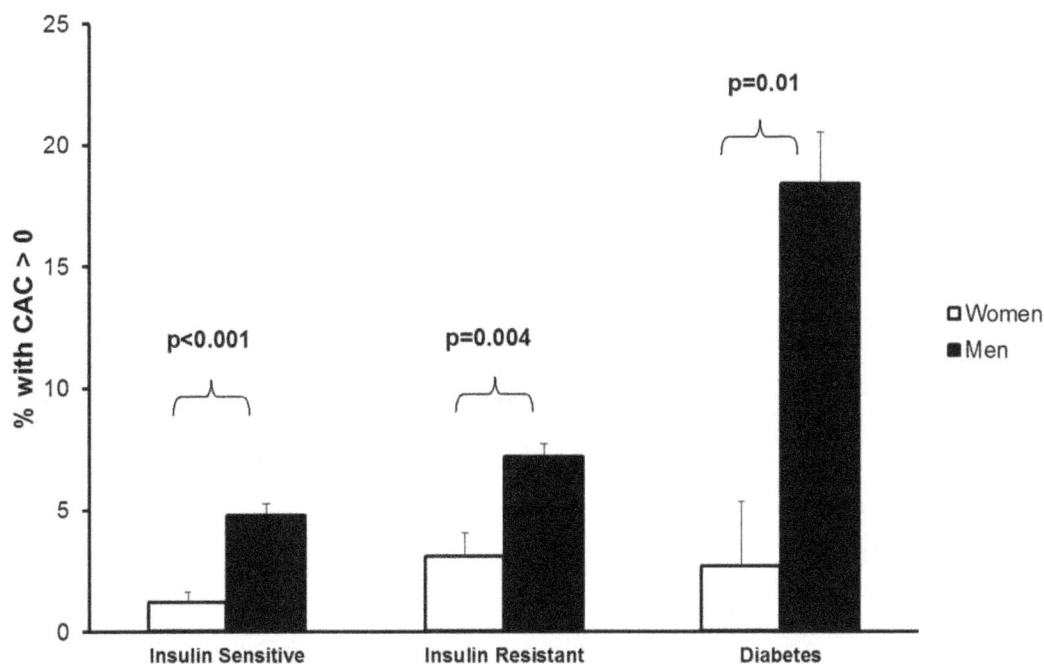

Figure 1. Proportion with detectable CAC by insulin resistance and diabetes status in young women and men. Regardless of the classification, men were significantly more likely to have CAC. P refers to difference in proportion between genders. Error bars represent standard error.

to the small sample of women with diabetes in this cohort. In addition, some of the differential impact of diabetes by gender may relate to the observation that men with diabetes had greater CVD risk factors compared with men without diabetes (e.g., greater smoking). Finally, the immediate impact of diabetes on CVD risk may be low in young women because of their low baseline risk.

Compared with older cohorts, the majority of individuals with CAC had low calcium scores (<100), which were lower than the threshold that were previously shown to predict future coronary artery disease [31,32]. Therefore, the significance of CAC in this young cohort could be debated. On the other hand, it is remarkable that insulin resistance and diabetes were significantly associated with CAC in men, even at this young age. In addition, since baseline presence of CAC is a strong predictor of rate of

progression of coronary calcification [33], individuals with early CAC are likely to be at the highest risk for future coronary artery disease compared with their cohorts without CAC.

There are several limitations of this study. First, we had more men than women. However, our cohort had more women than in previous studies that have measured CAC in young cohorts [3,18,19,20]. Second, men in our cohort smoked more than women, which could partially explain the disparity in CAC prevalence between genders. However, the prevalence of current smokers was similar between insulin sensitive and resistant groups within genders; therefore, smoking status is unlikely to be responsible for the observed differences between insulin sensitive and resistant groups. Third, we did not ascertain a family history of premature coronary artery disease in our cohort, which could

Table 3. Odds ratio (OR) for coronary artery calcium by insulin resistance and diabetes status in young men and women.

	Univariate			Multivariate Model 1*			Multivariate Model 2**		
	OR	95% CI	p	OR	95% CI	p	OR	95% CI	p
Men									
HOMA-IR, log	1.50	1.31, 1.73	<0.001	1.22	1.05, 1.41	0.01	1.19	1.01, 1.41	0.04
Upper Quartile of HOMA-IR (yes, no)	1.57	1.31, 1.87	<0.001	1.25	1.03, 1.52	0.03	1.20	0.97, 1.48	0.09
Diabetes (yes, no)	3.60	2.68, 4.82	<0.001	2.23	1.64, 3.04	<0.001	2.19	1.61, 2.98	<0.001
Women									
HOMA-IR, log	1.48	0.84, 2.62	0.18	0.86	0.47, 1.58	0.63	0.83	0.43, 1.61	0.59
Upper Quartile of HOMA-IR (yes, no)	2.28	1.05, 4.94	0.04	1.22	0.51, 2.89	0.66	1.25	0.49, 3.17	0.65
Diabetes (yes, no)	1.75	0.23, 13.2	0.59	0.79	0.10, 6.31	0.83	0.78	0.10, 6.42	0.82

*Model 1 is adjusted for age, smoking status, hypertension, LDL-C, HDL-C;
**Model 2 is adjusted for variables in Model 1 and BMI.

have increased the risk for CAC in this young adult population. Fourth, we used HOMA-IR as a surrogate measure of insulin resistance. Although significantly associated with direct measures of insulin resistance [34], HOMA-IR might have misclassified insulin sensitivity status. Finally, our study was a cross-sectional study and thus provides a snapshot of the association between insulin resistance and CAC, which is a reflection of calcified plaque burden in coronary arteries. Therefore, we cannot discount the impact of insulin resistance on future CVD in women and on noncalcified atherosclerosis.

In conclusion, young women have a lower risk for CVD and a lower CAC prevalence compared with men. This favorable CVD risk profile in women appears to occur regardless of insulin sensitivity. In addition, unlike men, insulin resistance was not a predictor of CAC in women. Therefore, insulin resistance has less impact on CVD risk and CAC in young women compared with men, and insulin resistance alone does not explain the gender disparity in CVD risk that is observed at an early age.

Acknowledgments

We would like to acknowledge the fine efforts of the members of the health-screening group at Kangbuk Samsung Hospital, Seoul, Republic of Korea.

Author Contributions

Performed the experiments: KCS HJK BSK. Analyzed the data: SHK. Contributed reagents/materials/analysis tools: JHC HCG SHC. Wrote the paper: KCS SHK.

References

1. Ho JE, Paultre F, Mosca L (2005) The gender gap in coronary heart disease mortality: is there a difference between blacks and whites? Journal of women's health 14: 117–127.
2. Kalin MF, Zumoff B (1990) Sex hormones and coronary disease: a review of the clinical studies. Steroids 55: 330–352.
3. Hoffmann U, Massaro JM, Fox CS, Manders E, O'Donnell CJ (2008) Defining normal distributions of coronary artery calcium in women and men (from the Framingham Heart Study). The American journal of cardiology 102: 1136–1141, 1141 e1131.
4. Larsson CA, Gullberg B, Merlo J, Rastam L, Lindblad U (2005) Female advantage in AMI mortality is reversed in patients with type 2 diabetes in the Skaraborg Project. Diabetes care 28: 2246–2248.
5. Huxley R, Barzi F, Woodward M (2006) Excess risk of fatal coronary heart disease associated with diabetes in men and women: meta-analysis of 37 prospective cohort studies. BMJ 332: 73–78.
6. Lee WL, Cheung AM, Cape D, Zinman B (2000) Impact of diabetes on coronary artery disease in women and men: a meta-analysis of prospective studies. Diabetes care 23: 962–968.
7. Rodriguez A, Muller DC, Metter EJ, Maggio M, Harman SM, et al. (2007) Aging, androgens, and the metabolic syndrome in a longitudinal study of aging. The Journal of clinical endocrinology and metabolism 92: 3568–3572.
8. Chen K, Lindsey JB, Khera A, De Lemos JA, Ayers CR, et al. (2008) Independent associations between metabolic syndrome, diabetes mellitus and atherosclerosis: observations from the Dallas Heart Study. Diabetes & vascular disease research: official journal of the International Society of Diabetes and Vascular Disease 5: 96–101.
9. Ervin RB (2009) Prevalence of metabolic syndrome among adults 20 years of age and over, by sex, age, race and ethnicity, and body mass index: United States, 2003–2006. National health statistics reports: 1–7.
10. Moran A, Jacobs DR Jr, Steinberger J, Steffen LM, Pankow JS, et al. (2008) Changes in insulin resistance and cardiovascular risk during adolescence: establishment of differential risk in males and females. Circulation 117: 2361–2368.
11. Regitz-Zagrosek V, Lehmkuhl E, Weickert MO (2006) Gender differences in the metabolic syndrome and their role for cardiovascular disease. Clinical research in cardiology: official journal of the German Cardiac Society 95: 136–147.
12. Chobanian AV, Bakris GL, Black HR, Cushman WC, Green LA, et al. (2003) The Seventh Report of the Joint National Committee on Prevention, Detection, Evaluation, and Treatment of High Blood Pressure: the JNC 7 report. JAMA: the journal of the American Medical Association 289: 2560–2572.
13. American Diabetes Association (2011) Diagnosis and classification of diabetes mellitus. Diabetes care 34 Suppl 1: S62–69.
14. Agatston AS, Janowitz WR, Hildner FJ, Zusmer NR, Viamonte M Jr, et al. (1990) Quantification of coronary artery calcium using ultrafast computed tomography. Journal of the American College of Cardiology 15: 827–832.
15. Matthews DR, Hosker JP, Rudenski AS, Naylor BA, Treacher DF, et al. (1985) Homeostasis model assessment: insulin resistance and beta-cell function from fasting plasma glucose and insulin concentrations in man. Diabetologia 28: 412–419.
16. Wilson PW, D'Agostino RB, Levy D, Belanger AM, Silbershatz H, et al. (1998) Prediction of coronary heart disease using risk factor categories. Circulation 97: 1837–1847.
17. Cavanaugh-Hussey MW, Berry JD, Lloyd-Jones DM (2008) Who exceeds ATP-III risk thresholds? Systematic examination of the effect of varying age and risk factor levels in the ATP-III risk assessment tool. Preventive medicine 47. 619–623.
18. Loria CM, Liu K, Lewis CE, Hulley SB, Sidney S, et al. (2007) Early adult risk factor levels and subsequent coronary artery calcification: the CARDIA Study. Journal of the American College of Cardiology 49: 2013–2020.
19. Mahoney LT, Burns TL, Stanford W, Thompson BH, Witt JD, et al. (1996) Coronary risk factors measured in childhood and young adult life are associated with coronary artery calcification in young adults: the Muscatine Study. Journal of the American College of Cardiology 27: 277–284.
20. Taylor AJ, Feuerstein I, Wong H, Barko W, Brazaitis M, et al. (2001) Do conventional risk factors predict subclinical coronary artery disease? Results from the Prospective Army Coronary Calcium Project. American heart journal 141: 463–468.
21. Sekikawa A, Ueshima H, Zaky WR, Kadowaki T, Edmundowicz D, et al. (2005) Much lower prevalence of coronary calcium detected by electron-beam computed tomography among men aged 40–49 in Japan than in the US, despite a less favorable profile of major risk factors. International journal of epidemiology 34: 173–179.
22. Newman AB, Naydeck BL, Whittle J, Sutton-Tyrrell K, Edmundowicz D, et al. (2002) Racial differences in coronary artery calcification in older adults. Arteriosclerosis, thrombosis, and vascular biology 22: 424–430.
23. Wannamethee SG, Papacosta O, Lawlor DA, Whincup PH, Lowe GD, et al. (2011) Do women exhibit greater differences in established and novel risk factors between diabetes and non-diabetes than men? The British Regional Heart Study and British Women's Heart Health Study. Diabetologia.
24. Jeppesen J, Hansen TW, Rasmussen S, Ibsen H, Torp-Pedersen C, et al. (2007) Insulin resistance, the metabolic syndrome, and risk of incident cardiovascular disease: a population-based study. Journal of the American College of Cardiology 49: 2112–2119.
25. Reilly MP, Wolfe ML, Rhodes T, Girman C, Mehta N, et al. (2004) Measures of insulin resistance add incremental value to the clinical diagnosis of metabolic syndrome in association with coronary atherosclerosis. Circulation 110: 803–809.
26. Arad Y, Newstein D, Cadet F, Roth M, Guerci AD (2001) Association of multiple risk factors and insulin resistance with increased prevalence of asymptomatic coronary artery disease by an electron-beam computed tomographic study. Arteriosclerosis, thrombosis, and vascular biology 21: 2051–2058.
27. Grundy SM, Cleeman JI, Daniels SR, Donato KA, Eckel RH, et al. (2005) Diagnosis and management of the metabolic syndrome: an American Heart Association/National Heart, Lung, and Blood Institute Scientific Statement. Circulation 112: 2735–2752.
28. Wong ND, Sciammarella MG, Polk D, Gallagher A, Miranda-Peats L, et al. (2003) The metabolic syndrome, diabetes, and subclinical atherosclerosis assessed by coronary calcium. Journal of the American College of Cardiology 41: 1547–1553.
29. Lee KK, Fortmann SP, Fair JM, Iribarren C, Rubin GD, et al. (2009) Insulin resistance independently predicts the progression of coronary artery calcification. American heart journal 157: 939–945.
30. Colhoun HM, Rubens MB, Underwood SR, Fuller JH (2000) The effect of type 1 diabetes mellitus on the gender difference in coronary artery calcification. Journal of the American College of Cardiology 36: 2160–2167.
31. Arad Y, Goodman KJ, Roth M, Newstein D, Guerci AD (2005) Coronary calcification, coronary disease risk factors, C-reactive protein, and atherosclerotic cardiovascular disease events: the St. Francis Heart Study. Journal of the American College of Cardiology 46: 158–165.
32. Polonsky TS, McClelland RL, Jorgensen NW, Bild DE, Burke GL, et al. (2010) Coronary artery calcium score and risk classification for coronary heart disease prediction. JAMA: the journal of the American Medical Association 303: 1610–1616.
33. Yoon HC, Emerick AM, Hill JA, Gjertson DW, Goldin JG (2002) Calcium begets calcium: progression of coronary artery calcification in asymptomatic subjects. Radiology 224: 236–241.
34. Yeni-Komshian H, Carantoni M, Abbasi F, Reaven GM (2000) Relationship between several surrogate estimates of insulin resistance and quantification of insulin-mediated glucose disposal in 490 healthy nondiabetic volunteers. Diabetes Care 23: 171–175.

7

The Relationship between BMI and Glycated Albumin to Glycated Hemoglobin (GA/A1c) Ratio According to Glucose Tolerance Status

Ji Hye Huh[1,9], Kwang Joon Kim[2,9], Byung-Wan Lee[1]*, Dong Wook Kim[3], Eun Seok Kang[1], Bong Soo Cha[1], Hyun Chul Lee[1]

1 Division of Endocrinology and Metabolism, Department of Internal Medicine, Yonsei University College of Medicine, Seoul, Korea, 2 Severance Executive Healthcare Clinic, Severance Hospital, Seoul, Korea, 3 Division of Medical Statistics, Yonsei University College of Medicine, Seoul, Korea

Abstract

Glycated albumin to glycated hemoglobin (GA/A1c) ratio is known to be inversely related with body mass index (BMI) and insulin secretory capacity. However, the reasons for this association remain unknown. We aimed to investigate whether BMI directly or indirectly influences GA/A1c by exerting effects on insulin secretion or resistance and to confirm whether these associations differ according to glucose tolerance status. We analyzed a total of 807 subjects [242 drug-naïve type 2 diabetes (T2D), 378 prediabetes, and 187 normal glucose tolerance (NGT)]. To assess the direct and indirect effects of BMI on GA/A1c ratio, structural equation modeling (SEM) was performed. GA/A1c ratio was set as a dependent variable, BMI was used as the independent variable, and homeostasis model assessment-pancreatic beta-cell function (HOMA-β), homeostasis model assessment-insulin resistance (HOMA-IR), glucose level were used as mediator variables. The estimates of a direct effect of BMI on GA/A1c to be the strongest in NGT and weakest in T2D (−0.375 in NGT, −0.244 in prediabetes, and −0.189 in T2D). Conversely, the indirect effect of BMI on GA/A1c exerted through HOMA-β and HOMA-IR was not statistically significant in NGT group, but significant in prediabetes and T2D groups (0.089 in prediabetes, −0.003 in T2D). It was found that HOMA-β or HOMA-IR indirectly influences GA/A1c in T2D and prediabetes group through affecting fasting and postprandial glucose level. The relationship between GA/A1c and BMI is due to the direct effect of BMI on GA/A1c in NGT group, while in T2D and prediabetes groups, this association is mostly a result of BMI influencing blood glucose through insulin resistance or secretion.

Editor: Marta Letizia Hribal, University of Catanzaro Magna Graecia, Italy

Funding: The authors have no support or funding to report.

Competing Interests: The authors have declared that no competing interests exist.

* E-mail: bwanlee@yuhs.ac

9 These authors contributed equally to this work and are co-first authors.

Introduction

Until now, the gold standard parameter for monitoring glycemic excursion has been glycated hemoglobin (A1c). However, A1c does not provide accurate information following earlier changes in glycemic control after drug intervention or in various conditions affecting the lifespan of red blood cells [1–3]. Although glycated albumin (GA), a useful glycemic index for intermediate periods over 2–4 weeks, may be viewed as an adjunct to A1c, it is gaining popularities during the transition between medications for intensive treatment or for diabetes management at a monthly level [4–6]. In addition, serum GA has been shown to be a superior indicator for plasma glucose variability to A1c [7].

Recently, not only GA but also the ratio of GA to A1c (GA/A1c) is expected to be a new glucose control marker [8]. However, notwithstanding the pathologic condition affecting albumin metabolism such as thyroid dysfunction, nephrotic syndrome, or liver cirrhosis [4], the physiologic variables such as age or body mass index (BMI) [9] make the GA/A1c ratio a little unpredictable in clinical practice. Among them, several studies have suggested a negative correlation between BMI and serum GA in non-diabetic children, as well as in adult diabetic patients [9–11]. However, conflicting result was observed in Kyushu and Okinawa Population Study, which reported no significant association between GA and BMI in type 2 diabetic subjects [12]. In spite of the discordant results on the association between GA/A1c ratio and BMI in especially diabetic patients, there has been no study in the literature to date focusing on the relationship between GA/A1c ratio and BMI according to glucose tolerance status. Moreover, we have demonstrated that insulin secretory functions, such as homeostasis model assessment-pancreatic beta-cell function (HOMA-β) and insulinogenic index, but not insulin resistance, are negatively associated with GA/A1c ratio in patients with type 2 diabetes (T2D) [13]. Increase in BMI generally leads to not only insulin resistance but also compensatory elevated insulin secretion, and insulin secretion is inversely associated with GA/A1c; therefore, a decrease in GA/A1c is expected following elevated BMI. In other words, it could be hypothesized that the influence of BMI on GA/A1c level might be mediated through elevated insulin secretion. However, there are few studies reporting the relationship between GA/A1c ratio and BMI in association with insulin secretory function, insulin resistance, and serum glucose level. Therefore, this study aimed to observe the association between BMI, insulin secretion, resistance, blood glucose, and GA/A1c according to glucose tolerance; furthermore, it employed structural equation modeling (SEM), which can differentiate direct and indirect effects, to identify whether the characteristics of aforementioned associations are different among subjects with normal glucose tolerance, prediabetes, and T2D.

Materials and Methods

Ethics Statement

The study was carried out according to the Declaration of Helsinki and the International Conference on Harmonization Good Clinical Practice Principles. The protocol was approved by the independent institutional review board at Yonsei University College of Medicine. All enrolled subjects provided written informed consent.

Study population and design

In this clinical, cross-sectional study, we analyzed patients who satisfied certain criteria based on their medical records. We included patients enrolled in the diabetes registry of Severance Diabetes Center between June 2008 and February 2012; only first-time visitors to the center and subjects who had been tested for GA, HbA1c, plasma glucose and C-peptide were included. Exclusion criteria included a history of use of hypoglycemic or lipid-lowering agents, severe liver or kidney disease (chronic kidney disease $\geq$ stage 3), active thyroid disorders, pregnancy, steroid therapy, heavy alcohol usage, Type 1 diabetic patients (C-peptide <0.5 ng/mL) and malignant disease.

To investigate the relationship between BMI and GA/A1c ratio stratified by degree of insulin secretory function and insulin resistance, patients were classified into 3 groups based on the American Diabetes Association 2011 guidelines: T2D (A1c$\geq$6.5%), increased risk for diabetes (A1c = 5.7–6.4%, described as prediabetes hereon), and normal glucose tolerance (NGT) (A1c$\leq$5.6%) [3,14]. Anthropometric measurements were taken with patients wearing light clothing and no shoes. Waist circumference was measured with the tape measure placed horizontally at the level of the umbilicus while the participant gently exhaled. BMI was calculated as weight in kilograms divided by the square of height in meters. The study protocol was approved by the Ethics Committee of Yonsei University College of Medicine.

Laboratory measurements

Blood samples were collected at 0 and 90 mins (postprandial) for glucose, insulin and C-peptide analyses. Plasma glucose levels were measured using the glucose oxidase method (Hitachi 747 automatic analyzer, Hitachi Instruments Service, Tokyo, Japan). Serum GA levels were measured using the enzymatic method and a Hitachi 7699 P module autoanalyzer (Hitachi Instruments Service). A1c levels were measured by high-performance liquid chromatography using a Variant II Turbo (Bio-Rad Laboratories, Hercules, CA, USA). Serum insulin and C-peptide levels were measured in duplicate by immunoradiometric assay (Beckman Coulter, Fullerton, CA, USA).

Basal β-cell function and insulin resistance were assessed by HOMA-β and insulin resistance was assessed by homeostasis model assessment-insulin resistance (HOMA-IR).

$$HOMA\text{-}\beta = \frac{fasting\ insulin(\mu IU/mL) \times 20}{0.055551 \times fasting\ glucose(mg/dL) - 3.5}$$

$$HOMA\text{-}IR = \frac{fasting\ insulin(\mu IU/mL) \times 20}{0.055551 \times fasting\ glucose(mg/dL) - 3.5}$$

Statistical analyses

All continuous variables are shown as mean $\pm$ standard deviation. Analysis of variance (ANOVA) followed by post hoc analysis using Bonferroni correction was used to compare variables across multiple groups. The relationships between clinical and laboratory variables were evaluated using univariate Pearson's correlation analysis. To correct for skewed distributions, HOMA-β, HOMA-IR were logarithmically transformed. Then SEM analyses were performed to assess the direct and indirect effects of between variables. Values of variables used in SEM were standardized due to the wide ranges encountered for these variables. The standardization method for a dataset of size k with mean value μ and variance σ^2 is as follows:

$$X_1, X_2, \cdots, X_K \sim (\mu, \sigma^2)$$

$$Z_1 = \frac{X_i - \mu}{\sigma}, i = 1, 2, \cdots, K.$$

Z_i is a standardized value based on the mean and standard deviation.

To assess the direct effect of BMI on GA/A1c ratio independent of the indirect effect of BMI on GA/A1c ratio mediated by other variables, a statistical analysis was performed using SEM and path diagram analysis by IBM® SPSS® Amos (Figure S1) [15]. Briefly, GA/A1c ratio was set as a dependent variable, and BMI was set as an independent variable. HOMA-β, HOMA-IR, fasting glucose and postprandial glucose were used as mediator variables which are associated with each other and with GA/A1c ratio, respectively. The purpose of this analysis was to observe whether the independent variables—in this case, BMI—have direct or indirect effects (through mediator variables) on GA/A1c ratio, the dependent variable. In other words, although one independent variable may seem to directly influence GA/A1c ratio, a path diagram analysis may reveal that this relationship is in fact due to another independent variable that acts as a mediator between the first independent variable and GA/A1c ratio. For this study, we proposed the following path diagrams (Figure 1) which was examined for each group. P values less than 0.05 were considered statistically significant. All data were analyzed using PASW Statistics version 18 (SPSS Inc, Chicago, IL, USA).

Results

Baseline Characteristics of Patients

A total of 807 patients (242 with T2D, 378 with prediabetes, and 187 with NGT) satisfied the inclusion criteria of this study. Table 1 summarizes the demographic and clinical characteristics of the patients. The mean age of all patients was 55.26 years, and the mean GA/A1c ratio was 2.20±0.41. BMI, waist-hip ratio, and body weight were significantly higher in the T2D group, followed by the prediabetes and the NGT groups. GA and GA/A1c ratio were significantly higher in the T2D group than other two groups. HOMA-β (%) was significantly higher ($P<0.001$) in the prediabetes group (80.55±54.17), followed by the NGT (76.96±54.10)

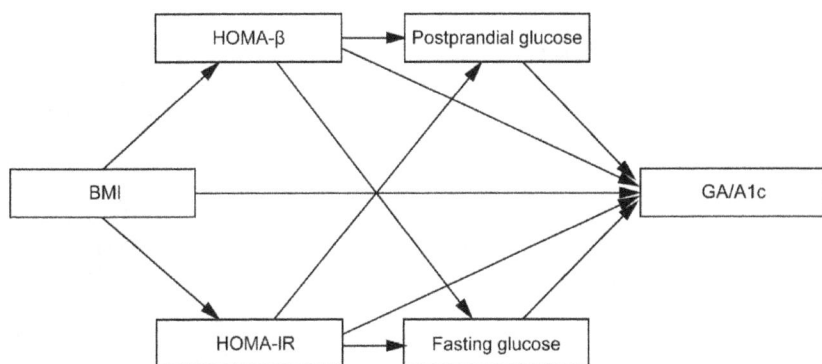

Figure 1. Structural equation models for the GA/A1c ratio.

Table 1. Baseline characteristics.

	Total N = 807	NGT n = 187	Prediabetes n = 378	Diabetes n = 242	P value
Sex: M/F (male %)	432/375 (53.5%)	93/94 (49.7%)	198/180 (52.4%)	141/101 (58.3%)	0.177
Age (year)	55.26±11.51	49.02±11.92[†‡]	58.19±9.84[†#]	55.53±11.76[‡#]	<0.001
Height (cm)	165.04±8.52	166.05±8.58	164.80±8.15	164.62±9.01	0.171
Weight (Kg)	67.19±12.48	63.85±11.92[†‡]	67.09±12.31[†#]	69.93±12.55[‡#]	<0.001
BMI (kg/m2)	24.58±3.45	23.05±2.96[†‡]	24.60±3.40[†#]	25.75±3.41[‡#]	<0.001
WHR	0.89±0.06	0.86±0.08[†‡]	0.89±0.05[†#]	0.91±0.05[‡#]	<0.001
SBP (mmHg)	126.14±16.68	119.16±13.91[†‡]	125.63±15.92[†#]	132.29±17.53[‡#]	<0.001
DBP (mmHg)	78.41±11.15	76.44±10.23[‡]	78.21±11.06	80.21±11.72[‡]	0.002
HbA1c (%)	6.55±1.52	5.47±0.16[†‡]	5.98±0.22[†#]	8.27±1.81[‡#]	<0.001
GA (%)	14.76±6.28	11.27±1.48[†‡]	12.34±1.77[†#]	21.10±8.07[‡#]	<0.001
GA/A1c	2.20±0.41	2.06±0.28[‡]	2.06±0.27[#]	2.52±0.52[‡#]	<0.001
Glucose at 0 min (mg/dL)	111.57±36.93	88.98±8.14[†‡]	99.30±11.27[†#]	147.34±49.25[‡#]	<0.001
Glucose at 90 min (mg/dL)	164.32±78.34	112.79±33.61[†‡]	135.21±44.55[†#]	241.04±81.96[‡#]	<0.001
C-peptide at 0 min (μg/L)	2.26±1.12	1.83±0.92[†‡]	2.24±1.08[†#]	2.56±1.19[‡#]	<0.001
C-peptide at 90 min (μg/L)	7.15±3.66	6.63±4.08[†]	7.75±3.77[†#]	6.52±3.12[#]	<0.001
Insulin at 0 min (μIU/mL)	7.98±5.91	5.55±3.60[†‡]	7.71±5.13[†#]	9.83±7.39[‡#]	<0.001
Insulin at 90 min (μIU/mL)	50.63±46.97	35.28±40.39[†‡]	52.56±50.24[†]	55.41±43.47[‡]	<0.001
HOMA-β (%)	71.49±55.85	76.96±54.10[‡]	80.55±54.17[#]	53.86±55.61[‡#]	<0.001
HOMA-IR	2.34±2.20	1.27±0.84[†‡]	1.93±1.40[†#]	3.61±3.04[‡#]	<0.001
Cholesterol (mg/dL)	188.83±38.92	186.17±35.10	188.90±38.84	190.74±41.74	0.488
LDL (mg/dL)	110.23±35.19	109.82±30.74	112.68±34.94	106.69±38.47	0.117
HDL (mg/dL)	51.26±19.27	52.18±13.67	50.82±17.39	51.23±25.00	0.735
Fasting TG (mg/dL)	131.32±98.59	105.75±69.75[‡]	117.80±57.77[#]	172.37±145.27[‡#]	<0.001
Postprandial TG (mg/dL)	156.86±117.63	104.43±84.12[‡]	124.45±63.15[#]	206.91±147.97[‡#]	<0.001
Hb (g/dL)	14.21±1.49	14.13±1.42	14.10±1.49[#]	14.47±1.54[#]	0.01
Protein (g/dL)	6.95±0.42	6.80±0.37[†‡]	6.92±0.41[†#]	7.11±0.43[‡#]	<0.001
Albumin (g/dL)	4.37±0.33	4.30±0.32[‡]	4.33±0.29[#]	4.49±0.35[‡#]	<0.001
Creatinine (mg/dL)	0.84±0.31	0.77±0.17[†‡]	0.86±0.40[†]	0.87±0.22[‡]	0.003

Data presented as n (%) or mean ± standard deviation.
[†]: The difference between NGT and Prediabetes : p<0.05 after Bonferroni correction.
[‡]: The difference between NGT and Diabetes : p<0.05 after Bonferroni correction.
[#]: The difference between Prediabetes and Diabetes : p<0.05 after Bonferroni correction.
Abbreviations: NGT, normal glucose tolerance; BMI, body mass index; WHR, waist-to-hip ratio; SBP, systolic blood pressure; DBP, diastolic blood pressure; HbA1c, glycated hemoglobin; GA, glycated albumin; GA/A1c, ratio of glycated albumin to glycated hemoglobin; HOMA-β, homeostasis model assessment- pancreatic beta-cell function; HOMA-IR, homeostatsis model assessment-insulin resistance; LDL, low-density lipoprotein; HDL, high-density lipoprotein; TG, triglyceride.

Table 2. Correlations between GA/A1c ratio and other variables.

| Variables | GA/A1c | | |
	NGT (*n*=187)	Prediabetes (*n*=378)	Diabetes (*n*=242)
Age	NS	0.151(0.003)	NS
WHR	NS	−0.178(0.001)	NS
BMI	−0.383(<0.001)	−0.221(<0.001)	−0.181(0.005)
A1c	−0.183(0.015)	0.188(<0.001)	0.423(<0.001)
Glycated albumin	0.971 (<0.001)	0.963 (<0.001)	0.807(<0.001)
Glucose at 0 min	NS	0.293(<0.001)	0.459(<0.001)
Glucose at 90 min	NS	0.258(<0.001)	0.463(<0.001)
LN HOMA-β	NS	−0.342 (<0.001)	−0.332(<0.001)
LN HOMA-IR	NS	−0.138 (0.007)	NS

Values are Pearson correlation coefficients between variables and GA/A1c ratio. Abbreviations: NGT, normal glucose tolerance; BMI, body mass index; WHR, waist-to-hip ratio; A1c, hemoglobin A1c; GA/A1c, ratio of glycated albumin to glycated hemoglobin; LN HOMA-β, log transformed homeostasis model assessment-pancreatic beta-cell function; LN HOMA-IR, log transformed homeostatis model assessment-insulin resistance; NS, not significant.

and the T2D (53.86±55.61) groups. HOMA-IR was significantly higher ($P<0.001$) in the T2D group (3.61±3.04), followed by the prediabetes (1.93±1.40) and the NGT (1.27±0.84) groups.

Correlation of GA/A1c Ratio and BMI in Diabetic, Prediabetic, and NGT Patients

To assess the correlation between GA/A1c ratio and BMI according to glucose tolerance status, we performed Pearson correlation analysis (Table 2). The negative association between GA/A1c ratio and BMI was the most prominent in the NGT group. (NGT: R = −0.383, $P<0.001$; prediabetes: R = −0.221, $P<0.01$; T2D: R = −0.181, $P<0.001$). There was a significant positive correlation between fasting, postprandial glucose and GA/A1c ratio in the prediabetes and the T2D groups. Moreover, a negative relationship between GA/A1c ratio and HOMA-β was significant in the T2D group and the prediabetes groups but not in the NGT group (prediabetes: R = −0.342, $P<0.001$; and T2D: R = −0.322, $P<0.001$). The relationship between insulin resistance and GA/A1c ratio was statistically significant only in the prediabetes groups (R = −0.138, $P=0.007$).

Decomposition of Direct and Indirect Effect of BMI on GA/A1c Ratio

SEM was employed to separately analyze the direct effects of BMI on GA/A1c ratio (Figure 1). Figure 2 depicts the SEM for GA/A1c ratio in each glucose tolerance group. Using this model, the estimates of a direct effect of BMI on GA/A1c were −0.375 ($P<0.001$) in the NGT group, −0.244 ($P<0.001$) in the prediabetes group, and −0.189 ($P=0.002$) in the T2D group. In the NGT group, there was no significant indirect effect of BMI on GA/A1c ratio. In contrast, in prediabetes and T2D group, the indirect effects of BMI on GA/A1c ratio which is mediated by HOMA-β→fasting glucose or postprandial glucose and HOMA-IR→fasting glucose or postprandial glucose were significant. However, in the prediabetes and the T2D groups, these indirect effects of BMI on GA/A1c ratio were relatively weak (0.089 in the

prediabetes group; −0.003 in the T2D group). In each group, the variables which were significantly associated with GA/A1c ratio was only BMI in the NGT group (estimate of effect: −0.375, $P<0.001$), while fasting glucose, postprandial glucose, and BMI in the prediabetes and T2D groups. In addition, in prediabetes and T2D group, the influence of fasting and prostprandial glucose parameters on GA/A1c was greater than that of BMI. (BMI→GA/A1c: −0.244, Postprandial glucose→ GA/A1c: 0.173, Fasting glucose→ GA/A1c: 0.499 in prediabtes group; BMI→GA/A1c: −0.189, Postprandial glucose→ GA/A1c: 0.300, Fasting glucose→ GA/A1c: 0.220 in T2D group). The degree of effect of BMI on HOMA-β was the most prominent in NGT, followed by the prediabetes and the T2D groups, in that order. However, a direct effect of HOMA-β or HOMA-IR on GA/A1c was not observed in any groups.

Discussion

The present study represents the first of its kind to investigate the relation between BMI and GA/A1c according to glucose tolerance status. Our results indicated that inverse association between BMI and GA/A1c ratio was observed in all glucose tolerance status, which was strongest in NGT group, followed by the prediabetes and the T2D groups, in that order. Furthermore, using SEM, we found that the variables influencing GA/A1c ratio was different according to glucose tolerance status; only BMI in the NGT group, BMI, postprandial glucose and fasting glucose in the prediabetes and T2D groups. The results suggested that although it is true that BMI is inversely related to GA/A1c ratio, the ratio is under greater influence by glucose parameters than by BMI in prediabetes or T2D; therefore, this suggests that while GA/A1c cannot be an accurate index of glycemic control status in NGT, it may be a significant index in prediabetes or diabetes regardless of BMI.

Previous studies have indicated that obesity is negatively associated with GA and GA/A1c ratio. However, the underlying mechanisms of this relationship remain to be answered, and they were not fully evaluated in subjects with prediabetes or NGT. Koga et al. demonstrated that obesity and its related chronic inflammation are involved in lower serum GA levels [16]. On the other hand, other studies have suggested that the negative association of obesity with GA is due to abnormal albumin concentrations in obese subjects [17]. However, Nishimura et al indicated that obese children had higher serum albumin than non-obese children, and Koga et al. found no correlation between BMI and albumin concentrations [9,16]. Based on these unclear answers for the mechanism of the association between BMI and GA/A1c ratio, we tried to explain this mechanism with respect to BMI, a representative parameter for obesity, and insulin secretory function. In accordance with the increase of BMI, insulin secretory function might be also increased to overcome the insulin resistance. However, the degree of increase of insulin secretory function required to overcome insulin resistance would differ according to various glucose tolerance status. Therefore, the effect of BMI on GA/A1c, which is negatively associated with insulin secretory function [18], would also differ according to glucose tolerance status. Based on these findings, we hypothesized that the magnitude of negative influence of BMI on GA/A1c ratio might be dependent on gluco-insulin homeostasis, especially on insulin secretory function compensating for insulin resistance. Therefore, we investigated the association between BMI and GA/A1c ratio according to glucose tolerance status. To address these questions, we recruited drug-naive subjects with NGT, prediabetes, and T2D. The present study represents the first of its kind to

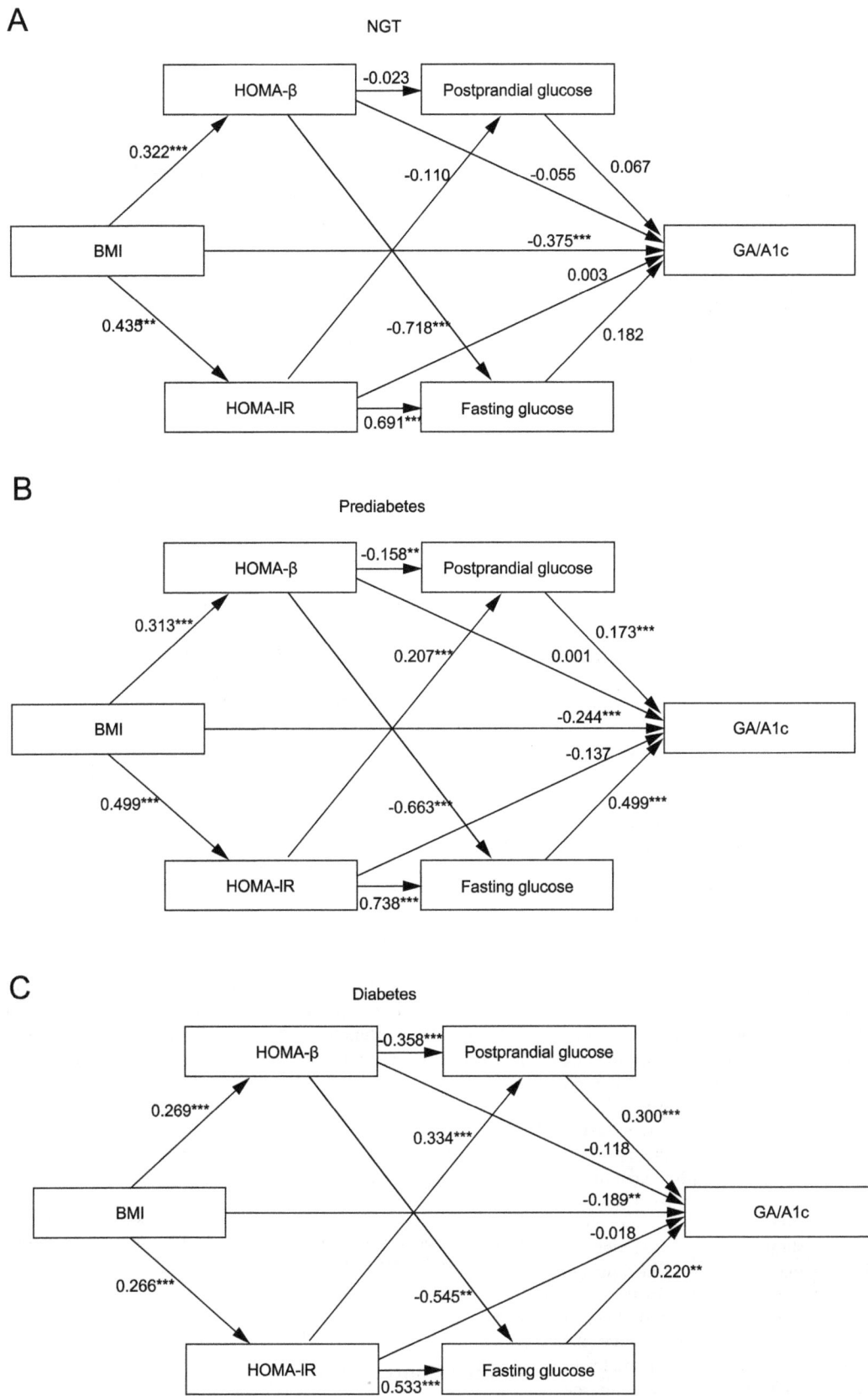

Figure 2. Structural equation models for the GA/A1c ratio in NGT (A), prediabetes (B) and diabetes group (C). *$P<0.05$; **$P<0.01$;*** $P<0.001$.

investigate the relation between BMI and GA/A1c ratio according to glucose tolerance status. The results demonstrated four main findings with respect to correlations with the GA/A1c ratio.

First, the inverse association between BMI and GA/A1c ratio was observed in all glucose tolerance status, which was strongest in NGT group, followed by the prediabetes and the T2D groups. The reason for the different degrees of effect of BMI on GA/A1c ratio by glucose tolerance status groups may be a greater influence of BMI on factors other than GA/A1c ratio in the prediabetes and the T2D groups. A recent, large population-based study [12] showed that BMI had no effect on GA levels in subject with T2D, even when including patients with high BMI. This unexpected result suggests that BMI exerts influence on other factors besides GA; consequently, the association between BMI and GA may seem to have been weakened especially in subjects with T2D. Second, using SEM analysis, we found that HOMA-β does not significantly affect GA/A1c. Similar to previous studies [14], a simple correlation analysis found a negative correlation between HOMA-β and GA/A1c ratio. However, when we analyzed SEM which excluded other factors that influences GA/A1c ratio, we observed that HOMA- β does not directly affect GA/A1c ratio. These findings explain that the negative association between HOMA-β and GA/A1c ratio shown in previous studies [13,14] may be attributed to the indirect effect of the glucose variability of fasting and postprandial glucose mainly caused by the decline of insulin secretory function [19] Third, the variables influencing GA/A1c ratio were different according to glucose tolerance status groups. In the NGT group, only BMI significantly influenced GA/A1c ratio, whereas in the prediabetes and the T2D groups, fasting glucose and postprandial glucose also influenced GA/A1c ratio. The absence of influence of glucose level in the NGT group may be explained by the following. The pathophysiology of T2D is characterized by insulin resistance and impaired compensatory insulin secretion. Therefore, in T2D, insulin secretion is unable to quickly compensate for insulin resistance, leading to increased postprandial sugar levels and greater elevation of GA (known to be an index reflecting postprandial glycemic status) compared to A1c. However, in patients with NGT with intact insulin secretory function, excessive postprandial elevation of blood glucose is not observed, and a disproportionate increase of GA compared to A1c does not occur, resulting in loss of association between GA/A1c ratio and insulin secretory function. Furthermore, we have confirmed that only BMI held a significant influence over GA/A1c ratio in NGT while in prediabetes and T2D, both glucose parameters and BMI significantly inflenced GA/A1c ratio, with the former providing a greater influence. These findings may be the basis of explaining the clearer effect of BMI on GA/A1c ratio in NGT group. Fourth, the effect of HOMA-β on fasting glucose was the most prominent in the NGT group, followed by the prediabetes group and the T2D groups. Also, the effect of HOMA-β on postprandial glucose was the most prominent in the T2D group, followed by the prediabetes and the NGT groups. This result is consistent with the previous study because early-phase insulin secretion and glucose-stimulated insulin secretion are decreased in the NGT and the prediabetes groups, which mainly contribute to the increase of fasting glucose [20]. On the other hand, because the overall insulin secretory function declines in T2D group, the insulin secretory function might influence the postprandial glucose as well as the fasting glucose compared with other groups. These findings provide important clues to the greater understanding of the concept of GA/A1c ratio with reference to glucose parameter.

A recent study has demonstrated that GA may be lower than the actual plasma glucose levels in NGT patients who have elevated body fat content; furthermore, the actual plasma glucose levels may be underestimated in obese patients when monitoring glycemic control with GA alone [21]. These data corresponded well to our result, which showed a strong association between BMI and GA/A1c ratio in NGT patients. However, in our study, the association between BMI and GA/A1c ratio was relatively weak in the prediabetes and the T2D groups. Instead, GA/A1c ratio was more strongly related with increasing glucose level. Therefore, when monitoring glycemic control with GA, it is necessary to consider the effect of BMI on GA/A1c ratio. Nonetheless, because the effect of BMI on GA/A1c ratio is relatively weaker than those of the glucose parameters in the T2D group, GA/A1c ratio well reflect the status of glucose control even in high BMI.

Our study has some limitations. First, we could not measure body composition, such as fat mass, or inflammatory cytokines (e.g. CRP), which may explain the mechanism of the negative association between BMI and GA/A1c ratio. Second, the cross-sectional study design precluded observations of future variations. Third, we could not adjust for known independent influencing factors of GA, such as triglyceride, smoking status, and age. Despite all these weaknesses, however, this study has found that the direct effect of HOMA-β alone on GA/A1c ratio is not significant in diabetic patients, contrary to the findings of previous studies which suggested an inverse association between GA/A1c ratio and HOMA-β. The previously found association between these two factors is more likely to be mediated through fasting and/or postprandial glucose. Furthermore, the factors influencing GA/A1c ratio is different according to glucose tolerance status. Insulin secretory function is preserved in the NGT, resulting in less glucose excursion; consequently, GA does not increase compared to A1c, which explains the fact that the ratio is not associated with other glucose parameters (fasting/postprandial glucose, HOMA-β, etc.) in the NGT group. Fasting glucose exerted the greatest influence on GA/A1c ratio in the prediabetes group, whereas postprandial glucose was the greatest contributing factor to GA/A1c ratio in the T2D group.

In conclusion, the inverse association between GA/A1c and BMI is the result of different mechanisms according to glucose tolerance status: in the NGT group, it is due to the direct association between BMI and GA/A1c, while in the prediabetes and T2D group, GA/A1c ratio was influenced by glucose parameters in addition to BMI, resulting in less influence of BMI on the ratio compared to NGT. These findings suggest that GA may underestimate the actual glycemic status in obese patients; however, this discrepancy tends to disappear as the subject reaches closer to T2D.

Acknowledgments

We are grateful thank to Dong-Su Jang, B.A. (Research Assistant, Department of Anatomy, Yonsei University College of Medicine, Seoul, Korea) for figure assistance

Author Contributions

Analyzed the data: JHH KJK DWK. Contributed reagents/materials/analysis tools: DWK. Wrote the paper: JHH KJK. Theory development: BWL. Helped write and revise the manuscript: BWL ESK BSC HCL.

References

1. Koenig RJ, Peterson CM, Jones RL, Saudek C, Lehrman M, et al. (1976) Correlation of glucose regulation and hemoglobin A1c in diabetes mellitus. N Engl J Med 295: 417–420.

2. Goldstein DE, Little RR, Lorenz RA, Malone JI, Nathan D, et al. (2004) Tests of glycemia in diabetes. Diabetes Care 27: 1761–1773.

3. Kim JH, Kim GW, Lee MY, Shin JY, Shin YG, et al. (2012) Role of HbA1c in the screening of diabetes mellitus in a Korean rural community. Diabetes Metab J 36: 37–42.

4. Kim KJ, Lee BW (2012) The roles of glycated albumin as intermediate glycation index and pathogenic protein. Diabetes Metab J 36: 98–107.

5. Won HK, Kim KJ, Lee BW, Kang ES, Cha BS, et al. (2011) Reduction in glycated albumin can predict change in HbA1c: comparison of oral hypoglycaemic agent and insulin treatments. Diabet Med 29: 74–79.

6. Lee YH, Lee BW, Chun SW, Cha BS, Lee HC (2011) Predictive characteristics of patients achieving glycaemic control with insulin after sulfonylurea failure. Int J Clin Pract 65: 1076–1084.

7. Yoshiuchi K, Matsuhisa M, Katakami N, Nakatani Y, Sakamoto K, et al. (2008) Glycated albumin is a better indicator for glucose excursion than glycated hemoglobin in type 1 and type 2 diabetes. Endocr J 55: 503–507.

8. Koga M, Kasayama S (2010) Clinical impact of glycated albumin as another glycemic control marker. Endocr J 57: 751–762.

9. Miyashita Y, Nishimura R, Morimoto A, Matsudaira T, Sano H, et al. (2007) Glycated albumin is low in obese, type 2 diabetic patients. Diabetes Res Clin Pract 78: 51–55.

10. Nishimura R, Kanda A, Sano H, Matsudaira T, Miyashita Y, et al. (2006) Glycated albumin is low in obese, non-diabetic children. Diabetes Res Clin Pract 71: 334–338.

11. Koga M, Matsumoto S, Saito H, Kasayama S (2006) Body mass index negatively influences glycated albumin, but not glycated hemoglobin, in diabetic patients. Endocr J 53: 387–391.

12. Furusyo N, Koga T, Ai M, Otokozawa S, Kohzuma T, et al. (2011) Utility of glycated albumin for the diagnosis of diabetes mellitus in a Japanese population study: results from the Kyushu and Okinawa Population Study (KOPS). Diabetologia 54: 3028–3036.

13. Kim D, Kim KJ, Huh JH, Lee BW, Kang ES, et al. (2012) The ratio of glycated albumin to glycated haemoglobin correlates with insulin secretory function. Clin Endocrinol (Oxf) 77: 679–683.

14. Koga M, Murai J, Saito H, Kasayama S (2010) Glycated albumin and glycated hemoglobin are influenced differently by endogenous insulin secretion in patients with type 2 diabetes. Diabetes Care 33: 270–272.

15. Stein CM, Morris NJ, Nock NL (2012) Structural equation modeling. Methods Mol Biol 850: 495–512.

16. Koga M, Otsuki M, Matsumoto S, Saito H, Mukai M, et al. (2007) Negative association of obesity and its related chronic inflammation with serum glycated albumin but not glycated hemoglobin levels. Clin Chim Acta 378: 48–52.

17. Salas-Salvado J, Bullo M, Garcia-Lorda P, Figueredo R, Del Castillo D, et al. (2006) Subcutaneous adipose tissue cytokine production is not responsible for the restoration of systemic inflammation markers during weight loss. Int J Obes (Lond) 30: 1714–1720.

18. Ko SH, Kim SR, Kim DJ, Oh SJ, Lee HJ, et al. (2011) 2011 clinical practice guidelines for type 2 diabetes in Korea. Diabetes Metab J 35: 431–436.

19. Lee EY, Lee BW, Kim D, Lee YH, Kim KJ, et al. (2011) Glycated albumin is a useful glycation index for monitoring fluctuating and poorly controlled type 2 diabetic patients. Acta Diabetol 48: 167–172.

20. Abdul-Ghani MA, Matsuda M, Jani R, Jenkinson CP, Coletta DK, et al. (2008) The relationship between fasting hyperglycemia and insulin secretion in subjects with normal or impaired glucose tolerance. Am J Physiol Endocrinol Metab 295: E401–406.

21. Wang F, Ma X, Hao Y, Yang R, Ni J, et al. (2012) Serum glycated albumin is inversely influenced by fat mass and visceral adipose tissue in Chinese with normal glucose tolerance. PLoS One 7: e51098.

8

Is Serum Zinc Level Associated with Prediabetes and Diabetes?

Md. Rafiqul Islam[1], Iqbal Arslan[3], John Attia[1], Mark McEvoy[1], Patrick McElduff[1], Ariful Basher[2], Waliur Rahman[3], Roseanne Peel[1], Ayesha Akhter[4], Shahnaz Akter[5], Khanrin P. Vashum[1], Abul Hasnat Milton[1]*

1 Centre for Clinical Epidemiology and Biostatistics (CCEB), School of Medicine and Public Health, The University of Newcastle, New Lambton Heights, New South Wales, Australia, 2 Department of Medicine, Mymensingh Medical College, Ministry of Health and Family Welfare, Government of Bangladesh, Mymensingh, Bangladesh, 3 Department of Biochemistry, Bangobondhu Sheikh Mujib Medical University (BSMMU), Dhaka, Bangladesh, 4 Department of Obstetrics and Gynaecology, Tairunnessa Memorial Medical College, Gazipur, Dhaka, Bangladesh, 5 Department of Paediatrics, Institute of Child and Mother Health (ICMH), Dhaka, Bangladesh

Abstract

Aims: To determine serum zinc level and other relevant biological markers in normal, prediabetic and diabetic individuals and their association with Homeostasis Model Assessment (HOMA) parameters.

Methods: This cross-sectional study was conducted between March and December 2009. Any patient aged ≥30 years attending the medicine outpatient department of a medical university hospital in Dhaka, Bangladesh and who had a blood glucose level ordered by a physician was eligible to participate.

Results: A total of 280 participants were analysed. On fasting blood sugar results, 51% were normal, 13% had prediabetes and 36% had diabetes. Mean serum zinc level was lowest in prediabetic compared to normal and diabetic participants (mean differences were approximately 65 ppb/L and 33 ppb/L, respectively). In multiple linear regression, serum zinc level was found to be significantly lower in prediabetes than in those with normoglycemia. Beta cell function was significantly lower in prediabetes than normal participants. Adjusted linear regression for HOMA parameters did not show a statistically significant association between serum zinc level, beta cell function (P = 0.07) and insulin resistance (P = 0.08). Low serum zinc accentuated the increase in insulin resistance seen with increasing BMI.

Conclusion: Participants with prediabetes have lower zinc levels than controls and zinc is significantly associated with beta cell function and insulin resistance. Further longitudinal population based studies are warranted and controlled trials would be valuable for establishing whether zinc supplementation in prediabetes could be a useful strategy in preventing progression to Type 2 diabetes.

Editor: Yiqing Song, Brigham & Women's Hospital, and Harvard Medical School, United States of America

Funding: The study was funded by the Directorate General Health Services, Ministry of Health and Family Welfare, Government of the People's Republic of Bangladesh. The funders had no role in study design, data collection and analysis, decision to publish, or preparation of the manuscript.

Competing Interests: The authors have declared that no competing interests exist.

* E-mail: milton.hasnat@newcastle.edu.au

Introduction

Diabetes Mellitus is a major public health problem for both developed and developing countries [1]. Considering the differences in risk factors across countries, it is estimated that the number of diabetics will be more than double by the year 2030 compared to 2000 [2,3]. Most non insulin dependent diabetics and patients with impaired glucose tolerance are resistant to insulin stimulated glucose uptake [4].

Molecular and cellular studies in animal models have demonstrated that zinc (Zn) plays a key role in the synthesis and action of insulin under normal physiological conditions, and that zinc supplementation can be protective in rodent models of type 2 diabetes. In 1980, Coulston & Dandona demonstrated that zinc (II) chloride stimulated lipogenesis in rat adipocytes, similarly to insulin [5]. In another study of ob/ob mice, insulin secretion was potentiated following zinc supplementation [6]. Dietary zinc supplementation in young db/db mice for 6 weeks reduced fasting hyperglycemia and hyperinsulinemia [7].

In humans, there is a paucity of data about the role of zinc in insulin resistance. It is documented that diabetes patients have low serum zinc levels but this is likely to be due to hyperzincuria (losing zinc in the urine secondary to nephropathy in diabetes) and impaired zinc absorption [8]. Evidence for the causal role of zinc in the development of diabetes is circumstantial. In the islet cells of type 2 diabetes patients, Human Islet Amyloid Polypeptide (hIAPP) causes β cell loss and low insulin secretion; zinc significantly inhibits hIAPP amyloid fibrillogenesis and has been shown to prevent hIAPP mediated β cell loss [9]. Other studies in humans document the need for zinc in the synthesis and release of insulin from β cells [10,11]. An observational study reported a lower incidence of type 2 diabetes in women who had higher intakes of dietary zinc [11]. Also, oxidative stress is relatively common in diabetes and zinc supplementation reduces oxidative stress [12]. Despite these data, a recent Cochrane review concluded that there was insufficient evidence to determine if zinc supplementation in adults is efficacious for prevention of insulin resistance [13]; another recent study suggested more detailed investigations of zinc supplementation on glucose metabolism [14].

Prediabetes often preceeds diabetes mellitus, and is characterized by impaired fasting glucose (IFG) and or impaired glucose tollerance (IGT) [15]. The condition is prevalent in many populations, especially among the middle aged and elderly [4,16,17]. Data from the United States estimates a prediabetic state among 40% of adults between 40 and 74 years [18], while an Australian study shows a 16.4% prevalence of prediabetes among adults 25 years of age or over [15]. The natural history of impaired fasting glucose (IFG) and impaired glucose tolerance (IGT) is variable; progression to diabetes occurs in approximately 25%, the abnormal glycemic state remains in 50%, and reversion to normal glucose tolerance (NGT) occurs in 25% over 3–5 years of observation [14]. Compared to normo-glycemic individuals, prediabetics are 5–15 times more likely to develop type 2 diabetes [18]. IFG and IGT also carry an increased risk of cardio vascular disease [19].

Given this existing data, it is reasonable to hypothesize that low zinc may predispose to insulin resistance and consequently, that zinc supplementation in prediabetes may prevent or delay progression to type 2 diabetes. Our study primarily aimed to evaluate whether serum zinc levels are associated with glycemic status, HbA_1c, and HOMA parameters, i.e. β cell efficiency, insulin sensitivity and insulin resistancein normal, prediabetic and diabetic individuals

Methods

This cross-sectional study was conducted in Bangobandu Sheikh Mujib Medical University (BSMMU), Dhaka, Bangladesh between March and December 2009. We obtained necessary ethics approval from the Ethics Committee, Director General Health Services, Ministry of Health and Family Welfare, Government of Bangladesh. Potential participants were approached by trained Study Medical Officers to participate in the study. After obtaining informed verbal consent the participants were recruited. With the low literacy rate noted in the planning phase of the study, we decided to obtain verbal consent from prospective participants and this was approved by the ethics committee. The Study Medical Officers maintained a register for those who consented verbally to participate in the study. In addition, at least 5% of the recruited participants were re-interviewed by the study investigators for quality control to cross check that verbal consent was properly obtained. Study participants were recruited from adults aged 30 or above attending the medicine outpatient department (MOPD) of the university hospital in weekly daytime business hours (9am to 2pm) for blood glucose testing and presented with or without any comorbidity other than signs and symptoms of glycemic conditions. After obtaining verbal consent and considering the participant's status (random or fasting), patients were screened by glucometer for their initial group allocation (Normal, Prediabetes and Diabetes) to aim for roughly equal numbers of participants in each group. The medical officers requested that participants come to the hospital on the following day for determination of their fasting blood glucose level in the laboratory. Subsequent analysis and group allocation in this paper are based on laboratory results of fasting blood glucose levels although we have taken out 25 participnats from normal and 25 participants from prediabetes group as they were on hypoglycemic agents at the time of fasting blood glucose measurement. The Study Medical Officers completed the data collection form on each participant on the day of screening by glucometer. A trained laboratory technician collected a blood sample (10 mls) from each study participant to analyse their fasting blood glucose, serum zinc, serum insulin, and serum HbA_1C level.

Exposure definitions and measurements

Considering the laboratory fasting blood glucose measurements, participants were categorized into three groups using American Diabetic Association (ADA) guidelines:

Normal (normoglycemic): fasting blood glucose level was <5.6 mmol/l,

Prediabetes: fasting blood glucose level was 5.6–6.9 mmol/l, and

Diabetes: fasting blood glucose level was ≥7 mmol/l.

Measurement of other exposure variables. Participants' self-reported socio-economic characteristics, smoking status, diabetes, hypertension, family history, medications (esspecially steroids), and anthropometric measurements were collected.

Outcome measurement

Serum zinc measurement. Serum zinc level was measured using Atomic Absorption Spectro Photometry (AAS) (Shimadzu Corporation, Japan). Calibration curves for zinc were prepared using stock standard solution (1000 mg/l = 1000 ppm) with analytical grade zinc salt preserved in polypropylene bottles. There was a linear relationship between absorbance and concentration (r = 0.9993) throughout the calibration curve, and all results were obtained from the linear range. The samples were analyzed by graphite furnace Atomic Absorption Spectrometry (AAS) using the following settings: 213.9 nm of wavelength, 0.5 nm of slit width, BCG-D2 lamp mode, 8 mA of lamp with low current and 0 mA of lamp with high current.

Statistical Analysis

Based on previous studies we assumed a mean difference of 2 mmol/L (±5 mmol/L) in serum zinc levels among three groups (normal, pre-diabetes and diabetes) and calculated a sample size of 300 with 95% confidence interval and 80% power. Assuming a 10% refusal and drop-out rate, recruiting a total of 330 eligible participants was estimated to be sufficient to observe the differences for this study, i.e. 110 in each group. Data were entered and analysed using STATA version 10.0 supplied by STATA Corporation, Texas, USA. Summary statistics were calculated and presented as mean, standard deviation and proportion by groups. Non parametric tests were performed for variables that did not follow a normal distribution. Scatter plots, simple and multiple linear regression analyses were performed to observe associations between serum zinc levels and glycemic status. Associations with zinc were undertaken with zinc treated as a continuous variable, and as a dichotomous variable ("normal" ≥700 ppb/L and "low" <700 ppb/L [20,21]). Univariate regression analysis was performed to identify factors that were associated with participants' serum zinc status. Any factor that provided a univariate p value <0.25 was entered into a multiple regression model. Homeostasis Model Assesment (HOMA2) calculator (University of Oxford, UK website; http://www.dtu.ox.ac.uk/homacalculator/index.php) was used to calculate steady state beta cell function (%B), insulin sensitivity (%S) and insulin resistance (IR) for normal and prediabetes participants and multiple linear regression analysis was performed for all three

Table 1. Characteristics of study participants by their glycemic status (N = 280).

Indicators	Normal (n = 143)	Prediabetic (n = 36)	Diabetic (n = 101)
Age (mean, ±SD):	45.5 (10.7)	46.7 (10.6)	47.4 (11.5)
Sex (n, %):			
Male	81 (56.6)	17 (47.2)	53 (52.5)
Female	62 (43.4)	19 (52.8)	48 (47.5)
Education (n, %):			
No education	18 (12.6)	8 (22.2)	10 (9.9)
Primary	17 (11.9)	4 (11.1)	11 (10.9)
Secondary/Higher secondary	67 (46.8)	15 (41.7)	52 (51.5)
Graduate/Masters	40 (28.0)	9 (25.0)	27 (26.7)
Others and missing	1 (0.7)	0 (0.0)	1 (1.0)
Household income/m (n, %):			
0–5000	36 (25.1)	3 (8.3)	10 (9.9)
5001–10000	39 (27.3)	16 (44.5)	32 (31.7)
10001–20000	43 (30.1)	10 (27.8)	35 (34.6)
>20000	24 (16.8)	7 (19.4)	22 (21.8)
No information	1 (0.7)	0 (0.0)	2 (2.0)
Smoking status (n, %):			
Smoked never	106 (74.1)	31 (86.1)	75 (74.3)
Previous smoker	19 (13.3)	1 (2.8)	18 (17.8)
Current smoker	18 (12.6)	3 (8.3)	8 (7.9)
No information	0 (0.0)	1 (2.8)	0 (0.0)
Diabetes in family (n, %):			
Yes	22 (15.4)	8 (22.2)	31 (30.7)
No	121 (84.6)	28 (77.8)	70 (69.3)
Hypertension status (n, %):			
Yes	43 (30.1)	17 (47.2)	32 (31.7)
No	80 (55.9)	13 (36.1)	52 (51.5)
Don't know	19 (13.3)	6 (16.7	16 (15.8)
No information	1 (0.7)	0 (0.0)	1 (1.0)
BMI (n,%):			
<18.5	15 (10.5)	1 (2.8)	8 (7.9)
18.5–25	77 (53.8)	24 (66.6)	55 (54.5)
>25	51 (35.7)	11 (30.6)	38 (37.6)
Taking any medicines (n, %):			
Yes	85 (59.4)	20 (55.6)	75 (74.3)
No	57 (39.9)	16 (44.4)	25 (24.7)
No information	1 (0.7)	0 (0.0)	1 (1.0)
Taking antihypertensive (n,%):			
Yes	43 (30.1)	17 (47.2)	28 (27.7)
No	85 (59.4)	11 (30.6)	65 (64.4)
No information	15 (10.5)	8 (22.2)	8 (7.9)
Taking hypoglycaemics (n, %)			
Yes	0 (0.0)	0 (0.0)	53 (52.5)
No	128 (89.5)	27 (75.0)	41 (40.6)
No information	15 (10.5)	9 (25.0)	7 (6.9)

HOMA parameters (beta cell function, insulin sensitivity and insulin resistance) to determine factors associated with each outcome.

Results

Based on the laboratory fasting blood glucose levels, a total of 330 participants were initially recruited for this study; however, 25 participants from the normal group and 25 participants from the prediabetic group were dropped from subsequent analyses as they were already on hypoglycemic agents at the time of recruitment. Of the remaining 280 participants, 51% were normal, 13% had prediabetes and 36% had diabetes; charateristics of the participants are listed in Table 1. Participants were predominantly middle-aged, male, had at least high school education and were never smokers. Overall 22% of the participants had a positive family history of diabetes, 34% were hypertensive and 36% were obese. Approximately, 31% of the participants were on anti-hypertensive medications and 19% were taking any form of hypoglycemic agent. Mean fasting blood sugar levels were 4.3, 6.3 mmol/L and 11.9 mmol/L in normal, prediabetic and diabetic participants, respectively (Table 2).

Zinc was significantly different between the disease groups, with the difference reaching statistical significance for the comparison between normal and pre-diabetes groups (P = 0.02, Table 2). This comparison remained statistically significant after adjusting for multiple possible confounders in a linear regression (Table 3), with the pre-diabetes group on average having a zinc level lower by about 66.7 ppb/l (P = 0.02) than normals. The results also remained consistent in multiple logistic regression when zinc levels were dichotomised at 700 ppb/l, a threshold used previously. We found that prediabetes and diabetes individuals were 78% (p = 0.008) and 54% (P = 0.01) less likely to have a normal serum zinc levels (≥700 ppb/L) compared to normal participants, respectively (data not shown). In all regression analysis, we included participants' gender and smoking status in the final model based on the findings from other studies [22,23] although they were not associated in univariate analysis.

In order to explore these associations more finely, we calculated the HOMA parameters. The HOMA is not suitable for use in frank diabetes and so these parameters were not calculated for the diabetes group.

We found that all these biochemical and HOMA parameters (Table 2) were non-normally distributed; therefore, the non-parametric Kruskal-Wallis test was used to test differences by glycaemic status. Mean serum zinc and mean serum insulin levels were significantly different between normoglycemic and prediabetes participants. Moreover, beta-cell function was significantly lower in prediabetic than in normal participants (P<0.001); however, there was no statistically significant difference in insulin sensitivity and insulin resistance levels between normoglycemic and prediabetic participants (P = 0.4) (Table 2).

All the HOMA parameters were then regressed against serum zinc levels as continuous values, stratified by the participant's glycaemic status (Normal and prediabetes). We found that in normal people the higher the zinc the higher the insulin sensitivity and the lower the insulin resistance; as a result the less the beta cells have to function (hence the negative coefficient). These results are consistent whether zinc is analysed as a continuous or a dichotomised variable (Tables 4, 5, 6, 7). In prediabetic participants, similar stratified analysis did not show any significant association between HOMA parameters and serum zinc (Tables 5, 7)

Given the strong effect of BMI on diabetes risk, we also explored the effect of BMI on HOMA parameters and zinc. Figures 1, 2, 3 indicates that serum zinc as a dichotomous variable has an interaction with BMI; we observed a significant interaction between dichotomized serum zinc and BMI for insulin resistance in multivariate analysis (P for interaction = 0.005) (Figure 3). At the same high BMI, participants with low serum zinc levels were more likely to have higher insulin resistance than those with high serum zinc levels (Figure 3).

Table 2. Laboratory findings of blood/serum analysis and Homeostasis Model Assessment (HOMA) using HOMA-2 calculator for beta cell efficiency of the participants in different groups (N = 280, Normoglycemic = 143, Prediabetic = 36 and Diabetic = 101).

Patient status	Laboratory findings				Beta cell efficiency using HOMA-2 calculator		
	Mean fasting blood glucose mmol/l ± SD (Median, IQR*)	Mean serum zinc, ppb/l ± SD (Median, IQR*)	Mean serum insulin, μu/ml ± SD (Median, IQR*)	Mean HbA₁C level, % ± SD (Median, IQR*)	Mean % of beta cell function ± SD (Median, IQR*)	Mean % of insulin sensitivity ± SD (Median, IQR*)	Mean insulin resistance ± SD (Median, IQR*)
Normal (n = 143)	4.3±0.60 (4.4, 4.0 to 4.8)	585.31±160.63 (600, 500 to 700)	10.47±6.45 (9.3, 6.2 to 14.0)	6.03±0.85 (6.0, 5.3 to 6.5)	154.69±78.24 (135.3, 99.6 to 185.2)	108.38±67.95 (88.1, 57.2 to 131.7)	1.30±0.76 (1.10, 0.8 to 1.7)
Prediabetic (n = 36)	6.3±0.38 (6.3, 6.0 to 6.6)	520.55±161.36 (500, 400 to 650)	11.33±9.15 (7.95, 6.65 to 12.15)	6.36±0.98 (6.3, 5.7 to 6.85)	75.52±38.29 (63.65, 51.25 to 85.05)	90.27±43.95 (90.95, 60.8 to 107.95)	1.53±1.18 (1.10, 0.90 to 1.65)
Diabetic (n = 101)	11.87±5.3 (10.5, 8.3 to 13.7)	553.96±148.44 (550, 450 to 650)	15.89±19.0 (10.0, 6.8 to 17.6)	8.39±2.43 (8.0, 6.3 to 9.7)	-	-	-
Non-parametric Kruskal-Wallis P value	φ<0.001, ⁵<0.001, ψ<0.001	φ0.03, ⁵0.02, ψ0.07	φ0.08, ⁵0.8, ψ0.03	φ<0.001, ⁵0.1, ψ<0.001	<0.001	0.4	0.4

*IQR = Interquartile range,
φacross all groups;
⁵between normal and prediabetic only;
ψbetween normal and diabetic only.

Table 3. Adjusted linear regression for serum zinc levels by participant's glycemic status ((N = 278, Normoglycemic = 142, Prediabetic = 35 and Diabetic = 101).

Exposure parameters	Serum Zinc		
	Coefficient	**95% Confidence Interval**	**P Value**
Glycemic status:			
Normoglycemic	Ref	Ref	Ref
Prediabetic	−66.69	−125.15 to −8.24	0.02
Diabetic	−25.60	−66.20 to 14.98	0.21
Age	−1.14	−2.96 to 0.67	0.21
Sex	−42.16	−86.37 to 2.04	0.06
Education	−2.44	−5.60 to 0.72	0.13
Smoking History	0.04	−31.26 to 31.34	0.99
BMI	2.24	−2.00 to 6.49	0.30
Constant	665.92	489.02 to 842.83	<0.001

Discussion

Our study clearly indicates that mean serum zinc levels were the lowest in the prediabetes participants and this remained significant even when adjusted for multiple potential confounders. Even though this is a cross-sectional study, we recruited participants at different stages in the diabetic spectrum; the results suggest that low zinc precedes the development of diabetes and that low zinc is not simply an epiphenomenon of increased renal loss of zinc in diabetics. This has not been evident in previous cross-sectional studies. To further explore the role of low zinc in this process, we calculated the HOMA parameters. We found that higher zinc was associated with lower beta cell function and lower insulin resistance, and this was statistically significant regardless of whether zinc was treated as a continuous or a dichotomized variable. There was also an interaction between dichotomized zinc and BMI, indicating that at any given BMI, those with low zinc had higher insulin resistance than those with high zinc.

Other results were more puzzling. Stratified analyses in the prediabetic group did not show any effect of BMI or zinc, in contrast to the results in the normoglycaemic group. This may simply be due to insufficient power in our analysis or may be a genuine

Table 4. Adjusted linear regression analysis for HOMA parameters with serum zinc as continuous value in normal participants (N = 142).

Exposure indicators	HOMA2 Parameters								
	Beta Cell function			**Insulin Sensitivity**			**Insulin Resistance**		
	Coefficient	**95% CI[†]**	**P value**	**Coefficient**	**95% CI[†]**	**P value**	**Coefficient**	**95% CI[†]**	**P value**
Serum Zinc	−0.77	−0.15 to −0.00	0.05	0.040	−.02 to 0.10	0.19	−0.0008	−0.001 to −0.0001	0.02
Age	−0.90	−2.14 to 0.33	0.15	1.00	0.007 to 1.99	0.048	−0.006	−0.17 to 0.005	0.29
Gender	−6.54	−36.15 to 23.07	0.66	−15.38	−39.17 to 8.40	0.20	−0.067	−0.34 to 0.20	0.62
Education	−1.31	−4.12 to 1.50	0.36	−2.82	−5.07 to −0.56	0.015	0.002	−0.02 to 0.02	0.84
Smoking History	−1.36	−20.47 to 17.75	0.89	3.53	−11.82 to 18.88	0.65	−0.06	−0.23 to 0.11	0.49
BMI	7.17	4.29 to 10.05	<0.001	−6.13	−8.44 to −3.81	<0.001	0.08	0.05 to 0.11	<0.001
Constant	91.83	−40.97 to 224.64	0.17	229.13	122.45 to 335.82	<0.001	0.20	−1.02 to 1.44	0.74

[†]CI: Confidence Interval.

Table 5. Adjusted linear regression analysis for HOMA parameters with serum zinc as continuous value in prediabetic participants (N = 35).

Exposure indicators	HOMA2 Parameters								
	Beta Cell function			**Insulin Sensitivity**			**Insulin Resistance**		
	Coefficient	**95% CI[†]**	**P value**	**Coefficient**	**95% CI[†]**	**P value**	**Coefficient**	**95% CI[†]**	**P value**
Serum Zinc	−0.01	−0.09 to 0.06	0.78	0.02	−0.07 to 0.12	0.66	0.000	−0.002 to 0.002	0.89
Age	−0.45	−1.75 to 0.85	0.48	0.39	−1.24 to 2.03	0.62	−0.12	−0.05 to 0.02	0.55
Gender	0.83	−30.11 to 31.77	0.96	−4.12	−43.15 to 34.79	0.82	0.000	−0.97 to 0.97	1.00
Education	0.009	−2.55 to 2.56	0.99	−0.02	−3.24 to 3.20	0.98	−0.001	−0.08 to 0.07	0.97
Smoking History	−8.56	−32.28 to 15.15	0.46	13.24	−16.62 to 43.11	0.37	−0.28	−1.02 to 0.46	0.45
BMI	3.64	0.68 to 6.61	0.018	−2.57	−6.30 to 1.16	0.17	0.11	0.01 to 0.20	0.02
Constant	22.20	−108.91 to 153.31	0.73	114.45	−50.67 to 279.58	0.17	−0.33	−4.47 to 3.80	0.87

[†]CI: Confidence Interval.

Table 6. Adjusted linear regression analysis for HOMA parameters with serum zinc as category in normal participants (N = 142).

Exposure parameters	HOMA2 Parameters								
	Beta cell function			Insulin sensitivity			Insulin resistance		
	Coeff.*	95% CI*	P value	Coeff.*	95% CI*	P value	Coeff.*	95% CI*	P value
Zinc categories (≥700 ppb/L)	−28.51	−54.47 to −2.56	0.03	16.13	−4.72 to 36.99	0.12	−0.35	−0.59 to −0.11	0.004
Age	−0.88	−2.1 to 0.34	0.16	0.99	0.005 to 1.98	0.049	−0.006	−0.01 to 0.005	0.28
Gender	−4.50	−33.76 to 24.75	0.76	−16.36	−39.88 to 7.15	0.17	−0.05	−0.32 to 0.21	0.71
Education	−1.52	−4.35 to 1.29	0.28	−2.68	−4.95 to −0.41	0.02	−0.000	−0.02 to 0.02	0.97
Smoking History	−0.08	−19.18 to 19.01	0.99	2.80	−12.55 to 18.15	0.72	−0.04	−0.22 to 0.13	0.60
BMI	7.45	4.54 to 10.36	<0.001	−6.30	−8.64 to −3.96	<0.001	0.08	0.06 to 0.11	<0.001
Constant	46.70	−76.36 to 169.78	0.45	252.91	153.99 to 351.83	<0.001	−0.27	−1.40 to 0.86	0.63

*Coeff: Coefficient,
*CI: Confidence Interval.

difference due to the fact that in prediabetes, participants may have reached to a metabolic break point.

Globally, zinc deficiency is widespread and 33% of the world's population are affected [24]. Studies report that diets rich in phytates and dietary fibers which contain low sources of readily bioavailable zinc can cause zinc deficiency in individuals and populations [25,26]. In rural Bangladesh, predominant consumption of rice based diet with a few animal foods are the main risk factors for zinc deficiency [27]. Our finding of low zinc among pre-diabetes participants without significant renal disease argues that low zinc precedes the diabetes state and is not simply a result of renal loss of zinc, indicating that zinc may play a substantial role in the progression of this disease. There are many potential mechanisms for this; zinc is important in regard to metabolic diseases (insulin resistance, metabolic syndrome and diabetes) mainly because it is required for insulin storage in pancreas and stabilizing of insulin hexamers. Its anti-oxidative properties may delay progression of insulin resistance and diabetes [28]. Besides, reduction in some particular forms of zinc such as zinc-α2-glycoprotein (ZAG), an adipokine, plays a role in the development of metabolic diseases [29].

In previous studies, higher body mass index was found to be related with insulin resistance with or without other associated conditions [30,31,32]. Release of chemokines and inflammatory cytokines from adipose tissue in obesity may cause chronic systemic low grade inflammation, thus insulin resistance may develop [30]. In obesity, blood zinc levels were found to be lower and inversely related to obesity [22] and the level was significantly lower than controls [20]. One study demonstrates that, alteration in the concentration of zinc in obesity may contribute to the development of insulin resistance as zinc improves the solubility of insulin in the beta cells of pancreas and increases the capacity of the receptor for binding this hormone. They also recommend further research on the metabolic role of zinc in the insulin resistance syndrome [21] and short term metabolic disorders may not be associated with low plasma zinc in obesity [23].

Our study has a number of potential limitations:

- We do not consider other trace elements such as iron and copper that may influence participant's zinc status.
- In this study we used a glucometer to screen adults who attended for blood sugar analysis in the study hospital's medicine outpatient department. Our aim for screening was to obtain an equal number of participants in each group. The use of a glucometer for measuring blood sugar levels has previously been found to have a low sensitivity for correctly detecting an individual's blood sugar level [33,34] and laboratory venous blood sugar measurement has since been recommended over

Table 7. Adjusted linear regression analysis for HOMA parameters with serum zinc as category in prediabetic participants (N = 35).

Exposure parameters	HOMA2 Parameters								
	Beta cell function			Insulin sensitivity			Insulin resistance		
	Coeff.*	95% CI*	P value	Coeff.*	95% CI*	P value	Coeff.*	95% CI*	P value
Zinc categories (≥700 ppb/L)	−20.86	−59.33 to 17.6	0.27	16.84	−32.33 to 66.02	0.48	−0.55	−1.77 to 0.66	0.35
Age	−0.44	−1.72 to 0.83	0.48	0.39	−1.24 to 2.02	0.62	−0.01	−0.05 to 0.02	0.56
Gender	0.17	−29.94 to 30.29	0.99	−3.07	−41.57 to 35.43	0.87	0.002	−0.95 to 0.95	0.99
Education	−0.12	−2.62 to 2.37	0.92	0.12	−3.07 to 3.32	0.93	−0.003	−0.08 to 0.07	0.92
Smoking History	−7.70	−30.66 to 15.24	0.49	11.94	−17.39 to 41.39	0.41	−0.27	−1.00 to 0.44	0.43
BMI	3.62	0.72 to 6.52	0.01	−2.57	−6.28 to 1.13	0.16	0.10	0.016 to 0.20	0.02
Constant	20.20	−102.18 to 142.60		122.59	−33.86 to 279.06	0.12	−0.16	−4.03 to 3.71	0.93

*Coeff: Coefficient,
*CI: Confidence Interval.

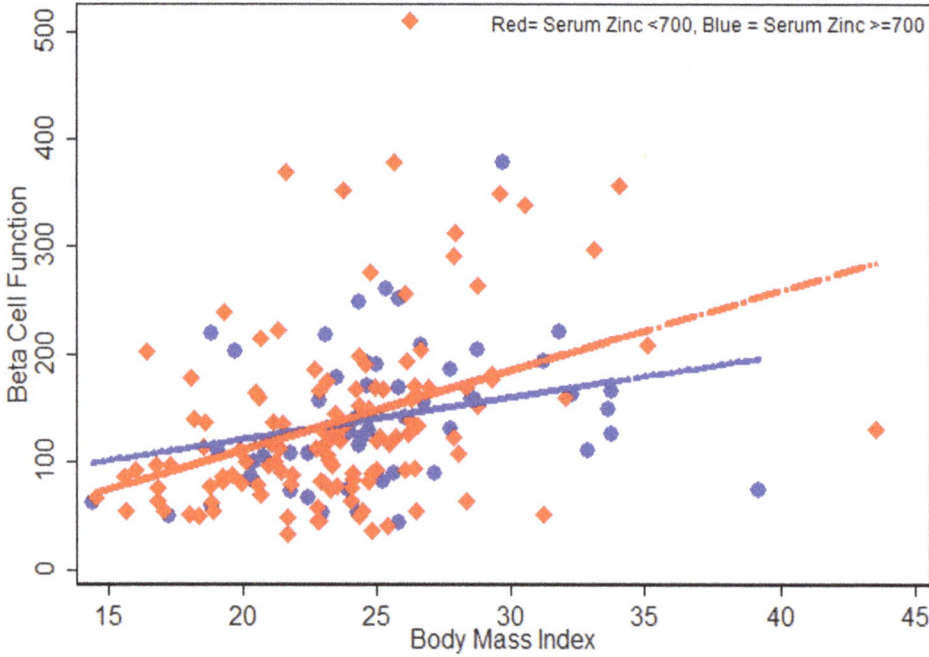

Figure 1. Scatter plots for HOMA-Beta Cell Function against Serum Zinc levels (<700, ≥700) by participants Body Mass Index (n = 179; normal = 143 and prediabetic = 36).

the preference of bedside capillary blood sugar measurement using a glucometer [35]. Similarly, our study also observed differences in the results of blood sugar levels using glucometer and laboratory measurements and therefore, the number of participants recruited was different across groups.

- Our study is cross-sectional and we infer progression from the results of those in various groups, i.e. normal, pre-diabetic, and diabetic. These results need to be replicated in longitudinal studies.

In conclusion, prediabetic individuals are more likely to be zinc deficient and zinc deficiency in turn is associated with poorer beta-

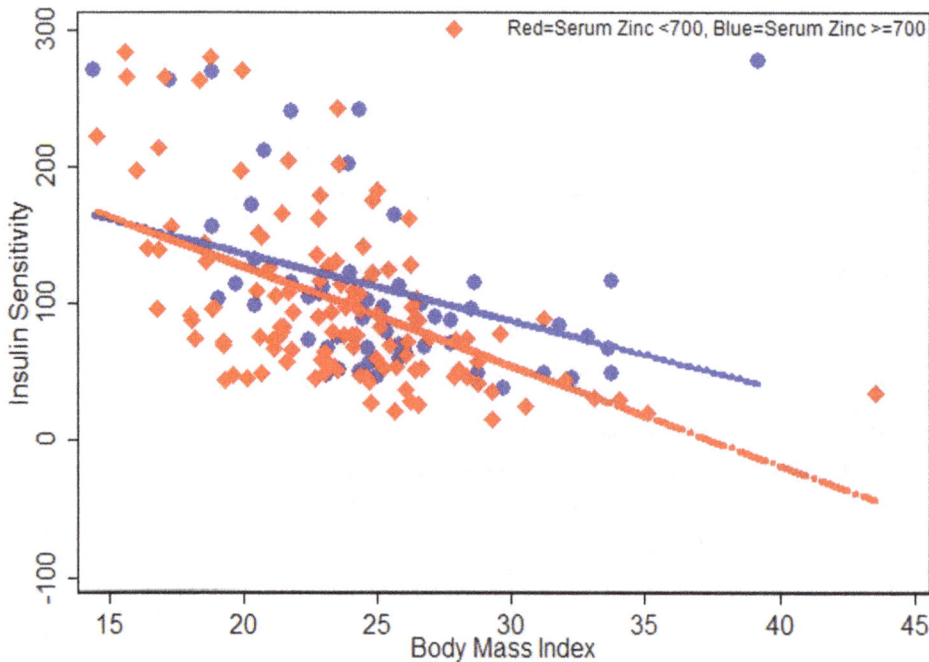

Figure 2. Scatter plots for HOMA-Insulin Sensitivity against Serum Zinc levels (<700, ≥700) by participants Body Mass Index (n = 179; normal = 143 and prediabetic = 36).

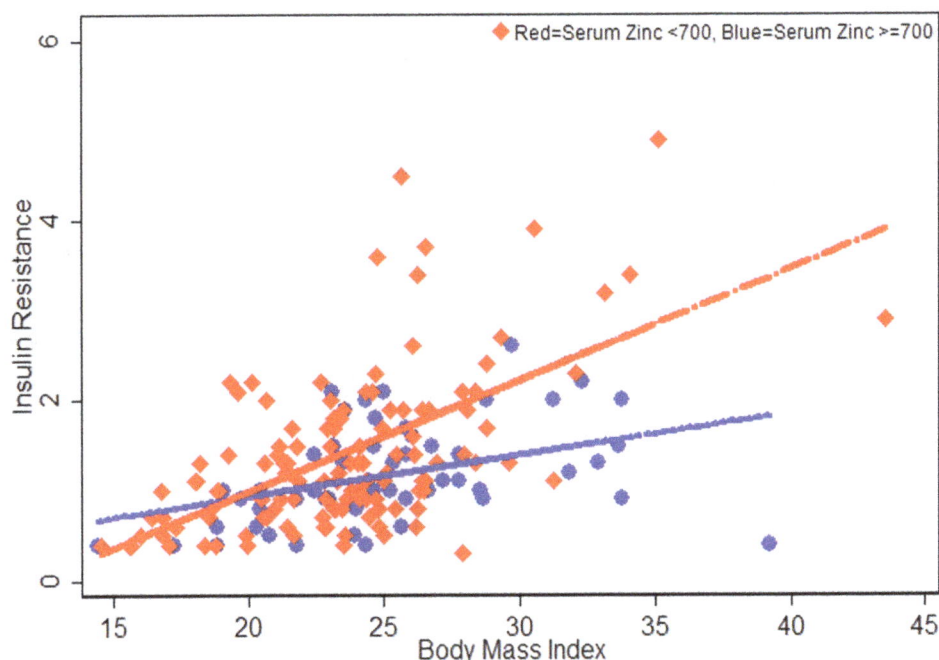

Figure 3. Scatter plots for HOMA-Insulin Resistant against Serum Zinc levels (<700, ≥700) by participants Body Mass Index (n = 179; normal = 143 and prediabetic = 36).

cell function and greater insulin resistance. There is an interaction with BMI in that for any given BMI, those with low zinc are more insulin resistant than those with high zinc. The results suggest the potential of targeting zinc supplementation for those with pre-diabetes or who have high BMI to prevent or impede the progression to diabetes. Further population based research and prospective controlled trials are required to clarify these findings.

Acknowledgments

We greatly acknowledge the contribution of the Research Team who worked very hard to collect quality data in timely manner.

Author Contributions

Conceived and designed the experiments: MRI IA JA MM PM RP KPV AHM. Performed the experiments: MRI IA AB WR AA SA AHM. Analyzed the data: MRI JA MM PM RP AA SA AHM. Contributed reagents/materials/analysis tools: MRI AHM IA AB WR AA SA. Wrote the paper: MRI IA JA PM MM RP AA SA KPV AB WR AHM.

References

1. Berry C, Tardif J-C, Bourassa MG (2007) Coronary Heart Disease in Patients With Diabetes. J Am Coll Cardiol 49: 631–642.
2. Wild S, Roglic G, Green A, Sicree R, King H (2004) Global prevalence of diabetes: estimates for the year 2000 and projections for 2030. Diabetes Care 27: 1047–1053.
3. Rathmann W, Giani G (2004) Global prevalence of diabetes: estimates for the year 2000 and projections for 2030. Diabetes Care 27: 2568–2569; author reply 2569.
4. Benjamin SM, Valdez R, Geiss LS, Rolka DB, Venkat Narayan KM (2003) Estimated Number of Adults With Prediabetes in the U.S. in 2000: Opportunities for prevention. Diabetes Care 26: 645–649.
5. Reaven GM (1988) Role of Insulin Resistance in Human Disease. Diabetes 37: 1595–1607.
6. Coulston L, Dandona P (1980) Insulin-like effect of zinc on adipocytes. Diabetes 29: 665–667.
7. Begin-Heick N, Dalpe-Scott M, Rowe J, Heick HM (1985) Zinc supplementation attenuates insulin secretory activity in pancreatic islets of the ob/ob mouse. Diabetes 34: 179–184.
8. Simon SF, Taylor CG (2001) Dietary zinc supplementation attenuates hyperglycemia in db/db mice. Exp Biol Med (Maywood) 226: 43–51.
9. Chausmer AB (1998) Zinc, insulin and diabetes. J Am Coll Nutr 17: 109–115.
10. Brender JR, Hartman K, Nanga RP, Popovych N, Bea dlS, et al. (2010) Role of zinc in human islet amyloid polypeptide aggregation. J Am Chem Soc 132: 8973–8983.
11. Huang XF, Arvan P (1995) Intracellular transport of proinsulin in pancreatic beta-cells. Structural maturation probed by disulfide accessibility. J Biol Chem 270: 20417–20423.
12. Sun Q, van Dam RM, Willett WC, Hu FB (2009) Prospective study of zinc intake and risk of type 2 diabetes in women. Diabetes Care 32: 629–634.

13. Roussel AM, Kerkeni A, Zouari N, Mahjoub S, Matheau JM, et al. (2003) Antioxidant effects of zinc supplementation in Tunisians with type 2 diabetes mellitus. J Am Coll Nutr 22: 316–321.
14. Haase H, Overbeck S, Rink L (2008) Zinc supplementation for the treatment or prevention of disease: current status and future perspectives. Exp Gerontol 43: 394–408.
15. Beletate V, El Dib RP, Atallah AN (2007) Zinc supplementation for the prevention of type 2 diabetes mellitus. Cochrane Database Syst Rev: CD005525.
16. Wenying Y, Juming L, Jianping W, Weiping J, Linong J, et al. (2010) Prevalence of Diabetes among Men and Women in China. N Engl J Med 362: 1090–1101.
17. Nathan DM, Davidson MB, DeFronzo RA, Heine RJ, Henry RR, et al. (2007) Impaired fasting glucose and impaired glucose tolerance: implications for care. Diabetes Care 30: 753–759.
18. Twigg SM, Kamp MC, Davis TM, Neylon EK, Flack JR (2007) Prediabetes: a position statement from the Australian Diabetes Society and Australian Diabetes Educators Association. Med J Aust 186: 461–465.
19. Ukropec J, Radikova Z, Huckova M, Koska J, Kocan A, et al. (2010) High prevalence of prediabetes and diabetes in a population exposed to high levels of an organochlorine cocktail. Diabetologia 53: 899–906.
20. Di Martino G, Matera MG, De Martino B, Vacca C, Di Martino S, et al. (1993) Relationship between zinc and obesity. J Med 24: 177–183.
21. Marreiro DN, Geloneze B, Tambascia MA, Lerario AC, Halpern A, et al. (2004) Role of zinc in insulin resistance. Arq Bras Endocrinol Metabol 48: 234–239.
22. Chen MD, Lin PY, Lin WH (1991) Investigation of the relationships between zinc and obesity. Gaoxiong Yi Xue Ke Xue Za Zhi 7: 628–634.
23. Ming-Der C, Pi-Yao L, Sheu Wayne H-H (1997) Zinc status in plasma of obese individuals during glucose administration. Biological Trace Elements Research 60: 123–129.

24. Usha D, Girish H, Venugopal PM, Pratibha D, Archana S, et al. (2009) Zinc Deficiency: Descriptive Epidemiology and Morbidity among Preschool Children in Peri-urban Population in Delhi, India. Journal of Health Population and Nutrition 27: 632–639.

25. Sandstead H (1991) Zinc deficiency. A public health problem? Am J Dis Child 145: 853–859.

26. Katja K, Mohammed AW, Henrik F, Shakuntala HT (2006) Acute Phase Protein Levels, T. trichiura, and Maternal Education Are Predictors of Serum Zinc in a Cross-Sectional Study in Bangladeshi Children. J Nutr 136: 2262–2268.

27. Arsenault JE, Yakes EA, Hossain MB, Islam MM, Ahmed T, et al. (2010) The current high prevalence of dietary zinc inadequacy among children and women in rural Bangladesh could be substantially ameliorated by zinc biofortification of rice. J Nutr 140: 1683–1690.

28. Nicolas Wiernsperger, Rapin J (2010) Trace elements in glucometabolic disorders: an update. Wiernsperger and Rapin Diabetology & Metabolic Syndrome 2.

29. Balaz M, Ukropcova B, Kurdiova T, Penesova A, Skyba P, et al. (2012) Prediabetes in adult GH deficiency is associated with a substantial reduction in serum and adipose tissue expression levels of zinc-α2-glycoprotein. ICE/ECE 2012. Florence, Italy: Bioscientifica. pp. 1196.

30. Ognjanovic S, Jacobs DR, Steinberger J, Moran A, Sinaiko AR (2012) Relation of chemokines to BMI and insulin resistance at ages 18–21. Int J Obes (Lond).

31. Ferrannini E, Natali A, Bell P, Cavallo-Perin P, Lalic N, et al. (1997) Insulin resistance and hypersecretion in obesity. European Group for the Study of Insulin Resistance (EGIR). J Clin Invest 100: 1166–1173.

32. Luisa Trirogoff M, Shintani A, Himmelfarb J, Alp Ikizler T (2007) Body mass index and fat mass are the primary correlates of insulin resistance in nondiabetic stage 3–4 chronic kidney disease patients. Am J Clin Nutr 86: 1642–1648.

33. Benja M, Pattara S, Pongdech S, Worawitaya T, Mantana T, et al. (2012) Use of glucometer and fasting blood glucose as screening tools for diabetes mellitus type 2 and glycated haemoglobin as clinical reference in rural community primary care settings of a middle income country. BMC Public health 12.

34. Baig A, Siddiqui I, Jabbar A, Azam SI, Sabir S, et al. (2007) Comparision between bed side testing of blood glucose by glucometer vs centralized testing in a tertiary care hospital. J Ayub Med Coll Abbottabad 19: 25–29.

35. Boyd R, Leigh B, Stuart P (2005) Capillary versus venous bedside blood glucose estimations. Emerg Med J 22: 177–179.

9

MAP3K8 (TPL2/COT) Affects Obesity-Induced Adipose Tissue Inflammation without Systemic Effects in Humans and in Mice

Dov B. Ballak[1,2,3◊], Peter van Essen[1,2◊], Janna A. van Diepen[1,2], Henry Jansen[1], Anneke Hijmans[1], Tetsuya Matsuguchi[4], Helmut Sparrer[5], Cees J. Tack[1], Mihai G. Netea[1,3], Leo A. B. Joosten[1,3¶], Rinke Stienstra[1,2,6*¶]

1 Department of Medicine, Radboud University Medical Centre, Nijmegen, The Netherlands, 2 Institute for Genomic and Metabolic Disease, Radboud University Medical Centre, Nijmegen, The Netherlands, 3 Nijmegen Institute for Infection Inflammation and Immunity, Radboud University Medical Centre, Nijmegen, The Netherlands, 4 Department of Oral Biochemistry, Field of Developmental Medicine, Kagoshima University, Graduate School of Medical and Dental Sciences, Sakuragaoka, Kagoshima, Japan, 5 Novartis Pharma AG, Basel, Switzerland, 6 Department of Human Nutrition, Wageningen University and Research Centre, Wageningen, The Netherlands

Abstract

Chronic low-grade inflammation in adipose tissue often accompanies obesity, leading to insulin resistance and increasing the risk for metabolic diseases. MAP3K8 (TPL2/COT) is an important signal transductor and activator of pro-inflammatory pathways that has been linked to obesity-induced adipose tissue inflammation. We used human adipose tissue biopsies to study the relationship of MAP3K8 expression with markers of obesity and expression of pro-inflammatory cytokines (IL-1β, IL-6 and IL-8). Moreover, we evaluated obesity-induced adipose tissue inflammation and insulin resistance in mice lacking MAP3K8 and WT mice on a high-fat diet (HFD) for 16 weeks. Individuals with a BMI >30 displayed a higher mRNA expression of MAP3K8 in adipose tissue compared to individuals with a normal BMI. Additionally, high mRNA expression levels of IL-1β, IL-6 and IL-8, but not TNF -α, in human adipose tissue were associated with higher expression of MAP3K8. Moreover, high plasma SAA and CRP did not associate with increased MAP3K8 expression in adipose tissue. Similarly, no association was found for MAP3K8 expression with plasma insulin or glucose levels. Mice lacking MAP3K8 had similar bodyweight gain as WT mice, yet displayed lower mRNA expression levels of IL-1β, IL-6 and CXCL1 in adipose tissue in response to the HFD as compared to WT animals. However, MAP3K8 deficient mice were not protected against HFD-induced adipose tissue macrophage infiltration or the development of insulin resistance. Together, the data in both human and mouse show that MAP3K8 is involved in local adipose tissue inflammation, specifically for IL-1β and its responsive cytokines IL-6 and IL-8, but does not seem to have systemic effects on insulin resistance.

Editor: Yan Chen, Institute for Nutritional Sciences, China

Funding: The funders had no role in study design, data collection and analysis, decision to publish, or preparation of the manuscript. MGN was supported by a Vici grant of the Netherlands Organization for Scientific Research. RS was supported by a Ruby Grant of the Dutch Diabetes Research Foundation.

Competing Interests: One of the authors is an employee of the Novartis Pharma AG, Basel, Switzerland. However, neither he or the company have any competing interests in this study. Additionally, no patents or marketing products have been used in the current study, nor will the company benefit from the results reported in this manuscript. Helmut Sparrer has provided the authors with the unique MAP3K-deficient mouse model. and contributed to writing and revising of the manuscript. Novartis does not conduct any research on MAP3K and has no intellectual or financial interests.

* E-mail: rinke.stienstra@radboudumc.nl

◊ These authors contributed equally to this work.

¶ These authors share senior authorship.

Introduction

Obesity is characterized by chronic low-grade inflammation arising from the adipose tissue [1]. This inflammatory trait mainly results from resident or infiltrating immune cells into the adipose tissue and is associated with insulin resistance and metabolic diseases such as type 2 diabetes mellitus [2]. In response to pro-inflammatory stimuli, immune receptors activate signalling pathways, such as protein kinase like IκB kinase (IKK) and extracellular signal-regulated kinase (ERK). Stimulation of these pathways leads to activation of NF-κB and JNK transcription factors, resulting in transcription of pro-inflammatory genes including TNF-α, IL-6, IL-1β, and CCL2 [3]. These pathways have been recognized to play a pivotal role in instigating a local inflammatory reaction in the adipose tissue of obese patients, secondarily affecting the insulin signalling pathway [4–6].

Serine threonine mitogen activated protein kinase kinase kinase 8 (MAP3K8), in mice also called tumor progression locus 2 (TPL2) and in humans called Cancer Osaka Thyroid (COT), activates ERK-1/2 [7,8]. In quiescent state, MAP3K8 forms a complex with A20-binding inhibitor of NF-κB (ABIN-2) and p105 NF-κB, precursor of the NF-κB transcription factor. It can be activated by pro-inflammatory stimuli, such as TNF-α, IL-1β and LPS. MAP3K8 knockout mice that are exposed to LPS/D-galactosamine-induced pathology are protected against endotoxin shock,

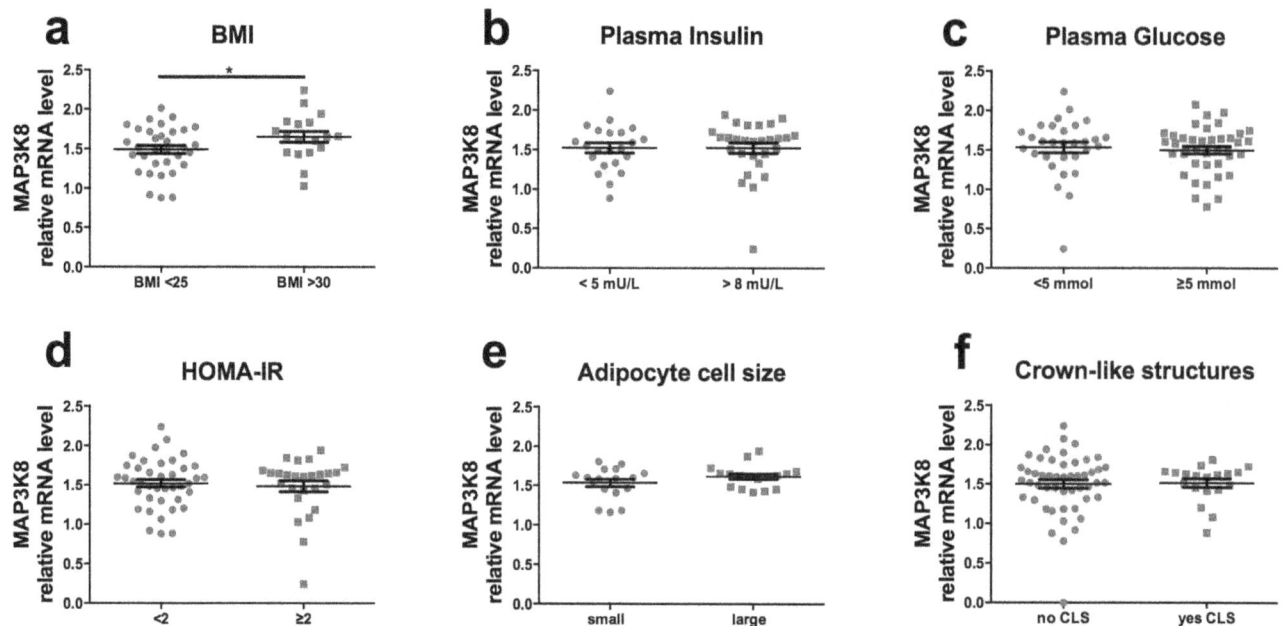

Figure 1. MAP3K8 in humans is associated with higher BMI and cytokine expression. MAP3K8 mRNA expression in human subcutaneous adipose tissue, associated with (a) BMI, (b) plasma insulin values, (c) plasma glucose levels, (d) HOMA-IR, (e) adipocyte sell size cell size and (f) crown-like structures. *p<0.05. n = 51, 50, 71, 70 respectively. HOMA-IR = Homeostatic Model Assessment for insulin resistance.

showing that MAP3K8 is an essential protein in directing inflammatory responses [9]. The role of MAP3K8 in regulating the inflammatory trait of obesity is not fully clear. The function of MAP3K8 in obesity-induced inflammation has been studied previously.

One study reported that MAP3K8 is upregulated in adipose tissue in response to IL-1ß and TNF-α and mediates lipolysis induced by these cytokines [10]. Another study reported that MAP3K8 regulates obesity-associated inflammation and insulin resistance. MAP3K8 deficient mice showed a reduction of high fat diet (HFD)-induced adipose tissue inflammation and a reduced expression of inflammatory markers, as well as improved insulin sensitivity [11]. These results were not confirmed in a study that found contradictory results after conducting a similar high fat diet intervention study. The authors showed that MAP3K8 deficient mice were not protected against the detrimental effects of diet-induced obesity [12]. No differences in mRNA levels of several markers of adipose tissue inflammation or whole body glucose or insulin tolerance were observed in mice. Moreover, MAP3K8 was not up-regulated in adipose tissue due to HFD-feeding.

Considering these contradictory data in the literature, we aimed to illuminate the role of MAP3K8 using a complementary approach combining murine studies with assessment of the role of MAP3K8 in human adipose tissue. We found that human MAP3K8 expression in adipose tissue is indeed associated with obesity. However, using mice lacking MAP3K8, our data show a redundant role for MAP3K8 in obesity-associated metabolic dysfunction. Local adipose tissue inflammation was only mildly influenced. Moreover, human adipose tissue biopsies show that MAP3K8 expression in adipose tissue associates with mRNA levels of IL-1β, IL-6 and IL-8, but not with systemic metabolic parameters. Together these data suggest that MAP3K8 partially affects pro-inflammatory gene expression in adipose tissue, yet does not play an important role in the development of insulin resistance during obesity.

Material and Methods

Human subjects

Subcutaneous adipose tissues were obtained from 70 healthy donors subjects with a broad range of BMI. The measurements were carried out in the first and last quartile. The group was divided in low BMI and high BMI (BMI <25, n = 33, BMI >30, n = 18), low and high plasma insulin levels (concentration < 5 mU/L, n = 22, >8 mU/L, n = 28); low and high plasma glucose levels (concentration <5 mM, n = 30, >5 mM, n = 40); low and high HOMA-IR levels (<2, n = 40, >2 n = 26); adipocyte cell size (diameter in µM, smallest and largest quartile n = 36). HOMA-IR was calculated by: (glucose * insulin plasma levels)/22.5. For association with mRNA levels of IL-1β, IL-6, IL-8 and TNFα to MAP3K8 lowest and highest quartile were compared (n = 36). Similarly, highest en lowest quartile of serum amyloid A (SAA) and C-reactive protein (CRP) levels were associated with MAP3K8 expression (n≥30) (SAA: Q1≤0.7 mg/L, Q4≥1.6 mg/L; CRP. Q1≤0.5 mg/L, Q4≥2.0 mg/L). All subjects gave written informed consent. The study was approved by the ethical committee of the Radboud University Medical Centre, Nijmegen.

Animals

MAP3K8-ko mice [13] and WT mice on a C57Bl/6 background were housed in a pathogen-free environment in the animal facility from the Radboud University Nijmegen. All animal procedures were conducted under protocols approved by the animal experimentation committee of Radboud University Nijmegen Medical Centre. Bodyweight of the animals was recorded weekly. After a 2 weeks run-in period on low fat diet, mice were given low fat diet (LFD) or high fat diet (HFD) feeding for 16 weeks, containing 10% or 45% of energy derived from palm oil fat (D125450B or 12451; Research Diets, Inc).

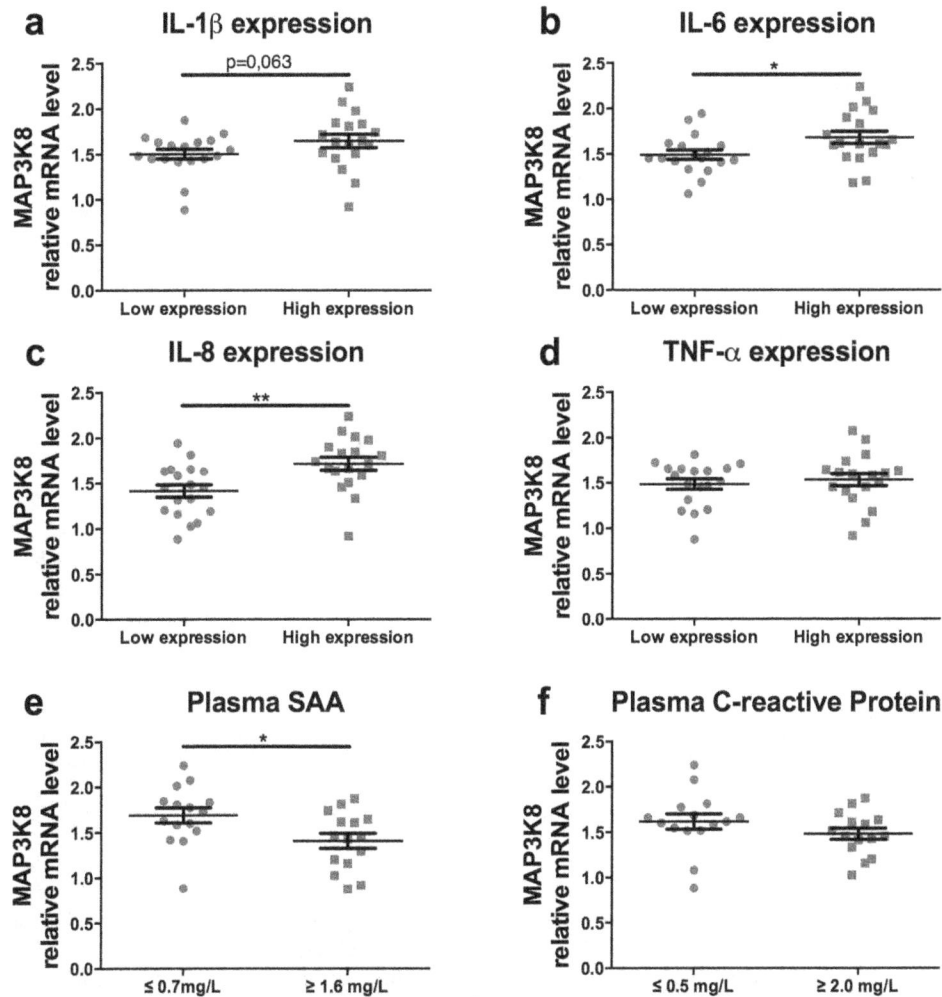

Figure 2. MAP3K8 in humans is associated with IL-1β, IL-6 and IL-8 cytokine expression. Biopsies from subcutaneous adipose tissue were obtained from healthy subjects with varying levels of obesity. Association of MAP3K8 mRNA expression in human subcutaneous adipose tissue with mRNA expression of (a) IL-1ß, (b) IL-6, (c) IL-8, (d) TNF-α, (e) serum amyloid A levels (SAA: Q1≤0.7 mg/L, Q4≥1.6 mg/L), (f) C-reactive protein (CRP: Q1≤0.5 mg/L, Q4≥2.0 mg/L). *p<0.05, **p<0.01.

Oral glucose and insulin tolerance tests

Oral glucose tolerance (OGTT) and insulin tolerance tests (ITT) were performed. Prior to the OGTT, animals were fasted overnight (9 hours) and 2 g/kg glucose (D-glucose, Gibco, Invitrogen) was orally administered. Prior to the ITT, mice were fasted 6 hours and insulin (0,75 U/kg) was injected intraperitoneally. Blood glucose levels were determined with an Accu-chek glucosemeter (Roche Diagnostics, Almere, The Netherlands) at indicated time points after glucose administration.

Histochemistry

For detection of macrophages/monocytes, an F4/80[+] antibody (product code: MCA497G, AbD Serotec, Düsseldorf, Germany) was used for mice samples, a CD68-monoclonal antibody (Clone EBM11, Dako, Denmark) was used for human samples. Visualization of the complex was done using 3,3'-diaminobenzidene for 5 min. Negative controls were used by omitting the primary antibody. Morphometry of individual fat cells was assessed using digital image analysis. Microscopic images were digitized in 24-bit RGB (specimen pixel size $1.28 \times 1.28 \ \mu m^2$). Recognition of fat cells was initially performed by applying a region-growing algorithm on manually indicated seed points, and minimum Feret diameter was calculated.

qPCR

Total RNA was isolated from adipose tissue using TRIzol (Invitrogen, Carlsbad, CA), according to manufacturer's instructions. RNA was reverse-transcribed (iScript cDNA Synthesis Kit, Bio-Rad Laboratories). RT-PCR was performed using specific primers (see Table S1), power SYBR green master mix (Applied Biosystems, Foster City, CA) using the Step-one Real-Time PCR system (Applied Biosystems, Foster City, CA). For mice samples, we used both 36B4 and GAPDH as housekeeping genes. For human samples we used B2M as a housekeeping gene.

Western blot analysis

Lysis buffer (50 mM Tris (pH 7.4), 150 mMNaCl, 2 mMEDTA, 1% Nonidet P-40, 50 mMNaF, and 0.25% sodium deoxycholate) with phosstop phosphatase-inhibitor cocktail tablet (Roche) and complete, EDTA-free protease-inhibitor cocktail tablet (Roche) was used to prepare adipose tissue lysates. The homogenized lysate was then centrifuged at 4°C for 10 min at

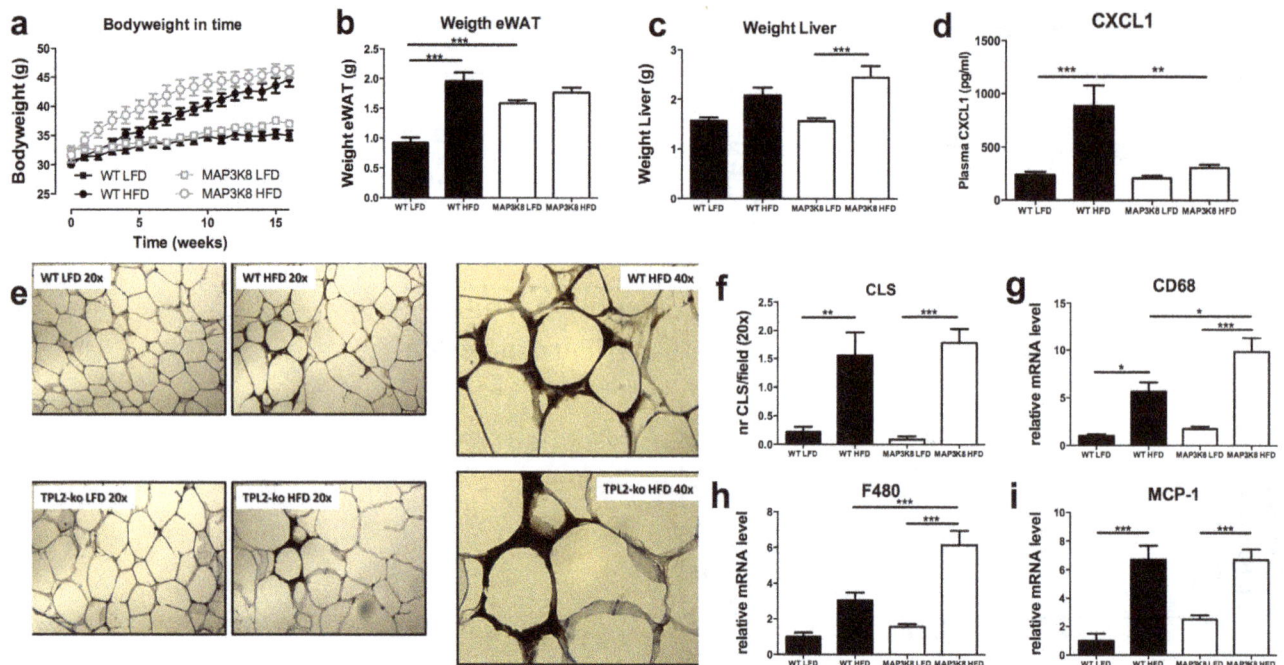

Figure 3. Obesity and macrophage influx in adipose tissue of HFD-fed WT and MAP3K8-ko animals. MAP3K8-ko and WT mice were fed a LFD or HFD during 16 weeks. (a) Bodyweight development upon LFD or HFD feeding. (b) Epididymal white adipose tissue (eWAT) weight after 16 weeks of LFD or HFD. (c) Liver weight after 16 weeks of LFD or HFD. (d) Plasma CXCL1 levels after 16 weeks of LFD or HFD (e) Macrophage influx into the adipose tissue as determined by immunohistochemistry, F4/80 (serotec) staining: 20× magnification or 40× as indicated: (f) Number of crown-like structures per field. (g–i) qPCR analysis for macrophage infiltration markers, (g) CD68, (h) F4/80, (i) MCP-1 in adipose tissue of MAP3K8-ko and WT animals. * p<0.05, ** p<0.01, *** p<0.001.

18.000 rcf. Subsequently, the supernatant was used for Western Blot. Equal amounts of protein as determined by a BCA protein assay (Thermo FisherScientific, Rockford, IL) were loaded, and separated using a polyacrylamide SDS page gel. After SDS-PAGE, proteins were transferred to a nitrocellulose membrane using Trans-Blot Turbo Transfer System (Biorad) following manufacturer's instructions. The membrane was blocked for 1 h at room temperature with 5% (wt/vol) milk powder in Tris-buffered saline (TBS)/Tween 20. Subsequently, the membrane was incubated overnight at 4°C with a phospho-p65 (Cell Signaling, 93H1) or pan-p65 antibody (Cell Signaling, D14E12), phospho-ERK (Promega, V8031) or pan-ERK antibody (Promega, V1141) and a tubulin antibody (Santa Cruz Biotechnology, 2–28–33) in 5% (wt/vol) milk powder/TBS/0.1% Tween 20. Hereafter, the blots were incubated with horseradish peroxidase-conjugated secondary antibodies (dilution of 1:5000) in 5% (wt/vol) milk powder in TBS/0.1% Tween-20 for 1 h at room temperature and subsequently developed with Clarity reagent (Biorad) according to the manufacturer's instructions. Bands were visualized using a ChemiDoc System (Biorad) and quantified using Image lab software (Biorad).

Plasma proteins

Plasma concentrations of insulin (ultra sensitive mouse insulin ELISA kit, Crystal Chem Inc., IL, USA; detection limit: 5 pg/ml) were measured by ELISA according to the manufacturer's instructions. Mice CXCL-1 concentrations were determined according to manufacturer's instructions (Duoset, R&D systems, MN, USA; detection limit 16 pg/ml). High sensitive C-reactive protein (hsCRP) was measured by enzyme-immunoassay according to the instructions from the manufacturer (Dako, Glastrup,

Denmark; detection limit 3.1 ng/ml). SAA was measured using the N Latex SAA test (Siemens Healthcare Diagnostic, Germany, detection limit: 0.02 ng/ml) according to the instructions from the manufacturer.

Plasma glucose

Glucose (Liquicolor, Human GmbH, Wiesbaden, Germany) was measured enzymatically following manufacturers' protocols.

Statistical analysis

Data are shown as means ± SEM. Differences between groups were analyzed using Student's t test, differences among 4 groups were analyzed with ANOVA followed by post-hoc Bonferroni tests in Graphpad Prism 5.0. p-values <0.05 were considered significant.

Results

BMI, IL-6 and IL-8 expression are associated with higher MAP3K8 expression in human adipose tissue

First, we determined the association of MAP3K8 (TPL2/COT) expression in human adipose tissue with measures of obesity (BMI), adipose tissue inflammation (cytokine expression) and insulin resistance (plasma insulin). Human subcutaneous tissue biopsies were acquired from healthy subjects with a wide range in BMI. As shown in **Figure 1a**, mRNA expression levels of MAP3K8 were significantly higher in individuals with a BMI higher than 30, compared to subjects with a normal BMI (between 20–25 kg/m²). However, no differences in MAP3K8 expression were observed between persons with low versus high plasma insulin and glucose levels (**Fig. 1b/c**). In line with this, no

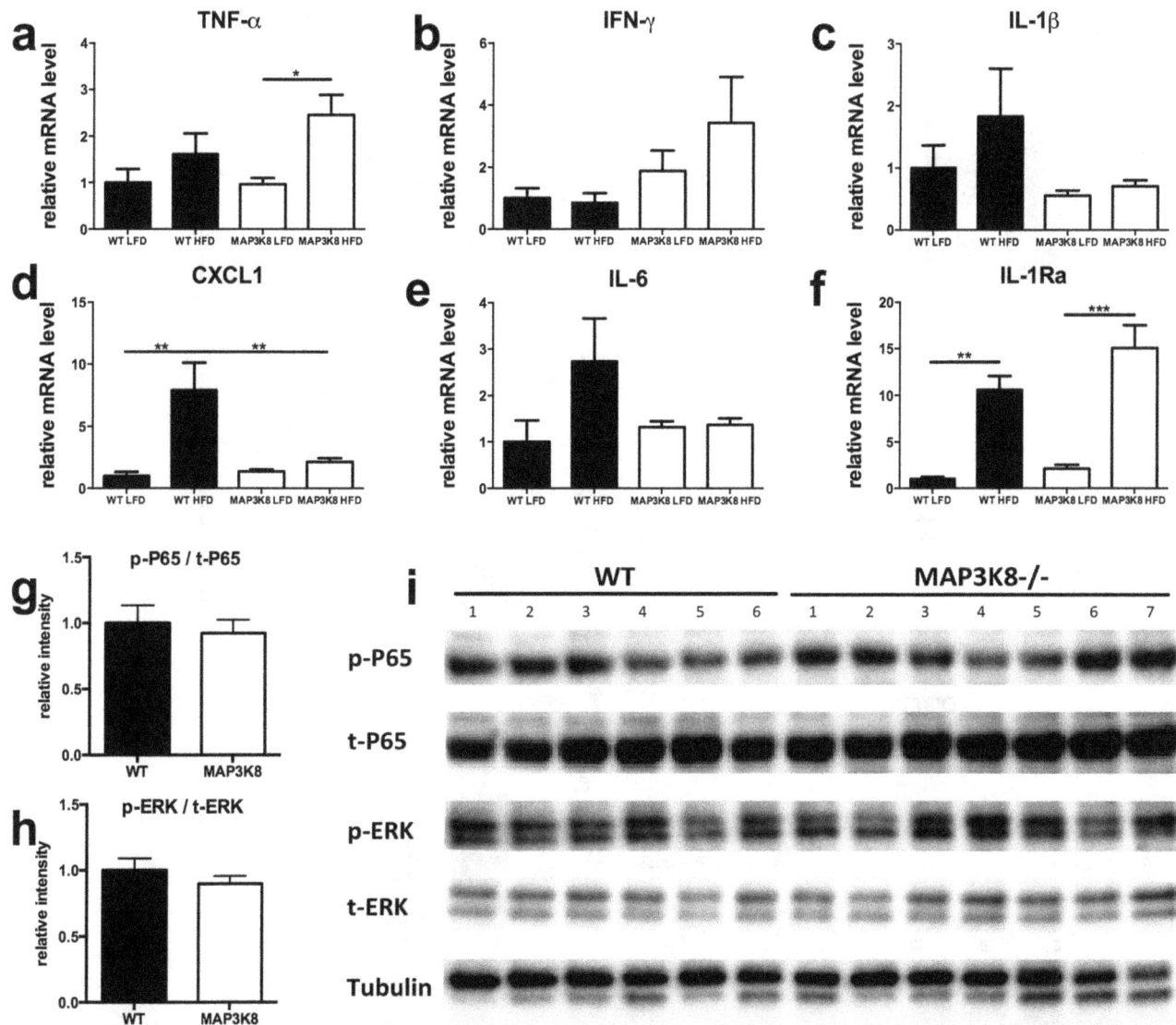

Figure 4. Inflammatory profile of the adipose tissue of HFD-fed WT and MAP3K8-ko animals. MAP3K8-ko and WT mice were fed a LFD or HFD during 16 weeks. (a–f) qPCR analysis for cytokines (a) TNF-α, (b) IFNγ, (c) IL-1β, (d) CXCL-1, (e) IL-6 and (f) IL-1Ra. n = 9 mice per group. Relative phosphorylation of NFκB p65 (g) and ERK 1/2 (h) in eWAT of MAP3K8-ko and WT animals after HFD-feeding (i). * p<0.05, ** p<0.01, *** p<0.001.

differences were observed for MAP3K8 expression in subjects with increased insulin resistance, as calculated by the homeostatic model for insulin resistance (**Fig. 1d**). Moreover, we did not see an increased expression of MAP3K8 in subjects with small versus large adipocyte size (**Fig. 1e**) or in subjects with crown-like structures (CLS) formed by infiltrating CD68 positive macrophages in adipose tissue compared to subjects with no CLS (**Fig. 1f**).

Interestingly, we found that higher mRNA expression of IL-1ß in human adipose tissue was associated with higher mRNA levels of MAP3K8, although this difference did not reach statistical significance, p = 0.063 (**Fig. 2a**). Moreover, mRNA expression levels of IL-1ß responsive cytokines, IL-6 and IL-8, were significantly associated with higher MAP3K8 expression (**Fig. 2b/c**). In contrast, TNFα mRNA levels did not associate with MAP3K8 expression (**Fig. 2d**). Moreover, systemic inflammatory markers were measured in the plasma and related to MAP3K8 expression in adipose tissue. Higher levels of serum amyloid A (SAA) were negatively associated with MAP3K8

expression in adipose tissue (**Fig. 2e**). In contrast, no relation was measured for MAP3K8 expression and plasma C-reactive protein (CRP) levels (**Fig. 2f**).

MAP3K8-ko mice show similar body weight compared to WT mice

Based on the association of higher MAP3K8 expression with both BMI and enhanced levels of IL-1ß responsive genes in human adipose tissue, we set out to determine if MAP3K8 causally affects obesity and adipose tissue inflammation in vivo. Therefore, 12-week old MAP3K8 deficient or WT mice, were fed a high-fat diet (HFD, 45% calories by energy content derived from fat) or low-fat diet (LFD, 10%) for 16 weeks. Although MAP3K8-ko mice gained bodyweight faster during the initial phase of the diet intervention, at the end of the study there were no differences in bodyweight between MAP3K8-ko and WT mice (**Figure 3a**). At the end of the intervention period, both genotypes gained approximately 9–10 grams more bodyweight due to the HFD-

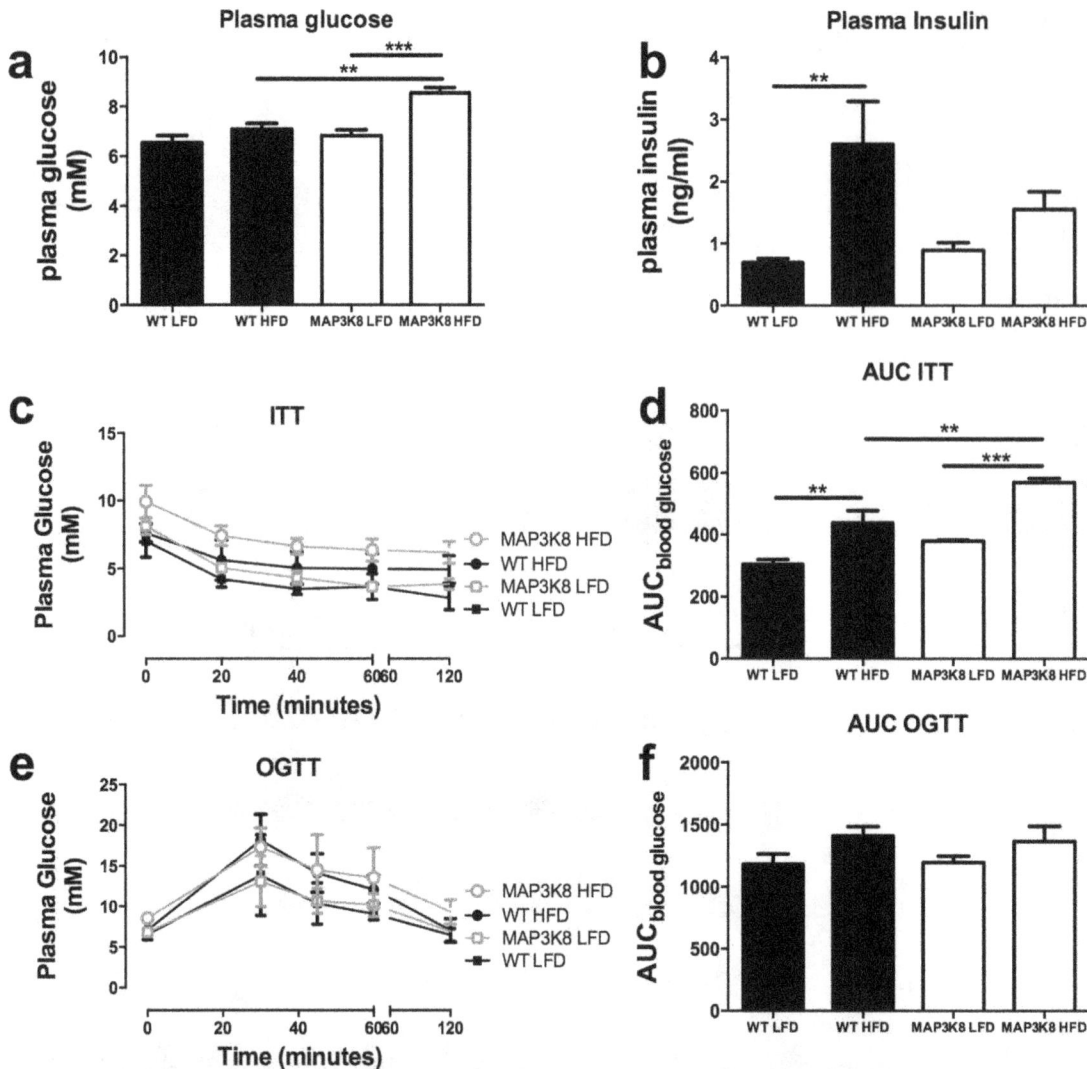

Figure 5. MAP3K8-ko mice display similar bodyweight and insulin sensitivity compared to WT mice. MAP3K8-ko and WT mice were fed a LFD or HFD during 16 weeks. (a) Plasma insulin and (b) plasma glucose levels after diet intervention. Insulin (itt) and oral glucose (ogtt) tolerance tests after 16 weeks of diet intervention. (c) itt after 16 weeks of HFD and (d) area under the curve itt. (e) ogtt after 16 weeks of HFD and (f) area under the curve of ogtt. n = 9 mice per group. * p<0.05, ** p<0.01, *** p<0.001.

feeding, compared to the LFD intervention. Moreover, MAP3K8-ko and WT mice had a similar epididymal white adipose tissue (eWAT) and liver weight after HFD feeding (**Fig. 3b/c**). Interestingly, MAP3K8-ko mice had a significant higher eWAT weight after LFD.

Different mRNA expression profile of inflammatory in adipose tissue

Next, we investigated whether MAP3K8-deficiency affected inflammation in response to HFD feeding. Indeed, in WT mice systemic CXCL-1 levels were increased after HFD-feeding. However, this effect was blunted in MAP3K8ko mice (**Fig. 3d**). Adipose tissue sections were stained for F4/80 and the amount of crown-like structures (CLS) in the adipose tissue was counted (**Fig. 3e**). HFD feeding significantly increased the amount of CLS in adipose tissue similarly, in both MAP3K8-ko and WT mice (**Fig. 3f**). Interestingly, mRNA expression levels of the macrophage markers CD68 and F4/80 were significantly higher in

MAP3K8-ko mice, while expression of MCP-1 was similar between both genotypes upon HFD feeding (**Fig. 3g–i**).

In line with an increased expression of macrophage markers, TNF-α and IFNγ mRNA levels tended to be increased in MAP3K8-ko mice fed a HFD, although this change did not reach statistical significance for IFNγ (**Fig. 4a/b**). In contrast, HFD-feeding did not upregulate expression of IL-1β and IL-1 effector cytokines IL-6 and CXCL-1 in MAP3K8-ko mice (**Fig. 4c–e**). Furthermore, mRNA IL-1Ra levels were not changed in MAP3K8-ko mice as compared to WT animals (**Fig. 4f**). To determine whether intracellular downstream targets of inflammatory pathways were affected in MAP3K8-ko versus WT mice, western blots were performed to measure the presence of phosphorylated ERK1/2 and NF-κB p65 in adipose tissue of both genotypes after HFD-feeding. No changes were observed in relative phosphorylation of both ERK1/2 and NF-κB p65 (**Fig. 4g/h**) as shown in **Figure 4i**.

MAP3K8-ko and WT display similar glucose and insulin tolerance after HFD

Next, we investigated whether the changes in adipose tissue inflammation in MAP3K8-ko and WT mice influence systemic insulin sensitivity. HFD-feeding increased fasting plasma insulin levels in WT, but not MAP3K8-ko mice (**Fig. 5a**). In contrast, basal plasma glucose levels were increased in MAP3K8-ko mice after HFD compared to WT on the same diet (**Fig. 5b**). To investigate whether insulin and glucose homeostasis was different in MAP3K8-ko and WT mice, we subjected the mice to an oral glucose tolerance test (ogtt) and insulin tolerance test (itt). As shown in **Figures 5c–f** MAP3K8 deficiency did not affect glucose or insulin tolerance upon LFD or HFD feeding. Notably, MAP3K8-ko mice fed a HFD even displayed a worsening if insulin tolerance as determined by the area under the curve (AUC), although this finding is partially explained by the elevated basal plasma glucose level.

Discussion

Inflammation plays a pivotal role in the development of insulin resistance associated with obesity. MAP3K8 (TPL2/COT) has been suggested to be an interesting therapeutic target in order to reduce inflammation, as it regulates activation of NF-κB and JNK transcription factors. Indeed, we observed that the mRNA expression of pro-inflammatory cytokines IL-1ß, IL-6 and IL-8 are associated with expression of MAP3K8 mRNA in human adipose tissue. However, our results do not reveal any association of MAP3K8 expression with markers of insulin sensitivity in human subjects and do not support a crucial role for MAP3K8 as an important regulator in the development of insulin resistance during obesity in mice. The results of this study show that human MAP3K8 adipose tissue expression is positively associated with BMI and expression of several pro-inflammatory cytokines in adipose tissue, but not with systemic inflammatory- or metabolic parameters such as plasma SAA, CRP, insulin or glucose levels. Similarly, although absence of MAP3K8 in mice induced mild changes in inflammation in adipose tissue, there were no differences in systemic insulin resistance even after 16 weeks of a HFD intervention. Therefore, these findings suggest that other inflammatory pathways or kinases may play a more dominant role in the development of obesity induced inflammation and insulin resistance. Hence, MAP3K8 may restrict its role to mediating local cytokine secretion as a downstream kinase of pivotal inflammatory receptors, but without affecting systemic metabolic parameters.

Although MAP3K8 has been reported to be an important regulator of inflammatory pathways in other diseases [14], the effect of MAP3K8 on obesity-induced chronic low-grade inflammation has been a point of debate. Three prior studies have provided contradictory evidence for the role of MAP3K8 in obesity-induced inflammation and metabolic dysfunction [10–12]. We found that MAP3K8 is upregulated in human adipose tissue in obese individuals. Moreover, we demonstrate an association between higher MAP3K8 mRNA expression and both IL-1ß and the IL-1ß -responsive cytokines IL-6 and IL-8 in the adipose tissue. MAP3K8 expression levels are not associated with a general enhancement in the inflammatory status of the adipose tissue as mRNA levels of the pro-inflammatory cytokine TNF-α are not changed between the low and high MAP3K8 expressing groups. Although TNF-α is known to be dependent on MAP3K8 in macrophages [9,15], TNF-α can also be produced independently of MAP3K8 [15,16]. Moreover, systemic inflammatory markers SAA and CRP were not positively associated with increased

MAP3K8 adipose tissue levels, suggestive of a redundant role of MAP3K8 in obesity-induced low-grade systemic inflammation.

Furthermore, we show that MAP3K8-ko and WT mice do not differ in weight after 16 weeks of high fat diet feeding, and that liver weight is similar as well, which is in accordance with earlier studies ([11] [12]). In the present study, the MAP3K8-ko mice did not show ameliorated inflammation in the adipose tissue in response to HFD, which is similar to findings of Lancaster et al. but opposed to the study of Perfield et al. In fact, expression levels of several macrophage markers (F480, CD68) were higher in adipose tissue of MAP3K8-ko mice compared to WT mice, suggesting increased macrophage infiltration. Interestingly, we observed that expression levels of IL-1ß and IL-1ß effector cytokines (CXCL1 and IL-6) were downregulated, leading to a reduction in circulating plasma CXCL1 levels. Since these cytokines are known to be activated via NFκB and ERK signaling, the reduction in cytokine expression could be secondary to a reduced activation of NFκB or ERK that are downstream molecules of MAP3K8 [14,16,17]. However, no difference in activation of NFκB or ERK 1/2 was found, suggesting that these downstream mediators of MAP3K8 were not differently regulated after HFD in both genotypes, hence other molecules downstream of MAP3K8 may be of more importance. The enhanced expression of macrophage markers in absence of MAP3K8 may be a compensatory mechanism for the inhibited cytokine expression by adipose tissue macrophages. Moreover, the increase of TNF-α and IFN-γ expression in adipose tissue in the MAP3K8-ko mice, might explain that no differences are seen on systemic metabolic parameters via compensatory mechanisms, as indicated by unchanged insulin or glucose tolerance in the MAP3K8-ko mice. Together, these results show that absence of MAP3K8 may affect certain inflammatory pathways and macrophage infiltration, but does not affect the presence of crown-like structures or systemic insulin sensitivity. Interestingly, our current results show that insulin levels in the MAP3K8-ko mice are lower, probably explaining a higher fasting glucose level, as was reported before. It may be worthwhile in the future to investigate the effect of MAP3K8 on insulin secretion of the pancreas. Hence, in line with the lower expression levels of IL-1ß that is known to affect beta-cell function [18] the absence of MAP3K8 may affect insulin production.

Parts of our results differ from earlier findings, which may be explained by different experimental or housing conditions. Gut microbiota is suggested to contribute to adipose tissue inflammation and metabolic disease [19]. Therefore, differences in microbiota composition may exist between facilities and could contribute to opposing. In addition, some studies used different types of high fat diets. Another possible explanation is that in the study of Perfield et al., mice were given a high fat diet from 6 weeks of age, while in this study and the study of Lancaster, the mice were several weeks older at the start of the diet intervention. Importantly, in our study, data from mice experiments were in agreement with data derived from human adipose tissue biopsies, confirming a positive association of MAP3K8 expression with local cytokine expression, but not with systemic metabolic parameters.

In summary, these data show that MAP3K8 has a limited role in obesity-induced inflammation and support earlier results by Lancaster et al. [12], who did not see protection against obesity-induced metabolic disease in knock-out mice. Altogether, the findings argue against MAP3K8 to be a central kinase in regulating pro-inflammatory signals leading to insulin resistance. For the first time, we show an association between adipose tissue expression of MAP3K8 and IL-1ß, IL-6 and IL-8 in humans. In line with this, our data reveal that MAP3K8 deficiency in HFD-fed mice reduces adipose tissue expression of IL-1ß, IL-6 and IL-8. Therefore, we propose that MAP3K8 may affect production of specific cytokines in adipose tissue inflammation during development of obesity, but that these changes do not translate to profound systemic effects. Although we cannot rule out an effect on insulin sensitivity upon specific inhibition of the MAP3K8 signalling pathway during obesity, future studies should rather illuminate the role of other inflammatory pathways and kinases in adipose tissue affecting systemic metabolic health.

Author Contributions

Conceived and designed the experiments: DB PvE HS CT MN LJ RS. Performed the experiments: DB PvE JvD HJ AH. Analyzed the data: DB JvD CT MN LJ RS. Contributed reagents/materials/analysis tools: TM HS. Wrote the paper: DB JvD CT MN LJ RS.

References

1. Gregor MF, Hotamisligil GS (2011) Inflammatory Mechanisms in Obesity. Annu Rev Immunol.

2. Donath MY, Shoelson SE (2011) Type 2 diabetes as an inflammatory disease. Nat Rev Immunol 11: 98–107.

3. Olefsky JM, Glass CK (2010) Macrophages, inflammation, and insulin resistance. Annu Rev Physiol 72: 219–246.

4. Tanti JF, Jager J (2009) Cellular mechanisms of insulin resistance: role of stress-regulated serine kinases and insulin receptor substrates (IRS) serine phosphorylation. Curr Opin Pharmacol 9: 753–762.

5. Jager J, Gremeaux T, Cormont M, Le Marchand-Brustel Y, Tanti JF (2007) Interleukin-1beta-induced insulin resistance in adipocytes through down-regulation of insulin receptor substrate-1 expression. Endocrinology 148: 241–251.

6. Bost F, Aouadi M, Caron L, Even P, Belmonte N, et al. (2005) The extracellular signal-regulated kinase isoform ERK1 is specifically required for in vitro and in vivo adipogenesis. Diabetes 54: 402–411.

7. Chiariello M, Marinissen MJ, Gutkind JS (2000) Multiple mitogen-activated protein kinase signaling pathways connect the cot oncoprotein to the c-jun promoter and to cellular transformation. Mol Cell Biol 20: 1747–1758.

8. Salmeron A, Ahmad TB, Carlile GW, Pappin D, Narsimhan RP, et al. (1996) Activation of MEK-1 and SEK-1 by Tpl-2 proto-oncoprotein, a novel MAP kinase kinase kinase. EMBO J 15: 817–826.

9. Dumitru CD, Ceci JD, Tsatsanis C, Kontoyiannis D, Stamatakis K, et al. (2000) TNF-alpha induction by LPS is regulated posttranscriptionally via a Tpl2/ERK-dependent pathway. Cell 103: 1071–1083.

10. Jager J, Gremeaux T, Gonzalez T, Bonnafous S, Debard C, et al. (2010) Tpl2 kinase is upregulated in adipose tissue in obesity and may mediate interleukin-1beta and tumor necrosis factor-{alpha} effects on extracellular signal-regulated kinase activation and lipolysis. Diabetes 59: 61–70.

11. Perfield JW 2nd, Lee Y, Shulman GI, Samuel VT, Jurczak MJ, et al. (2011) Tumor progression locus 2 (TPL2) regulates obesity-associated inflammation and insulin resistance. Diabetes 60: 1168–1176.

12. Lancaster GI, Kowalski GM, Estevez E, Kraakman MJ, Grigoriadis G, et al. (2012) Tumor progression locus 2 (Tpl2) deficiency does not protect against obesity-induced metabolic disease. PLoS One 7: e39100.

13. Sugimoto K, Ohata M, Miyoshi J, Ishizaki H, Tsuboi N, et al. (2004) A serine/threonine kinase, Cot/Tpl2, modulates bacterial DNA-induced IL-12 production and Th cell differentiation. J Clin Invest 114: 857–866.

14. Vougioukalaki M, Kanellis DC, Gkouskou K, Eliopoulos AG (2011) Tpl2 kinase signal transduction in inflammation and cancer. Cancer Lett 304: 80–89.

15. Mielke LA, Elkins KL, Wei L, Starr R, Tsichlis PN, et al. (2009) Tumor progression locus 2 (Map3k8) is critical for host defense against Listeria monocytogenes and IL-1 beta production. J Immunol 183: 7984–7993.

16. Gantke T, Sriskantharajah S, Ley SC (2011) Regulation and function of TPL-2, an IkappaB kinase-regulated MAP kinase kinase kinase. Cell Res 21: 131–145.

17. Raman M, Chen W, Cobb MH (2007) Differential regulation and properties of MAPKs. Oncogene 26: 3100–3112.

18. Dinarello CA (2010) How interleukin-1beta induces gouty arthritis. Arthritis Rheum 62: 3140–3144.

19. Chassaing B, Aitken JD, Gewirtz AT, Vijay-Kumar M (2012) Gut microbiota drives metabolic disease in immunologically altered mice. Adv Immunol 116: 93–112.

10

High Dietary Magnesium Intake is Associated with Low Insulin Resistance in the Newfoundland Population

Farrell Cahill[1][9], **Mariam Shahidi**[1][9], **Jennifer Shea**[1], **Danny Wadden**[1], **Wayne Gulliver**[1], **Edward Randell**[2], **Sudesh Vasdev**[1], **Guang Sun**[1]*

1 Division of Medicine, Faculty of Medicine, Memorial University of Newfoundland, St. John's, Canada, 2 Discipline of Laboratory Medicine, Faculty of Medicine, Memorial University of Newfoundland, St. John's, Canada

Abstract

Background: Magnesium plays a role in glucose and insulin homeostasis and evidence suggests that magnesium intake is associated with insulin resistance (IR). However, data is inconsistent and most studies have not adequately controlled for critical confounding factors.

Objective: The study investigated the association between magnesium intake and IR in normal-weight (NW), overweight (OW) and obese (OB) along with pre- and post- menopausal women.

Design: A total of 2295 subjects (590 men and 1705 women) were recruited from the CODING study. Dietary magnesium intake was computed from the Willett Food Frequency Questionnaire (FFQ). Adiposity (NW, OW and OB) was classified by body fat percentage (%BF) measured by Dual-energy X-ray absorptiometry according to the Bray criteria. Multiple regression analyses were used to test adiposity-specific associations of dietary magnesium intake on insulin resistance adjusting for caloric intake, physical activity, medication use and menopausal status.

Results: Subjects with the highest intakes of dietary magnesium had the lowest levels of circulating insulin, HOMA-IR, and HOMA-ß and subjects with the lowest intake of dietary magnesium had the highest levels of these measures, suggesting a dose effect. Multiple regression analysis revealed a strong inverse association between dietary magnesium with IR. In addition, adiposity and menopausal status were found to be critical factors revealing that the association between dietary magnesium and IR was stronger in OW and OB along with Pre-menopausal women.

Conclusion: The results of this study indicate that higher dietary magnesium intake is strongly associated with the attenuation of insulin resistance and is more beneficial for overweight and obese individuals in the general population and pre-menopausal women. Moreover, the inverse correlation between insulin resistance and dietary magnesium intake is stronger when adjusting for %BF than BMI.

Editor: Yiqing Song, Brigham & Women's Hospital, and Harvard Medical School, United States of America

Funding: None of the authors had a personal or financial conflict of interest. This study was supported in part by the Canadian Foundation for Innovation (CFI) and the Canadian Institute for Health Research (operating grant: OOP-77984 to Guang Sun). The funders had no role in study design, data collection and analysis, decision to publish, or preparation of the manuscript.

Competing Interests: The authors have declared that no competing interests exist.

* E-mail: gsun@mun.ca

[9] These authors contributed equally to this work.

Introduction

Type 2 diabetes comprises 90% of all diabetic cases and has become an ever increasing healthcare challenge as the number of people affected reaches epidemic proportions [1]. The prevalence of this condition is expected to reach over 438 million people globally by the year 2030 and carries with it a significant fiscal burden [2]. This is especially relevant to the Canadian province of Newfoundland and Labrador considering it has one the highest rates of diabetes and obesity in Canada. Currently, 9% of the population of Newfoundland and Labrador struggle with diabetes which corresponds to an annual cost of $254 million dollars [3]. The Canadian Diabetes Association has projected that by the year 2020 over 15% of Newfoundland and Labradorean's will be diabetic with an annual health care cost exceeding $360 million dollars [3]. Although there is currently no medical intervention capable of preventing the development of diabetes, simple lifestyle modifications (such as increased physical activity, moderate weight loss, and eating behavior modifications) have been shown to attenuate the onset of type 2 diabetes [1,4]. However few studies to date have investigated the association between dietary micronutrient intake and insulin function in the general population.

Magnesium, a cofactor required in over 300 enzymatic reactions, is the fourth most abundant cation in the human body involved with both glucose metabolism and insulin homeostasis [5,6]. Although recent evidence has suggested that dietary magnesium intake may play an important role in enhancing insulin sensitivity, population based studies have found conflicting evidence regarding the potential benefit of dietary magnesium intake. Several studies have correlated low dietary magnesium intake [7–9] and serum magnesium [10] with increased insulin resistance [11–13]. However, other studies do not support the proposed protective effect that dietary magnesium can attenuate the development of diabetes [14–16]. Of note, most studies have not adequately controlled for adiposity in their analysis. Instead of controlling for relative body fat, the majority of studies have utilized the body mass index (BMI) which cannot accurately distinguish fat mass from and fat-free mass [17]. Since adiposity is the parameter most closely linked with the development of insulin resistance [18], controlling for this important confounding factor is critical. Therefore we designed the present study to investigate the association between magnesium intake and insulin resistance in the Canadian province of Newfoundland and Labrador, taking into consideration age, gender, caloric intake, physical activity, medication use, smoking status, menopause and adiposity.

Methods

Ethics Statement

Ethics approval was obtained from the Human Investigation Committee, Faculty of Medicine, Memorial University, St. John's, Newfoundland, Canada. All subjects provided written and informed consent before participation in this study.

Subjects

All 2330 subjects (600 men 1725 women) from the current study are volunteers from the general population of Newfoundland and Labrador and the cohort for our ongoing CODING (Complex Diseases in the Newfoundland Population: Environment and Genetics) Study. The CODING study is a large-scale nutrige-nomics investigation [17,19,20]. Eligibility of participants for the CODING study are based upon the following inclusion criteria: 1) ≥19 yrs of age; 2) at least a third generation Newfoundlander; and 3) healthy, without any serious metabolic, cardiovascular, or endocrine diseases. The primary method of subject recruitment for the CODING study was the use of posters and handouts. This literature was distributed throughout public facilities (offices, hospitals, and gyms) in the city of St. John's, Newfoundland and Labrador. All subjects completed screening questionnaires providing information about physical characteristics, physical activity, health status, and dietary practices. Anthropometrics, body composition, and biochemical measurements were collected following a 12 hour fast.

Physical Activity

Physical activity patterns were measured using the ARIC-Baecke Questionnaire, which consists of a Work Index, Sports Index, and Leisure Time Activity Index [21].

Dietary Magnesium Assessment

Dietary intake patterns of each participant were assessed using a 124 item semi-quantitative Willett Food Frequency Questionnaire (FFQ) [22]. The Willett FFQ is one of the most commonly used dietary questionnaires for large-scale epidemiologic studies [23]. The Willett FFQ obtains from subjects, the number of weekly servings consumed of specific food item(s). NutriBase Clinical Nutrition Manager (version 8.2.0; CybersoftInc, Phoenix, AZ) software package was used to convert weekly serving values into mean daily serving values to calculate the total daily intake of magnesium (mg/day) for each individual. The nutritional information, including dietary magnesium intake, was computed for all subjects in the CODING study [19].

Anthropometric and Body Composition Measurements

Subjects were weighed (Health O Meter, Bridgeview, IL) to the nearest 0.1 kg in standardized clothing (hospital gown). Height was measured using a fixed stadiometer (nearest 0.1 cm). Body mass index (kg/m^2) was calculated as weight in kilograms divided by participants' height in meters squared. Whole body composition measurements including fat mass, lean body mass, and bone mineral densities were measured using dual-energy X-ray absorptiometry (DXA) Lunar Prodigy (GE Medical Systems, Madison, WI). DXA can produce an accurate measurement of adipose tissue within the body with a low margin of error. For this reason, DXA is considered to be one of the most accurate measurements of adiposity. DXA measurements were performed on subjects following the removal of all metal accessories, while lying in a supine position as previously described by us [17,19,20]. Body fat percentage (%BF) is determined as a ratio of fat mass to total body mass (Version 12.2 of the enCORE software). Quality assurance was performed on our DXA scanner daily and the typical CV was 1.3% during the study period.

Biochemical Measurements

Serum concentrations of glucose and magnesium were measured on an Lx20 analyzer (Beckman Coulter Inc., Fullerton, CA) using Synchron reagents. Serum insulin was measured on an Immulite Immunoassay analyzer. Insulin resistance and beta cell function were determined with the homeostasis model assessment (HOMA), as described by Matthews et al [24].

$$HOMA-IR = ((Fasting\_Insulin[mU/L] \times Fasting\_Glu\cos e[mmol/L])/22.5)$$

$$HOMA-\beta = ((20 \times Fasting\_Insulin[mU/L] /(Fasting\_Glu\cos e[mmol/L]-3.5))$$

Smoking, Medication and Menopausal Status

A self-administered screening questionnaire was used to collect information about the subjects' demographics, personal and family medical history, medication use (yes or no), and smoking status (yes or no). Women completed an additional questionnaire regarding menstrual history and menopausal status (pre- or post-menopausal) [17,19].

Statistical analysis

All data are reported as mean ± standard deviation (SD) unless otherwise stated. Participants with daily total caloric intake (kcal/day) falling outside the range of ±3SDs were considered outliers and excluded from further analyses to account for possible errors associated with over- or under-reporting of food intake on the FFQ. Insulin, HOMA-IR, and HOMA-β were log-transformed to normalize distributions and meet the assumptions of statistical tests. The sample size for the study was 2295 participants (590 men, 1705 women). Differences in physical, biochemical, and dietary patterns between men and women were assessed using one-way ANOVA. Subjects were subdivided by adiposity into Normal-Weight (NW), Overweight (OW), and Obese (OB) groups based on %BF measured by DXA according to the age and gender-specific criteria recommended by Bray [25]. Differences in physical, biochemical, and dietary patterns among adiposity groups was assessed using a one-way ANCOVA controlling for age, gender, total caloric intake, physical activity, medication use and smoking and menopause. As the number of underweight subjects was too low (n = 28) to perform effective statistical analysis, they were excluded from these analyses. To initially explore the relationship between dietary magnesium and IR (fasting glucose (mmol/l), insulin (pmol/l), HOMA-IR, HOMA-β), participants were divided into a tertile (low, medium, or high) based upon dietary magnesium intake (mg/day) which were assessed using an ANCOVA controlling for age, gender, total caloric intake, physical activity, medication use, smoking, menopause and %BF. Subsequently, multiple regression analyses were used to more rigorously explore the potential association of dietary magnesium intake (g/kg body weight) with insulin resistance (HOMA-IR) within the entire cohort and among men and women adjusting for age, gender, caloric intake, physical activity, medication use, smoking, menopause and %BF or BMI. However, only caloric intake, physical activity, medication use, menopause and %BF or BMI were statistically considered as confounding variables within the regression models. In addition, due to the significant interaction of adiposity and menopause on the association between dietary magnesium intake and insulin resistance, multiple regression analysis was performed among normal-weight, overweight and obese subjects along with pre-menopausal (n = 834) and post-menopausal (n = 577) women. Multiple regression analyses were performed on subjects stratified into tertiles (low, medium, or high) based upon both BMI and %BF measured from DXA to assess the difference in their adjustments on the relationship between dietary magnesium intake and insulin resistance. Lastly, Binary logistic analysis was also performed to explore the association between magnesium intake (g/kg/day) and diabetes status. Diabetes status was defined by a fasting glucose cutoff (glucose >7.0 mmol/L) together with those individuals who reported they were diabetics. Under the aforementioned definition, 102 subjects were labeled as diabetics for this analysis. Age, gender, caloric intake, physical activity, medication use, menopausal status, and smoking status were used as covariates. However, only caloric intake, medication status and age were statistically considered as confounding variables within the binary logistic model. Some subjects had missing data in one or more measurements. Five subjects did not disclose their smoking status and eight subjects did not respond to the medication use question. 1981 participants had all complete dataset for all variables measured to be used for the ANCOVA and multiple regression analysis. All statistical analyses were performed with and without diabetic subjects; however none of the results were not affected. All statistical analyses were performed using PASW 19.0 (SPSS Inc., Chicago, IL). All tests were two-sided and a p-value <0.05 was considered to be statistically significant.

Results

Physical, Biochemical, and Dietary Characteristics of Normal-weight, Overweight, and Obese participants

Physical, biochemical, and dietary characteristics for men and women along with those for normal-weight, overweight and obese participants are presented in **Table 1**. Glucose, insulin, and HOMA-IR were significantly greater for men than women, but HOMA-β was significantly greater among women. In terms of dietary intake, male participants had a significantly higher total daily caloric and magnesium intake than females. However, women had significantly greater magnesium intake (mg/day/kg) per kilogram body weight than men. Insulin, glucose, HOMA-β, and HOMA-IR values were greater among overweight and obese

subjects, which we have previously described [17,19,20]. Individuals with the highest insulin, HOMA-IR and HOMA-β had the highest levels of adiposity. In addition, subjects with highest levels of adiposity had the lowest levels of magnesium intake (mg/day), and magnesium intake per kilogram of body weight (mg/day/kg). The findings remained significant after controlling for total age, gender, caloric intake, physical activity, medication use, menopausal status and smoking status. Serum magnesium was not significantly different among adiposity groups (**Table 1**).

Insulin Resistance Among Low, Medium, and High Dietary Magnesium Intake Groups

Physical, biochemical, and dietary characteristics were assessed among a tertile (low, medium, or high) based upon dietary magnesium intake (mg/day) (**Table 2**). Those individuals with the highest magnesium intake had the lowest insulin, HOMA-IR and HOMA-ß. Individuals with the lowest magnesium intake had the highest fasting insulin levels, HOMA-IR, and HOMA-ß. The findings remained significant after accounting for age, gender, caloric intake, physical activity, medication use, smoking, menopause and %BF. The dietary magnesium intake ranged from; 33.06 to 270.83 mg/day in the low dietary magnesium intake group, 270.84 to 393.66 mg/day in the medium dietary magnesium intake group, and 394.07 to 2493.01 mg/day in the high dietary magnesium intake group. Dietary magnesium intake per kilogram of body weight ranged from; 0.43 to 5.3 mg/kg/day in the low dietary magnesium intake group, 2.0 to 8.18 mg/kg/day in the medium dietary magnesium intake group, and 3.17 to 44.84 mg/kg/day in the high dietary magnesium intake group.

Relationship between Dietary Magnesium and Insulin Resistance

Unadjusted and adjusted linear regression analysis results of dietary magnesium intake on insulin resistance are shown in **Table 3**. There was a significant negative association between dietary magnesium intake (g/day/kg) with HOMA-IR in the entire cohort before and after adjusting for caloric intake, physical activity, medication use, menopausal status and %BF or BMI. In addition, the negative association between magnesium intake and insulin resistance was greater having adjusted for adiposity (%BF) over adjusting for BMI (**Table 3**). Multiple regression analysis of the entire study cohort also revealed a significant interaction of adiposity (%BF & BMI) with the negative association of magnesium intake with insulin resistance. Therefore, multiple regression analysis was performed on NW, OW and OB groups based upon %BF according to the Bray Criteria (**Table 3**). Magnesium intake was found to be significantly negatively associated with HOMA-IR among all adiposity groups. This inverse relationship was greater among overweight and obese subjects and pre-menopausal women.

Relationship between Dietary Magnesium and Insulin Resistance Among Low, Medium and High %BF and BMI

Unadjusted and adjusted linear regression analysis results of dietary magnesium intake (g/day/kg) on insulin resistance among low, medium and high BMI and %BF groups are shown in **Table 4**. Magnesium intake was increasingly more negatively associated with HOMA-IR the greater the adiposity (%BF) or body mass index (BMI). Moreover, the negative association between dietary magnesium intake and insulin resistance was more prevalent according to a %BF classification than a BMI classification (**Table 4**).

Table 1. Physical, Biochemical, and Dietary Intake Characteristics of Normal-weight, Overweight, and Obese Participants.

	Entire Cohort	Gender Male	Female	Percent Body Fat - Bray Criteria Normal Weight	Overweight	Obese	p
	(n = 2295)	(n = 590)	(n = 1705)	(n = 547)	(n = 600)	(n = 781)	
Age (yr) [3]	43.16±13	41.04±14.4	43.92±12.4	40.96±14.34	45.02±12.53	44.14±12.3	<0.001
Weight (kg)[2]	74.72±16.5	86.86±15.8	70.5±14.5	64.63±10.47	71.22±11.37	86.12±16.53	<0.001
Height (cm)[2]	165.8±8.6	176.09±6.5	162.24±5.9	166.68±8.5	165.32±8.2	165.98±9.0	NS
Waist (cm)[2]	93.07±15	98.68±13.9	91.13±14.9	82.35±9	90.8±10.3	103.68±14.5	<0.001
Hip (cm)[3]	101.66±11.9	100.8±10.4	101.94±12.4	92.76±6.6	99.48±7.2	110.25±11.8	<0.001
Waist-Hip Ratio[2]	0.91±0.1	0.98±0.1	0.89±0.1	0.89±0.1	0.91±0.1	0.93±0.1	<0.001
BMI (kg/m²)[2]	27.1±5.2	27.98±4.6	26.79±5.4	23.17±2.6	25.97±2.9	31.19±5.0	<0.001
Total Body Fat (%)[3]	35.17±9.1	26.31±7.7	38.22±7.5	26.86±6.5	34.86±5.7	42.12±6.6	<0.001
Glucose (mmol/L)[2]	5.16±0.9	5.35±1	5.09±0.9	4.98±0.7	5.15±0.8	5.33±1.1	<0.001
Insulin (pmol/L)[2]	68.86±67.7	73.53±63	67.2±69.3	50.58±59.3	64.16±72.8	84.74±73.2	<0.001
HOMA-IR[2]	2.39±3.3	2.65±3.4	2.3±3.3	1.72±3.4	2.21±3.6	3.0±3.4	<0.001
HOMA-β[3]	133.99±165	127.24±129.4	136.25±175.8	111.98±176.3	122.75±102.65	153.38±204.4	<0.001
Magnesium intake (mg/day)[2]	368.57±210.4	394.29±228.7	359.66±203.3	415.96±253.78	354.06±171.3	351.5±208.7	0.003
Magnesium intake (mg/day/kg)[3]	5.15±3.1	4.68±2.8	5.3±3.26	6.51±3.9	5.05±2.5	4.2±2.4	<0.001
Serum Magnesium (mmol/L)[2]	0.88±0.1	0.9±0.09	0.87±0.08	0.88±0.08	0.88±0.08	0.87±0.08	NS
Calories (kcal/day)[2]	1985.8±878.6	2246.5±982.7	1896.1±821.7	2118.6±937.1	1885.9±764.62	1958±897.4	<0.001

[1]Data presented as mean ± SD. Homeostasis model assessment of insulin resistance (HOMA-IR) and β-cell function (HOMA-β). Gender differences were assessed with a one-way ANOVA. Subjects were also stratified into normal-weight, overweight and obese based upon %BF according to the Bray criteria (25). Adiposity differences were assessed with an ANCOVA controlling for caloric intake, physical activity, medication use, and menopause. [2]Significantly greater for men compared to women. [3]Significantly greater for women compared to men. [4]Statistical significance for one-way ANOVA and ANCOVA were set to p<0.05 (IBM SPSS Statistics 19).

Table 2. Physical, Biochemical, and Dietary Intake Characteristics According to Magnesium Intake.

	Dietary Magnesium Intake (mg/day) Low Mg Intake	Medium Mg Intake	High Mg Intake	p
	(n = 765)	(n = 765)	(n = 765)	–
Age (yr)	43.78±12.1	43.49±12.3	42.22±14.5	–
Weight (kg)	74.63±16.7	74.46±15.9	75.04±16.8	NS
Height (cm)	164.7±8.2	165.65±8.3	167.07±9.0	NS
Waist (cm)	94.3±15.0	92.94±15.4	91.93±14.5	NS
Hip (cm)	102.99±11.8	101.78±11.9	100.18±11.9	NS
Waist-Hip Ratio	0.91±0.08	0.91±0.08	0.92±0.09	NS
BMI (kg/m²)	27.4±5.3	27.08±5.1	26.79±5.2	NS
Total Body Fat (%)	36.68±8.3	35.3±9.1	33.5±9.7	–
Glucose (mmol/L)	5.18±0.8	5.18±1.0	5.17±1.0	NS
Insulin (pmol/L)	72.82±68.6	71.45±91.3	60.57±42.9	<0.001
HOMA-IR	2.49±2.5	2.59±5.2	2.07±1.8	0.003
HOMA-β	142.37±213.3	135.7±182.0	116.24±89.9	<0.001
Magnesium intake (mg/day)	201.57±48.6	328.85±36.3	575.98±224.1	<0.001
Magnesium intake (mg/day/kg)	2.83±0.9	4.59±1.0	7.99±3.6	<0.001
Serum Magnesium (mmol/L)	0.88±0.08	0.88±0.07	0.89±0.08	0.023
Calories (kcal/day)	1299.11±409.9	1904.21±440.42	2747.22±928.49	–

[1]Data presented as mean ± SD. Homeostasis model assessment of insulin resistance (HOMA-IR) and β-cell function (HOMA-β).
[2]Subjects were stratified into a tertile (low, medium and high) based upon magnesium intake (mg/day).
[3]Magnesium intake group differences were assessed with an ANCOVA controlling for caloric intake, physical activity, medication use, menopause and %BF.
[4]Statistical significance for one-way ANCOVA was set to p<0.05 (IBM SPSS Statistics 19).

Table 3. Regression Models of Magnesium Intake on Insulin Resistance.

	Unadjusted			Adjusted			Adjusted+%BF			Adjusted+BMI		
	β	β*	p	β	β*	p	β	β*	p	β	β*	p
HOMA-IR												
Entire Cohort	−21.03 (1.8)	−0.232 (0.02)	<0.0001	−33.75 (2.9)	−0.374 (0.03)	<0.0001	−19.33 (2.9)	−0.214 (0.03)	<0.0001	−11.65 (2.9)	−0.129 (0.03)	<0.0001
Normal-weight	−7.68 (2.6)	−0.085 (0.03)	0.003	−10.92 (4.0)	−0.120 (0.05)	<0.0001	–	–	–	–	–	–
Overweight	−12.84 (3.9)	−0.141 (0.04)	0.001	−30.13 (6.9)	−0.332 (0.08)	<0.0001	–	–	–	–	–	–
Obese	−23.79 (4.0)	−0.262 (0.04)	<0.0001	−45.97 (6.5)	−0.506 (0.07)	<0.0001	–	–	–	–	–	–
Pre-Menopause	−15.07 (2.5)	−0.188 (0.03)	<0.0001	−35.32 (4.4)	−0.439 (0.05)	<0.0001	−20.4 (4.6)	−0.254 (0.05)	<0.001	−13.57 (4.4)	−0.169 (0.05)	0.002
Post-Menopause	−18.91 (3.5)	−0.208 (0.04)	<0.0001	−27.44 (4.6)	−0.311 (0.05)	<0.0001	−16.89 (4.8)	−0.191 (0.05)	<0.001	−7.32 (4.6)	−0.083 (0.05)	NS

[1]Regression model adjusted for caloric intake, physical activity, medication use and menopausal status.
[2]β = Unstandardized Beta (standard error), β* = Standardized Beta (standard error), Magnesium intake (g/day/kg).
[3]Normal-weight, overweight and obese groups are based upon %BF according to the Bray criteria (25).
[4]Magnesium intake (Pre-Menopause 360.63±209.8 mg/day, Post-Menopause 353.82±192.9 mg/day) (Entire cohort, Normal-weight, Overweight, & Obese – See Table.1).
[5]Statistical significance was set to p<0.05 (IBM SPSS Statistics 19).

Relationship between Dietary Magnesium and Diabetes Status

Binary logistic analysis, performed to explore the association between magnesium intake (g/kg/day) with diabetes status, revealed that magnesium intake (g/kg/day) was significantly negatively associated with diabetes status (n = 102, Unstandardized β = −499.80, standard error 79.45, p<0.0001). Caloric intake, medication status and age were statistically considered as confounding variables within the binary logistic model.

Serum Magnesium and Markers of Insulin Resistance

The relationship between serum magnesium and insulin resistance was also explored. Although serum magnesium concentration concomitantly increased with dietary magnesium intake, it was not found to be significantly associated with insulin resistance in the Newfoundland population (data not shown).

Discussion

The noteworthy finding of the present investigation was a beneficial dose dependent relationship between dietary magnesium intake and insulin resistance, independent of age gender, total caloric intake, physical activity, medication use, menopause, and adiposity. However, this favorable association was more significant in overweight and obese subjects suggesting that this population may be more sensitive to the beneficial effects of dietary magnesium intake. Obesity, as a disorder, is a well-known

Table 4. Regression Models of Magnesium Intake on Insulin Resistance based upon %BF and BMI.

	Body Fat Percentage								
	Low			Medium			High		
	β	β*	p	β	β*	p	β	β*	p
Entire Cohort									
Unadjusted	−14.98 (2.5)	−0.165 (0.03)	<0.0001	−17.36 (3.4)	−0.191 (0.04)	<0.0001	−20.98 (4.1)	−0.231 (0.05)	<0.0001
Adjusted	−14.30 (4.1)	−0.157 (0.04)	0.001	−23.39 (6.0)	−0.258 (0.07)	0.0002	−45.59 (6.48)	−0.502 (0.07)	0.000
	Body Mass Index								
Entire Cohort									
Unadjusted	−3.89 (2.1)	−0.043 (0.02)	NS	−12.4 (3.5)	−0.137 (0.04)	0.0004	−24.27 (4.7)	−0.267 (0.05)	<0.0001
Adjusted	−9.97 (3.5)	−0.110 (0.04)	0.004	−12.8 (6.4)	−0.141 (0.07)	0.047	−57.6 (7.9)	−0.446 (0.08)	0.000

[1]Regression model adjusted for caloric intake, physical activity, medication use and menopausal status.Subjects were also stratified into a tertiles(Low, Medium and High) based upon %BF and BMI.
[2]β = Unstandardized Beta (standard error), β* = Standardized Beta (standard error), Magnesium intake (g/day/kg).
[3]Magnesium intake (Low BMI 409.78±243.5 mg/day, Medium BMI 353.24±180.9 mg/day, High BMI 342.76±196.1 mg/day) (Low %BF 387.5±230.3 mg/day, Medium %BF 360.54±187.5 mg/day, High %BF 357.68±210.7 mg/day).
[4]Statistical significance was set to p<0.05 (IBM SPSS Statistics 19).

condition which can place individuals at a significantly elevated risk for impaired insulin action [26] and various metabolic abnormalities such as hypertension, dyslipidemia, and a reduction in glucose tolerance [26]. The functional relationship between various hormones and obesity-related conditions is a significant focus of obesity research, however diet composition has become increasingly recognized and studied [2,4]. One study specifically demonstrated that an increase in dietary magnesium can significantly improve insulin sensitivity [27]. Magnesium has been proposed to be functionally related to glucose metabolism through an interaction with tyrosine-kinase activity on the insulin receptor which is associated with the development of insulin resistance and type 2 diabetes [28]. Studies have suggested that the effect of dietary magnesium on decreasing markers of IR [11,12] and development of type 2 diabetes is more pronounced in overweight patients [11,12]. However, body fat percentage was not measured in these studies. This is an especially important point to consider when the relative amount and distribution of adipose tissue, both important determinants of insulin sensitivity, cannot be determined by the body mass index [29–31].

In fact the majority of studies evaluating the association between dietary magnesium and insulin resistance have only utilized BMI when attempting to control for adiposity, bearing in mind that percent body fat and BMI likely represent different physiological entities. Having adjusted for the influence of %BF and BMI on the association of dietary magnesium intake with insulin resistance, we observed that this inverse association was stronger after having adjusted for %BF than for BMI which further supports our hypothesis. Considering that our laboratory and others have revealed that BMI is not an accurate measure of body fat due to its inability to differentiate fat mass from fat free mass [20,32,33], it is implicit that BMI cannot represent adiposity. We found that overweight and obese individuals, defined by a high resolution adiposity measurement, are more sensitive to the beneficial effect of magnesium intake on insulin resistance. Our current findings, taken together with others of others [11,12] provides strong evidence that overweight individuals, classified by either %BF or BMI, could potentially benefit from an increase in magnesium intake. It is possible that overweight and obese individuals are better able to absorb and metabolize magnesium, thereby enhancing its action at the insulin receptor and promoting insulin sensitivity. To our knowledge, this study is the first large cross-sectional study to systematically control for major confounding factors including %BF when analyzing the relationship between dietary magnesium intake and markers of insulin resistance. This study is also the first investigation to observe that dietary magnesium is more strongly associated with insulin resistance when adjusting for %BF than BMI.

The association between dietary magnesium intake and insulin resistance was examined with regards smoking [34], menopause [12] and medication [35,36] as possible confounding factors for this relationship. Evidence suggests that nicotine intake may increase insulin resistance, however we did not find a significant association of smoking status with HOMA-IR or magnesium intake. In addition, during the regression model development smoking status failed to reach statistical significance and was not included in the regression model. Our data would suggest that smoking is not a critical confounding factor regarding the beneficial effect of dietary magnesium intake on insulin resistance in the Newfoundland population. However, this finding may be due to the significantly smaller sample size of smokers (n = 222) to non-smokers (n = 1754) in our study cohort. Further study is needed to elucidate the potential interaction of smoking on the relationship of dietary magnesium intake and insulin resistance.

Medication status was significantly associated with insulin resistance and there is evidence to suggest that various medications inhibit magnesium re-absorption in the kidney which can result in magnesium deficiency [35,36]. However, we were unable to find a significant interaction of medication use on the inverse association with magnesium intake and insulin resistance. Pre-menopausal women were more significantly associated the beneficial effects of magnesium intake on insulin resistance than post-menopausal women. This finding is strengthened by the Shanghai Women's Health Study, designed to assess the prospective risk of type 2 diabetes, which found a statistically significant negative correlation between magnesium intake and type 2 diabetes risk in pre-menopausal women only [12]. We considered, since over 68% of our post-menopausal women are medication users, that the lack of association of magnesium intake with insulin resistance could be drug related interference. However, this relationship remained absent among post-menopausal women whether or not medication status was included in the regression model. Therefore, our data would suggest that the beneficial effects of magnesium intake are less sensitive among post-menopausal women and further study is needed to explore the physiological mechanism involved. Lastly, we discovered that magnesium intake was significantly negatively associated with diabetes. Considering that insulin resistance is a significant clinical symptom of diabetes and that insulin resistance was significantly inversely associated with magnesium intake this, finding was not surprising. Our results suggest that the potential beneficial influence of magnesium intake exists in a wide range of populations from the general population to insulin resistance and to those people struggling with struggling with diabetes in Newfoundland and Labrador.

Aside from investigating the influence of %BF and BMI on the association between magnesium intake and insulin resistance in the general population and the influence that an adiposity status defined by %BF has on this relationship, we also investigated whether an adiposity status defined by BMI would have a different effect than %BF on this association.

Considering that the adiposity status criteria for the World Health Organization (WHO) [1] is considerably different from that developed by Bray et al. [25], the association between dietary magnesium intake and insulin resistance was examined among low, medium and high tertiles according to %BF and BMI. Our data revealed that the inverse relationship between dietary magnesium intake and insulin resistance was progressively stronger the greater the %BF or BMI. However, the aforementioned association was more significantly pronounced for concomitant increases in %BF over BMI. Consider that %BF is a more direct measure of adiposity than BMI, together with our current findings, we recommend that %BF be used when considering adiposity as a factor.

The apparent protective role of magnesium on IR and type 2 diabetes has not been fully explained but is likely due to enhanced insulin sensitivity through multiple mechanisms. For example, phosphorylation of the tyrosine kinase enzyme of the insulin receptor, required for post-receptor insulin sensitivity and subsequent insulin-mediated glucose uptake, is dependent on adequate intracellular concentrations of magnesium [37]. As such, we also chose to investigate the relationship between serum magnesium and markers of IR; no significant association between them was observed. Inconsistencies have been present in previous studies examining this relationship, some supporting a negative correlation [38,39] and others not [10]. One possible explanation for these differences is that serum magnesium may not accurately reflect intracellular magnesium levels, which may be low, even when serum levels are within the normal range [14]. Additional studies are warranted to further clarify the relationship between serum magnesium and markers of IR.

Our study had certain limitations, many of which were due to its cross-sectional design. Firstly, our use of a FFQ to evaluate patterns of dietary intake raises the possibility of recall bias by subjects. However, the Willett FFQ chosen for this study is one of the most commonly applied tool for the evaluation of dietary intake in epidemiologic population-based studies [22,23]. In addition, dietary magnesium is highly correlated with other micronutrients and dietary components believed to affect insulin sensitivity, such as vegetables, fruits, potassium, calcium, and fiber. Thus, it is very difficult to separate their independent effects [7,12]. In addition, to avoid over-adjustment, we opted not to control for every available nutrient in our analysis. We did not measure or account for magnesium supplementation regarding daily magnesium intake, which could have potentially reduced the strength of the inverse association found between magnesium intake and IR makers. Furthermore, the reliability of serum magnesium levels in recognizing total body magnesium deficiency is unclear. Although intracellular magnesium concentrations are believed to provide a more accurate estimation of magnesium status, they are not generally easily measured [38]. Finally, our study enrolled Caucasian Newfoundlanders, so our findings may not be applicable to those from other ethnicities [16,40].

In summary, our cross-sectional study investigated the relationship between dietary magnesium intake and insulin resistance among 2295 Newfoundlanders and Labradoreans. To our knowledge this study is the most comprehensive of its kind having controlled for major confounding factors, most specifically being

dual energy x-ray absorptiometry (DXA) determined body fat percentage. Our findings suggest that higher dietary magnesium intake is associated with improved insulin sensitivity and this effect is particularly beneficial for overweight and obese individuals in the general population along with pre-menopausal women.

We also provide the first evidence that the association between dietary magnesium and insulin resistance is more strongly associated with %BF than BMI and the concomitant increase in %BF over BMI. Due to the fact that %BF more accurately represents adiposity than BMI, caution should be taken when attempting to utilize BMI as a measure of adiposity. Further large-scale prospective studies, where body fat is adequately accounted for and which enroll various ethnic groups, are needed to further elucidate the role of dietary magnesium in improving insulin function and preventing diabetes.

Acknowledgments

We would like to thank all of the volunteers who participated in the present study. We would also like to thank the following people for their contributions to the collection of data: Hong Wei Zhang, Peyvand Amini, and Andrew Lee.

Author Contributions

Assisted with insulin measurements: SV. Assisted with magnesium measurements: ER. Conceived and designed the experiments: FC MS JS WG GS. Performed the experiments: FC JS DW. Analyzed the data: FC MS JS DW. Contributed reagents/materials/analysis tools: ER SV WG. Wrote the paper: FC MS.

References

1. Organization WH (2011) World Health Organization Diabetes Fact Sheet No 312 World Health Organization. Geneva.
2. Canadian Diabetes Association (2009) The prevalence and costs of diabetes facts. Toronto: Canadian Diabetes Association.
3. Canadian Diabetes Association (2010) The Cost of Diabetes in Newfoundland and Labrador. Canadian Diabetes Association1–20 p.
4. Ur E, Ransom T, Chiasson J (2008) Prevention of Diabetes. Canadian Journal of Diabetes (suppl 1): S17–19.
5. Fox C, Ramsoomair D, Carter C (2001) Magnesium: its proven and potential clinical significance. South Med J 94: 1195–1201.
6. He K, Liu K, Daviglus ML, Morris SJ, Loria CM, et al. (2006) Magnesium intake and incidence of metabolic syndrome among young adults. Circulation 113: 1675–1682.
7. Rumawas ME, McKeown NM, Rogers G, Meigs JB, Wilson PW, et al. (2006) Magnesium intake is related to improved insulin homeostasis in the framingham offspring cohort. J Am Coll Nutr 25: 486–492.
8. McKeown NM, Jacques PF, Zhang XL, Juan W, Sahyoun NR (2008) Dietary magnesium intake is related to metabolic syndrome in older Americans. Eur J Nutr 47: 210–216.
9. Ma B, Lawson AB, Liese AD, Bell RA, Mayer-Davis EJ (2006) Dairy, magnesium, and calcium intake in relation to insulin sensitivity: approaches to modeling a dose-dependent association. Am J Epidemiol 164: 449–458.
10. Simmons D, Joshi S, Shaw J (2010) Hypomagnesaemia is associated with diabetes: Not pre-diabetes, obesity or the metabolic syndrome. Diabetes Res Clin Pract 87: 261–266.
11. Kim DJ, Xun P, Liu K, Loria C, Yokota K, et al. (2010) Magnesium intake in relation to systemic inflammation, insulin resistance, and the incidence of diabetes. Diabetes Care 33: 2604–2610.
12. Villegas R, Gao YT, Dai Q, Yang G, Cai H, et al. (2009) Dietary calcium and magnesium intakes and the risk of type 2 diabetes: the Shanghai Women's Health Study. Am J Clin Nutr 89: 1059–1067.
13. Song Y, Manson JE, Buring JE, Liu S (2004) Dietary magnesium intake in relation to plasma insulin levels and risk of type 2 diabetes in women. Diabetes Care 27: 59–65.
14. Kao WH, Folsom AR, Nieto FJ, Mo JP, Watson RL, et al. (1999) Serum and dietary magnesium and the risk for type 2 diabetes mellitus: the Atherosclerosis Risk in Communities Study. Arch Intern Med 159: 2151–2159.
15. Hodge AM, English DR, O'Dea K, Giles GG (2004) Glycemic index and dietary fiber and the risk of type 2 diabetes. Diabetes Care 27: 2701–2706.
16. Nanri A, Mizoue T, Noda M, Takahashi Y, Kirii K, et al. (2010) Magnesium intake and type II diabetes in Japanese men and women: the Japan Public Health Center-based Prospective Study. Eur J Clin Nutr 64: 1244–1247.
17. Shea JL, King MT, Yi Y, Gulliver W, Sun G (2011) Body fat percentage is associated with cardiometabolic dysregulation in BMI-defined normal weight subjects. Nutr Metab Cardiovasc Dis.
18. Buse J, Polonsky K, Burant C (2008) Type 2 Diabetes Mellitus; Williams K, editor. Philadelphia: Saunders Elsevier.
19. Green K, Shea J, Vasdev S, Randell E, Gulliver W, et al. (2010) Higher Dietary Protein Intake is Associated with Lower Body Fat in the Newfoundland Population. Clinical Medicine Insights: Endocrinology and Diabetes 3: 1–11.
20. Kennedy AP, Shea JL, Sun G (2009) Comparison of the classification of obesity by BMI vs. dual-energy X-ray absorptiometry in the Newfoundland population. Obesity (Silver Spring) 17: 2094–2099.
21. Baecke JA, Burema J, Frijters JE (1982) A short questionnaire for the measurement of habitual physical activity in epidemiological studies. Am J Clin Nutr 36: 936–942.
22. Willett WC, Sampson L, Stampfer MJ, Rosner B, Bain C, et al. (1985) Reproducibility and validity of a semiquantitative food frequency questionnaire. Am J Epidemiol 122: 51–65.
23. Subar AF, Thompson FE, Kipnis V, Midthune D, Hurwitz P, et al. (2001) Comparative validation of the Block, Willett, and National Cancer Institute food frequency questionnaires : the Eating at America's Table Study. Am J Epidemiol 154: 1089–1099.
24. Matthews DR, Hosker JP, Rudenski AS, Naylor BA, Treacher DF, et al. (1985) Homeostasis model assessment: insulin resistance and beta-cell function from fasting plasma glucose and insulin concentrations in man. Diabetologia 28: 412–419.
25. Bray G (2003) Contemporary diagnosis and management of obesity and the metabolic syndrome. Newtown: Handbooks in Health Care.
26. Gallagher EJ, Leroith D, Karnieli E (2010) Insulin resistance in obesity as the underlying cause for the metabolic syndrome. Mt Sinai J Med 77: 511–523.
27. Guerrero-Romero F, Tamez-Perez HE, Gonzalez-Gonzalez G, Salinas-Martinez AM, Montes-Villarreal J, et al. (2004) Oral magnesium supplementation improves insulin sensitivity in non-diabetic subjects with insulin resistance. A double-blind placebo-controlled randomized trial. Diabetes Metab 30: 253–258.
28. Kolterman OG, Gray RS, Griffin J, Burstein P, Insel J, et al. (1981) Receptor and postreceptor defects contribute to the insulin resistance in noninsulin-dependent diabetes mellitus. J Clin Invest 68: 957–969.
29. Leslie WD, Ludwig SM, Morin S (2010) Abdominal fat from spine dual-energy x-ray absorptiometry and risk for subsequent diabetes. J Clin Endocrinol Metab 95: 3272–3276.
30. Paradisi G, Smith L, Burtner C, Leaming R, Garvey WT, et al. (1999) Dual energy X-ray absorptiometry assessment of fat mass distribution and its

association with the insulin resistance syndrome. Diabetes Care 22: 1310–1317.

31. Rattarasarn C, Leelawattana R, Soonthornpun S, Setasuban W, Thamprasit A, et al. (2003) Relationships of body fat distribution, insulin sensitivity and cardiovascular risk factors in lean, healthy non-diabetic Thai men and women. Diabetes Res Clin Pract 60: 87–94.

32. Frankenfield DC, Rowe WA, Cooney RN, Smith JS, Becker D (2001) Limits of body mass index to detect obesity and predict body composition. Nutrition 17: 26–30.

33. Romero-Corral A, Somers VK, Sierra-Johnson J, Thomas RJ, Collazo-Clavell ML, et al. (2008) Accuracy of body mass index in diagnosing obesity in the adult general population. Int J Obes (Lond) 32: 959–966.

34. Bergman BC, Perreault L, Hunerdosse D, Kerege A, Playdon M, et al. (2012) Novel and Reversible Mechanisms of Smoking-Induced Insulin Resistance in Humans. Diabetes.

35. Dyckner T, Wester PO (1985) Renal excretion of electrolytes in patients on long-term diuretic therapy for arterial hypertension and/or congestive heart failure. Acta Med Scand 218: 443–448.

36. Rob PM, Lebeau A, Nobiling R, Schmid H, Bley N, et al. (1996) Magnesium metabolism: basic aspects and implications of ciclosporine toxicity in rats. Nephron 72: 59–66.

37. Barbagallo M, Dominguez LJ (2007) Magnesium metabolism in type 2 diabetes mellitus, metabolic syndrome and insulin resistance. Arch Biochem Biophys 458: 40–47.

38. Lima Mde L, Cruz T, Rodrigues LE, Bomfim O, Melo J, et al. (2009) Serum and intracellular magnesium deficiency in patients with metabolic syndrome-evidences for its relation to insulin resistance. Diabetes Res Clin Pract 83: 257–262.

39. Aguilar MV, Saavedra P, Arrieta FJ, Mateos CJ, Gonzalez MJ, et al. (2007) Plasma mineral content in type-2 diabetic patients and their association with the metabolic syndrome. Ann Nutr Metab 51: 402–406.

40. Hopping BN, Erber E, Grandinetti A, Verheus M, Kolonel LN, et al. (2010) Dietary fiber, magnesium, and glycemic load alter risk of type 2 diabetes in a multiethnic cohort in Hawaii. J Nutr 140: 68–74.

11

Advanced Glycation End Products in Infant Formulas do not Contribute to Insulin Resistance Associated with their Consumption

Kristína Simon Klenovics[1,2], Peter Boor[3,4], Veronika Somoza[5,6], Peter Celec[3], Vincenzo Fogliano[7], Katarína Šebeková[1,3]*

1 Department of Clinical and Experimental Pharmacotherapy, Medical Faculty, Slovak Medical University, Bratislava, Slovakia, 2 Institute of Physiology, Medical Faculty, Comenius University, Bratislava, Slovakia, 3 Institute of Molecular BioMedicine, Medical Faculty, Comenius University, Bratislava, Slovakia, 4 Division of Nephrology and Institute of Pathology, RWTH University of Aachen, Aachen, Germany, 5 German Research Center for Food Chemistry, Garching, Germany, 6 Department of Nutritional and Physiological Chemistry, University of Vienna, Vienna, Austria, 7 Department of Food Science, University of Naples Federico II, Naples, Italy

Abstract

Introduction: Infant formula-feeding is associated with reduced insulin sensitivity. In rodents and healthy humans, advanced glycation end product (AGE)-rich diets exert diabetogenic effects. In comparison with human breast-milk, infant formulas contain high amounts of AGEs. We assessed the role of AGEs in infant-formula-consumption-associated insulin resistance.

Methods: Total plasma levels of N^{ε}-(carboxymethyl)lysine (CML), AGEs-associated fluorescence ($\lambda_{ex} = 370$ nm/ $\lambda_{em} = 445$ nm), soluble adhesion molecules, markers of micro- binflammation (hsCRP), oxidative stress (malondialdehyde, 8-isoprostanes) and leptinemia were determined, and correlated with insulin sensitivity in a cross-sectional study in 166 healthy term infants aged 3-to-14 months, subdivided according to feeding regimen (breast-milk- vs. infant formula-fed) and age (3-to-6-month-olds, 7-to-10-month-olds, and 11-to-14-month-old infants). Effects of the consumption of low- vs. high-CML-containing formulas were assessed. 36 infants aged 5.8 ± 0.3 months were followed-up 7.5 ± 0.3 months later.

Results: Cross-sectional study: 3-to-6-month-olds and 7-to-10-month-old formula-fed infants presented higher total plasma CML levels and AGEs-associated fluorescence ($p < 0.01$, both), while only the 3-to-6-month-olds displayed lower insulin sensitivity ($p < 0.01$) than their breast-milk-fed counterparts. 3-to-6-month-olds fed low-CML-containing formulas presented lower total plasma CML levels ($p < 0.01$), but similar insulin sensitivity compared to those on high-CML-containing formulas. Markers of oxidative stress and inflammation, levels of leptin and adhesion molecules did not differ significantly between the groups. Follow-up study: at initial investigation, the breast-milk-consuming infants displayed lower total plasma CML levels ($p < 0.01$) and AGEs-associated fluorescence ($p < 0.05$), but higher insulin sensitivity ($p < 0.05$) than the formulas-consuming infants. At follow-up, the groups did not differ significantly in either determined parameter.

Conclusions: In healthy term infants, high dietary load with CML does not play a pathophysiological role in the induction of infant formula-associated insulin resistance. Whether a high load of AGEs in early childhood affects postnatal programming remains to be elucidated.

Editor: Michael Müller, Wageningen University, The Netherlands

Funding: This study was supported by the grant from 6th FP of EC of EU (ICARE, No. COLL-CT-2005-516415), and from Slovak Research and Development Agency (No. VMSP-II-0027-09). The funders had no role in study design, data collection and analysis, decision to publish, or preparation of the manuscript.

Competing Interests: The authors have declared that no competing interests exist.

* E-mail: kata.sebekova@gmail.com

Introduction

In recent years, there has been a worldwide rise in the incidence of type 2 diabetes mellitus (T2DM) in children and adolescents, albeit T2DM was along back thought to be unique to adults [1]. The initial step in the development of T2DM is a decrease in insulin sensitivity, frequently associated with obesity [2]. In infants, the risk of insulin resistance is particularly high for newborns who are small for their gestational age and undergo rapid postnatal weight gain to obesity [3]. Much less attention is paid to decreased insulin sensitivity in infants appropriate for gestational age, although it has been well documented that formula feeding is associated with reduced insulin sensitivity and increased insulin secretion [4–6]. The composition of human breast milk differs profoundly from that of infant formulas, and to accommodate the infant's needs best it changes dynamically during breast-feeding period [7–9]. Higher protein content, lower concentrations of long-chain polyunsaturated fatty acids, and presumably the lack of insulin-sensitizing hormones as well as numerous other biologically active substances in infant formulas in comparison with breast-milk, are thought to play a pathophysiological role in formula-feeding-associated decreased insulin sensitivity [10–12]. Recently, it has been suggested that food-derived advanced glycation end-products (AGEs) in AGE-rich infant formulas might precondition the infants to insulin resistance via induction of inflammation and oxidative stress [13].

Industrial processing of infant formulas requires heat-treatment. This results in the formation of substantial amounts of AGEs, which may exceed those present in human breast-milk up to 670-fold [14–17]. We have shown previously that AGEs from formulas are at least partially absorbed and contribute to the circulating pool of AGEs [14]. Vast majority of studies in rodents and in adult humans suggest that an excessive intake of highly thermally processed foods, rich in AGEs, may affect circulating AGE levels and may thus play a role in a wide range of harmful health effects, e.g. diabetogenic, pro-oxidative and pro-inflammatory events [13,18–20]. However, some other studies evidenced beneficial effects, as reviewed in [21]. Interaction of AGEs with their specific cell surface receptors RAGE may result, among others, in the production of reactive oxygen species and induction of micro-inflammation, which may in turn accelerate the formation of AGEs, and exacerbate insulin resistance [2,22,23]. However, some studies have disputed these findings: there are still controversies on the identity of the actual AGEs that initiate the RAGE-mediated reactions, and questions regarding evidence that endotoxin contamination of AGE protein preparations compromised the results of some studies [24,25]. Experimental studies show that AGEs *per se* may initiate the insulin-resistant state in skeletal muscle and adipocytes [26–28], or decrease the insulin content and secretion in pancreatic islets [29–31]. In line with the experimental data, a direct relationship between circulating AGE levels and insulin resistance was documented in non-obese non-diabetic adults [32–34].

Recent clinical data suggest that soluble RAGE (sRAGE) and vascular adhesion protein-1 (sVAP-1) may affect circulating AGE levels, and, thus, may play a role in insulin resistance. Circulating sRAGE bears the extracellular ligand binding domain but lacks the transmembrane and cytoplasmic domain. By removing or neutralizing circulating RAGE ligands, it acts as a natural competitive inhibitor of signal transducing metabolic pathways [35]. In humans, low sRAGE levels are associated with insulin resistance [36–38]. Endothelial VAP-1 represents an adhesion molecule, possessing the enzyme activity of semicar-bazide-sensitive aminooxidase (SSAO) [39]. SSAO degrades primary amines into corresponding aldehydes, producing hydrogen peroxide and ammonia [40]. Reactive aldehydes are potent glycating agents, while hydrogen peroxide contributes to oxidative stress, thus may accelerate formation of AGEs. In diabetic rats, SSAO/VAP-1 imposes antidiabetic action via activation of glucose metabolism in adipocytes and muscle cells [41]. In humans, hyperglycemia induces a rise in circulating sVAP-1, which directly correlates with plasma AGE levels [42,43].

The cross-sectional and follow-up study described in this work was aimed at elucidating whether formula-feeding-induced rise in circulating AGE levels may play a role in the induction of formula-feeding associated insulin resistance in healthy infants. Our data suggest that increased levels of circulating CML and/or the levels of AGE-associated fluorescence of plasma imposed by infant formulas consumption do not play a role in formula-consumption-associated insulin resistance, either directly or indirectly by induction of oxidative stress, micro-inflammation, hyperleptine-mia, or decline in circulating sVAP-1 levels.

Research Design and Methods

The study was carried out according to the Declaration of Helsinki, after the approval of the protocol by the Ethics Board (Slovak Medical University, Bratislava) and after obtaining the written informed consent from the mothers/legal guardians of the children.

The present cross-sectional study includes data from one hundred and sixty-six 3-to-14-month-old healthy term infants of Central European descent, infants of apparently healthy mothers residing in Bratislava and surroundings, examined from March 2006 to December 2008 in frames of ICARE (Impeding neoformed Contaminants Accumulation to Reduce their health Effects) study. From among 231 recruited 3–14-month-old infants, 65 met the exclusion criteria (pathology during physical examination, elevated inflammatory markers, acute/recurrent inflammatory or chronic diseases including allergies, positivity for antibodies against HCV/HIV, prematurity, being born small for their gestational age, and infant's feeding regimen not compliant with Slovak recommendations for their age; and/or diagnosis of chronic disease or gestational diabetes in the mother) and were excluded from the present evaluation.

Subjects

Cross-sectional study. Cohort characteristics are given in Table 1. Infant's feeding regimen was recorded into the questionnaire filled in by mothers/legal guardians of the infants under supervision of pediatricians/educated nurses. If the child had received infant formula, the brand and the age at which formula feeding had started were recorded. Infants were allocated according to their age into 3 groups: 3-to-6-month-old infants (n = 69), 7-to-10-month-old weaning infants (n = 78), and older infants aged 11-to-14 months (n = 19). Each age-group was divided according to feeding regimen into breast-milk- and formula-receiving subgroup. Formula-fed infants consumed 17 different types of infant formulas. From among these, CML content was determined in 16 (marketed in Slovakia), as published elsewhere [14]. Based on these data [14], formula consuming groups were subdivided according to the CML content of the formulas. Formulas containing roughly 5-to-11 mg CML/100 g protein were considered as low CML-containing formulas, while those with 16-to-63 mg CML/100 g protein as high CML-containing formulas. Eight low CML-containing formulas were non-hydrolyzed and two were hydrolyzed formulations, while within the high CML-containing formulas one out of six was non-hydrolyzed [14]. Flow-chart depicting allocation of the infants according to age and feeding regimen is given in Figure 1.

In Slovakia, the recommendation is to not introduce solid foods before 6 month of age. Thus, 33 included 3-to-6-month-old infants were exclusively breast-fed. From among their 36 formula/mixed-fed counterparts, 27 were exclusively formula-fed, in 6 infants fruits or vegetables (raw or cooked) were added to one daily portion of formula, or a portion was replaced with this serving, and 3 were mixed-fed, i.e. received concurrently breast-milk and infant formula since their birth. The exclusion of mixed-fed infants, or those consuming fruits or vegetables, from the analysis did not alter the results (data not given).

In seventy-eight 7-to-10-month-old weaning infants, fruits, vegetables, flour, fish and lean meat were stepwise introduced to replace either breast-milk (n = 41), or infant formula (n = 37).

All 11-to-14 month-olds infants consumed a mixed diet. Six of them still received breast-milk (1–2-times/day) as a supplement to diversified diet, while 13 drunk formula (2–3-times/day).

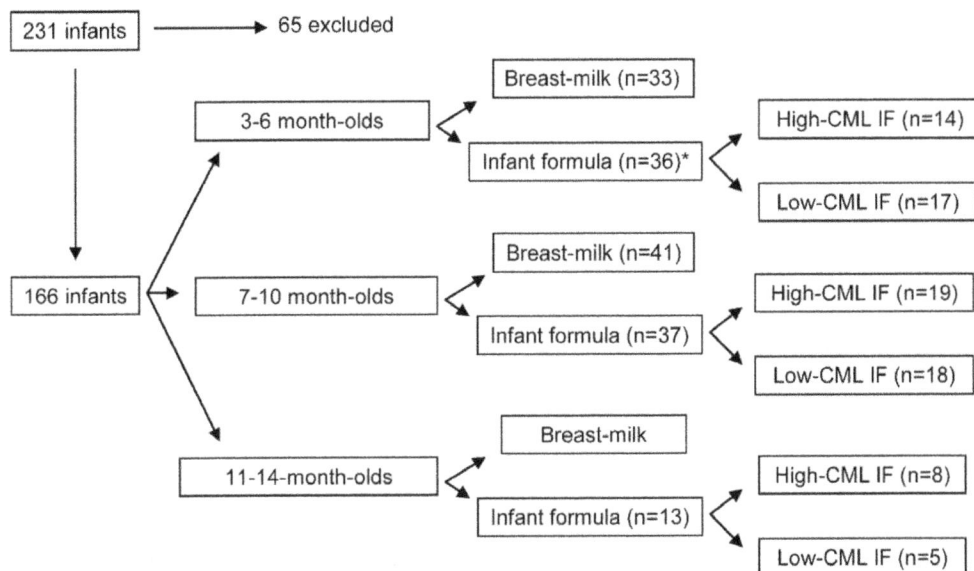

Figure 1. Recruitment and allocation of the infants according to age and feeding regimen. IF: infant formula; CML: N^{ε}-(carboxymethyl)lysine; *: Five infants could not be unequivocally assigned to any group (four due to concurrent administration or just recent switch from low- to high-CML-containing formula, one child consumed formula not analyzed for CML content).

Follow-up study. Thirty-six infants from the cross-sectional study, aged 5.8±0.3 months, were followed-up for another 7.5±0.3 months. Eleven out of them still received breast-milk as a supplement to the infant's mixed diet at follow-up. Twenty-five infants were formula-fed at basal check-up, and received formulas as a supplement to infants' mixed diet at follow-up. Only the initial sampling values of the infants participating in a follow-up study were included into the evaluation of the cross-sectional data. Cohort characteristics are given in Table 2.

Methods

Mother's age, her actual weight, height, and weight gain during the pregnancy were recorded, and body mass index (BMI, kg/m²) was calculated.

Mothers were asked not to feed the infants 3 hours prior to blood sampling. If mother confirmed the child was fasting at least 3 hours, 4-to-5 ml of blood were collected from infant's antecubital vein in the morning hours (between 7.30 and 9.30 a.m.). Plasma was obtained by standard centrifugation procedure. Hemolytic samples were excluded from analyses. Spot urine obtained on the day of blood sampling (around the time of blood collection) from 23 breast-milk- and 21 formula-fed 3-to-6-month-old infants was analyzed for 8-isoprostanes.

Standard blood and urine chemistry. Plasma glucose and creatinine (Vitros 250 analyzer, J&J, Rochester, USA) were determined. Commercial radioimmunoassay was used to analyze immunoreactive insulin (Immunotech, Prague, Czech Republic). Insulin sensitivity was evaluated by Quantitative insulin-sensitivity check index (QUICKI) [44].

Special analyses. Total CML concentration in plasma was determined using an ELISA assay (MicroCoat Biotechnologie GmbH, Bernried, Germany), after pretreatment of the samples with proteinase K (Roche, Mannheim, Germany) according to manufacturer's instructions. ELISA kits, performed according to manufacturers' instructions, were also used to determine plasma concentration of sRAGE (R&D, Minneapolis, MN, USA), high-sensitivity C-reactive protein (hsCRP, ImmunDiagnostik, Ben-

sheim, Germany), leptin, soluble intercellular adhesion molecule-1 (sICAM-1), soluble vascular cell adhesion molecule-1 (sVCAM-1), sVAP-1, leptin (all BenderMedSystem Inc., Vienna, Austria), and urinary 8-isoprostanes (Cayman Chemicals, MI, USA). Plasma malondialdehyde (MDA) levels were determined employing HPLC method with fluorimetric detection [45], plasma AGE-associated fluorescence ($\lambda_{ex} = 370$ nm/$\lambda_{em} = 445$ nm) was determined [46]. For technical reasons (insufficient biological material), plasma MDA levels were determined only in 33 breast-milk- and 18 infant-formula-receiving infants, and plasma leptin levels were not determined in the 11-to-14-month-olds infants. Renal excretion of 8-isoprostanes was expressed as a ratio to urinary creatinine.

Statistical analyses. Sample size was calculated using OpenEpi statistical program on the assumption that 3-to-6-month-olds breast-milk- versus formula-fed infants differ in plasma AGE levels by 50%, and SD represents 50% of the mean [14]; with confidence interval 95%, power 80%, and sample size ratio 1, calculated sample size was 16. Normally distributed data are given as mean ± SEM, those not fitting to normal distribution as median, and interquartile range. Two-sided Student's t-test (paired or unpaired, as appropriate), or Wilcoxon and Mann-Whitney U-test were used to compare 2 sets of data, as appropriate. Three sets of data (fitting to normal distribution) were compared using ANOVA with Scheffe's post-hoc test. Data displaying non-parametric distribution were compared using Kruskal-Wallis test with post-hoc Mann-Whitney U-test with Bonferonni correction for target alpha. Categorical data were compared using chi-square. Pearson's (indicated in results as "r") or Spearman's (if the correlated data did not fit to normal distribution) correlation coefficients were calculated. Multiple regression analyses were performed using General linear model (GLM). P<0.05 was considered significant. For evaluation, SPSS v. 16 statistical program was used.

Table 1. Cohort characteristics and blood chemistry data – cross-sectional study.

	3–6 month-olds	7–10 month-olds	11–14 month-olds
Age (months)			
BM	5.2±0.2	8.4±0.2	12.3±0.5
IF	5.0±0.1	8.3±0.2	12.1±0.4
Low-CML IF	4.8±0.2	8.0±0.3	11.5±0.4
High-CML IF	5.2±0.2	8.4±0.3	$13.1±0.4^{+}$
Gender (Female/Male)			
BM	11/22	15/26	3/3
IF	17/19	20/17	7/6
Low-CML IF	6/11	10/8	3/2
High-CML IF	6/8	10/9	4/4
Gestational age (weeks)			
BM	39.6±0.2	39.2±0.2	39.4±0.4
IF	39.6±0.2	39.6±0.2	39.6±0.3
Low-CML IF	39.8±0.3	39.5±0.4	39.9±0.3
High-CML IF	39.3±0.4	39.6±0.3	39.0±0.7
Birth weight (g)			
BM	3632±76	3323±87	3252±275
IF	$3143±89^{***}$	3305±80	3370±160
Low-CML IF	2937±122	3300±144	3308±241
High-CML IF	3227±136	3309±98	3470±178
Body weight (g)			
BM	7551±172	8417±179	9474±552
IF	$6768±179^{**}$	$7883±164^{*}$	9206±326
Low-CML IF	6581±278	7771±210	8981±456
High-CML IF	6859±270	7984±258	9567±440
Mean daily weight gain (g)			
BM	25±1	20±1	17±1
IF	25±1	19±1	16±1
Low-CML IF	26±1	20±1	17±1
High-CML IF	24±2	19±1	16±1
Creatinine (µmol/l)			
BM	30; 25–38	30; 27–35	27; 26–37
IF	$27; 23–30^{*}$	29; 24–48	34; 26–48
Low-CML IF	26; 23–31	35; 24–49	34; 25–48
High-CML IF	28; 24–30	26; 24–33	27; 24–32
AGE-FI (AU)			
BM	92±8	$128±6^{\#\#}$	$161±19^{\#\#}$
IF	$123±6^{**}$	$155±6^{**,\#\#}$	$162±9^{\#\#}$
Low-CML IF	$109±6^{*}$	$149±9^{\#\#}$	$159±11^{\#\#}$
High-CML IF	$132±9^{**,+}$	$158±8^{**}$	166±19
sRAGE (pg/ml)			
BM	1899±142	2076±131	2229±339
IF	1807±115	1904±119	1802±170
Low-CML IF	1838±196	1930±166	1721±302
High-CML IF	1840±181	1813±175	1852±216
Glucose (µmol/l)			
BM	4.6; 4.3–4.8	4.5; 4.1–4.9	4.1; 3.6–4.4
IF	$4.1; 3.6–4.7^{**}$	4.4; 4.0–4.9	$4.7; 4.3±5.0^{*,\#}$
Low-CML IF	4.0; 3.6–5.1	4.4; 4.0–4.9	$4.7; 4.5–5.3^{*}$

Table 1. Cont.

	3–6 month-olds	7–10 month-olds	11–14 month-olds
High-CML IF	4.4; 4.0–4.7	4.3; 3.8–4.8	4.4; 3.8–4.9
Insulin (μIU/ml)			
BM	2.8; 1.5–5.7	3.7; 2.4–5.1	2.4; 1.6–3.5
IF	8.1; 3.2–15.4***	4.1; 2.7–7.7	3.9; 1.7–9.4
Low-CML IF	9.0; 4.6–15.1**	4.5; 2.7–8.8	4.6; 1.5–9.0
High-CML IF	4.2; 2.5–11.3	3.6; 2.6–5.9	2.9; 1.9–15.4
hsCRP (mg/l)			
BM	0.2; 0.2–0.3	0.2; 0.2–0.3	0.2; 0.9–2.0
IF	0.2; 0.2–0.4	0.2; 0.2–0.7*	0.8; 0.2–2.3
Low-CML IF	0.2; 0.2–0.6	0.3; 0.2–1.9+	0.6; 0.2–3.9
High-CML IF	0.2; 0.2–0.4	0.2; 0.2–0.4	0.8; 0.5–2.3
sICAM-1 (ng/ml)			
BM	432±31	411±14	524±106
IF	419±26	414±21	435±13
Low-CML IF	377±25	363±17	446±14
High-CML IF	484±52	441±32	419±25
sVCAM-1 (ng/ml)			
BM	2263±215	1930±151	1436±252
IF	2093±175	1761±106	1431±144
Low-CML IF	1919±120	1631±103	1529±201
High-CML IF	2383±413	1847±183	1274±200
sVAP-1 (ng/ml)			
BM	542±22	555±20	580±65
IF	546±20	537±28	563±38
Low-CML IF	498±31	562±48	598±53
High-CML IF	579±29	520±33	506±46
Leptin (ng/ml)			
BM	3.1; 2.5–5.3	2.4; 1.8–3.0##	ND
IF	2.9; 2.4–4.0	2.1; 1.5–3.0##	ND
Low-CML IF	3.1; 2.7–3.9	2.3; 1.4–3.0	ND
High-CML IF	2.7; 2.0–5.1	1.9; 1.6–3.1	ND

Infants were allocated according to their age and feeding regimen. From among 69 infants 3-to-6-month-olds, 33 were exclusively breast-fed (BM) and 36 received infant formula (IF): 17 consumed formulas with high- and 14 with low-CML-content. Fourty-one 7-to-10-month-old infants were weaned from breast-milk, while 37 from formulas: 18 infants consumed low-CML- and 19 high-CML-containing formulas. Six older infants aged 11-to-14 months still received breast-milk as a supplement to diversified diet, while 13 drunk formula (5 consumed low-CML- and 8 high-CML-containing formulas). AGE-FI: plasma advanced glycation end-products specific fluorescence; AU: arbitrary units; sRAGE: soluble receptor for advanced glycation end products; hsCRP: high-sensitive C-reactive protein; sICAM-1: soluble intercellular adhesion molecule-1; sVCAM-1: soluble vascular adhesion molecule-1; sVAP-1: soluble vascular adhesion protein-1;
*: p<0.05 vs. the corresponding age-group consuming breast-milk;
**: p<0.01 vs. the corresponding age-group consuming BM;
***: p<0.001 vs. the corresponding age-group consuming BM;
+: p<0.05 vs. the corresponding age-group consuming infant formula with low-CML content;
#: p<0.05 vs. the 3-to-6-month-old infants on the same feeding regimen;
##: p<0.01 vs. the 3-to-6-month-old infants on the same feeding regimen; results are given as mean±sem or median and interquartile range;
ND: not determined.

Results

The mothers of the breast- and formula-fed infants did not differ significantly by age, BMI, and the weight gain during the pregnancy (Table 3).

Cross-sectional Study

Basic cohort characteristics. Anthropometric data of the infants at birth and at investigation are presented in Table 1.

Within the 3 age-groups, infants receiving breast-milk did not differ significantly from those receiving formulas by age, gestational age, mean daily weight gain, and plasma creatinine concentration. Proportion of girls and boys in the breast-milk- and formula-fed groups of corresponding age did not differ significantly (chi square: n.s., all). Formula-fed 3-to-6-month-old infants had lower birth weight and body weight at investigation when compared with their breast-milk-fed counterparts. Although the mean birth weights of the cohorts differed significantly, they

Table 2. Characteristics of the followed-up infants.

	Basal data	Follow-up
Gestational age (weeks)		
BM	39.4±0.5	–
IF	39.4±0.4	–
Birth weight (g)		
BM	3562±125	–
IF	2956±113**	–
Weight (g)		
BM	7964±239	10549±295
IF	6879±228*	9440±286*
Mean daily weight gain (g)		
BM	22±1	16±1
IF	24±1	18±1
Creatinine (μmol/l)		
BM	28; 24–34	30; 28–35
IF	28; 24–31	27; 24–33
Glucose (mmol/l)		
BM	4.5; 4.2–4.9	4.3; 4.1–4.7
IF	4.0; 3.7–4.4*	4.2; 4.0–4.59
Insulin (μIU/ml)		
BM	3.1; 1.3–5.8	3.1; 2.6–5.1
IF	6.1; 3.8–10.9*	5.1; 3.1–7.8
QUICKI		
BM	0.425±0.022	0.411±0.020
IF	0.373±0.008*	0.385±0.009
CML (ng/ml)		
BM	711; 513–879	839; 624–1024++
IF	1218; 867–1404**	1129; 820–1427
AGE-Fl (AU)		
BM	101±13	171±9++
IF	132±10*	162±9
sRAGE (pg/ml)		
BM	1888±234	1897±152
IF	2034±143	1977±161
hsCRP (mg/l)		
BM	0.2; 0.2–0.4	0.2; 0.2–0.3
IF	0.2; 0.2–0.6	0.3; 0.2–0.6
sICAM-1 (ng/ml)		
BM	434±31	422±25
IF	403±23	441±31
sVCAM-1 (ng/ml)		
BM	2655±470	1924±394
IF	1922±90	1706±155
sVAP-1 (ng/ml)		
BM	530±33	266±42++

Table 2. Cont.

	Basal data	Follow-up
IF	539±32	296±21++

Thirty-six infants aged 5.8±0.3 (Basal data) months were followed-up 7.5±0.3 months later (Follow-up). BM: 11 infants exclusively breast-fed at basal sampling and receiving breast-milk as a supplement to infants' mixed diet at follow-up; IF: 25 infants consuming infant formulas at basal investigation as well as at follow-up; QUICKI: Quantitative insulin-sensitivity check index; CML: plasma N^ε-(carboxymethyl)lysine; AGE-fl: plasma advanced glycation end products specific fluorescence; sRAGE: soluble receptor for advanced glycation end products; hsCRP: high-sensitive C-reactive protein; sICAM-1: soluble intercellular adhesion molecule-1; sVCAM-1: soluble vascular adhesion molecule-1; sVAP-1: soluble vascular adhesion protein-1;
*: p<0.05 vs. the breast-milk consuming group at corresponding time interval;
**: p<0.01 vs. the breast-milk consuming group at corresponding time interval;
+: p<0.05 vs. the basal sampling in the same feeding regimen group;
++: p<0.001 vs. the basal sampling in the same feeding regimen group; results are given as mean±sem or median and interquartile range;
–: not applicable.

were within the "normal" birth weight range of eutrophic term-infants (2500–4000 g). The same holds true for the age-adjusted body weight at investigation. Formula-fed 7-to-10-month-olds displayed similar birth weight, but lower body weight if compared with the breast-milk-fed infants. Again, the means differed significantly, despite that the age-adjusted body weights were within the normal range. 11-to-14-month-old breast-milk- and formula-fed infants did not differ by the birth and body weight significantly.

Infants consuming low- vs. high-CML-containing formulas did not differ significantly in either characteristics, except for the fact that 11-to-14-month-olds infants consuming low-CML-containing formulas were younger (by 6 weeks in mean, p = 0.03) than those on high-CML-containing formulas (Table 1).

Theoretical daily dietary CML burden. From among 56 breast-milk samples analyzed for CML content [14], 21 were donated by the mothers of 3-to-6-month-old herein evaluated infants. The calculated daily burden of CML in the 3-to-6-month-old breast-fed infants did not exceed 0.03 mg CML/day, thus was less than 0.004 mg CML/kg body weight/day. From among 36 formula-fed 3-to-6-month-old infants, 17 consumed formulas with high-CML content and 14 were fed low-CML-containing formulas (Table 1). Five infants could not be unequivocally assigned to any group (concurrent administration/recent switch from low- to high-CML-containing formula, consumption of formula not analyzed for CML content). The theoretical daily burden of CML ingested from formulas, calculated on the basis of determined CML content of formula [14] and daily dosage specified by the manufacturers, ranged from 8.8 mg/day to 10.3 mg/day in infants consuming high-CML-containing formulas, while those on low-CML-containing formulas ingested amounts from 1.8 mg/day to 2.2 mg/day. Taking into account the estimated mean body weight at the time of investigation, infants on low-CML-containing formulas ingested daily 0.27–0.33 mg CML/kg body weight, e.g. up-to 83-fold higher (0.33 mg/kg body weight/day) amounts in comparison with their breast-milk-fed counterparts. Those on high-CML-containing formulas consumed 1.3–1.5 mg CML/kg body weight/day, thus

Table 3. Characteristics of the mothers of included infants.

	Infants' age		
	3-6 month-olds	7-10 month-olds	11-14 month-olds
Age (years)			
BM	30.4±1.0	28.7±0.7	28.6±1.1
IF	29.6±1.4	28.6±1.3	32.8±2.8
BMI (kg/m^2)			
BM	23.4±0.7	22.6±4.9	22.3±0.8
IF	26.5±1.7	22.9±0.9	25.7±1.6
Pregnancy weight gain (kg)			
BM	13.8±1.1	14.0±0.8	14.3±3.5
IF	14.4±1.1	14.4±1.4	13.5±2.0

BM: mothers of exclusively breast-fed infants; IF: mothers of infant formulas recieving infants; BMI: body mass index.

even 375-fold higher amounts of CML/kg/day than the corresponding breast-milk-fed infants.

As calculated on the basis of 19 breast-milk samples obtained from the mothers of 7-to-10-month-old infants, the maximal amounts of ingested CML corresponded to those in 3-to-6-month-olds. Eighteen 7-to-10-month-old infants were administered formulas with low-CML contents, and 19 received high-CML-containing formulas (Table 1). The calculated mean daily burden of CML arising from low-CML-containing formulas ranged between 1.0 mg/d to 1.3 mg/day, i.e. 0.13–0.17 mg CML/kg body weight/day (up-to 43-fold higher than the corresponding breast-milk-fed infants), while consumption of high-CML-containing formulas represented an intake between 3.7 mg and 6.4 mg CML/day, corresponding to 0.46–0.80 mg CML/kg body weight/day (e.g. up-to 200-fold more CML per kg body weight in comparison with breast-milk fed counterparts).

Five 11-to14-month-old infants received high-CML-containing formulas as a supplement to a mixed infant diet, while 8 consumed low-CML formulas. Since the manufacturers do not indicate the dosage of formula for this age-group, and the breast-milk from mothers of 11-to-14-month-old infants was not available, the theoretical CML dietary burden coming from the milk drunken was not calculated. In any case, the vast majority (i.e. 97%) of ingested AGEs in this age-group does come from the solid foods [13] in which CML content was not determined in present study.

CML. Compared with breast-fed infants, 3-to-6-month-olds and 7-to-10-month-old formula-fed infants displayed higher plasma total CML concentrations (Figure 2a). Total CML levels were higher in the 11-to-14-month-old breast-milk fed infants if compared with the 2 younger breast-milk-fed groups. Since the birth weight and/or body weight of the formula- and breast-fed 3-to-6-month-old and 7-to-10-month-old infants differed significantly, multivariate analysis was employed to elucidate whether the weights independently and significantly affected the total CML levels. GLM confirmed that feeding regimen was a single independent significantly contributing factor (data not given). Total CML levels showed an age-dependent rise if all breast-milk-consuming infants were evaluated together (Fig. 2b).

3-to-6-month-olds on the low-CML-containing formulas presented significantly lower total plasma CML levels (Figure 2a) in comparison with the group fed by high-CML-containing formulas. Total plasma CML levels were higher in the 3-to-6-month-olds and 7-to-10-month-olds on low-CML-as well as high-CML-containing formulas than in the corresponding breast-milk-fed

infants (Figure 2a). While in the infants fed high-CML-containing formulas, total plasma CML concentration decreased by age (Fig. 2b), no significant relationship was observed in those on low-CML-containing formulas (Fig. 2c).

Plasma AGE-associated fluorescence (λ_{ex} = 370 nm/ λ_{em} = 445 nm). 3-to-6-month-olds and 7-to-10-month-old formula-fed infants displayed higher plasma fluorescence than their breast-milk-fed counterparts (Table 1). It showed an age-dependent rise if either all breast-milk-consuming infants (y = 9.09x+47.45, r = 0. 547, p = 0.001), or the formula-fed infants (y = 5.68x+100.24, r = 0.446, p = 0.001) were evaluated together.

3-to-6-month-olds on the low-CML-containing formulas presented significantly lower plasma fluorescence (Table 1) in comparison with the group fed by high-CML-containing formulas.

Insulin sensitivity. Breast-milk-fed 3-to-6-month-old infants presented higher plasma glucose concentration in comparison with their formula-fed counterparts but they maintained glycemia with lower insulin levels (Table 1), resulting in higher insulin sensitivity (Figure 2d). In the 7-to-10-month-olds and 11-to-14-month-olds glycemia, insulinemia and insulin sensitivity did not differ significantly between the breast-milk- and formula-consuming groups. Correction for the birth or body weight did not alter the results, and General linear model did not indicate these parameters as independent significant contributors (data not given). However, correction for mean daily weight gain revealed that both, feeding regimen (p<0.001) and mean daily weight gain (p = 0.003) significantly affect insulin sensitivity (corrected model: p<0.001), contributing to 12.2% of its variability. In the whole cohort insulin sensitivity displayed significant inverse relationship to mean daily weight gain (y = −0.002x+0.453, r = −0.200, p = 0.014). This relationship was on the account of the formula-fed infants (y = −0.003x+0.452, r = −0.333, p = 0.003), since the correlation in the breast-milk-fed cohort was not significant (data not given). When the 3 age-groups were analyzed separately, GLM indicated concurrent significant independent impact of feeding regimen (p<0.001) and the mean daily weight gain (p = 0.003) only in the 3-to-6-month olds (corrected model: p<0.001; R^2: 0.266). In this age group the simple correlation between insulin sensitivity and the mean daily weight gain was inverse both in the breast- (r = −0.385, p = 0.033) and formula-fed-infants (r = −0.387, p = 0.026). No significant relationship between QUICKI and total plasma CML or AGEs-associated fluorescence was revealed in either group, and total plasma CML or AGEs-associated fluorescence showed no impact on insulinemia

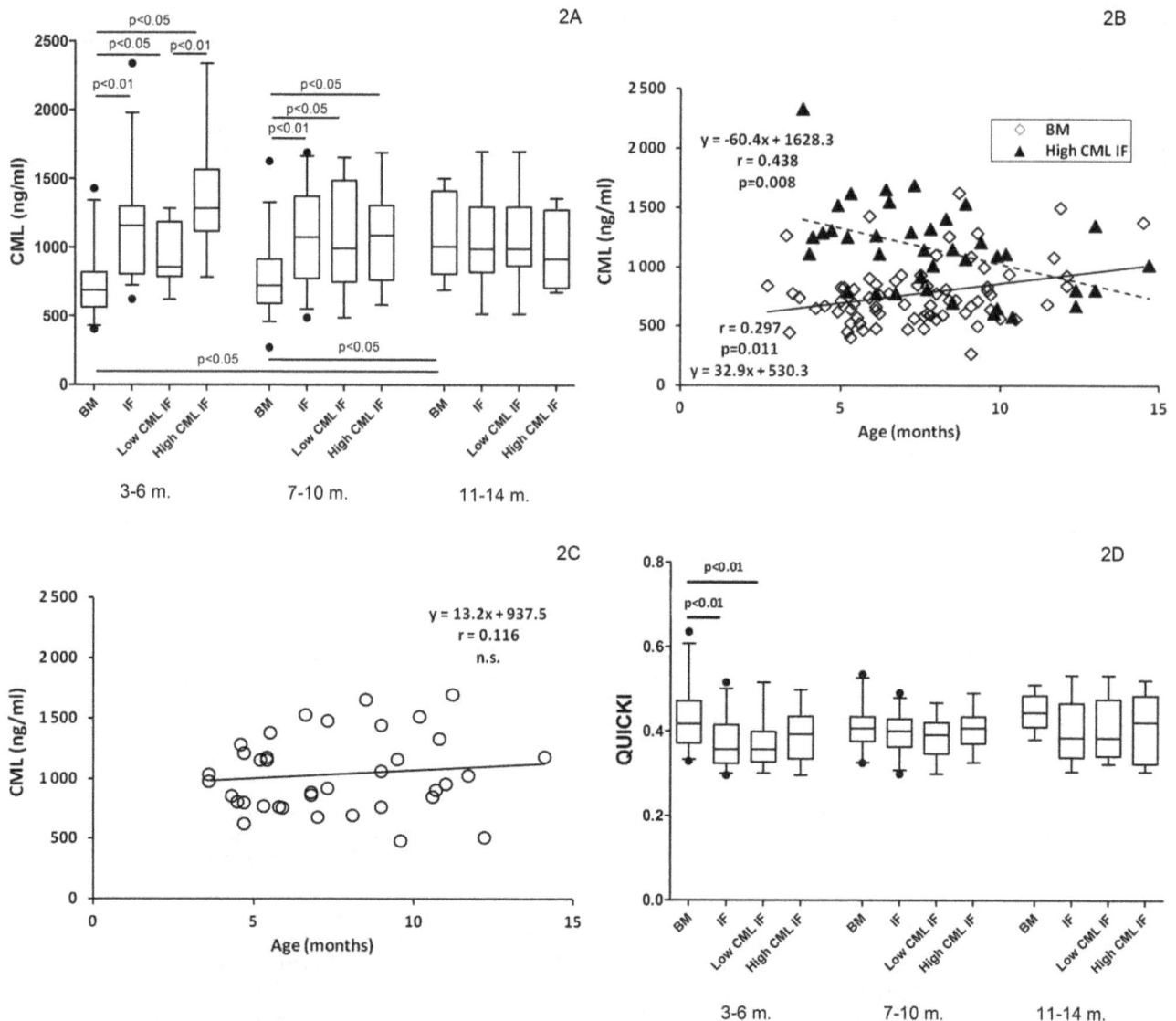

Figure 2. Total plasma N$^\varepsilon$-(carboxymethyl)lysine (CML) levels and insulin sensitivity in breast-milk- and formula-fed infants included in the cross-sectional study. 2A/Plasma total CML concentration in relation to feeding regimen and age. Box-plots represent median, interquartile range and 5th–95th percentile; 2B/Age-dependence of plasma total CML concentration in the breast-milk-fed infants (BM) and those consuming high-CML-containing infant formulas (IF); 2C/Relationship between plasma total CML concentration and age in the low-CML-containing infant formulas fed healthy infants; 2D/Insulin sensitivity assessed by Quantitative insulin-sensitivity check index (QUICKI) in the breast-milk- (BM) and infant formula-fed (IF) infants, low-CML-containing formulas (Low-CML IF) and high-CML-containing formulas (High-CML IF) consuming infants aged 3-to-6-months (m.), 7-to-10-months, and 11-to-14-months. Box-plots represent median, interquartile range and 5th–95th percentile.

or insulin sensitivity in multiple correlation model (data not shown).

Infants consuming low- versus high-CML-containing formulas did not differ significantly either by plasma glucose, insulin (Table 1), or insulin sensitivity (Figure 2d) in either age-group. 3-to-6-month-old infants consuming low- (but not high-) CML-containing formulas displayed higher concentrations of insulin and lower insulin sensitivity if compared with the breast-milk-fed counterparts (Table 1 and Figure 2d).

Soluble RAGE. No significant difference was revealed between the breast-milk- and formula-consuming infants in either age-group (Table 1). In the formula-consuming group plasma sRAGE levels correlated directly with those of total CML ($y = 0.13x+863.7$, $r = 0.243$, $p = 0.031$).

Consumption of high- or low-CML-containing infant formulas was not reflected by significant difference in sRAGE levels (Table 1). In the infants consuming high-CML-containing formulas plasma sRAGE levels showed direct relationship to total CML ($y = 0.072x+1051.4$, $r = 0.337$, $p = 0.024$).

hsCRP and adhesion molecules. The breast-milk- and formula-consuming infants did not differ significantly by hsCRP, sICAM-1, sVCAM-1 and sVAP-1 levels in either age-group (Table 1). No significant relationship between total plasma CML, glycemia, insulinemia or QUICKI, and sVAP-1 was revealed in either feeding-regimen group (data not given). However, sVAP-1 levels correlated directly with those of sRAGE in the both cohorts (mother-milk-fed: $y = 0.052x+446.4$, $r = 0.337$, $p = 0.002$; formula-fed: $y = 0.063x+427.9$, $r = 0.300$, $p = 0.006$).

Infants consuming low-CML-containing formulas did not differ significantly from those fed high-CML-containing formulas by plasma hsCRP, sICAM-1, sVCAM-1 and sVAP-1 levels (Table 1). No significant relationship between total plasma CML, glycemia, insulinemia or QUICKI, and sVAP-1 levels was revealed in either group (data not given). sVAP-1 and sRAGE levels correlated directly in both cohorts (low-CML-containing formula-fed group: $y = 0.091x+376.5$, $r = 0.386$, $p = 0.044$; high-CML-containing formula-fed group: $y = 0.052x+443.5$, $r = 0.326$, $p = 0.045$).

Oxidative stress markers. In the 3-to-6-month-old infants, plasma MDA levels did not differ significantly between the groups: breast-milk-fed: 1.3 ± 0.1 μmol/l; formula-fed: 1.1 ± 0.1 μmol/l; $p = 0.08$. Correspondingly, no significant difference in urinary excretion of 8-isoprostanes was revealed: breast-milk-fed: 52 ± 4 ng/mmol creatinine; formula-fed: 54 ± 4 ng/mmol creatinine; $p = 0.68$.

Leptin. The breast-milk- and formula-consuming infants did not differ significantly in leptinemia (Table 1). However, in both, the breast-milk- and formulas-consuming groups, 7-to-10-month-olds infants displayed lower leptin concentrations than the 3-to-6-month olds. To elucidate whether this decline was associated with ageing or change in body weight, GLM was performed entering the feeding regimen as fixed factor and age and mean daily weight gain as covariates. Mean daily weight gain appeared as a single significant independent contributor (corrected model: $p<0.001$; R^2: 0.332). This relationship was confirmed in the whole cohort by a single regression model ($y = 216x - 1650$; $r = 0.577$, $p<0.001$). Correlation remained significant even if the breast- and formula-fed infants were evaluated separately ($r = 0.617$, and $r = 0.571$, respectively; both: $p<0.001$). No significant relationship between insulin, QUICKI, total plasma CML or AGEs-associated fluorescence and leptin levels was revealed in either feeding-regimen group (data not shown).

Infants consuming low- vs. high-CML-containing formulas did not differ significantly by plasma leptin levels in either age-group (Table 1).

Effects of birth weight or actual body weight. Multivariate analysis (GLM) did not indicate any significant independent impact of birth weight or body weight on plasma AGE-associated fluorescence, sRAGE, markers of inflammation, oxidative stress, or leptin levels (data not given).

Effect of mothers' weight gain during pregnancy. Neither of determined blood chemistry parameters in the infants displayed significant relationship with the mothers' weight gain during her pregnancy either in the simple or in multiple regression models (data not given).

Follow-up Study

CML. At baseline, the breast-milk-fed infants had significantly lower total plasma CML levels than the formula-receiving group. At the end of the follow-up period, no significant differences were observed between the groups: in the breast-milk-consuming infants the total plasma CML levels were higher than at baseline (Table 2).

Plasma AGEs-associated fluorescence ($\lambda_{ex} = 370$ nm/ $\lambda_{em} = 445$ nm). At baseline, but not at follow up, the breast-milk-fed infants displayed significantly lower plasma AGEs-associated fluorescence than the formula-receiving group. In the breast-milk-consuming infants the baseline plasma fluorescence was lower than at follow-up (Table 2).

Insulin sensitivity. At baseline, formula-fed infants displayed significantly lower glycemia and higher insulinemia, resulting in lower insulin sensitivity if compared with their breast-milk-fed counterparts. Neither of these parameters differed significantly at follow-up (Table 2).

Soluble RAGE. No significant difference was revealed between the breast-milk- and formula-consuming infants (Table 2).

hsCRP and adhesion molecules. The breast-milk- and formula-fed infants did not differ significantly by hsCRP, sICAM-1, sVCAM-1 and sVAP-1 levels (Table 2). In both cohorts the circulating sVAP-1 levels were significantly lower at follow-up in comparison with the baseline data. In the formula-consuming infants a direct relationship between sRAGE and sVAP-1 was revealed ($y = 0.034x+269.5$, $r = 0.303$, $p = 0.034$).

Leptin. In correspondence with the cross-sectional study data, the breast-milk- and formula-fed infants did not differ significantly by baseline leptinemia (3.2; 2.2–5.7 ng/ml, and 2.7; 1.8–3.8 ng/ml, respectively).

Discussion

Breast-milk- versus formula-feeding represents a unique long-term human model of AGE-poor versus AGE-rich diets consumption, in which the adherence to the diet is doubtless. We show that, in healthy term infants, high dietary intake of AGEs in form of infant formulas is reflected by a rise in circulating total plasma CML levels, and AGEs-associated fluorescence, but it is neither involved in formula-consumption-associated reduced insulin sensitivity, nor accompanied by enhanced oxidative stress and micro-inflammation. Trends in total plasma levels of CML and AGE-associated fluorescence seem not to be the same over time.

Plasma CML Levels

Lactose, a main milk sugar in mammals, is a potent glycating agent modifying lysine residues into CML and other Maillard reaction products [47]. In our study milk prepared from infant formulas contained 5.3%–8.3% lactose, 6.6% in mean. Human breast milk contains 6.9–7.2% lactose [48]. Thus, we postulate that the amount of ingested lactose in form of infant formula was similar to that ingested in breast milk; and the difference in lactose intake could not underlie observed differences in total plasma CML levels between the formula- and breast-fed infants.

Mericq et al. showed that in comparison with exclusively breast-fed newborns, in 12-month-olds on a mixed diet the daily intake of AGEs is 7.5-fold higher, reflected by an age-dependent rise in serum CML [13]. We confirmed this data: in infants weaned from breast-milk total plasma CML levels rise age-dependently, reflecting an increased dietary CML load imposed by a mixed diet. However, introduction of a mixed diet to high-CML-containing formulas-consuming infants is associated with an age-dependent decline in total plasma CML concentrations, implying that mixed diet imposes a lower dietary CML-load than formula consumption. Replacement of low-CML-containing formula with a mixed diet is not associated with apparent changes in circulating CML levels, indicating that the diet provides a similar oral CML-load to that of low-CML-containing formulas. When consuming a mixed diet, formerly breast-milk- and formula-fed infants present comparable total plasma CML levels.

Oxidative stress and inflammation may also lead to AGE formation [13,49–51]. Our data do not suggest that these mechanisms contribute to elevation of circulating CML and AGEs-associated fluorescence in formula-consuming infants, since these infants neither present increased levels of markers of lipid peroxidation (MDA, 8-isoprostanes), nor of microinflammation (hsCRP, adhesion molecules), if compared with their breast-milk-fed counterparts.

In adults, an increase in serum SSAO/VAP-1 is mirrored by a rise in circulating AGEs, and oxidative stress markers [43].

Formula-fed infants neither present alterations in circulating levels of sVAP-1 and oxidative stress markers, nor significant correlation between plasma AGE and sVAP-1 levels. Thus, SSAO pathway is probably not involved in formula-consumption-associated rise in plasma AGE levels.

Exogenously administered sRAGE blocks the harmful effects of AGEs in animals by acting as a decoy receptor [52]. Endogenous sRAGE probably does not exert the same biological effect since serum levels of sRAGE in humans are 1000-fold lower than needed for binding to AGEs [52], and in healthy adults circulating AGEs positively, rather than inversely, correlate with sRAGE levels [53]. Although groups on different dietary regimen did not differ significantly in sRAGE levels, formula-consuming infants, particularly those administered high-CML-containing formulas, presented a positive relationship between total plasma CML and sRAGE concentrations, probably reflecting the enhanced cleavage of sRAGE from the cell surface RAGE. Correlation between sRAGE and sVAP-1 levels, both shed from cell surface by matrix metalloproteinases [41,54], supports this assumption. Our data suggest that under long-term high-AGE diet endogenous sRAGE is not the determinant of total circulating CML levels.

Thus, during the period when milk represents a sole or major source of nutrition absorbed dietary infant formulas-derived AGEs account for elevated total plasma CML and AGE-associated fluorescence levels.

Insulin Sensitivity

Exclusively breast-fed infants presented higher insulin sensitivity, and lower total plasma CML levels and plasma fluorescence than their formulas-consuming counterparts. This could support the presumption that an AGE-rich-diet-induced rise in AGEs might be involved in the induction of insulin resistance. However, several lines of evidence point against this assumption. First, in comparison with low-CML-containing-formulas, consumption of high-CML-containing formulas resulting in higher total circulating CML levels does not aggravate insulin resistance. Second, 7-to-10-month-olds weaned either from formula or breast-milk presented comparable insulin sensitivity, despite approximately 40-to-200-fold difference in the dietary CML burden imposed, reflected accordingly by higher total plasma CML levels in the formula-consuming group. Third, the introduction of a mixed diet, with substantially higher AGE contents than that in breast-milk [13], to exclusively breast-fed infants was not associated with a decrease in insulin sensitivity in our study. Fourth, in contrast to data from healthy adults [32–34], we did not reveal any significant relationship between total plasma CML levels or plasma AGEs-associated fluorescence and insulin sensitivity. A recent well-controlled study in healthy young adults also documented that ingestion of highly thermally processed food, in comparison with steamed diet, results in rise in plasma CML levels and decline of insulin sensitivity, without any correlation between these two parameters [19]. Although Mericq et al. [13] demonstrated a concomitant rise in plasma AGE levels and insulin resistance in healthy infants weaned from mother milk, no correlation between the two parameters was presented, preventing a direct comparison of our data with their findings. Fifth, in contrast to studies in adults, we did not observe an induction of oxidative stress- and microinflammatory-markers, which could contribute to the induction of insulin resistance [13,49] during formula-feeding. Sixth, since high AGE-diet did not affect sVAP-1 levels, insulin resistance could not be elicited by sVAP-1 decline. VAP-1 has been found to have an antidiabetic function in the rats [41], and might contribute to lactation-associated insulin sensitivity in humans [55]. Seventh, the formula-feeding-induced rise in total

plasma CML and AGEs-associated fluorescence was not accompanied by hyperleptinemia, which could participate in the induction of insulin resistance [56,57]. Similar leptinemia between the breast-milk- and formula-fed infants was reported also by others [58]. And eighth, markers of oxidative stress and inflammation neither differed significantly between formula- and mother-milk-consuming infants, nor showed significant relationship to total plasma CML, or to insulin sensitivity. This contradicts the suggestion that formula-derived AGEs might precondition the infants to insulin resistance via induction of inflammation and oxidative stress [13]. Eventually, in our study either unspecified AGEs present in infant formulas possessing an antioxidant capacity, or fortification of formulas with antioxidant vitamins counteracted the AGEs-induced oxidative stress. High levels of antioxidant vitamins seem to exert similar protective effects in vegetarians, who, despite of high plasma AGE levels, present higher insulin sensitivity than omnivores [59].

A rapid growth in early childhood in infants born small for gestational age is considered as a risk factor for development of insulin resistance and metabolic syndrome in later life [3,60]. However, Kerkhof et al. recently suggested that a gain in weight during the first 3 months of life, not the birth weight per se, was the most important determinant of prevalence of metabolic syndrome, and its signs, in young adults [12]. Our data showing that mean daily weight gains in 3-to-6-month-olds show inverse relation to insulin sensitivity regardless of the feeding regimen, are in line with the above mentioned observation, although Kerkhof et al. [12] did not investigate the effects of breast- versus formula-feeding. Our data also suggest that in the case of formula feeding this effect might not be restricted to early infancy, as indicated by inverse relationship between the mean weight gain and insulin resistance in infant formula-fed group generally. In addition, we revealed a tight relationship between leptin levels (a regulator of food intake and energy metabolism, [56]) and mean daily weight gain. Changes in circulating leptin levels are thought to be related to insulin-mediated glucose metabolism in adipose tissue [57]. In light of these facts the associations observed in our study in healthy, term and appropriate for gestational age infants require attention, and their potential clinical relevance remains to be confirmed in larger and prospective studies.

Although industrial heat-processing of infant formulas results in a substantial rise of early and advanced glycation end-products [17], in contrast to thermally processed foods consumed by adults, infant formulas generally contain only traces of, if any, other heat-born toxic substances [61–63]. Thus, as far as the ongoing debate whether dietary AGEs are harmful to human health or not is concerned [18,21,49,50,64], our data favor the assumption that the negative health effects of thermally processed foods do not result from ingestion of CML *per se*, but rather from other AGEs, or additive effects of different heat-processing-derived substances.

Relatively high proportion of the formula-fed infants was administered high-CML-containing (e.g. hypoallergenic, hydrolyzed) formulas, despite that food or other allergy was an exclusion criterion. In so far these formulas were not administered therapeutically. The intentional prescription of hydrolyzed formulas to infants with lower normal birth weight can be excluded, since the infants on high-CML-containing formulas tended to have higher birth weight. However, the high proportion of infants on hydrolyzed formulas did not stem purely from implementation of preventive measures, often applied if a sibling suffered from allergy. Some infants were shifted from non-hydrolyzed to hydrolyzed formulas if they did not accept the new formula well, or did not thrive well, e.g. during weaning or introduction of follow-on formula. In light of rising prevalence of allergies [65,66] mothers are often convinced that hydrolyzed formulas are better, thus feed their baby with these despite being explained by the pediatrician that it is not indicated.

Limitations

Some of the age-matched groups of formula- and breast-milk-fed infants differed by the body weight, due to the higher birth weights of the breast-fed infants. We suppose that this was a coincidence, since the infants were not randomly assigned to feeding-regimen groups. Other studies reporting higher birth weights of the breast-fed infants suggest that mothers who intend to breast feed are more conscious of their lifestyle during pregnancy, resulting in a higher birth weight of their child [67,68]. Sample size was calculated to detect 50% difference in plasma AGEs in 3-to-6-month-olds infants, and thus could be underpowered to assess significant differences in some other studied parameters. Blood chemistry parameters were not analyzed after overnight fasting. In infants, the duration of fasting should be selected as a compromise between avoiding postprandial blood sampling and obtaining a reasonable fasting interval not harming/endangering the child. The fasting time employed in our study (3 hours) fits well with that applied in other studies on insulin sensitivity in toddlers, e.g. fasting intervals of 2-to-4 hours [6,69]. Exact duration of fasting prior to blood sampling was not recorded, thus the data could not be corrected for this parameter. Malondialdehyde, a widely used marker of oxidative stress [13,32,33], was determined only in 3-to-6-month-olds, not allowing the detailed analysis of the relationships to plasma AGE levels and markers of microinflammation. Although the total interference of low-molecular-weight fluorophores naturally occurring in plasma under physiological conditions with plasma fluorescence ($\lambda_{ex} = 370$ nm/$\lambda_{em} = 445$ nm) is low (up to 1%) [46], the interference of non-AGE-modified proteins cannot be excluded. The daily burden of ingested CML was not expressed upon determination of CML content in individual samples taken from each child's formula. Planning the study we considered this approach, but we concluded that analysis of CML in individual formulas collected from each child's household could bias the results substantially, since the collection of powder formula samples, their handling and storage between sampling in each household and hand-over in our laboratory, as well as the storage period prior to sending the samples for CML analyses to central laboratory (Garching, Germany in frames of ICARE project) could not be adequately standardized. Thus, we gave a priority to the approach described previously [14]: the formulas consumed by the enrolled infants were purchased in the pharmacy and analyzed for CML content, also assuming a standardized procedure for the processing of each formula which in general is aimed at low intra-individual variances. Our results are pertinent to the consumption of 17 different infant formulas produced by 5 different world renowned companies. It might not be excluded that other infant formulas contain different amounts of CML, or exert different effects on parameters determined herein. However, our data on the CML content of infant formulas, as well as the estimated

difference in CML content between mother milk and infant formula, are in excellent accordance with those reported by Delatour et al. [14,16]. It might be argued that inclusion of infants consuming 17 different formulas might have confounded the results. Taking into account that human milk composition changes during the lactation, and displays particular inter-individual differences, our formula-fed infants might represent even more homogenous group than the breast-milk-fed infants. We determined a single chemically defined AGE – CML. Data on CML urinary excretion are not presented, since CML levels in random spot urines neither reflect accurately the daily CML-load, nor can be used for calculation of dietary CML exposure. In the pilot study we showed that infant formula-fed infants excrete roughly 60-fold more CML than their breast-milk-fed counterparts [14]. In non-proteinuric subjects free CML adducts account for urinary CML excretion. Extremely large inter-individual variability of CML in random spot urines from formula-fed infants suggests a rapid elimination after the absorption [14]. This fits with the experimental data showing that the half-life of i.v. administered labeled fluorobenzylated-CML is very short (about 20 min) [70]. However, the biodistribution and elimination profile of this i.v. administered derivatized free adduct may differ from that of underivatized CML administered orally. At least but not at last, pre-pregnancy BMI of the mothers (not recorded in our study) could adversely affect the insulin sensitivity of the infant.

Taken together, our data support our previous hypothesis that high circulating AGEs in formula-consuming infants arise from high dietary intake of AGEs [14], and are in line with results from a recent study of Mericq et al. [13]. We confirmed that formula feeding is associated with the development of transient insulin resistance. In healthy infants, AGEs absorbed from infant formulas do not play a role in formula-consumption-associated insulin resistance, either directly or indirectly by induction of oxidative stress, micro-inflammation, hyperleptinemia or decline in sVAP levels. It remains to be elucidated whether the formula-feeding-associated high dietary load with AGEs in early infancy could exert negative health effects in vulnerable, sensitive, or diseased children; or predispose them to earlier, accelerated, or more serious manifestation of chronic degenerative diseases in later life.

Acknowledgments

Authors wish to express their gratitude to the mothers/legal guardians and their children for participation; pediatricians of first contact, Drs.: Bradiak F, Chramcová N, Holanová E, Kollárová E, Kadlíčková A, Križanová E, Lásková J, Lukyová M, Petríková I, Polláková V, Prokopová E, Rapošová R, Salcerová J, Sláviková E, Šimeková L, Špániková M, Vicianová K, and their nurses for cooperation in recruitment and collection of the samples.

Author Contributions

Conceived and designed the experiments: KŠ VS VF. Performed the experiments: KSK KŠ. Analyzed the data: KSK KŠ PC. Contributed reagents/materials/analysis tools: KSK PB VS PC VF KŠ. Wrote the paper: KSK VS KŠ.

References

1. Dabelea D (2009) The accelerating epidemic of childhood diabetes. Lancet 373: 1999–2000.

2. Dandona P, Aljada A, Bandyopadhyay A (2004) Inflammation: the link between insulin resistance, obesity and diabetes. Trends Immunol 25: 4–7.

3. Mericq V, Ong KK, Bazaes R, Pena V, Avila A, et al. (2005) Longitudinal changes in insulin sensitivity and secretion from birth to age three years in small- and appropriate-for-gestational-age children. Diabetologia 48: 2609–2614.

4. Lucas A, Boyes S, Bloom SR, Aynsley-Green A (1981) Metabolic and endocrine responses to a milk feed in six-day-old term infants: differences between breast and cow's milk formula feeding. Acta Paediatr Scand 70: 195–200.

5. Ginsburg BE, Lindblad BS, Lundsjo A, Persson B, Zetterstrom R (1984) Plasma valine and urinary C-peptide in breast-fed and artificially fed infants up to 6 months of age. Acta Paediatr Scand 73: 213–217.

6. Madsen AL, Schack-Nielsen L, Larnkjaer A, Molgaard C, Michaelsen KF (2010) Determinants of blood glucose and insulin in healthy 9-month-old term Danish infants; the SKOT cohort. Diabet Med 27: 1350–1357.

7. Heird WC (2007) Progress in promoting breast-feeding, combating malnutrition, and composition and use of infant formula, 1981–2006. J Nutr 137: 499S–502S.

8. Leung AKC, Sauve RS (2005) Breast is best for babies. J Natl Med Assoc 97: 1010–1019.

9. Schack-Nielsen L, Michaelsen KE (2007) Advances in our understanding of the biology of human milk and its effects on the offspring. J Nutr 137: 503S–510S.

10. Das UN (2002) The lipids that matter from infant nutrition to insulin resistance. Prostaglandins Leukot Essent Fatty Acids 67: 1–12.

11. Savino F, Fissore MF, Liguori SA, Oggero R (2009) Can hormones contained in mothers' milk account for the beneficial effect of breast-feeding on obesity in children? Clin Endocrinol (Oxf) 71: 757–765.

12. Kerkhof GF, Leunissen RW, Hokken-Koelega AC (2012) Early origins of the metabolic syndrome: role of small size at birth, early postnatal weight gain, and adult IGF-I. J Clin Endocrinol Metab 8: 2637–2643.

13. Mericq V, Piccardo C, Cai W, Chen X, Zhu L, et al. (2010) Maternally transmitted and food-derived glycotoxins: a factor preconditioning the young to diabetes? Diabetes Care 33: 2232–2237.

14. Sebekova K, Saavedra G, Zumpe C, Somoza V, Klenovicsova K, et al. (2008) Plasma concentration and urinary excretion of N epsilon-(carboxymethyl)lysine in breast milk- and formula-fed infants. Ann N Y Acad Sci 1126: 177–180.

15. Birlouez-Aragon I, Pischetsrieder M, Leclére J, Morales FJ, Hasenkopf K, et al. (2004) Assessment of protein glycation markers in infant formulas. Food Chemistry 87: 253–259.

16. Delatour T, Hegele J, Parisod V, Richoz J, Maurer S, et al. (2009) Analysis of advanced glycation endproducts in dairy products by isotope dilution liquid chromatography-electrospray tandem mass spectrometry. The particular case of carboxymethyllysine. J Chromatogr A 1216: 2371–2381.

17. Pischetsrieder M, Henle T (2012) Glycation products in infant formulas: chemical, analytical and physiological aspects. Amino Acids 42: 1111–1118.

18. Sebekova K, Somoza V (2007) Dietary advanced glycation endproducts (AGEs) and their health effects–PRO. Mol Nutr Food Res 51: 1079–1084.

19. Birlouez-Aragon I, Saavedra G, Tessier FJ, Galinier A, Ait-Ameur L, et al. (2010) A diet based on high-heat-treated foods promotes risk factors for diabetes mellitus and cardiovascular diseases. Am J Clin Nutr 91: 1220–1226.

20. Uribarri J, Cai W, Sandu O, Peppa M, Goldberg T, et al. (2005) Diet-derived advanced glycation end products are major contributors to the body's AGE pool and induce inflammation in healthy subjects. Ann N Y Acad Sci 1043: 461–466.

21. Van Nguyen C (2006) Toxicity of the AGEs generated from the Maillard reaction: On the relationship of food-AGEs and biological-AGEs. Mol Nutr Food Res 50: 1140–1149.

22. Bierhaus A, Humpert PM, Morcos M, Wendt T, Chavakis T, et al. (2005) Understanding RAGE, the receptor for advanced glycation end products. J Mol Med (Berl) 83: 876–886.

23. Yan SF, Ramasamy R, Naka Y, Schmidt AM (2003) Glycation, inflammation, and RAGE: a scaffold for the macrovascular complications of diabetes and beyond. Circ Res 93: 1159–1169.

24. Buetler TM, Latado H, Leclerc E, Weigle B, Baumeyer A, et al. (2011) Glycolaldehyde-modified beta-lactoglobulin AGEs are unable to stimulate inflammatory signaling pathways in RAGE-expressing human cell lines. Mol Nutr Food Res 55: 291–299.

25. Buetler TM, Leclerc E, Baumeyer A, Latado H, Newell J, et al. (2008) N(epsilon)-carboxymethyllysine-modified proteins are unable to bind to RAGE and activate an inflammatory response. Mol Nutr Food Res 52: 370–378.

26. Cassese A, Esposito I, Fiory F, Barbagallo AP, Paturzo F, et al. (2008) In skeletal muscle advanced glycation end products (AGEs) inhibit insulin action and induce the formation of multimolecular complexes including the receptor for AGEs. J Biol Chem 283: 36088–36099.

27. Miele C, Riboulet A, Maitan MA, Oriente F, Romano C, et al. (2003) Human glycated albumin affects glucose metabolism in L6 skeletal muscle cells by impairing insulin-induced insulin receptor substrate (IRS) signaling through a protein kinase C alpha-mediated mechanism. J Biol Chem 278: 47376–47387.

28. Unoki H, Bujo H, Yamagishi S, Takeuchi M, Imaizumi T, et al. (2007) Advanced glycation end products attenuate cellular insulin sensitivity by increasing the generation of intracellular reactive oxygen species in adipocytes. Diabetes Res Clin Pract 76: 236–244.

29. Zhao Z, Zhao C, Zhang XH, Zheng F, Cai W, et al. (2009) Advanced glycation end products inhibit glucose-stimulated insulin secretion through nitric oxide-dependent inhibition of cytochrome c oxidase and adenosine triphosphate synthesis. Endocrinology 150: 2569–2576.

30. Puddu A, Storace D, Odetti P, Viviani GL (2010) Advanced glycation end-products affect transcription factors regulating insulin gene expression. Biochem Biophys Res Commun 395: 122–125.

31. Shu TT, Zhu YX, Wang HD, Lin Y, Ma Z, et al. (2011) AGEs Decrease Insulin Synthesis in Pancreatic beta-Cell by Repressing Pdx-1 Protein Expression at the Post-Translational Level. PLoS One 6.

32. Tan KC, Shiu SW, Wong Y, Tam X (2011) Serum advanced glycation end products (AGEs) are associated with insulin resistance. Diabetes Metab Res Rev 27: 488–492.

33. Uribarri J, Cai W, Ramdas M, Goodman S, Pyzik R, et al. (2011) Restriction of advanced glycation end products improves insulin resistance in human type 2 diabetes: potential role of AGER1 and SIRT1. Diabetes Care 34: 1610–1616.

34. Tahara N, Yamagishi S, Matsui T, Takeuchi M, Nitta Y, et al. (2012) Serum Levels of Advanced Glycation End Products (AGEs) are Independent Correlates of Insulin Resistance in Nondiabetic Subjects. Cardiovascular Therapeutics 30: 42–48.

35. Yonekura H, Yamamoto Y, Sakurai S, Petrova RG, Abedin MJ, et al. (2003) Novel splice variants of the receptor for advanced glycation end-products expressed in human vascular endothelial cells and pericytes, and their putative roles in diabetes-induced vascular injury. Biochem J 370: 1097–1109.

36. Boor P, Celec P, Klenovicsova K, Vlkova B, Szemes T, et al. (2010) Association of biochemical parameters and RAGE gene polymorphisms in healthy infants and their mothers. Clin Chim Acta 411: 1034–1040.

37. Basta G, Sironi AM, Lazzerini G, Del Turco S, Buzzigoli E, et al. (2006) Circulating soluble receptor for advanced glycation end products is inversely associated with glycemic control and S100A12 protein. J Clin Endocrinol Metab 91: 4628–4634.

38. Koyama H, Yamamoto H, Nishizawa Y (2007) Endogenous Secretory RAGE as a Novel Biomarker for Metabolic Syndrome and Cardiovascular Diseases. Biomark Insights 2: 331–339.

39. Smith DJ, Salmi M, Bono P, Hellman J, Leu T, et al. (1998) Cloning of vascular adhesion protein 1 reveals a novel multifunctional adhesion molecule. J Exp Med 188: 17–27.

40. Lyles GA, Chalmers J (1992) The metabolism of aminoacetone to methylglyoxal by semicarbazide-sensitive amine oxidase in human umbilical artery. Biochem Pharmacol 43: 1409–1414.

41. Abella A, Marti L, Camps M, Claret M, Fernandez-Alvarez J, et al. (2003) Semicarbazide-sensitive amine oxidase/vascular adhesion protein-1 activity exerts an antidiabetic action in Goto-Kakizaki rats. Diabetes 52: 1004–1013.

42. Li HY, Wei JN, Lin MS, Smith DJ, Vainio J, et al. (2009) Serum vascular adhesion protein-1 is increased in acute and chronic hyperglycemia. Clin Chim Acta 404: 149–153.

43. Li HY, Lin MS, Wei JN, Hung CS, Chiang FT, et al. (2009) Change of serum vascular adhesion protein-1 after glucose loading correlates to carotid intima-medial thickness in non-diabetic subjects. Clin Chim Acta 403: 97–101.

44. Katz A, Nambi SS, Mather K, Baron AD, Follmann DA, et al. (2000) Quantitative insulin sensitivity check index: a simple, accurate method for assessing insulin sensitivity in humans. J Clin Endocrinol Metab 85: 2402–2410.

45. Wong SH, Knight JA, Hopfer SM, Zaharia O, Leach CN Jr, et al. (1987) Lipoperoxides in plasma as measured by liquid-chromatographic separation of malondialdehyde-thiobarbituric acid adduct. Clin Chem 33: 214–220.

46. Munch G, Keis R, Wessels A, Riederer P, Bahner U, et al. (1997) Determination of advanced glycation end products in serum by fluorescence spectroscopy and competitive ELISA. Eur J Clin Chem Clin Biochem 35: 669–677.

47. Meltretter J, Pischetsrieder M (2008) Application of mass spectrometry for the detection of glycation and oxidation products in milk proteins. In: Schleicher E, Somoza V, Shieberle P, editors. Maillard Reaction: Recent Advances in Food and Biomedical Sciences. 134–140.

48. Jenness R (1979) The composition of human milk. Semin Perinatol 3: 225–239.

49. Vlassara H, Striker G (2007) Glycotoxins in the diet promote diabetes and diabetic complications. Curr Diab Rep 7: 235–241.

50. Ames JM (2007) Evidence against dietary advanced glycation endproducts being a risk to human health. Mol Nutr Food Res 51: 1085–1090.

51. Miyata T, Kurokawa K, van Ypersele de Strihou C (2000) Relevance of oxidative and carbonyl stress to long-term uremic complications. Kidney Int Suppl 76: S120–125.

52. Park L, Raman KG, Lee KJ, Lu Y, Ferran LJ Jr, et al. (1998) Suppression of accelerated diabetic atherosclerosis by the soluble receptor for advanced glycation endproducts. Nat Med 4: 1025–1031.

53. Nakamura K, Yamagishi SI, Matsui T, Adachi H, Takeuchi M, et al. (2007) Serum levels of soluble form of receptor for advanced glycation end products (sRAGE) are correlated with AGEs in both diabetic and non-diabetic subjects. Clin Exp Med 7: 188–190.

54. Zhang L, Bukulin M, Kojro E, Roth A, Metz VV, et al. (2008) Receptor for advanced glycation end products is subjected to protein ectodomain shedding by metalloproteinases. J Biol Chem 283: 35507–35516.

55. Klenovicsova K, Krivosikova Z, Gajdos M, Sebekova K (2011) Association of sVAP-1, sRAGE, and CML with lactation-induced insulin sensitivity in young non-diabetic healthy women. Clin Chim Acta 412: 1842–1847.

56. Havel PJ (1998) Leptin production and action: relevance to energy balance in humans. Am J Clin Nutr 67: 355–356.

57. Mueller WM, Gregoire FM, Stanhope KL, Mobbs CV, Mizuno TM, et al. (1998) Evidence that glucose metabolism regulates leptin secretion from cultured rat adipocytes. Endocrinology 139: 551–558.

58. Lonnerdal B, Havel PJ (2000) Serum leptin concentrations in infants: effects of diet, sex, and adiposity. Am J Clin Nutr 72: 484–489.

59. Sebekova K, Krajcovicova-Kudlackova M, Schinzel R, Faist V, Klvanova J, et al. (2001) Plasma levels of advanced glycation end products in healthy, long-term vegetarians and subjects on a western mixed diet. Eur J Nutr 40: 275–281.

60. Fabricius-Bjerre S, Jensen RB, Faerch K, Larsen T, Molgaard C, et al. (2011) Impact of Birth Weight and Early Infant Weight Gain on Insulin Resistance and Associated Cardiovascular Risk Factors in Adolescence. PLoS One 6.

61. Erkekoglu P, Baydar T (2010) Toxicity of acrylamide and evaluation of its exposure in baby foods. Nutr Res Rev 23: 323–333.

62. Felton JS, Knize MG, Wu RW, Colvin ME, Hatch FT, et al. (2007) Mutagenic potency of food-derived heterocyclic amines. Mutat Res 616: 90–94.

63. Fohgelberg P, Rosen J, Hellenas KE, Abramsson-Zetterberg L (2005) The acrylamide intake via some common baby food for children in Sweden during their first year of life–an improved method for analysis of acrylamide. Food Chem Toxicol 43: 951–959.

Advanced Glycation End Products in Infant Formulas do not Contribute to Insulin Resistance Associated...

99

64. Heizmann CW (2007) The mechanism by which dietary AGEs are a risk to human health is via their interaction with RAGE: arguing against the motion. Mol Nutr Food Res 51: 1116–1119.

65. Lack G (2012) Update on risk factors for food allergy. J Allergy Clin Immunol 129: 1187–1197.

66. DaVeiga SP (2012) Epidemiology of atopic dermatitis: a review. Allergy Asthma Proc 33: 227–234.

67. Agostoni C, Grandi F, Gianni ML, Silano M, Torcoletti M, et al. (1999) Growth patterns of breast fed and formula fed infants in the first 12 months of life: an Italian study. Arch Dis Child 81: 395–399.

68. Bulk-Bunschoten AM, van Bodegom S, Reerink JD, de Jong PC, de Groot CJ (2002) Weight and weight gain at 4 months (The Netherlands 1998): influences of nutritional practices, socio-economic and ethnic factors. Paediatr Perinat Epidemiol 16: 361–369.

69. Gupta M, Zaheer, Jora R, Kaul V, Gupta R (2010) Breast feeding and insulin levels in low birth weight neonates: a randomized study. Indian J Pediatr 77: 509–513.

70. Bergmann R, Helling R, Heichert C, Scheunemann M, Mading P, et al. (2001) Radio fluorination and positron emission tomography (PET) as a new approach to study the in vivo distribution and elimination of the advanced glycation endproducts N epsilon-carboxymethyllysine (CML) and N epsilon-carboxyethyl-lysine (CEL). Nahrung 45: 182–188.

12

The Relationship of the Anti-Oxidant Bilirubin with Free Thyroxine is Modified by Insulin Resistance in Euthyroid Subjects

Petronella E. Deetman*, Stephan J. L. Bakker, Arjan J. Kwakernaak, Gerjan Navis, Robin P. F. Dullaart, on behalf of the PREVEND Study Group[¶]

Department of Internal Medicine, University of Groningen, University Medical Center Groningen, The Netherlands

Abstract

Background: The strong anti-oxidative properties of bilirubin largely explain its cardioprotective effects. Insulin resistance is featured by low circulating bilirubin. Thyroid hormone affects both bilirubin generation and its biliary transport, but it is unknown whether circulating bilirubin is associated with thyroid function in euthyroid subjects. Aim is to determine relationships of bilirubin with TSH, free T_4 and free T_3 in euthyroid subjects without type 2 diabetes mellitus (T2DM), and to assess whether such a relationship would be modified by the degree of insulin resistance.

Methods: Total bilirubin, TSH, free T_4, free T_3, glucose, insulin, lipids and transaminases were measured in 1854 fasting euthyroid subjects without T2DM, recruited from the general population (PREVEND cohort). Insulin resistance was assessed by homeostasis model assessment.

Results: Bilirubin was positively related to free T_4 ($\beta = 0.116$, $P < 0.001$) and free T_3 ($\beta = 0.078$, $P = 0.001$), but bilirubin was unrelated to TSH. The relationship of bilirubin with free T_4 was modified by insulin resistance with a larger effect in more insulin resistant individuals (adjusted for age and sex: $\beta = 0.043$, $P = 0.056$ for interaction; additionally adjusted for smoking, alcohol intake, transaminases and total cholesterol ($\beta = 0.044$, $P = 0.044$ for interaction). The association of bilirubin with free T_4 was also modified by high density lipoprotein cholesterol (age- and sex-adjusted: $\beta = 0.040$, $P = 0.072$).

Conclusions: Low bilirubin relates to low free T_4 in euthyroid non-diabetic subjects. Low normal free T_4 may particularly confer low bilirubin in more insulin resistant individuals.

Editor: Harpal Singh Randeva, University of Warwick – Medical School, United Kingdom

Funding: The Dutch Kidney Foundation supported the infrastructure of the PREVEND program from 1997 to 2003 (Grant E.033). The University Medical Center Groningen supported the infrastructure from 2003 to 2006. Dade Behring, Ausam, Roche, and Abbott financed laboratory equipment and reagents by which various laboratory determinations could be performed. The Dutch Heart Foundation supported studies on lipid metabolism (Grant 2001–005). The funders had no role in study design, data collection and analysis, decision to publish, or preparation of the manuscript.

Competing Interests: The authors have declared that no competing interests exist.

* E-mail: p.e.deetman@umcg.nl

¶ Membership of the PREVEND Study Group is provided in the Acknowledgments.

Introduction

It is increasingly appreciated that endogenous bilirubin has strong anti-oxidative properties, which are attributed to its ability to scavenge peroxyl radicals and to inhibit low density lipoprotein (LDL) oxidation [1]. Hence, the concept is emerging that bilirubin is involved in the pathogenesis of cardiometabolic disorders in which oxidative-stress is considered to play an important role [1–3]. In this line, low circulating levels of bilirubin levels have been documented to be associated with increased severity of atherosclerosis [4] and higher risk of lower limb amputation [5]. Low levels of circulating bilirubin have also been associated with increased cardiovascular and all-cause mortality in men [6]. In addition, intima media thickness, an established marker of subclinical atherosclerosis, is smaller in subjects with isolated hyperbilirubinemia [7]. Conversely, increased intima media thickness relates to low bilirubin in middle-aged subjects [8].

The importance of bilirubin for the development of atherosclerotic cardiovascular diseases underscores the relevance to delineate the metabolic factors that affect its metabolism in more detail. Thyroid hormones stimulate heme oxygenase-1 activity (HO-1), which is the main enzyme responsible for bilirubin production [9,10]. Furthermore, thyroid hormones downregulate the enzymatic activity of uridine 5′-diphospho-glucuronosyltransferase (UDP-GT), which stimulates bilirubin conjugation, thereby facilitating bilirubin excretion [11,12]. In agreement with the hypothesis that thyroid function represents a clinically relevant determinant of serum bilirubin metabolism, we have recently shown that low free T_4 levels confer decreased bilirubin levels in euthyroid patients with type 2 diabetes mellitus (T2DM) [13]. Of further interest, insulin resistance and the metabolic syndrome

Table 1. Clinical characteristics, glucose, insulin, insulin resistance, lipids, transaminases, and thyroid hormones in 1854 subjects.

	Sex-stratified tertiles of bilirubin			β	P-value
	1	2	3		
	Men (n = 335)	Men (n = 324)	Men (n = 263)		
	<7 μmol/L	7–9 μmol/L	>9 μmol/L		
	Women (n = 354)	Women (n = 274)	Women (n = 291)		
	<6 μmol/L	6–7 μmol/L	>7 μmol/L		
Age (years)	48±12	48±13	46±13	−0.037	0.109
BMI (kg/m^2)	26.5±4.5	25.7±4.4	25.1±3.9	−0.114	<0.001
Alcohol				0.077	0.001
<10 gram per day (%)	76	69	72		
≥10 gram per day (%)	24	31	28		
Current smoker (%)	44	36	27	−0.163	<0.001
Waist circumference in men (cm)	95±12	92±11	92±12	−0.109	0.001
Waist circumference in women (cm)	83±13	82±13	80±11	−0.125	<0.001
Systolic blood pressure (mmHg)	129±21	129±19	126±20	0.022	0.338
Diastolic blood pressure (mmHg)	74±9	74±9	73±10	0.012	0.595
Glucose (mmol/L)	4.4 (4.0–4.9)	4.4 (4.0–4.8)	4.2 (3.9–4.6)	−0.028	0.234
Insulin (mU/L)	9.0 (6.1–13.2)	7.6 (5.5–11.1)	7.1 (5.1–10.0)	−0.133	<0.001
HOMA-IR	1.74 (1.15–2.76)	1.47 (1.03–2.26)	1.33 (0.92–1.94)	−0.122	<0.001
Total cholesterol (mmol/L)	5.82±1.16	5.60±1.16	5.41±1.08	−0.113	<0.001
HDL cholesterol (mmol/L)	1.32±0.39	1.35±0.39	1.43±0.43	0.031	0.189
Triglycerides (mmol/L)	1.24 (0.89–1.87)	1.12 (0.84–1.56)	1.01 (0.74–1.43)	−0.121	<0.001
Metabolic syndrome (%)	25	17	13	−0.101	0.001
TSH (mU/L)	1.34 (0.98–1.87)	1.28 (0.94–1.82)	1.37 (1.00–1.85)	−0.033	0.152
Free T$_4$ (pmol/L)	12.66±1.69	13.08±1.79	13.04±1.77	0.116	<0.001
Free T$_3$ (pmol/L)	3.69±0.62	3.72±0.61	3.80±0.62	0.078	0.001
AST (U/L)	24 (21–28)	24 (21–29)	25 (21–29)	0.154	<0.001
ALT (U/L)	20 (15–28)	20 (16–28)	20 (15–29)	0.115	<0.001

Data in mean ± SD or in median (interquartile range). BMI, body mass index; HOMA-IR, homeostasis model assessment-insulin resistance; HDL, high density lipoprotein; ALT, alanine aminotransferase; AST, aspartate aminotransferase; β, standardized regression coefficient. P-values for linear trend are shown. Bilirubin, glucose, insulin, HOMA-IR, triglycerides, TSH, AST and ALT were log transformed.

(MetS) are not only featured by low bilirubin levels, but also by low free T$_4$ [14,15]. In extension thereof, it may be hypothesized that a possible relationship of bilirubin with thyroid function among euthyroid subjects is influenced by insulin resistance.

Against this background, the present study was initiated to test whether low plasma bilirubin is related to a lower thyroid functional status in euthyroid non-diabetic subjects recruited from the general population. Second, we determined the extent to which such a relationship is modified by the degree of insulin resistance and MetS components.

Methods

Subjects

The population used for this study consisted of a random subset of participants of the PREVEND (Prevention of Renal and Vascular End Stage Disease) study, which are inhabitants, aged 28–75 yr, of the city of Groningen, The Netherlands. The protocol of this study has been described elsewhere [16,17]. The medical ethics committee of the University Medical Center Groningen approved the study, and all participants gave written informed consent. A health questionnaire indicated that the participants had no history of liver disease.

For the current analysis, we excluded subjects not being euthyroid, subjects using thyroid hormones, anti-thyroid drugs and amiodarone, subjects with diabetes mellitus (as indicated by self-reported questionnaire, a physician diagnosis of diabetes, the use of oral glucose-lowering medication and/or elevated plasma glucose), as well as subjects in whom blood was not taken in the fasting state. Euthyroidism was defined as TSH, free T$_4$ and free T$_3$ levels within the reference range as provided by the manufacturer (see Laboratory analyses). We additionally excluded subjects with positive anti-thyroid peroxidase auto-antibodies (cut-off value: see Laboratory analyses). Applying these selection criteria, 1854 subjects were eligible for the current analyses.

Patient characteristics, including age, sex, alcohol use, smoking status, body mass index (BMI), systolic and diastolic blood pressure, and waist circumference were obtained. Blood was drawn after an overnight fasting period for measurement of free T$_4$, free T$_3$, TSH, bilirubin, glucose, insulin, total cholesterol, high density lipoprotein (HDL) cholesterol, triglycerides, aspartate aminotransferase (AST), and alanine aminotransferase (ALT).

Body mass index was defined as weight (kg) by height (m) squared. Alcohol consumption was recorded with one drink being assumed to contain 10 grams of alcohol. Insulin resistance was estimated using the Homeostasis Model Assessment-Insulin Resistance (HOMA-IR): glucose (mmol/L) × insulin (mU/L)/ 22.5 [18]. Three or more of the following criteria were required for categorization of subjects with MetS: waist circumference > 102 cm for men and >88 cm for women, hypertension (blood pressure ≥130/85 mmHg or use of anti-hypertensive drugs), fasting triglycerides ≥1.70 mmol/L, fasting glucose ≥5.6 mmol/ L, and HDL cholesterol <1.03 mmol/L for men and < 1.29 mmol/L for women [19].

Laboratory analyses

Heparinized plasma and serum samples were stored at −80°C until analyses. Serum TSH (Architect; Abbott Laboratories, Abbott Park, IL, USA; reference range 0.35–4.94 mU/L), free T_4 (AxSYM; Abbott Laboratories, Abbott Park, IL, USA; reference range 9.14–23.81 pmol/L) and free T_3 (AxSYM; Abbott Laboratories, Abbott Park, IL, USA; reference range; 2.23–5.35 pmol/L) were measured by microparticle enzyme immunoassay. Anti-thyroid peroxidase autoantibodies were determined using commercially available automated enzyme linked immunoassays (Abbott Laboratories, Abbott Park, IL, USA; kit number 5F57). Anti-thyroid peroxidase autoantibodies were considered positive using a cutoff value as indicated by the supplier (≥12 kU/L). Plasma total bilirubin was measured by a colorimetric assay (2,4-dicholoraniline reaction; Merck MEGA, Darmstadt, Germany). In healthy subjects, bilirubin is most abundantly present in serum in its unconjugated form [20]. In a validation experiment (n = 80), a strong correlation between total bilirubin and unconjugated bilirubin (Spearman's r = 0.92, P< 0.001), as well as between total bilirubin and conjugated direct bilirubin (Spearman's r = 0.82, P<0.001) was observed. For the present study we only used total bilirubin in keeping with other

reports [21–23]. Serum ALT and AST were measured with pyridoxal phosphate activation (Merck MEGA, Darmstadt, Germany). Serum total cholesterol and plasma glucose were measured using Kodak Ektachem dry chemistry (Eastman Kodak, Rochester, NY, USA). Serum triglycerides were measured enzymatically. HDL cholesterol was measured with a homogeneous method (direct HDL, AEROSET system; Abbott Laboratories, Abbott Park, IL, USA; no. 7D67). Insulin was measured by microparticle enzyme immunoassay (AxSYM; Abbott Laboratories, Abbott Park, IL, USA).

Statistical analyses

Data analyses were performed using *SPSS* (version 20.0, SPSS Inc. Chicago, IL, USA). Normally distributed data are given as mean ± standard deviation (SD) and non-parametrically distributed data are presented as median (interquartile range, IQR). Categorical variables are given as percentages. Differences in bilirubin concentration between sexes were determined by Mann-Whitney U-test. Characteristics of the study population are presented according to sex-stratified tertiles of bilirubin. Univariable linear regression analysis was used to test for linear trends across tertiles of bilirubin. Multivariable linear regression analyses were used to determine the extent to which bilirubin is related to thyroid function, components of the metabolic syndrome, insulin, HOMA-IR and transaminases. To this end, logarithmically transformed values of bilirubin, glucose, insulin, HOMA-IR, triglycerides, TSH and transaminases were used. Multivariable models were all age- and sex-adjusted. Before calculating interaction terms, the continuous variable of interest were centered to the mean by subtracting the group mean value from individual values. This was done in order to avoid multicollinearity [24,25]. Interaction terms were considered statistically significant at *P*-values <0.10, as proposed by Selvin [26] and recommended by the Food and Drug Administration authorities [27]. Otherwise, two-sided *P*-values <0.05 were considered significant.

Results

A total of 1854 subjects (age 47±13, 50% men) participated in this study. Median bilirubin concentration was 8 (6–10) μmol/L in men and 6 (5–8) μmol/L in women (*P*<0.001). Clinical and laboratory characteristics of the study population are, therefore, shown according to sex-stratified tertiles of bilirubin (Table 1). Angiotensin converting enzyme inhibitors (ACEi) or angiotensin receptor blockers (ARB's) were used by 56 subjects (3%); 46 subjects (3%) used lipid lowering drugs (mainly statins).

In univariable analyses, bilirubin was inversely related to age, BMI, smoking status, waist circumference, insulin, HOMA-IR, total cholesterol, triglycerides, and the presence of metabolic syndrome (Table 1). We also found positive relationships of bilirubin with free T_4 and free T_3, alcohol use, ALT, and AST. Bilirubin was not associated with blood pressure, glucose, HDL cholesterol and TSH. There were no interactions of sex with free T_4, free T_3 and TSH on bilirubin (*P*>0.29 for all; data not shown). In age- and sex-adjusted linear regression analyses (Table 2), bilirubin was positively associated with free T_4, but there were no significant associations of bilirubin with free T_3 and TSH. Bilirubin was inversely associated with diastolic blood pressure, waist circumference, glucose, insulin, HOMA-IR, total cholesterol, HDL cholesterol and triglycerides in age- and sex-adjusted analyses (Table 2).

We then tested whether the relationship of bilirubin with free T_4 was modified by HOMA-IR, fasting insulin, individual MetS

Table 2. Age- and sex-adjusted linear regression analyses demonstrating relationships of bilirubin with thyroid hormones, components of the metabolic syndrome, insulin, insulin resistance and total cholesterol.

	Total bilirubin (μmol/L)	
	β	P-value
TSH (mU/L)	−0.015	0.510
Free T_4 (pmol/L)	0.086	<0.001
Free T_3 (pmol/L)	0.033	0.150
Systolic blood pressure (mmHg)	−0.028	0.296
Diastolic blood pressure (mmHg)	−0.058	0.026
Waist circumference (cm)	−0.116	<0.001
Glucose (mmol/L)	−0.055	0.022
Insulin (mU/L)	−0.144	<0.001
HOMA-IR	−0.143	<0.001
Total cholesterol (mmol/L)	0.121	<0.001
HDL cholesterol (mmol/L)	0.154	<0.001
Triglycerides (mmol/L)	−0.176	<0.001

HDL, high density lipoprotein; HOMA-IR, homeostasis model assessment-insulin resistance; β, standardized regression coefficient. Bilirubin, TSH, glucose, insulin and HOMA-IR and triglycerides were log transformed.

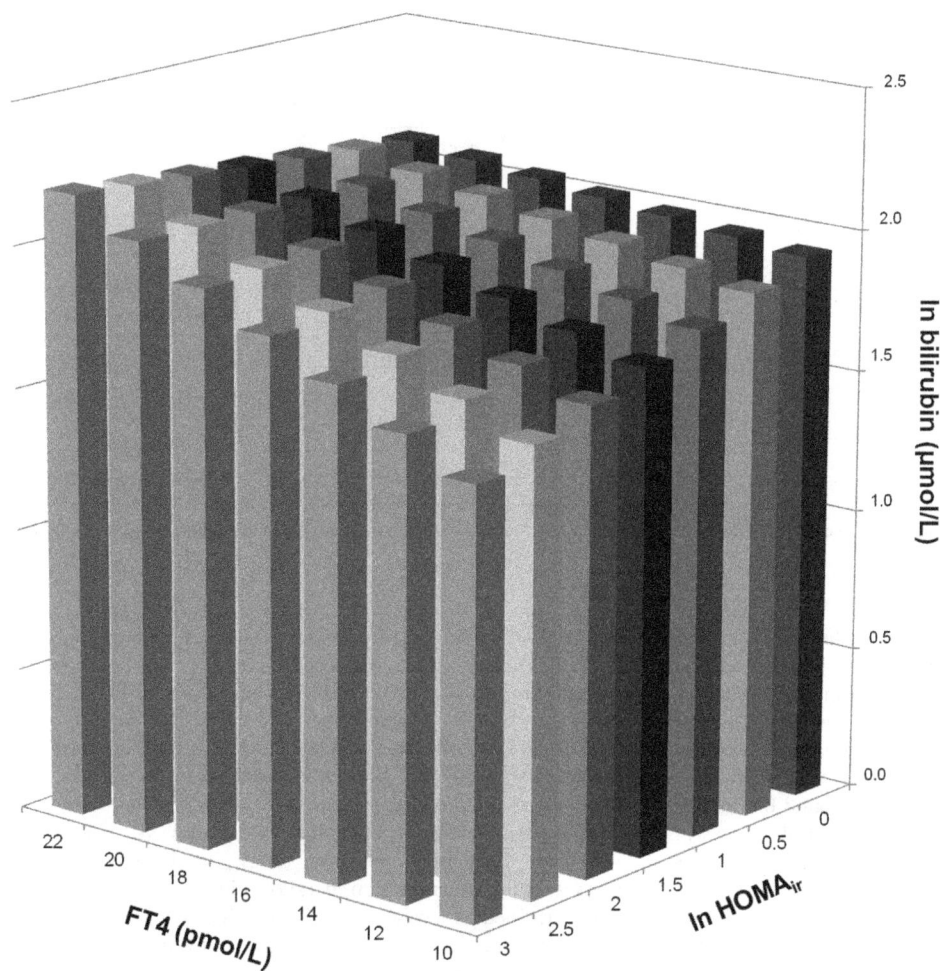

Figure 1. Graphical presentation of the interaction of free T$_4$ with insulin resistance on bilirubin. The standardized regression coefficients of the interaction term obtained by multivariable linear regression analysis as shown in Table 3, model 3 is used.

components, and total cholesterol. The relationship of bilirubin with free T$_4$ was significantly modified by HOMA-IR ($\beta = 0.043$, $P = 0.056$ for interaction; Table 3) and by plasma insulin ($\beta = 0.040$, $P = 0.072$ for interaction; Table S1). The effect-modification of free T$_4$ by HOMA-IR was independent of potential confounding factors including smoking, alcohol use $\geq$ 10 gram/day, AST, ALT and total cholesterol ($\beta = 0.044$, $P = 0.044$ for interaction; Table 3). Figure 1 provides a graphical presentation of the modification of the effect of free T$_4$ on bilirubin by HOMA-IR. As shown in Table S1, there were no significant modifications of the effect of free T$_4$ on bilirubin by systolic blood pressure, diastolic blood pressure, waist circumference, glucose, total cholesterol, or triglycerides in age- and sex-adjusted analyses ($P > 0.27$ for all), but there was a significant modification of the effect of free T$_4$ on bilirubin by HDL cholesterol ($\beta = 0.040$, $P = 0.072$). In addition, there were no significant modifications of a potential effect of free T$_3$ on bilirubin by HOMA-IR, fasting insulin, components of the metabolic syndrome, and total cholesterol ($P > 0.32$ for all; data not shown).

Secondary analyses were performed after exclusion of subjects using lipid lowering drugs, ACEi and ARB's. In the remaining subjects (n = 1759), there was again an age- and sex-adjusted positive relationship of bilirubin with free T$_4$ ($\beta = 0.094$, $P <$

0.001). Furthermore, the interaction of free T$_4$ with HOMA-IR on bilirubin was also significant in these analyses ($\beta = 0.050$, $P = 0.030$ for interaction), and remained significant after further adjustment for alcohol intake, transaminases and total cholesterol ($\beta = 0.056$, $P = 0.013$ for interaction).

Discussion

To our knowledge, this is the first report on an independent positive relationship of total bilirubin with free T$_4$ in a large group of euthyroid, non-diabetic individuals recruited from the general population. Of note, multivariable linear regression analyses demonstrated a significant positive modification of the effect of free T$_4$ on bilirubin by insulin resistance as quantified by HOMA-IR. This effect-modification remained essentially unaltered after controlling for potential confounders, including smoking, alcohol, transaminases, and total cholesterol. Our results, therefore, are in concert with the hypothesis that low-normal thyroid function may confer lower circulating bilirubin levels, especially in insulin resistant individuals. In addition, the effect of free T$_4$ on bilirubin was modified by the HDL cholesterol concentration.

We recently documented a positive relationship of circulating levels of bilirubin with free T$_4$ in euthyroid T2DM subjects [13]. In that report, bilirubin was not significantly correlated with free

Table 3. Multivariable linear regression models demonstrating the interaction between free T_4 and insulin resistance on bilirubin.

	Model 1		Model 2		Model 3	
	β	P-value	β	P-value	β	P-value
Age (years)	−0.030	0.196	−0.031	0.189	−0.004	0.864
Sex (men/women)	−0.250	<0.001	−0.251	<0.001	−0.213	<0.001
Free T_4 (pmol/L)	0.069	0.002	0.072	0.002	0.084	<0.001
HOMA-IR	−0.134	<0.001	−0.134	<0.001	−0.158	<0.001
Free T_4*HOMA-IR			0.043	0.056	0.044	0.044
Current smoker (yes/no)					−0.184	<0.001
Alcohol intake (≥10 gram/day)					0.026	0.250
Total cholesterol (mmol/L)					−0.101	<0.001
AST (U/L)					0.097	0.003
ALT (U/L)					0.015	0.675

HOMA-IR, Homeostasis model assessment-insulin resistance; AST, Aspartate aminotransferase; ALT, Alanine aminotransferase; β, standardized regression coefficient. Bilirubin, HOMA-IR, AST and ALT were log transformed.

T_4 in non-diabetic subjects, possibly due to the limited number of participants. Moreover, it could not be determined what was the driving force behind this association, i.e. insulin resistance or hyperglycemia resulting from β-cell dysfunction. Our previous findings [13], therefore, endorsed our main rationale to investigate the association between bilirubin and free T_4 in a large group of non-diabetic subjects. In the current study, we found bilirubin to be more strongly associated with HOMA-IR and insulin than with glucose in age- and sex-adjusted analysis. Furthermore, a positive modification of the effect of free T_4 on bilirubin by HOMA-IR was observed in such a way that the effect of free T_4 on bilirubin was most pronounced in the most insulin resistant subjects. This effect modification was not observed with plasma glucose, raising the possibility that insulin resistance rather than hyperglycemia *per se* could represent a mechanism linking low bilirubin to low normal thyroid function. In view of the strong anti-oxidative properties of the HDL fraction [28], and the modification of HDL anti-oxidative capacity by thyroid function [29], it is also of potential relevance that the effect of free T_4 on bilirubin was modified by HDL cholesterol.

The interaction of free T_4 with insulin resistance on bilirubin may have pathophysiological relevance since lower thyroid functional status, impaired insulin sensitivity, and low bilirubin are all characterized by enhanced oxidative stress [2,30–32]. The positive relationship of bilirubin with free T_4 may at least in part be explained by effects of thyroid function on bilirubin production, given the stimulatory effect of thyroid hormone on HO-1 expression, and the inhibitory effect on UDP-glucuronosyltransferase [10–12]. HO-1 expression is stimulated by insulin *in vitro* [33,34]. Furthermore, plasma levels of HO-1 are elevated in subjects with pre-diabetes and are strongly correlated with HOMA-IR [35]. Taken these findings together, it is plausible to hypothesize that effects of thyroid hormone on HO-1 expression could be more prominent in hyperinsulinemic and more insulin resistant individuals. On the other hand, it is obvious that stimulatory effects of insulin on HO-1 expression alone cannot explain the lower bilirubin levels in insulin resistant and MetS subjects [2]. Although little explored, insulin could also affect bilirubin metabolism, since insulin deficiency may result in

enhanced UDP-glucuronyltransferase activity and bilirubin excretion [36]. Further study is required to more precisely delineate the mechanisms responsible for the alleged effects of thyroid functional status on bilirubin metabolism. Moreover, it remains to be established why bilirubin was related to free T_4 (and in univariable analysis also to free T_3) but not to the TSH level, extending our previous report showing relationships of plasma lipids with free thyroid hormone levels rather than with TSH [13].

Several other methodological issues and limitations of the present study warrant consideration. First, euthyroidism was strictly defined as levels of free T_4, free T_3 and TSH within the assay-specific reference range as provided by the manufacturer. We also excluded subjects with positive anti-thyroid peroxidase auto-antibodies. This was done to reduce possible bias in the relationship of free thyroid hormone levels with TSH in subjects with very early stages of autoimmune thyroid dysfunction as much as possible. Second, we performed a cross-sectional study. Thus, cause-effect relationships cannot be established with certainty. However, bilirubin has been shown not to influence the set-point of the pituitary-thyroid axis [37], strongly suggesting that low bilirubin levels by themselves are unlikely to lower thyroid function. Third, statin treatment has been reported to decrease bilirubin levels [38], and to increase plasma glucose [39], whereas ACEi or ARB's are likely to inhibit oxidative stress [40] and to improve insulin sensitivity [41]. In primary analyses, we did not exclude subjects using lipid lowering drugs or individuals using ACEi or ARB's. Instead, we carried out a secondary analysis after exclusion of subjects using these medications. This secondary analysis showed an essentially unaltered relationship of bilirubin with free T_4 and a similar interaction of free T_4 with HOMA-IR on bilirubin.

In conclusion, the current study shows an independent relationship of low bilirubin with low free T_4 in euthyroid subjects. Low normal free T_4 may particularly confer low bilirubin in more insulin resistant individuals. Since bilirubin is a potent endogenous anti-oxidant, it is plausible to speculate that low normal thyroid functional status could enhance atherosclerosis susceptibility in the context of insulin resistance.

Acknowledgments

In addition to the authors, the PREVEND investigators are, from the university medical center Groningen, the Netherlands: de Jong PE, Gansevoort RT, Navis GJ, Bakker SJL (Dept. of Nephrology); van Veldhuisen DJ, van Voors AA, van der Harst P (Dept. of Cardiology); van Gilst WH, de Boer R (Dept. of Experimental Cardiology); Stolk RP, Hillege HL (Dept. of Clinical Epidemiology); de Zeeuw D (Dept. of Clinical Pharmacology); Dullaart RPF, Wolffenbuttel BHR (Dept. of Endocrinology); Slaets JPJ, Izaks G (Dept. of Geriatric Medicine) Gans ROB (Dept. of Internal Medicine); van de Berg PB, de Jong-van den Berg LT, Postma MJ, Visser ST (Dept. of Pharmacoepidemiology and Pharmacoeconomics). Lead author: Bakker SJL, s.j.l bakker @umcg.nl.

Author Contributions

Conceived and designed the experiments: PED SJLB GJN RPFD. Analyzed the data: PED AJK RPFD. Wrote the paper: PED AJK SJLB GJN RPFD. Initiation of the study: SJLB RPFD. Intellectual contributions: GJN. Supervision of data analyses, study planning: RPFD.

References

1. Vitek L, Schwertner HA (2007) The heme catabolic pathway and its protective effects on oxidative stress-mediated diseases. Adv Clin Chem 43: 1–57.
2. Vitek L (2012) The role of bilirubin in diabetes, metabolic syndrome, and cardiovascular diseases. Front Pharmacol 3: 55.
3. Oda E, Aizawa Y (2013) Total bilirubin is inversely associated with metabolic syndrome but not a risk factor for metabolic syndrome in japanese men and women. Acta Diabetol 50: 417–422.
4. Novotny L, Vitek L (2003) Inverse relationship between serum bilirubin and atherosclerosis in men: A meta-analysis of published studies. Exp Biol Med (Maywood) 228: 568–571.
5. Chan KH, O'Connell RL, Sullivan DR, Hoffmann LS, Rajamani K, et al. (2013) Plasma total bilirubin levels predict amputation events in type 2 diabetes mellitus: The fenofibrate intervention and event lowering in diabetes (FIELD) study. Diabetologia 56: 724–736.
6. Ajja R, Lee DC, Sui X, Church TS, Steven NB (2011) Usefulness of serum bilirubin and cardiorespiratory fitness as predictors of mortality in men. Am J Cardiol 108: 1438–1442.
7. Vitek L, Novotny L, Sperl M, Holaj R, Spacil J (2006) The inverse association of elevated serum bilirubin levels with subclinical carotid atherosclerosis. Cerebrovasc Dis 21: 408–414.
8. Dullaart RP, Kappelle PJ, de Vries R (2012) Lower carotid intima media thickness is predicted by higher serum bilirubin in both non-diabetic and type 2 diabetic subjects. Clin Chim Acta 414: 161–165.
9. Smith TJ, Drummond GS (1991) Retinoic acid can enhance the stimulation by thyroid hormone of heme oxygenase activity in the liver of thyroidectomized rats. Biochim Biophys Acta 1075: 119–122.
10. Li F, Lu S, Zhu R, Zhou Z, Ma L, et al. (2011) Heme oxygenase-1 is induced by thyroid hormone and involved in thyroid hormone preconditioning-induced protection against renal warm ischemia in rat. Mol Cell Endocrinol 339: 54–62.
11. Gartner LM, Arias IM (1972) Hormonal control of hepatic bilirubin transport and conjugation. Am J Physiol 222: 1091–1099.
12. Van Steenbergen W, Fevery J, De Vos R, Leyten R, Heirwegh KP, et al. (1989) Thyroid hormones and the hepatic handling of bilirubin. I. effects of hypothyroidism and hyperthyroidism on the hepatic transport of bilirubin mono- and diconjugates in the wistar rat. Hepatology 9: 314–321.
13. Deetman PE, Kwakernaak AJ, Bakker SJ, Dullaart RP (2013) Low normal free thyroxine confers decreased serum bilirubin in type 2 diabetes mellitus. Thyroid: In press.
14. Roos A, Bakker SJ, Links TP, Gans RO, Wolffenbuttel BH (2007) Thyroid function is associated with components of the metabolic syndrome in euthyroid subjects. J Clin Endocrinol Metab 92: 491–496.
15. Heima NE, Eekhoff EM, Oosterwerff MM, Lips PT, van Schoor NM, et al. (2012) Thyroid function and the metabolic syndrome in older persons: A population-based study. Eur J Endocrinol 168: 59–65.
16. Hillege HL, Janssen WM, Bak AA, Diercks GF, Grobbee DE, et al. (2001) Microalbuminuria is common, also in a nondiabetic, nonhypertensive population, and an independent indicator of cardiovascular risk factors and cardiovascular morbidity. J Intern Med 249: 519–526.
17. Pinto-Sietsma SJ, Janssen WM, Hillege HL, Navis G, De Zeeuw D, et al. (2000) Urinary albumin excretion is associated with renal functional abnormalities in a nondiabetic population. J Am Soc Nephrol 11: 1882–1888.
18. Matthews DR, Hosker JP, Rudenski AS, Naylor BA, Treacher DF, et al. (1985) Homeostasis model assessment: Insulin resistance and beta-cell function from fasting plasma glucose and insulin concentrations in man. Diabetologia 28: 412–419.
19. Expert Panel on Detection, Evaluation, and Treatment of High Blood Cholesterol in Adults (2001) Executive summary of the third report of the national cholesterol education program (NCEP) expert panel on detection, evaluation, and treatment of high blood cholesterol in adults (adult treatment panel III). JAMA 285: 2486–2497.
20. Tisdale WA, Klatskin G, Kinsella ED (1959) The significance of the direct-reacting fraction of serum bilirubin in hemolytic jaundice. Am J Med 26: 214–227.
21. Zelle DM, Deetman N, Alkhalaf A, Navis G, Bakker SJ (2011) Support for a protective effect of bilirubin on diabetic nephropathy in humans. Kidney Int 79: 686; author reply 686–7.
22. Katsiki N, Karagiannis A, Mikhailidis DP (2013) Diabetes, bilirubin and amputations: Is there a link? Diabetologia 56: 683–685.
23. Deetman PE, Zelle DM, Homan van der Heide JJ, Navis GJ, Gans RO, et al. (2012) Plasma bilirubin and late graft failure in renal transplant recipients. Transpl Int 25: 876–881.
24. Shieh G (2011) Clarifying the role of mean centring in multicollinearity of interaction effects. Br J Math Stat Psychol 64: 462–477.
25. Kraemer HC, Blasey CM (2004) Centring in regression analyses: A strategy to prevent errors in statistical inference. Int J Methods Psychiatr Res 13: 141–151.
26. Selvin S (1996) Statistical analysis of epidemiological data. New York: Oxford University Press.
27. Lu M, Lyden PD, Brott TG, Hamilton S, Broderick JP, et al. (2005) Beyond subgroup analysis: Improving the clinical interpretation of treatment effects in stroke research. J Neurosci Methods 143: 209–216.
28. Triolo M, Annema W, Dullaart RP, Tietge UJ (2013) Assessing the functional properties of high-density lipoproteins: An emerging concept in cardiovascular research. Biomark Med 7: 457–472.
29. Triolo M, de Boer JF, Annema W, Kwakernaak AJ, Tietge UJ, et al. (2013) Low normal free T4 confers decreased high-density lipoprotein antioxidative functionality in the context of hyperglycaemia. Clin Endocrinol (Oxf) 79: 416–423.
30. Ferder L, Inserra F, Martinez-Maldonado M (2006) Inflammation and the metabolic syndrome: Role of angiotensin II and oxidative stress. Curr Hypertens Rep 8: 191–198.
31. Duntas LH (2002) Thyroid disease and lipids. Thyroid 12: 287–293.
32. Chen SJ, Yen CH, Huang YC, Lee BJ, Hsia S, et al. (2012) Relationships between inflammation, adiponectin, and oxidative stress in metabolic syndrome. PLoS One 7: e45693.
33. Harrison EM, McNally SJ, Devey L, Garden OJ, Ross JA, et al. (2006) Insulin induces heme oxygenase-1 through the phosphatidylinositol 3-kinase/Akt pathway and the Nrf2 transcription factor in renal cells. FEBS J 273: 2345–2356.
34. Aggeli IK, Theofilatos D, Beis I, Gaitanaki C (2011) Insulin-induced oxidative stress up-regulates heme oxygenase-1 via diverse signaling cascades in the C2 skeletal myoblast cell line. Endocrinology 152: 1274–1283.
35. Bao W, Song F, Li X, Rong S, Yang W, et al. (2010) Plasma heme oxygenase-1 concentration is elevated in individuals with type 2 diabetes mellitus. PLoS One 5: e12371.
36. Tunon MJ, Gonzalez P, Garcia-Pardo LA, Gonzalez J (1991) Hepatic transport of bilirubin in rats with streptozotocin-induced diabetes. J Hepatol 13: 71–77.
37. Wassen FW, Moerings EP, van Toor H, Hennemann G, Everts ME (2000) Thyroid hormone uptake in cultured rat anterior pituitary cells: Effects of energy status and bilirubin. J Endocrinol 165: 599–606.
38. Ong KL, Wu BJ, Cheung BM, Barter PJ, Rye KA (2011) Association of lower total bilirubin level with statin usage: The united states national health and nutrition examination survey 1999–2008. Atherosclerosis 219: 728–733.
39. Preiss D, Seshasai SR, Welsh P, Murphy SA, Ho JE, et al. (2011) Risk of incident diabetes with intensive-dose compared with moderate-dose statin therapy: A meta-analysis. JAMA 305: 2556–2564.
40. Varin R, Mulder P, Tamion F, Richard V, Henry JP, et al. (2000) Improvement of endothelial function by chronic angiotensin-converting enzyme inhibition in heart failure: Role of nitric oxide, prostanoids, oxidant stress, and bradykinin. Circulation 102: 351–356.
41. Muscogiuri G, Chavez AO, Gastaldelli A, Perego L, Tripathy D, et al. (2008) The crosstalk between insulin and renin-angiotensin-aldosterone signaling systems and its effect on glucose metabolism and diabetes prevention. Curr Vasc Pharmacol 6: 301–312.

13

Pioglitazone Improves Cognitive Function via Increasing Insulin Sensitivity and Strengthening Antioxidant Defense System in Fructose-Drinking Insulin Resistance Rats

Qing-Qing Yin[1], Jin-Jing Pei[2], Song Xu[3], Ding-Zhen Luo[1], Si-Qing Dong[1], Meng-Han Sun[1], Li You[4], Zhi-Jian Sun[3], Xue-Ping Liu[1,3]*

1 Department of Senile Neurology, Provincial Hospital Affiliated to Shandong University, Jinan, Shandong, P. R. China, 2 Department of KI-Alzheimer Disease Research Center, Karolinska Institutet, Stockholm, Sweden, 3 Department of Anti-Ageing, Provincial Hospital Affiliated to Shandong University, Jinan, Shandong, P. R. China, 4 Department of Central Lab, Provincial Hospital Affiliated to Shandong University, Jinan, Shandong, P. R. China

Abstract

Insulin resistance (IR) links Alzheimer's disease (AD) with oxidative damage, cholinergic deficit, and cognitive impairment. Peroxisome proliferator-activated receptor γ (PPARγ) agonist pioglitazone previously used to treat type 2 diabetes mellitus (T2DM) has also been demonstrated to be effective in anti-inflammatory reaction and anti-oxidative stress in the animal models of AD and other neuroinflammatory diseases. Here, we investigated the effect of pioglitazone on learning and memory impairment and the molecular events that may cause it in fructose-drinking insulin resistance rats. We found that long-term fructose-drinking causes insulin resistance, oxidative stress, down-regulated activity of cholinergic system, and cognitive deficit, which could be ameliorated by pioglitazone administration. The results from the present study provide experimental evidence for using pioglitazone in the treatment of brain damage caused by insulin resistance.

Editor: Anthony E. Kline, University of Pittsburgh, United States of America

Funding: This study was supported by the fund from Research Program to Tackle Key problems of Shandong Province, P. R. China (2006GGB14630; 532 2011YD18081). The funders had no role in study design, data collection and analysis, decision to publish, or preparation of the manuscript.

Competing Interests: The authors have declared that no competing interests exist.

* E-mail: lxp6133@yahoo.com.cn

Introduction

Insulin resistance is one of the core defects in type 2 diabetes mellitus (T2DM) and this defect leads to hyperinsulinemia that compensates for the reduced efficacy of insulin in peripheral tissues. Insulin resistance may be manifested only by mild glucose intolerance for many years prior to the onset of frank diabetes, as the pancreas is able to generate sufficient levels of insulin to maintain glucose levels beneath the diabetic threshold. About 60–70% of T2DM patients have diabetic neuropathy in peripheral and central nervous systems (CNS) [1]. In CNS, deterioration of cognitive function such as learning and memory impairment has been proven to be associated with insulin resistance [2–4].

Oxidative damage plays an important role in the pathogenesis of T2DM, Alzheimer' disease (AD) and other neurological diseases [5,6]. Oxidative stress arises due to the imbalance of the production of free radicals and cellular antioxidant defense mechanism. The excessive production of free radicals in brain that has insulin resistance may attack many cellular components including membrane lipids and proteins, resulting in neuronal damage and dysfunction [7,8]. On the other hand, the antioxidant enzyme activities such as glutathione peroxidase (GPx), catalase (CAT), superoxide dismutase (SOD) as well as non-enzymatic antioxidants including reduced glutathione (GSH) were reduced in the brains of insulin resistance rats [9–13], suggesting that a declined antioxidant ability is induced by insulin resistance. Accumulating evidences have demonstrated the link between free radical and neuronal degeneration, which highlights the importance of antioxidants in the treatment of neurodegenerative disorders including diabetes-associated cognitive decline [5]. It is thought that oxidative damage contributes to learning and memory impairments in rat models with insulin resistance [7,14].

The deficit of cholinergic neurotransmission is an important mechanism in the pathogenesis of AD, and it correlates closely with the severity of cognitive impairment in AD patients, as well as in humans, rats, and mice with central insulin resistance [7,15,16]. The concentration of acetylcholine (Ach), the key neurotransmitter involved in cognitive process, is influenced by acetylcholinesterase (AChE) and choline acetrltransferase (ChAT) activities [16]. ACh is increased by inhibiting the activity of AChE or promoting the activity of ChAT, by which the impairment of cognitive function could be ameliorated [15,16]. AChE is responsible for degradation of ACh to acetate and choline in synaptic cleft [17]. Cholinergic replacement strategy is the only practiced treatment used for AD patients today. The mechanisms underlying the cholinergic deficit induced by insulin resistance in brain are still needed to be clarified.

Pioglitazone, a thiazolidinedione derivative, is a highly selective peroxisome proliferator-activated receptors (PPARγ) agonist. It is currently approved in the treatment of T2DM associated with insulin resistance. PPARγ agonists are known to improve insulin sensitization, modulate glucose and lipid metabolism [18], was also considered as candidate drug in the treatment of neurodegenerative disorders such as AD, Huntington's disease, and Parkinson's disease [19–21]. Besides the antioxidant ability, previous studies have shown that pioglitazone is beneficial to central cholinergic system, and ameliorates cognitive impairment in experimental dementia rats [22,23]. In our previous studies, we found that pioglitazone partly reversed the accumulation of β-amyloid and the activation of advanced glycosylation end products (AGEs)/receptors for AGEs (RAGE) system in brains of fructose-drinking insulin resistance rats [24,25]. So far, the precise molecular mechanisms as to how insulin resistance is induced by high fructose intake, resulting in cognitive impairment, and how the learning and memory deficit induced by high fructose intake is ameliorated by pioglitazone have not been completely understood.

In the present study, we tested if long-term fructose intake can induce insulin resistance, oxidative damage, and deficit in cholinergic function, and impairment in learning and memory ability in rats. We also investigated the potential therapeutic role of pioglitazone in these molecular events.

Materials and Methods

Animals and Grouping

Male Wistar rats, six-week-old, were obtained from the Experimental Animal Center of Shandong university, Jinan, China, and housed (3 rats/cage) at 22±2°C under diurnal cycle (light-dark: 08:00–20:00). The rats were given food and water ad libitum. The animals were cared in accordance with the Provisions and General Recommendation of Chinese Experimental Animals Administration Legislation. The experiment was approved by the Provincial Hospital Council on Animal Care Committee, Shandong University, China.

After adaptation for a week, the rats were randomly divided into 4 groups (10 in each group): a control group (control) and a control treatment group (Pioglitazone); a fructose group (fructose) and a fructose treatment group (Pioglitazone+fructose). Control rats were fed with plain water. Experimental rats received 10% fructose solution in drinking water for 16 weeks to develop insulin resistance. 10 mg/kg Pioglitazone (Actos™, Takeda Pharmaceuticals, Osaka, Japan) suspended in normal water was given to rats daily at a volume of 2 ml/kg/day by gavage for the last 12 weeks of the 16-week treatment period. Non-treated rats were administered with normal water at the same volume for the last 12 weeks [24].

Reagents

Immunoreagent kit used for fasting insulin (FINS) levels was from Beijing Furui Biotechnology (Beijing, China). The assay kit for total antioxidant capability (T-AOC) was from Nanjing Jiancheng Bioengineering Institute (Nanjing, China). All other chemicals for biochemical analysis were purchased from the Sigma-Aldrich (MO, USA) unless otherwise indicated.

Preparation of Homogenates or Supernatants

A total of 5 rats (one in control treatment group, two in fructose group, and two in fructose treatment group) were excluded from the study because they were dead or severely ill before the beginning of Morris water maze test, all other rats were killed by decapitation under anesthesia after behavioral experiments. The brains were immediately removed from each rat and washed with ice-cold normal saline, and the hippocampus and cerebral cortex were dissected. The hippocampus and cerebral cortex of the left hemisphere were weighed and homogenized in a 50 mM phosphate buffered saline (PBS) pH 7.0 containing 0.1 mmol/L ethylenediaminetetraacetic acid (EDTA). The half volume of homogenate was centrifuged at $1500 \times g$ for 15 min at 4°C to prepare supernatants for T-AOC, SOD, CAT, GPx, GSH, thibarbituric acid reactive substances (TABRS), ACh, and AChE assays. The other half of homogenate was further centrifuged at $12,000 \times g$ for 10 min at 4°C, and was prepared for protein carbonyl content (PCC) assay [26]. The hippocampus and cerebral cortex in the right hemisphere were weighed and homogenized in 50 mM PBS at PH 7.0 (10%, w/v) and centrifuged at $11,000 \times g$ for 15 min at 4°C for reactive oxygen species (ROS) assay [27].

Protein Concentration Measurement

The protein concentration in homogenates or supernatants prepared above was measured by the method of Lowry et al [28], using bovine serum albumin (BSA) as standard.

Detection of Fasting Glucose and Insulin (FINS) Levels in Plasma

Insulin sensitivity was assessed at the end of experiments by measuring insulin resistance index (IRI). The rats after behavior tests were fasted for 12 h, 3 ml blood samples collected from abdominal aorta for each case 2 days before animals were killed were centrifuged at $1200 \times g$ for detection of fasting blood glucose (FBG) and FINS levels. The FBG levels were determined by a glucose-oxidase biochemistry analyzer and FINS levels were measured by homogeneous phase competitive immunoradiometric assay with Immunoreagent kit using GC-911γ immunoradio-

Table 1. Effects of pioglitazone on plasma glucose and insulin in fructose-drinking insulin resistance rats.

Groups (n)	Body weight (g)	Fasting blood glucose (mmol/L)	Fasting insulin (mU/L)	Insulin resistance index
Control (10)	397.4±19.3	5.12±0.78	14.5±2.9	3.30±0.34
Pioglitazone (9)	401.5±15.9	4.83±0.39	13.9±3.3	2.98±0.28
Fructose (8)	409.3±12.9	5.54±0.58	34.6±4.5[a]	8.52±0.62[a]
Pioglitazone+fructose (8)	412.2±15.9	5.38±0.47	19.4±4.0[bc]	4.64±0.33[a,c]

Data are shown as mean ± S.E.M.
[a]$P<0.01$,
[b]$P<0.01$ versus control group;
[c]$P<0.05$ versus untreated fructose-drinking group.

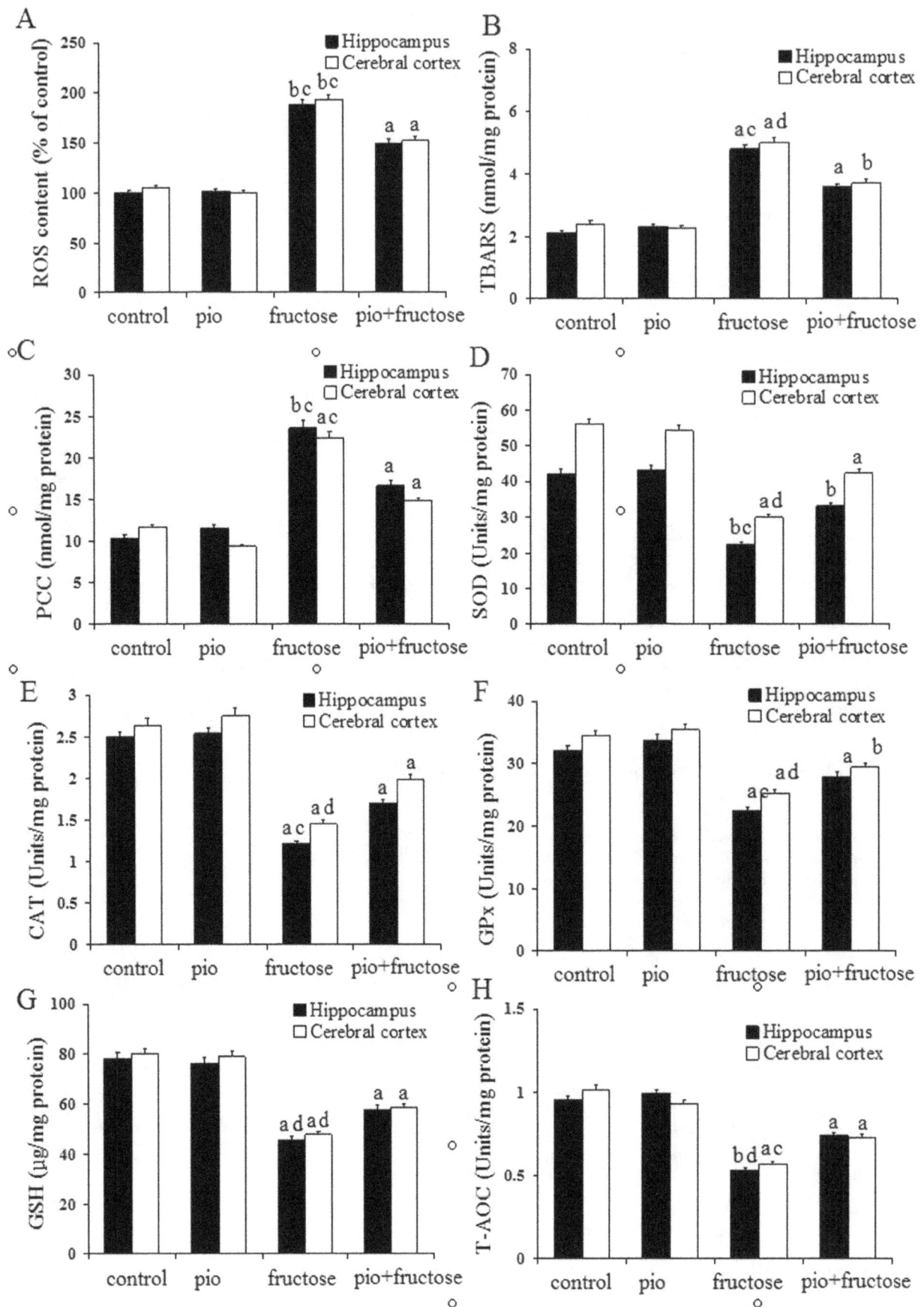

Figure 1. Effects of pioglitazone on the levels of ROS, TBARS, and contents of carbonyl proteins in the hippocampus and cerebral cortex of fructose-drinking insulin resistance rats (A–C); effects of pioglitazone on the activities of antioxidant enzymes (SOD, CAT and GPx) (D–F), the levels of GSH and T-AOC (G–H) in the hippocampus and cerebral cortex of fructose-drinking insulin resistance rats. The control group (control) and the control treatment group (pio: pioglitazone) were treated with normal drinking water while the fructose group (fructose) and fructose treatment group (pio+fructose: pioglitazone+fructose) were treated with 10% fructose solution for 16 weeks to develop insulin resistance. The fructose treatment group was orally administrated pioglitazone (10 mg/kg d) for the last 12 weeks of the 16-week period. Data are mean ± SEM. Data are mean ± SEM. The number of rats in groups control, pio, fructose and pio+fructose was 10, 9, 8, and 8, respectively. [a]$P<0.05$, [b]$P<0.01$ versus control group; [c]$P<0.05$, [d]$P<0.01$ versus untreated fructose-drinking group.

metric counter (Enterprises Group of USTC, Hefei, China). IRI was calculated as formula: IRI = FBG×FINS/22.5 [24,29].

ROS Determination

ROS levels were quantified by 2′-7′-dichlorofluorescein-diacetate (DCFH-DA) assay as previously described [27]. Briefly, 40 µl supernatant (4.5 mg/ml), 20 µl 100 µM DCFH-DA, and 140 µl 50 mM PBS (pH 7.0) were mixed, and the mixture was incubated for 30 min at 37°C. The reaction was stopped by placing it on ice, and the formation of oxidized fluorescent 2′-7′-dichlorofluorescein

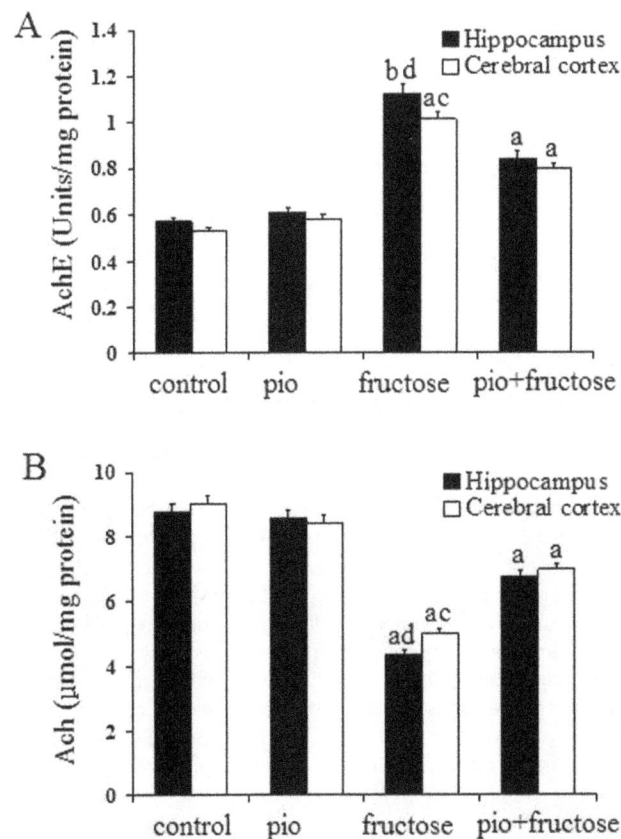

(DCF) was measured by fluorimeter (F96S; Lengguang, Shanghai, China) using excitation and emission wavelengths at 488 and 525 nm, respectively. The final results were corrected for protein concentration and then expressed as percentage of the corresponding values in control group. All steps were performed in the dark and DCF formation was also monitored immediately after DCFH-DA was added to the homogenate ($t = 0$ min) in order to subtract background autofluorescence.

TBARS Assay

The levels of lipid peroxidation were quantified by TBARS assay according to previously described [30]. 50 µl supernatant (8.5 mg/ml) was mixed with 1 ml 50 mM PBS (PH 7.0), 10 µl 0.375% thiobarbituric acid (TBA), 10 µl 15% trichloro acetic acid (TCA), 5 µl 0.25 M HCl, and 5 µl 6.8 mM 2,6-di-tert-butyl-4-methylphenol (BHT), was incubated at 95°C for 1 h. After cooling with tap water, the reaction was terminated with a mixture of 1.0 ml distilled water and 3.0 ml butyl alcohol and pyridine (15:1, v/v). The mixture was centrifuged at 2000×g for 10 min. The absorbance of the supernatant was determined at 532 nm by using 1,1,3,3-teraethoxypropane (TEP) as standard. The lipid peroxidation was expressed as TBARS in nanomoles per mg protein.

Protein Carbonyl Content Measurement

Protein carbonyl content (PCC), a marker of oxidized proteins, was measured spectrophotometrically [31]. Briefly, 300 µl mixture was prepared by adding 50 µl 5% streptomycin sulfate solution (w/v), 200 µl supernatant (9.5 mg/ml), and 50 µl 50 mM PBS (pH 7.0), and incubated for 15 min at 37°C. After centrifuged at 10,000 ×g for 10 min at 4°C, the pellet was dissolved in 100 µl 10 mM 2, 4-dinitrophenylhidrazine (DNPH) solved in 200 µl 2.5 M HCl. The re-suspended mixture was incubated in the dark for 1 h at 37°C. The proteins were precipitated by adding equal volume of 20% TCA (w/v), and subsequently washed three times with ethanol: ethyl acetate (1:1, v/v). The final protein pellet was dissolved in 400 µl of 6 M guanidine hydrochloride and the absorbance was read at 370 nm. The results were calculated as nM carbonyls groups mg of protein^{-1}, using the extinction coefficient of 22,000 M/cm for aliphatic hydrazones.

SOD Assay

SOD activity was measured basing on the method of Kono [32]. Stocking solution A was prepared by mixing 10 ml of 0.001 N NaOH comtaining 5 µM xanthine with 100 ml of 1 mM PBS (PH 7.0), containing 0.1 mM EDTA, and 2 µM cytochrome c. Stocking solution B (150 µl) was prepared by mixing 100 µl of 0.2 U xanthine oxidase/ml, and 50 µl of 0.1 mM EDTA. 50 µl supernatant (8.5 mg/ml) was mixed with 2.9 ml solution A and 50 µl solution B, the mixture was incubated for 30 min at 37°C. Reaction was stopped by adding 0.2 ml of 16% acetic acid (v/v) containing 2.6 mM sulfanilic and 38.6 µM naphthyl ethylenediamine. The absorbance at 550 nm was monitored. A blank was run by substituting 50 µl ultra pure water for the supernatant. SOD activity was expressed as units per milligram of protein.

Figure 2. Effects of pioglitazone on AChE (A) and ACh (B) in the hippocampus and cerebral cortex of fructose-drinking insulin resistance rats. The control group (control) and the control treatment group (pio: pioglitazone) were treated with normal drinking water while the fructose group (fructose) and fructose treatment group (pio+fructose: pioglitazone+fructose) were treated with 10% fructose solution for 16 weeks to develop insulin resistance. The fructose treatment group was orally administrated pioglitazone (10 mg/kg d) for the last 12 weeks of the 16-week period. Data are mean±SEM. Data are mean±SEM. The number of rats in groups control, pio, fructose and pio+fructose was 10, 9, 8, and 8, respectively. [a]$P<0.05$, [b]$P<0.01$ versus control group; [c]$P<0.05$, [d]$P<0.01$ versus untreated fructose-drinking group.

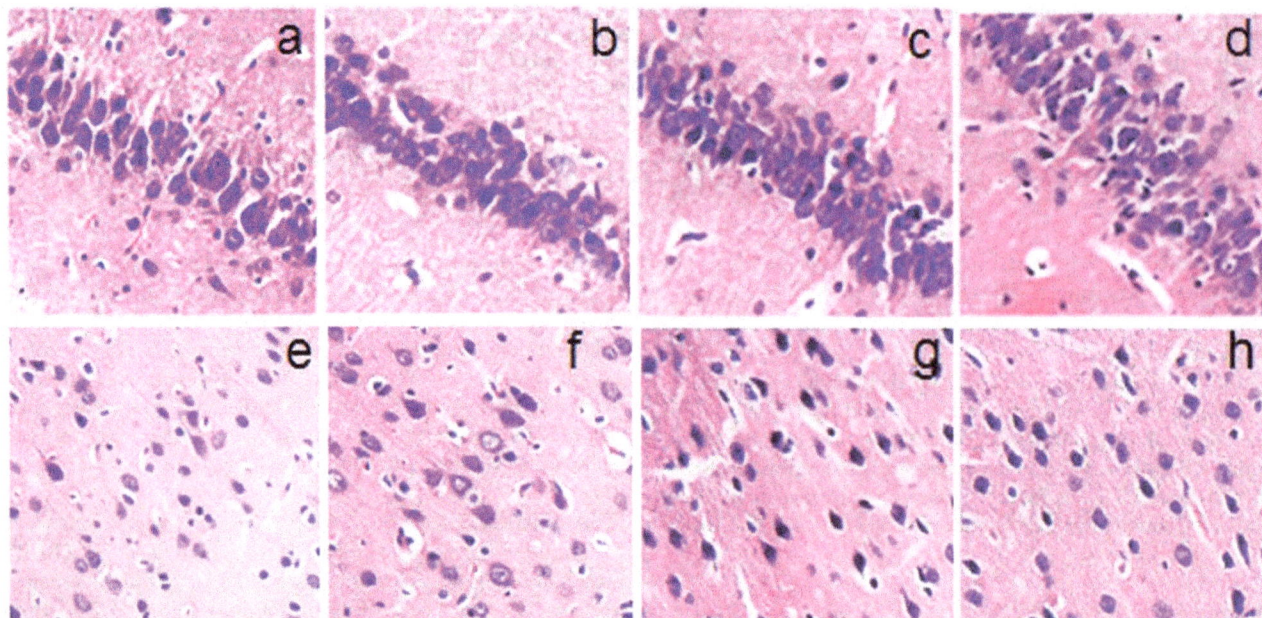

Figure 3. Effect of pioglitazone on histopathological changes in the hippocampus (a–d) and temporal cortex (e–h) of fructose-drinking insulin resistance rats. The hippocampal CA1 area (a,b) and temporal cortex (e,f) in the control, and the pioglitazone-treated control groups, rare damaged cells were seen. In the hippocampal CA1 area (c,d) and the temporal cortex (g,h) of the fructose-drinking insulin resistance control and the pioglitazone-treated groups, neurondegeneration was evident, but not difference was found between the two groups. The data were from five independent experiments. Magnification: ×200.

CAT Assay

CAT activity was measured by the method of Goth [33]. Briefly, 50 µl supernatant (8.5 mg/ml) was mixed with 50 µl of 6.5 µM hydrogen peroxide as substrate, and 100 µl of 50 mM PBS (PH 7.0), and incubated for 60 s at 37°C. The mixture was added with 100 µl of 32.4 mM ammonium molybdate to terminate the reaction. The absorbance was measured at 405 nm. One unit of the enzyme was defined as milli-moles of hydrogen peroxide degraded per min per mg protein.

GPx Assay

GPx activity was estimated according to the method of Hafemen [34]. Briefly, the 300 µl mixture contained 40 µl supernatant (8.5 mg/ml), 30 µl 3 µM GSH, 30 µl 6.5 µM hydrogen peroxide, and 200 µl 50 mM PBS (pH 7.0) was prepared, and incubated at 37°C for 3 min, followed by precipitating proteins with 100 µl 10% TCA (v/v). The resulting supernatant was collected and the reaction was stopped with 100 µl of 20 mM disodium hydrogen phosphate and 100 µl 0.025 mM 5, 5,-dithiobis (2-nitro-benzoic acid) (DTNB). The absorbance was measured at 412 nm. The unit of GPx activity was expressed as micromoles GSH oxidation per min per mg protein.

GSH Assay

GSH level was measured according to a previously described method [35]. 100 µl supernatant (8.5 mg/ml) was filled with 700 µl 0.1 mM PBS (pH 7.0), 100 µl 0.6 mM DTNB and 80 µl 0.2 mg/ml nicotinamide adenine dinucleotide phosphate (NADPH) to make a total volume of 980 µl, and the mixture was incubated at room temperature for 5 min. After mixing, glutathione reductase (20 U/ml, 20 µl) was added to stop the reaction. The formation of 5-thio-2-nitrobenzoic acid parallels the absorbance at 412 nm. GSH levels were expressed as µg per mg protein.

T-AOC Assay

The T-AOC was determined according to method described by Benzie and Strain. [36]. This method allows designing "total" reducing power of the electron donating antioxidants present in examined samples. In reaction mixture ions Fe^{3+} are reduced to Fe^{2+} and blue complex Fe^{2+}-TPTZ (2,4,6-Tri(2-pyridyl)-s-triazine) is produced. 20 µl supernatant (8.5 mg/ml) was added to 2.25 ml reaction buffer containing 130 mM acetate PH 3.6, 4.2 mM TPTZ prepared in 19 mM HCl, and 8.5 mM $FeCl_3 \cdot 6H_2O$), and incubated at room temperature for 5 min, then the reaction and the absorbance for reaction mixture was read at 593 nm immediately and 10 min after. Final readings were based on standard curve consisting of five to eight standard points, covering the entire range of expected concentrations which was prepared with aqueous solutions of known Fe^{2+} concentration (range 100–1000 µmol/ml). Data were expressed as U/mg protein.

AChE Assay

AChE activity was measured according to a previously described method [17]. 670 µl reaction mixture containing 33 µl supernatant (8.5 mg/ml), 470 µl 1 mM PBS (pH 8.0), and 167 µl 2% DTNB was incubated for 5 min at 37°C. Then, 280 µl 2 mM acetylcholine iodide were added to the mixture. After incubation for 5 min at 37°C, the reaction was terminated by adding 50 µl of 4 mM neostigmine. The absorbance was read at 412 nm at room temperature. 1 U AChE activity was defined as the number of hydrolyzed micromoles of acetylthiocholine iodide per min per microgram of protein. AChE activity was expressed as units per milligram of protein.

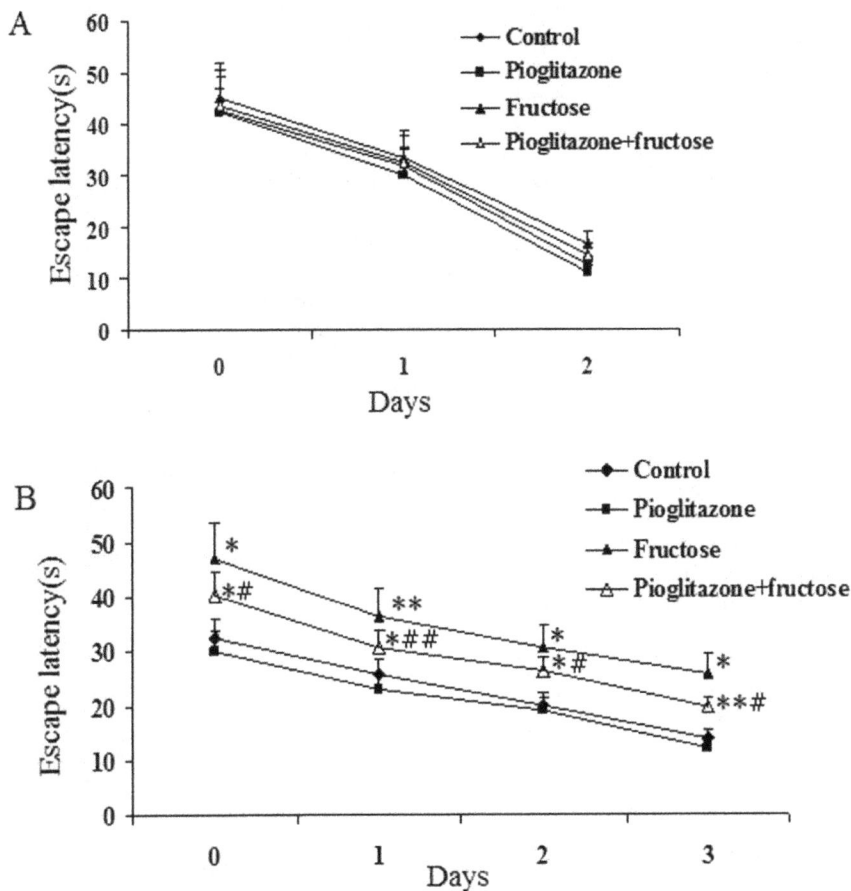

Figure 4. Effect of pioglitazone on memory impairment of fructose-drinking insulin resistance rats in MWM test. Day 0 represents performance on the first trial, and subsequent points indicate average of all daily trials. (A) No differences were found in the escape latency among four groups during the 2-day visible platform test. (B) Changes in escape latency to reach the hidden platform during the 3-day acquisition trials. Data are mean±SEM. The number of rats in groups control, pioglitazone, fructose and pioglitazone+fructose was 10, 9, 8, and 8, respectively. $^*P<0.05$, $^{**}P<0.01$ versus control group; $^\#P<0.05$, $^{\#\#}P<0.01$ versus untreated fructose-drinking group.

ACh Assay

The ACh content was estimated by the method of Yang [37]. Briefly, a total of 4.1 ml reaction mixture containing 0.8 ml (8.5 mg/ml) supernatant, 1 ml 2 M calabarine sulfate, 0.8 ml 1.85 M TCA, and 1.5 ml pure water was prepared, and incubated for 5 time at room temperature. After vortexing, the mixture was first centrifuged at 2000×g for 10 min, and the resulting supernatant was again centrifuged at 2000×g for 10 min. The collected supernatant (1 ml) was mixed with 2 M alkalinity hydroxylamine (1:1) for 10 min at room temperature. The reaction is stopped by adding 0.5 ml of 4 M HCl and 0.5 ml of 0.37 M ferric chloride. The absorbance was measured at 540 nm at room temperature. ACh content were expressed as μM per mg of protein.

Table 2. Comparison of learning and memory ability among the groups during the probe trial test.

Groups (n)	The times of swimming through the hidden escape platform	Proportion of path	Proportion of time
Control (10)	12.1±0.09	0.37±0.02	0.36±0.12
Pioglitazone (9)	12.4±1.21	0.37±0.08	0.36±0.06
Fructose (8)	5.73±1.34a	0.20±0.10a	0.16±0.09a
Pioglitazone+fructose (8)	9.35±0.45ab	0.31±0.01ac	0.31±0.06ac

Data are shown as mean ± S.E.M.
[a]P<0.01 versus control group;
[b]P<0.01 versus untreated fructose-drinking group;
[c]P<0.05 versus untreated fructose-drinking group.

Histopathological Examination

The cerebra (5 cases) were dehydrated and embedded in paraffin blocks after post-fixed with 4% paraformaldehyde. Four 10 μm coronal sections for each case taken from −4.0 mm posterior from bregma were stained with hematoxylin-eosin. Cells in the hippocampus and temporal coxtex were observed under a light microscope (Olympus, Japan) and pictures were taken at 200× magnification. The cells with a round or oval-shaped nuclei and no shrinkage or edema were regarded as undamaged.

Experiments of Behavioral Test

The Morris water maze (MWM) test, which consisted of 5-day training (visible and invisible platform training sessions) and a probe trial on day 6, was used to evaluate the learning and memory ability of the rats [38,39]. The maze is a circular pool (100 cm in diameter, 50 cm in height) which was painted black and filled with 22±2°C milk water to a depth of 30 cm with a platform (9 cm in diameter). It was placed in a dimly lit, sound-proof test room. The platform was placed in the center of the 4 quadrants and remained there throughout the experiment. Each rat was individually trained in both visible-platform (days 1–2) and hidden-platform (days 3–5) versions. Visible platform training was performed for baseline differences in vision and motivation; the platform was placed 1 cm below the surface of the water and was indicated by a small flag (5 cm in height). The hidden-platform trial evaluated the spatial learning and was used to determine the retention of memory to find the platform. During the training days, the platform was submerged 1 cm below the surface of the water and the flag was removed. On each day, the rat was subjected to 4 trials with a 1-h interval between trials. Each trial lasted for 90 seconds unless the animal reached the platform. The test was ended and the rat was gently placed to the platform for 30 seconds if a rat failed to find the platform within 90 seconds. On day 6, the platform was removed and the probe trial started, and rats had 90 seconds to search for the platform. The proportion of time and path that the rats had spent in the target quadrant, in which the hidden escape platform was previously located, was noted. In addition, the times of the rats swimming through the hidden escape platform were also noted by an overhead camera connected to a computerized tracking system (HVS Image, Hampton, UK).

Statistical Analyses

All results were reported as mean ± S.E.M. Statistical significance was assessed with one-way analysis of variance (ANOVA) followed by Tukey–Kramer test for post hoc comparisons between groups, except the statistical analysis for the acquisition phase of MWM test is repeated-measures ANOVA. The significance of differences was determined using two-way ANOVAs when two factors were assessed. The acceptable level for statistical significance was $P<0.05$.

Results

Pioglitazone Improves Insulin Sensitivity in Fructose-drinking Insulin Resistance Rats

As seen from **Table 1**, levels of plasma insulin and insulin resistance index, but not plasma glucose, in fructose-drinking insulin resistance rats were significantly higher than those in control rats (34.6±4.5 mU/L, 8.52±0.62 in fructose-drinking insulin resistance rats and 14.5±2.9 mU/L, 3.30±0.34 in control rats, respectively, $P<0.01$). Pioglitazone treatment significantly reduced the levels of plasma insulin and insulin resistance (19.4±4.0 mU/L and 4.64±0.33, respectively, $P<0.05$ for both)

compared to the level of the fructose-drinking insulin resistance rats. There were no significant difference in the levels of plasma insulin and insulin resistance index between control and pioglitazone-treated control rats (13.9±3.3 and 2.98±0.28, respectively, $P>0.05$).

Pioglitazone Up-regulates Anti-oxidant Defense System in Fructose-drinking Insulin Resistance Rats

As shown in the panels A, B, and C of Fig. 1, ROS overproduction (oxidative stress), TBARS (lipid peroxidation), and carbonyl content (protein oxidation, PCC) were measured. Fructose-drinking insulin resistance rats showed significant higher levels of ROS ($P<0.01$, $P<0.01$), TBARS ($P<0.05$, $P<0.05$) and carbonyl ($P<0.01$, $P<0.05$) in both the hippocampus and cerebral coxtex than control rats. Reduced levels of ROS ($P<0.05$, $P<0.05$), TBARS ($P<0.05$, $P<0.01$) and carbonyl ($P<0.05$, $P<0.05$) in both hippocampus and cerebral coxtex were observed in pioglitazone (pio)-treated fructose-drinking rats compared with fructose-drinking insulin resistance rats. There were no significant differences in the levels of the three oxidative damage markers for both brain regions between control and pioglitazone-treated control rats ($P>0.05$).

As shown in the panels D, E, and F of Fig. 1, SOD ($P<0.01$, $P<0.05$), CAT ($P<0.05$, $P<0.05$)and GPx ($P<0.05$, $P<0.05$) activities of both hippocampus and cerebral cortex in fructose-drinking insulin resistance rats were significantly lower than those of control rats, significant increase in SOD ($P<0.05$, $P<0.01$), CAT ($P<0.05$, $P<0.01$) and GPx ($P<0.05$, $P<0.01$) activities of both brain regions in pioglitazone–treated fructose-drinking insulin resistance rats were observed as compared to fructose-drinking insulin resistance rats, and no difference in SOD, CAT and GPx activities was observed between control and pioglitazone-treated control rats ($P>0.05$). Results showed that the levels of GSH in both brain regions of fructose-drinking insulin resistance rats were significantly lower than those of control animals ($P<0.05$, $P<0.05$), and pioglitazone administration increased the levels of GSH in both brain regions ($P<0.01$, $P<0.01$) (Fig. 2G). The level of T-AOC in the hippocampus and cerebral cortex were measured to assess overall antioxidative capacity. Both brain regions demonstrated a significant decline in T-AOC in fructose-drinking insulin resistance rats ($P<0.01$, $P<0.05$), and animals in pioglitazone-treated fructose-drinking insulin resistance group revealed a significant higher T-AOC than that in fructose-drinking insulin resistance group ($P<0.01$, $P<0.05$) (Fig. 2H). No significant difference was observed between control and pioglitazone-treated control rats ($P>0.05$).

Piogitazone Increases Cholinergic Activity in Fructose-drinking Insulin Resistance Rats

As shown in the panels A and B of Fig. 2, animals in fructose-drinking insulin resistance group showed significantly higher AChE activity in the hippocampus and cerebral cortex than control rats ($P<0.01$, $P<0.05$). Reduced AChE activity in both brain regions in pioglitazone-treated fructose-drinking insulin resistance rats were observed compared with fructose-drinking insulin resistance rats ($P<0.01$, $P<0.05$). The ACh content in hippocampus and cerebral cortex were significantly decreased in fructose-drinking insulin resistance rats compared with that in the controls ($P<0.05$, $P<0.05$). Pioglitazone administration considerably increased ACh content compared to those in the fructose-drinking insulin resistance rats ($P<0.01$, $P<0.05$), and no significant difference was found among both control group and the pioglitazone-treated control group ($P>0.05$).

Pioglitazone cannot Ameliorate the Irreversible Brain Damage in Fructose-drinking Insulin Resistance Rats

Fig. 3 is the representative photomicrograph of hematoxylin and eosin staining in the hippocampus CA1 area and temporal cortex of rats treated with fructose and pioglitazone. In the control group (a and e) and the pioglitazone-treated control group (b and f), rare damaged neurons were seen in the hippocampus and temporal cortex. However, neuronal degeneration and karyopycnosis were easily observed in the CA1 area of the hippocampus (c) and temporal cortex (g) in the fructose-drinking insulin resistance group. Pioglitazone administration showed similar pathological changes of neurons compared with the fructose-drinking insulin resistance control group.

Pioglitazone Improves Learning and Memory Ability in Fructose-drinking Insulin Resistance Rats

Morris water maze test was used to access the learning and memory functions in each group. As can be seen from Fig. 4A, rats in each group exhibited a similar escape latency in 2-day visible-platform test, suggesting no differences in vision or basal motivation ($P>0.05$). For 3-day spatial hidden-platform test, rats in the fructose-drinking insulin resistance group showed a significant increase in escape latency as compared to those controls (control group and pioglitazone-treated control group; $P<0.01$ for both, Fig. 4B), and the change observed in the fructose-drinking insulin resistance group was partially reversed by administration of pioglitazone (4 trials/day for 3 days, $P<0.05$). As shown in Table 2, in the probe trial, fructose-drinking insulin resistance rats had substantially decreased time of swimming through the hidden escape platform compared with both control rats (5.73 ± 1.34 and 12.1 ± 0.09 respectively, $P<0.01$) and pioglitazone-treated control rats (5.73 ± 1.34 and 12.4 ± 1.21 respectively, $P<0.01$). Pioglitazone-treated fructose-drinking insulin resistance rats had increased times of swimming through the hidden escape platform compared with fructose-drinking insulin resistance rats (9.35 ± 0.45 and 5.73 ± 1.34 respectively, $P<0.01$). Accordingly, fructose-drinking insulin resistance rats showed decreased proportion of path and time through the hidden escape platform, which were in sharp contrast with control and pioglitazone-treated control rats ($P<0.01$), pioglitazone-treated fructose-drinking insulin resistance rats showed increased proportion of path and time compared with fructose-drinking insulin resistance rats ($P<0.05$). Notably, there was no significant difference in all above-mentioned data between control and pioglitazone-treated control groups ($P>0.05$), suggesting that pioglitazone had little or no effect on the cognitive ability of healthy rats. The results indicate that our insulin resistance rat model manifested impaired learning and memory ability which was associated with fructose drinking, and pioglitazone partially improved the cognitive impairments.

Discussion

As a PPARγ agonist and an insulin sensitizer, pioglitazone is widely used for the treatment of T2DM, and has also been reported to be effective in a number of neurodegenerative disease models [19–21]. Higher dose of pioglitazone (including 10 mg/kg d) can cross the blood-brain barrier, and pioglitazone can be taken up and detected in the CNS [40], and exerts neuroprotective effect.

Differences in gender have been shown to influence the progression of insulin resistance. Studies using fructose-fed rats have demonstrated that the degree of insulin resistance developed in males is greater than females. Thus, we employed male rats for the present study [41–43]. Consistent to literatures [44,45], we

found that fructose had no influence on plasma glucose level. Although fructose does not appear to increase insulin level acutely, chronic exposure seems to cause hyperinsulinemia indirectly [45]. In the present study, we found that high-fructose feeding increased fasting insulin and insulin resistance index in plasma (Table 1), and the insulin resistance is likely mediated by altered activities of the enzymes that regulate hepatic carbohydrates metabolism, such as decreased glucokinase and increased glucose-6-phosphatase activities [46]. Despite the lack of obesity, a fat redistribution is suggested by the observation that enlarged adipose tissue is associated with increased size of adipocyte, which could be in part prevented by metformin [47,48]. In the present study, 12-week pioglitazone administration did not cause significant changes in weight and plasma glucose level. This is consistent with the data from the 18-month pioglitazone trial in patients with AD carried out by Geldmacher et al [49], in which pioglitazone was found to be well tolerated, without effect on blood glucose, hemoglobin A_{1C}, and other hematologic measures.

Oxidative stress is reported as one of the earliest events in the pathogenesis of neurodegenerative diseases including AD [5]. Insulin resistance can result in oxidative stress, leading to irreversible protein aggregation and neuronal degeneration [5–7]. In CNS, ROS was removed by antioxidant defense system that works as a complex team. In the present study, all of the three oxidative damage markers: ROS, TBARS and protein carbonyl were found significantly increased in the brains of fructose-drinking insulin resistance rats compared with control rats. SOD converts superoxide to hydrogen peroxide, GPx and CAT convert hydrogen peroxide to water, and they all are primary antioxidant enzymes [38]. GSH, an important non-enzymatic antioxidant, plays a critical role in antioxidant defense in CNS. GSH scavenges ROS by directly reacting with it or may prevent hydrogen peroxide-induced hydroxyl radical formation [17]. In the present study, the activities of SOD, GPx, and CAT were significantly decreased in the brains of fructose-drinking insulin resistance rats. These suggested that the brains in fructose-drinking insulin resistance rats were less efficient to convert hydrogen peroxide to water, and this might lead to the accumulation of hydrogen peroxide. The excessive hydrogen peroxide is also a harmful ROS that can induce cytotoxicity in the brain. Moreover, fructose-drinking insulin resistance rats also showed significant lower levels of GSH and T-AOC in brains. Taken together, it is suggested that insulin resistance induces ROS overproduction, lipid peroxidation, and protein oxidation, as well as decreased anti-oxidative capacity.

PPARγ agonists were used to suppress oxidative damage [7]. Pioglitazone could decrease lipid peroxidation and protein oxidation in the brain [22,23], and increase the antioxidant capacities in brains of the experimental dementia animal models, cardiomyopathy and nephrotoxicity [23,50,51]. In the present study, the markedly increased activities of SOD, CAT and GPx as well as significant higher levels of GSH and T-AOC suggested that pioglitazone administration might reduce the ROS production in fructose-drinking insulin resistance rats. Moreover, the higher T-AOC level also reflected the role of pioglitazone against oxidative stress. Thus, pioglitazone administration strengthens the overall antioxidant defense system.

We found an increased AChE activity and decreased ACh level in fructose-drinking insulin resistance rats in the present study. This is consistent with a previous study that AChE activity was decreased in some of the brain regions in streptozotocin-intracerebroventricularly treated central insulin resistance rats [7]. AChE was over-expressed in response to various oxidative stresses such as free radical and oxidative stress in the brain [17,52,53,54], thus it is possible that the significant increase of

AChE activity in the present study is due to oxidative damage induced by insulin resistance. The decreased ACh level in the brains of fructose-drinking insulin resistance rats may simply result from the increased AChE activity. Consistent with previous studies in experimental dementia and scopolamine-induced mice [22,53], pioglitazone could inhibit AChE activity and restore ACh level in fructose-drinking insulin resistance rats. In our previous studies, we showed that fructose-drinking insulin resistance promotes Aβ-amyloidosis in the brain [25], and AChE activity is increased within and around amyloid plaques [54]. Thus it is possible that the increase of AChE activity and impairment of cognitive function in the present study is due to Aβ induced by insulin resistance.

It is well known that the hippocampus and temporal cortex play important roles in learning and memory. Fructose feeding is used to induce fatty liver disease, and hippocampus-dependent memory function is impaired in this model [3,4,45,55,56]. Histopathological examination is important for evaluating neuronal damage and drug action [17]. In the present study, we demonstrated that

fructose can induce neurodegeneration in brains (Fig. 3). Furthermore, fructose-drinking insulin resistance rats exhibited obviously spatial learning and memory impairments assessed by Morris water maze test (Fig. 4), which supports that long-term fructose drinking impairs cognitive function. However, although pioglitazone cannot ameliorate the irreversible brain damage in fructose-drinking insulin resistance rats, pioglitazone administration indeed rescues learning and memory impairments induced by fructose-drinking, this rescuing effect of pioglitazone on cognition dysfunction is well correlated with its effect on the activities of cholinergic system (AChE and ACh).

Author Contributions

Conceived and designed the experiments: XPL QQY. Performed the experiments: QQY MHS SQD. Analyzed the data: ZJS SX XPL. Contributed reagents/materials/analysis tools: LY. Wrote the paper: QQY JJP XPL DZL.

References

1. Manschot SM, Biessels GJ, Rutten GE, Kessels RC, Gispen WH, et al. (2008) Peripheral and central neurologic complications in type 2 diabetes mellitus: no association in individual patients. J Neurol Sci 264: 157–162.

2. Craft S (2005) Insulin resistance syndrome and Alzheimer's disease: Age- and obesity-related effects on memory, amyloid, and inflammation. Neurobiol Aging 26: 65–69.

3. Gordon W, Carol EG, Gerardo GP, Claudia AG, Leah RR, et al. (2005) Memory impairment in obese Zucker rats: An investigation of cognitive function in an animal model of insulin resistance and obesity. Behav Neurosci 119(5): 1389–1395.

4. Stranahan AM, Norman ED, Roy G. Cutler KL, Telljohann RS, et al. (2008). Diet-induced insulin resistance impairs hippocampal synaptic plasticity and cognition in middle-aged rats, Hippocampus 18 (11): 1085–1088.

5. Reddy VP, Zhu XW, Perry G, Smith MA (2009) Oxidative stress in diabetes and Alzheimer' diaease. J Alzheimer Dis 16: 763–774.

6. Tinahones FJ, Murri-Pierri M, Garrido-Sánchez L, García-Almeida JM, García-Serrano S, et al. (2009) Oxidative stress in severely obese persons is greater in those with insulin resistance. Obesity 17(2): 240–246.

7. Salkovic-Petrisic M, Hoyer S (2007) Central insulin resistance as a trigger for sporadic Alzheimer-like pathology: an experimental approach, J Neural Transm 72: 217–233.

8. Ugochukwu NH, Mukes JD, Figgers CL (2006) Ameliorative effects of dietary caloric restriction on oxidative stress and inflammation in the brain of streptozotocin-induced diabetic rats. Clinica Chimica Acta 370: 165–173.

9. Sharma M, Gupta YK (2001) Intracerebroventricular injection of streptozptocin in rats produces both oxidative stress in the brain and cognitive impaiement. Life Sci 68: 1021–1029.

10. Sharma M, Gupta YK (2001) Effect of chronic treatment of melatonin on learning, memory, and oxidative deficiencies induced by intracerebroventricular streptozptocin in rats. Pharmacol Biochem Behav 70: 325–331.

11. Ramkumar KM, Latha M, Venkateswaran S, Pari L, Ananthan R, et al. (2004) Modulatory effect of gymnema montanum leaf extract on brain antioxidant status and lipid peroxidation in diabetic rats. J Medicinal Food 7(3): 366–371.

12. Hong JH, Lee IS (2009) Effects of artemisia capillaris ethyl acetate fraction on oxidative stress and antioxidant enzyme in high-fat diet induced obese mice. Chemico-Biological Interactions. 179: 88–93.

13. Thirunavukkarasu V, Anuradha CV (2004) Influence of α-lipoic acid on lipid peroxidation and antioxidant defence system in blood of insulin-resistant rats. Diabetes, Obesity and Metabolism. 6(3): 200–207.

14. De la Monte SM (2009) Insulin resistance and Alzheimer's disease. BMB Rep. 42(8): 475–481.

15. Terry Jr AV, Buccafusco JJ (2003) The cholinergic hypothesis of age and Alzheimer's disease-related cognitive deficits: recent challenges and their implications for novel drug development. J Pharmacol Exp Ther. 306: 821–827.

16. Ruan CJ, Si JY, Zhang L, Chen DH, Du GH, et al. (2009) Protective effect of stilbenes containing extract-fraction from Cajanus cajan L. on Aβ25–35-induced cognitive deficits in mice. Neurosci Lett 467: 159–163.

17. Zhong SZ, Ge QH, Qu R, Li Q, Ma SP (2009) Paeonol attenuates neurotoxicity and ameliorates cognitive impairment induced by D-galactose in ICR mice. J Neuro Sci 277: 58–64.

18. Sood V, Colleran K, Burge MR (2000) Thiazolidinediones: A comparative review of approved uses. Diabetes Technol Ther 2: 429–440.

19. Nicolakakis N, Hamel E (2010) The nuclear receptor PPARgamma as a therapeutic target for cerebrovascular and brain dysfunction in Alzheimer's disease. Front Aging Neurosci 2: 21–30.

20. Kalonia H, Kumar P, Kumar A (2010) Pioglitazone ameliorates behavioral, biochemical and cellular alterations in quinolinic acid induced neurotoxicity: Possible role of peroxisome proliferator activated receptor-γ (PPARγ) in Huntington's disease. Pharmacol Biochemis and Behav 96: 115–124.

21. Wahner AD, Bronstein JM, Bordelon YM, Ritz B (2007) Nonsteroidal anti-inflammatory drugs may protect against Parkinson disease. Neurology 69: 1836–1842.

22. Kaur B, Singh N, Jaggi AS (2009) Exploring mechanism of pioglitazone induced memory restorative effect in experimental dementia. Fund Clin Pharmacol 23: 557–566.

23. Pathan AR, Viswanad B, Sonkusare SK, Ramarao P (2006) Chronic administration of pioglitazone attenuates intracerebroventricular streptozotocin induced-memory impairment in rats, Life Sci 79: 2209–2216.

24. Liu X, Luo D, Zheng M, Hao Y, Hou L, et al. (2010) Effect of pioglitazone on insulin resistance in fructose-drinking rats correlates with AGEs/RAGE inhibition and block of NADPH oxidase and NF kappa B activation. Eur J Pharmacol 629: 153–158.

25. Luo D, Hao Y, Hou L, Wang M, Xu S, Dong C, et al. (2011) Effect of pioglitazone on altered expression of Aβ metabolism-associated molecules in the brain of fructose-drinking rats, a rodent model of insulin resistance. Eur J Pharmacol 664: 14–19.

26. Xu JQ, Rong S, Xie BJ, Sun Z, Zhang L, et al. (2009) Rejuvenation of antioxidant and cholinergic systems contributes to the effect of procyanidins extracted from the lotus seedpod ameliorating memory impairment in cognitively impaired rats. Euro Neuropsychopharmcol 19: 851–860.

27. Siqueira RI, Fochesatto C, Da Silva Torres IL, Dalmaz C, Netto CA (2005) Aging affects oxidative state in hippocampus, hypothalamus and adrenal glands of Wistar rats. Life Sci 78: 271–278.

28. Lowry OH, Rosebrough NJ, Farr AL, Randall RJ (1951) Protein measurement with the folin phenol reagent. J Biol Chem 193: 265–275.

29. Iwai H, Ohno Y, Aoki N (2003) The effect of leptin, tumor necrosis factor-alpha (TNFalpha), and nitric oxide (NO) production on insulin resistance in Otsuka Long–Evans fatty rats. J Endocr 50: 673–680.

30. Buege JA, Aust SD (1978) Microsomal lipid peroxidation. Methods Enzymol 52: 302–310.

31. Levine RL, Garland D, Oliver CN, Amici A, Climent I, et al. (1990) Determination of carbonyl content in oxidatively modified proteins. Methods Enzymol 186: 464–478.

32. Kono Y (1978) Generation of superoxide radical during autoxidation of hydroxylamine and an assay for superoxide dismutase. Arch Biochem Biophys 186: 189–195.

33. Goth L (1991) A simple method for determination of serum catalase activity and revision of reference range. Clin Chim Acta 196: 143–151.

34. Hafemen DG (1974) Effect of dietary selenium on erythrocyte and liver glutathione peroxidase in the rats. J Nutr 104: 580–587.

35. Griffith OW (1980) Determination of glutathione and glutathione disulfide using glutathione reductase and 2-vinylpyridine. Anal Biochem 106: 207–12.

36. Benzie IF, Strain JJ (1996) The ferric reducing ability of plasma (FRAP) as a measure of "antioxidant power": the FRAP assay. Anal Biochem 239: 70–76.

37. Yang HX, Wang WX, Ke JS (1995) Determine acetylcholine of whole blood by alkalinity hydroxylammonium and galactose chromatometry. J Clinic analy 13: 125–126.

38. Kumar P, Kumar A (2008) Prolonged pretreatment with carvedilol prevents 3-nitropropionic acid-induced behavioral alterations and oxidative stress in rats. Pharmacol Rep 60: 706–715.

39. Jiang LY, Tang SS, Wang XY, Liu LP, Long Y, et al. (2012) PPARγ Agonist Pioglitazone Reverses Memory Impairment and Biochemical Changes in a Mouse Model of Type 2 Diabetes Mellitus. CNS Neurosci & Ther 18: 659–666.

40. Maeshiba Y, Kiyota Y, Yamashita K, Yoshimura Y, Motohashi M, et al. (1997) Disposition of the new antidiabetic agent pioglitazone in rats, dogs, and monkeys. Arzneimittel Forsch 47: 29–35.

41. Galipeau D, Verma S, McNeill JH (2002) Female rats are protected against fructose-induced changes in metabolism and blood pressure. Am J Physiol Heart Circ Physiol 283: 2478–2484.

42. Vasudevan H, Xiang H, McNeill JH (2005) Differential regulation of insulin resistance and hypertension by sex hormones in fructose-fed male rats. Am J Physiol Heart Circ Physiol 289: 1335–1442.

43. Galipeau DM, Yao L, McNeill JH (2002) Relationship among hyperinsulinemia, insulin resistance, and hypertension is dependent on sex. Am J Physiol Heart Circ Physiol 283: 562–567.

44. Mehnert H (1976) Sugar substitutes in the diabetic diet. Int Z Vitam Ernahrungsforsch Beih 15: 295–324.

45. Basciano H, Federico L, Adeli K (2005) Fructose, insulin resistance, and metabolic dyslipidemia. Nutri & Metabol 2: 5–10.

46. Delbosc S, Paizanis E, Magous R, Araiz C, Dimo T, et al. (2005) Involvement of oxidative stress and NADPH oxidase activation in the development of cardiovascular complications in a model of insulin resistance, the fructose-fed rat. Atheroscler 179: 43–49.

47. Baret G, Peyronnet J, Grassi-Kassisse D, Dalmaz Y, Wiernsperger N, et al. (2002) Increased intraabdominal adipose tissue mass in fructose fed rats: correction by metformin. Exp Clin Endocrinol Diab 110(6): 298–303.

48. Juan CC, Au LC, Fang VS, Kang SF, Ko YH, et al. (2001) Suppressed Gene expression of adipocyte resistin in an insulin-resistant rat model probably by elevated free fatty acids. Biochem Biophys Res Commun 289 (5): 1328–1333.

49. Geldmacher DS, Fritsch T, McClendon MJ, Landreth G (2011) A randomized pilot clinical trial of the safety of pioglitazone in treatment of patients with Alzheimer's disease. Arch Neurol 68: 45–50.

50. Saraogi P, Pillai KK, Singh BK, Dubey K (2010) Rosiglitazone and pioglitazone aggravate doxorubicin-induced cardiomyopathy in Wistar rats. Biomed Pharmacother. Equb ahead of print.

51. Ozebek E, Ilbey YO, Simsek A, Cekmen M, Mete F, et al. (2010) Rosiglitazone, peroxisome proliferator receptor-gamma agonist, ameliorates gentamicin-induced nephrotoxicity in rats. Int Urol Nephrol 42: 579–587.

52. Schmatz R, Mazzanti CM, Spanevello R, Stefanello N, Gutierres J, et al. (2009) Resveratrol prevents memory deficits and the increase in acetylcholinesterase activity in streptozotocin-induced diabetic rats. Euro J Pharmacol 610: 42–48.

53. Xiang GQ, Tang SS, Jiang LY, Hong H, Li Q, et al. (2012) PPARγ agonist pioglitazone improves scopolamine-induced memory impairment in mice. J Pharm Pharmacol. Equb ahead of print.

54. Melo JB, Agostinho P, Oliveira CR (2003) Involvement of oxidative stress in the enhancement of acetylcholinesterase activity induced by amyloid beta-peptide. 45: 117–127.

55. Ross AP, Bartness TJ, Mielke JG, Parent MB (2009) A high fructose diet impairs spatial memory in male rats. Neurobiol Learn mem. 92(3), 410–416.

56. Ross AP, Bruggeman EC, Kasumu AW, Mielke JG, Parent MB (2012) Non-alcoholic fatty liver disease impairs hippocampal-dependent memory in male rats. Physiol & Behav 106(2): 133–141.

14

Erythropoietin Inhibits Gluconeogenesis and Inflammation in the Liver and Improves Glucose Intolerance in High-Fat Diet-Fed Mice

Ran Meng[1,2,3], Dalong Zhu[1]*, Yan Bi[1], Donghui Yang[1], Yaping Wang[2,3]*

1 Department of Endocrinology, Nanjing Drum Tower Hospital, Nanjing University School of Medicine, Nanjing, China, **2** Department of Medical Genetics, Nanjing University School of Medicine, Nanjing, China, **3** Jiangsu Key Laboratory of Molecular Medicine, Nanjing University, Nanjing, China

Abstract

Erythropoietin (EPO) has multiple biological functions, including the modulation of glucose metabolism. However, the mechanisms underlying the action of EPO are still obscure. This study is aimed at investigating the potential mechanisms by which EPO improves glucose tolerance in an animal model of type 2 diabetes. Male C57BL/6 mice were fed with high-fat diet (HFD) for 12 weeks and then treated with EPO (HFD-EPO) or vehicle saline (HFD-Con) for two week. The levels of fasting blood glucose, serum insulin and glucose tolerance were measured and the relative levels of insulin-related phosphatidylinositol 3-kinase (PI3K)/Akt, insulin receptor (IR) and IR substrate 1 (IRS1) phosphorylation were determined. The levels of phosphoenolpyruvate carboxykinase (PEPCK), glucose-6- phosphatase (G6Pase), toll like receptor 4 (TLR4), tumor necrosis factor (TNF)-α and IL-6 expression and nuclear factor-κB (NF-κB) and c-Jun N-terminal kinase (JNK), extracellular-signal-regulated kinase (ERK) and p38 MAPK activation in the liver were examined. EPO treatment significantly reduced the body weights and the levels of fasting blood glucose and serum insulin and improved the HFD-induced glucose intolerance in mice. EPO treatment significantly enhanced the levels of Akt, but not IR and IRS1, phosphorylation, accompanied by inhibiting the PEPCK and G6Pase expression in the liver. Furthermore, EPO treatment mitigated the HFD-induced inflammatory TNF-α and IL-6 production, TLR4 expression, NF-κB and JNK, but not ERK and p38 MAPK, phosphorylation in the liver. Therefore, our data indicated that EPO treatment improved glucose intolerance by inhibiting gluconeogenesis and inflammation in the livers of HFD-fed mice.

Editor: Jianping Ye, Pennington Biomedical Research Center, United States of America

Funding: This study was supported by National Natural Science Foundation of China (81070636), Natural Science Foundation of Jiangsu Province of China (BK2010110), Jiangsu Province's Key Discipline/Laboratory of Medicine (XK201105) and Program for the Talents in science and education of Jiangsu Province, China. The funders had no role in study design, data collection and analysis, decision to publish, or preparation of the manuscript.

Competing Interests: The authors have declared that no competing interests exist.

* E-mail: zhudldr@gmail.com (DLZ); wangyap@nju.edu.cn (YPW)

Introduction

Excessive caloric intake usually causes glucose intolerance and insulin resistance, the hallmarks of metabolic syndrome and type 2 diabetes (T2D), which are important health challenges in the world [1,2]. Currently, there are many medicines available and under the development for the treatment of glucose intolerance and insulin resistance. However, the therapeutic efficacy of these medicines and their safety profiles remain questionable. Therefore, the discovery and development of new medicines will be of great significance. Theoretically, glucose homeostasis is regulated by the balance of gluconeogenesis, glycogenesis, glyogenolysis and glucose metabolism. The gluconeogenesis is a critical process to convert non-carbohydrate carbon substrates, such as pyruvate, lactate, glycerol, and glucogenic amino acids, to glucose, regulating glucose metabolism in humans. Thus, inhibition of gluconeogenesis may be ideal for the improvement of glucose intolerance and insulin resistance, and a promising strategy for the treatment of metabolic syndrome and T2D.

Erythropoietin (EPO), a hematopoietic growth factor, is predominantly produced in the kidney, and has been widely used in patients with anemia from renal diseases and myelodysplasia

following chemotherapy or radiotherapy [3]. Interestingly, treatment with EPO has been shown to ameliorate insulin resistance in patients, who have end-stage renal disease (ESRD) and undergo hemodialysis therapy [4,5]. Furthermore, EPO transgenic mice display significantly lower levels of blood glucose, insulin and HA1C, and are resistant to high fat diet (HFD)-induced glucose intolerance and insulin resistance [6,7]. In contrast, EPO receptor (EPOR) null mice develop insulin resistant [8]. Accordingly, EPO may regulate glucose tolerance and insulin sensitivity. However, how EPO regulates glucose metabolism and whether EPO regulates gluconeogenesis have not been explored.

Insulin plays a crucial role in the regulation of glucose metabolism [9]. Insulin can bind to insulin receptor (IR) and activate IR tyrosine kinase, which activates IR substrate (IRS). Subsequently, the activated IRS recruits and activates the phosphatidylinositol 3-kinase (PI3K) and Akt, leading to glucose transportation, glucagon synthesis, and inhibiting gluconeogenesis in the liver [10–12]. Impairment in the PI3K/Akt pathway is associated with glucose intolerance and insulin resistance as well as increased expression of phosphoenolpyruvate carboxykinase (PEPCK) and glucose-6-phosphatase (G6Pase), two rate-limiting enzymes for hepatic glucose production [13,14]. Hence, enhancement of the PI3K/Akt activation may be a promising strategy for improving glucose tolerance and insulin sensitivity. Interestingly, EPO can activate, through the EPOR, the PI3K/Akt pathway in many organs [15–18]. Given that the EPOR is expressed in the liver, we hypothesize that EPO may activate the PI3K/Akt pathway to inhibit the PEPCK and G6Pase expression and gluconeogenesis in the liver, improving glucose tolerance and insulin sensitivity, even in obese animals.

Chronic low-grade inflammation contributes to the development of obesity-related glucose intolerance and insulin resistance [19]. The toll like receptor 4 (TLR4) recognizes endogenous free fat acid and exogenous pathogens [20,21] and engagement of TLR4 activates the nuclear factor κB (NF-κB) [22] and mitogen-activated protein kinase (MAPK) subfamily members [23], including the extracellular-signal-regulated kinase (ERK), c-Jun N-terminal kinases (JNK) and p38 MAPK, as well ascytokines [24], and stimulates the production of inflammatory cytokines, such as tumor necrosis factor (TNF)-α and interleukin (IL)-6, contributing to glucose intolerance and insulin resistance. Given that EPO treatment inhibits the NF-κB, ERK and JNK activation, and TNF-α and IL-6 production in animal models of hepatic injury [25–28], we hypothesize that EPO may also inhibit the HFD-induced chronic inflammation, contributing to the improvement of glucose intolerance and insulin resistance.

In the present study, we fed C57BL/6 mice with HFD to establish glucose intolerance and investigated the effects of EPO treatment on glucose tolerance and the potential molecular mechanisms underlying the action of EPO in regulating gluconeogenesis and inflammation in the liver.

Materials and Methods

Animals and experimental procedures

All experimental procedures were approved by the Animal Care and Use Committee of Nanjing University (Approval ID: 2008000027). Male C57BL/6 mice at 4 weeks of age were purchased from the Animal Center of Yangzhou University (Yangzhou, Jiangsu, China) and housed in a specific pathogen-free facility throughout the experimental period. The mice were fed with HFD (60% kcal fat, 20% kcal carbohydrates, 20% kcal protein, Guangzhou Animal Experiment Center, Guangzhou, China), or with normal chow diet (10% kcal fat, 70% kcal carbohydrates, 20% kcal protein) for 12 weeks. The HFD-fed mice were randomized and treated intraperitoneally with 1000 IU/kg recombinant human EPO (Sunshine Pharmaceutical, Shenyang, China) every other day for two weeks (HFD-EPO group) or with saline (HFD-Con group), respectively. The healthy control mice with normal chow diet were injected with saline (NC group). Their dietary intake and body weights were measured every other day. At the end of the experiment, their fasting blood samples were collected and the mice were sacrificed. Their liver tissues were harvested, weighed, snap frozen in liquid nitrogen, and stored at −80°C until use.

ELISA

The blood samples of individual mice were centrifuged at 1,500 ×g for 10 min for preparing plasma or serum samples. The concentrations of plasma TNF-α and IL-6 were measured using the cytokine-specific ELISA kits, according to the manufacturers' instruction (RayBiotech, Norcross, USA). Similarly, the concentrations of serum insulin in individual mice were determined using the mouse insulin ELISA kit, according to the manufacturer's instructions (Linco, Charles, USA). The detection limitation for TNF-α, IL-6 and insulin was 50 pg/ml, 2 pg/ml and 0.2 ng/ml, respectively.

Glucose tolerance test

After treatment with EPO or vehicle for two weeks, the mice were fasted for 6 h and injected intraperitoneally with glucose (1 g/kg body weight). The levels of tail venous blood glucose in individual mice were measured at 0, 30, 60 and 120 min post glucose challenge using test strips on an One Touch profile glucose meter (Johnson & Johnson, New Brunswick, USA). The area under the curve (AUC) for the levels of blood glucose over the experimental period was calculated.

Western blot analysis

The liver tissue samples were obtained from individual mice and lyzed in NP40 lysis buffer (140 mM NaCl, 10 mM Tris (pH 7.4), 1 mM CaCl2, 1 mM MgCl2, 10% glycerol, 1% Nonidet P-40, 1 mM dithiothreitol, 0.5 mM phenylmethylsulforyl fluoride, 2 ng/μl of aprotinin, 10 ng/μl of leupeptin), followed by centrifugation. After quantification of protein concentrations, the liver lysates (20 μg/lane) were separated by SDS-PAGE on 10% polyacrylamide gels, and electrotransferred onto polyvinylidene difluoride (PVDF) membranes (Millipore, Billerica, USA). The membranes were blocked with 5% fat-free milk and incubated with anti-IR, anti-IRS1 (Millipore, Billerica, USA), anti-JNK, anti-p-JNK (Thr183/Tyr185), anti-p-IRS1 (Ser307), anti-p-IR (Tyr1346), anti-Akt, anti-p-Akt (Ser473), anti-p38, anti-p-p38 (Thr180/Tyr182), anti-TLR4, anti-PEPCK, anti-G6Pase (Cell Signaling Technology, Danvers, USA), anti-GAPDH, anti-tubulin (Boster, Wuhan, China), respectively. The bound antibodies were detected using horseradish peroxidase (HRP)-conjugated anti-rabbit antibodies and visualized using enhanced chemiluminescence (ECL, Boster). The relative levels of target proteins to controls were determined by densimetric analysis using ImageJ software.

RT-PCR and quantitative PCR analysis

Total RNA was extracted from the liver samples of individual mice by Trizol (Takara Bio, Shiga, Japan) and reversely transcribed into cDNA using M-MLV reverse transcriptase (Toyobo, Osaka, Japan). The relative levels of EPO receptor mRNA transcription in individual liver samples was determined by RT-PCR using the specific primers of 5'-CTA TGG CTG TTG CAA CGC GA-3' (forward) and 5'-CCGAGG GCA CAG GAG CTT AG-3' (reverse). The kidney tissue samples from the same mice were used as positive controls for testing the EPO receptor expression. The amplification was performed at 94°C for 2 min and subjected to 30 cycles of 94°C for 30 seconds, 62°C for 30 seconds, and 72°C for 50 seconds, followed by a final extension at 72°C for 7 minutes. The PCR products were analyzed by 1% agarose gel electrophoresis and imaged.

In addition, the relative levels of target gene mRNA transcripts to β-actin in the liver tissues of individual mice were determined by quantitative real-time PCR using the SYBR Premix Ex Taq (Takara Bio, Shiga, Japan) and specific primers on a StepOne Real-Time PCR system, according to the manufacturer's instructions (Applied Biosystems, Foster City, USA). The sequences of primers are listed in Table 1. The relative levels of the target gene mRNA transcripts to the β-actin were calculated by $2^{-\Delta\Delta Ct}$.

Table 1. The sequences of the primers.

Gene	Forward Primer	Reverse Primer
IL-6	5'-TCCAGTTGCCTTCTTGGGAC-3'	5'-GTGTAATTAAGCCTCCGACTTG-3'
TNF-α	5'-CAGGAGGGAGAACAGAAACTCCA-3'	5'-CCTGGTTGGCTGCTTGCTT-3'
PEPCK	5'-GAACTGACAGACTCGCCCTATGT-3'	5'-GTTGCAGGCCCAGTTGTTG-3'
G6Pase	5'-GTGCAGCTGAACGTCTGTCTGT-3'	5'-TCCGGAGGCTGGCATTGT-3'
TLR4	5'-AGAAAATGCCAGGATGATGC-3'	5'-ATTTTGTCTCCACAGCCACC-3'
β-actin	5'-CATCCGTAAAGACCTCTATGCCAAC-3'	5'-ATGGAGCCACCGATCCACA-3'

The DNA-binding based ELISA for the measurement of NF-κB activity

Nuclear proteins were extracted from the liver tissue samples of individual mice using the nuclear protein extract kit, according to the manufacturers' instruction (Active Motif, Carlsbad, USA). The concentrations of proteins were quantified using a Bradford assay, and the activities of NF-κB p65 binding to the specific DNA oligonucleotides in individual samples were determined using the TransAM NF-κB p65 kit (Active Motif), as described previously [29,30].

Statistical analysis

Data are expressed as the means ± S.E.M. The different among groups was analyzed by one-way ANOVA and the least significant difference (LSD) using the SPSS 13.0 Program. A P value of <0.05 was considered statistically significant.

Results

Effects of EPO on body weights, food intakes, fasting blood glucose, fasting serum insulin and glucose tolerance in the HFD-fed mice

To test the effect of EPO on glucose tolerance, C57BL/6 mice were fed with HFD or normal chow (NC group) for 12 weeks. The HFD-fed mice were randomly treated with EPO (HFD-EPO group) or vehicle saline (HFD-Con group) every other day for two weeks and the body weights in the different groups of mice were monitored every other day through the experimental period. The body weights in the HFD-EPO and HFD-Con groups of mice were comparable within 4 days post treatment and were significantly greater than that of the NC group of mice (p<0.05, Fig. 1A). Subsequently, the body weights in the HFD-EPO group of mice gradually decreased and were significantly less than that of the HFD-Con group (p<0.05). At two weeks post treatment, the body weights in the HFD-EPO group of mice were similar to that in the NC group (p>0.05). There was no statistically significant difference in the amounts of food intakes among the different groups of mice throughout the experimental period (data not shown).

Analysis of fasting blood glucose and fasting serum insulin indicated that the concentrations of fasting blood glucose in the HFD-EPO group of mice were comparable with that in the NC group of mice and were significantly lower than that in the HFD-Con group of mice at the end of the experiment (p<0.01, Fig. 1B). Compared with that in the HFD-Con group, the concentrations of fasting serum insulin were significantly reduced by near 50% (p<0.05) although they were significantly higher than that in the NC group of mice (Fig. 1C).

Furthermore, we performed an intraperitoneal glucose tolerance test (IPGTT) in the different groups of mice and found that the dynamic changes in the levels of blood glucose in the HFD-EPO group of mice were similar to that in the NC group and the concentrations of blood glucose in the HFD-EPO group of mice were obviously lower than that in the HFD-Con group of mice following glucose challenge (Fig. 1D). Quantitative analysis revealed that the values of AUC for blood glucose in the HFD-EPO group of mice were similar to that in the NC group and significantly less than that in the HFD-Con group of mice (p<0.01, Fig. 1E). Collectively, these data clearly indicated that treatment with EPO after the establishment of obesity-related T2D significantly reduced the body weights, corrected hyperglycemia and glucose intolerance, and mitigated the HFD-induced hyperinsulinemia in HFD-fed mice.

The transcription of EPOR mRNA in the liver of mice

EPO binds to its receptor, EPOR, which mediates downstream signaling and biological function. To understand the mechanisms underlying the action of EPO, we first tested the levels of EPOR mRNA transcription in the livers of mice by semi-quantitative RT-PCR. We detected the EPOR mRNA transcripts in both the livers and kidneys of mice, suggesting that the EPOR was expressed and mediated its regulatory effect on gluconeogenesis in the livers of mice (Fig. 2).

EPO enhances the Akt, but not IR and IRS, activation in the livers of mice

Engagement of EPOR by EPO activates the PI3K/Akt pathway, which participates in the insulin and IR-mediated signaling [31]. To understand the mechanisms underlying the action of EPO in gluconeogenesis, we characterized the levels of total Akt, IR, IRS1 and phosphorylated Akt, IR and IRS1 in the livers of HFD-fed mice by Western blot assays. We found that there were similar levels of Akt, IR and IRS expression in the livers between the HFD-EPO and HFD-Con groups of mice (Fig. 3), suggesting that EPO treatment did not alter the levels of these event expression in the livers of mice. Furthermore, the ratios of the levels of phosphorylated Akt (p-Akt) to total Akt (t-Akt) in the liver tissues were significantly greater in the HFD-EPO group than that in the HFD-Con group of mice (p<0.05, Fig. 3A). However, there was no significant difference in the levels of phosphorylated IR and IRS1 in the livers between the HFD-EPO and HFD-Con groups of mice (Fig. 3B and C). Hence, treatment with EPO enhanced the Akt, but not IS and IRS1, activation in the livers of mice.

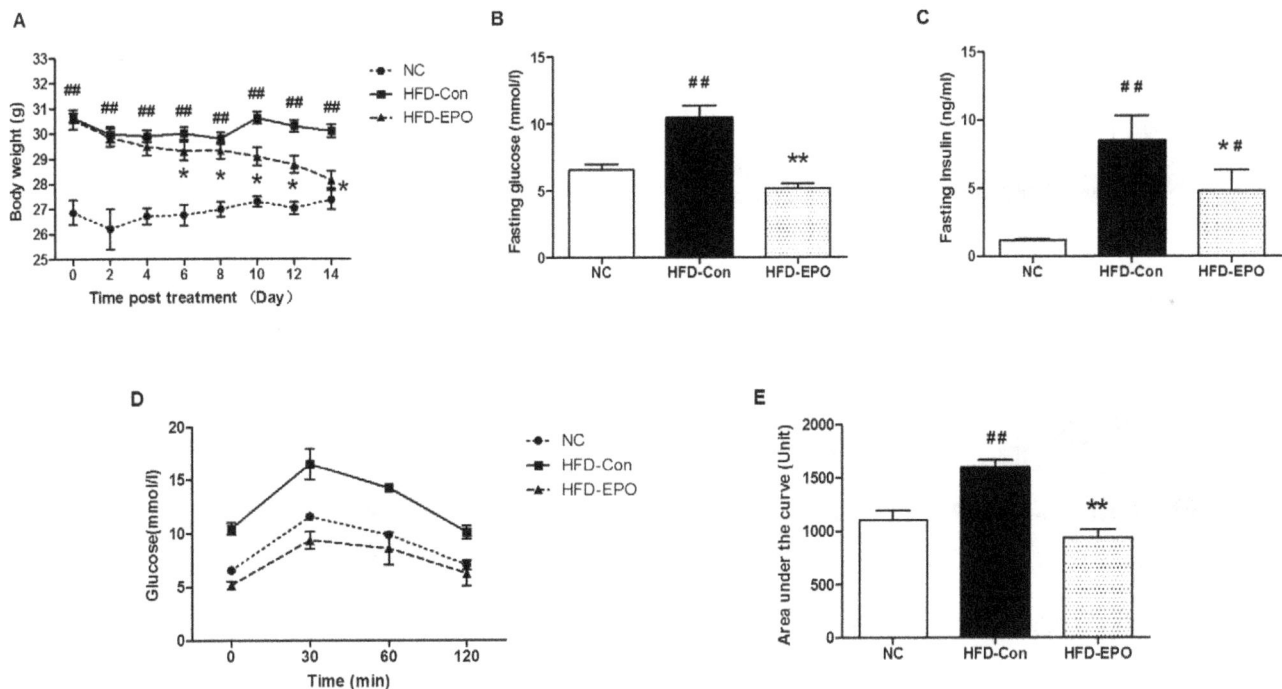

Figure 1. The effect of EPO on HFD-fed mice. C57BL/6 mice were fed with HFD for 12 weeks and treated with EPO (HFD-EPO) or injected with saline (HFD-Con) for two weeks. A control group (NC) of mice was fed with normal chow and injected with saline. The body weights and amounts of food consumed in individual mice were measured at the indicated time points. At the end of treatment, the mice were fasted and subjected to measurements of the levels of fasting blood glucose, fasting serum insulin and IPGTT. The AUC for blood glucose in individual mice was calculated. Data are present as the mean ± SEM of each group (n = 8) of mice from two-three separate experiments. (**A**) The body weights. (**B**) The levels of fasting blood glucose. (**C**) The levels of fasting serum insulin. (**D**) The glucose tolerance. (**E**) The values of AUC. There was no significant difference in the amounts of food intake among these groups of mice (data not shown). #$P < 0.05$ or ##$P < 0.01$ vs. the NC group, *$P < 0.05$ or **$P < 0.01$ vs. the HFD-Con group.

EPO inhibits the PEPCK and G6Pase expression in the liver of mice

The PI3K/Akt activation can regulate the PEPCK and G6Pase expression, which are two rate-limiting enzymes, controlling gluconeogenesis in hepatocytes [13,14]. Next, we examined whether EPO could modulate the PEPCK and G6Pase expression in the livers of HFD-fed mice by RT-PCR and Western blot assays. We found that the relative levels of PEPCK and G6Pase mRNA transcripts in the livers from the HFD-EPO groups of mice

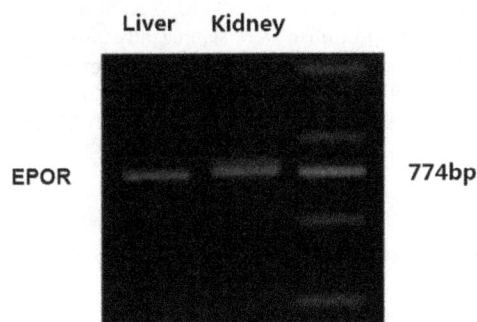

Figure 2. The EPOR mRNA transcription in the livers of mice. Total RNA was extracted from the liver and kidney samples of individual mice and reversely transcribed into cDNA. The EPOR mRNA transcripts were detected by semi-quantitative RT-PCR. Data shown are representative images of agarose gel electrophoresis from three separate experiments.

were significantly lower than that from the HFD-Con group although they were higher than that from the NC group of mice (Fig. 4A). Similarly, the relative levels of PEPCK and G6Pase proteins in the livers of HFD-EPO group of mice were significantly reduced, as compared with that in the HFD-Con group of mice (Fig. 4B and C). Thus, EPO treatment significantly inhibited the PEPCK and G6Pase expression in the livers of HFD-fed mice.

EPO mitigates obesity-related inflammatory signaling in the livers of mice

Chronic inflammation is associated with the development of glucose intolerance and insulin resistance. To further understand the mechanisms underlying the action of EPO, we examined the concentrations of serum inflammatory cytokines by ELISA. In comparison with that in the NC group of mice, we detected significantly higher levels of serum TNF-α and IL-6 in the HFD-Con group of mice, indicating that HFD feeding induced systemic inflammation in mice (Fig. 5A and B). In contrast, the levels of serum TNF-α and IL-6 in the HFD-EPO group of mice were significantly lower than that in the HFD-Con group of mice although the levels of IL-6, but not TNF-α, remained higher than that in the NC group of mice. A similar pattern of the relative levels of TNF-α and IL-6 mRNA transcripts in the livers was detected in the different groups of mice (Fig. 5C). Clearly, these data demonstrated that EPO treatment mitigated the HFD-up-regulated inflammatory cytokine expression in mice.

The NF-κB pathway is a central regulator of inflammation and controls inflammatory cytokine expression. We further investigated whether EPO treatment could alter the NF-κB activation in the

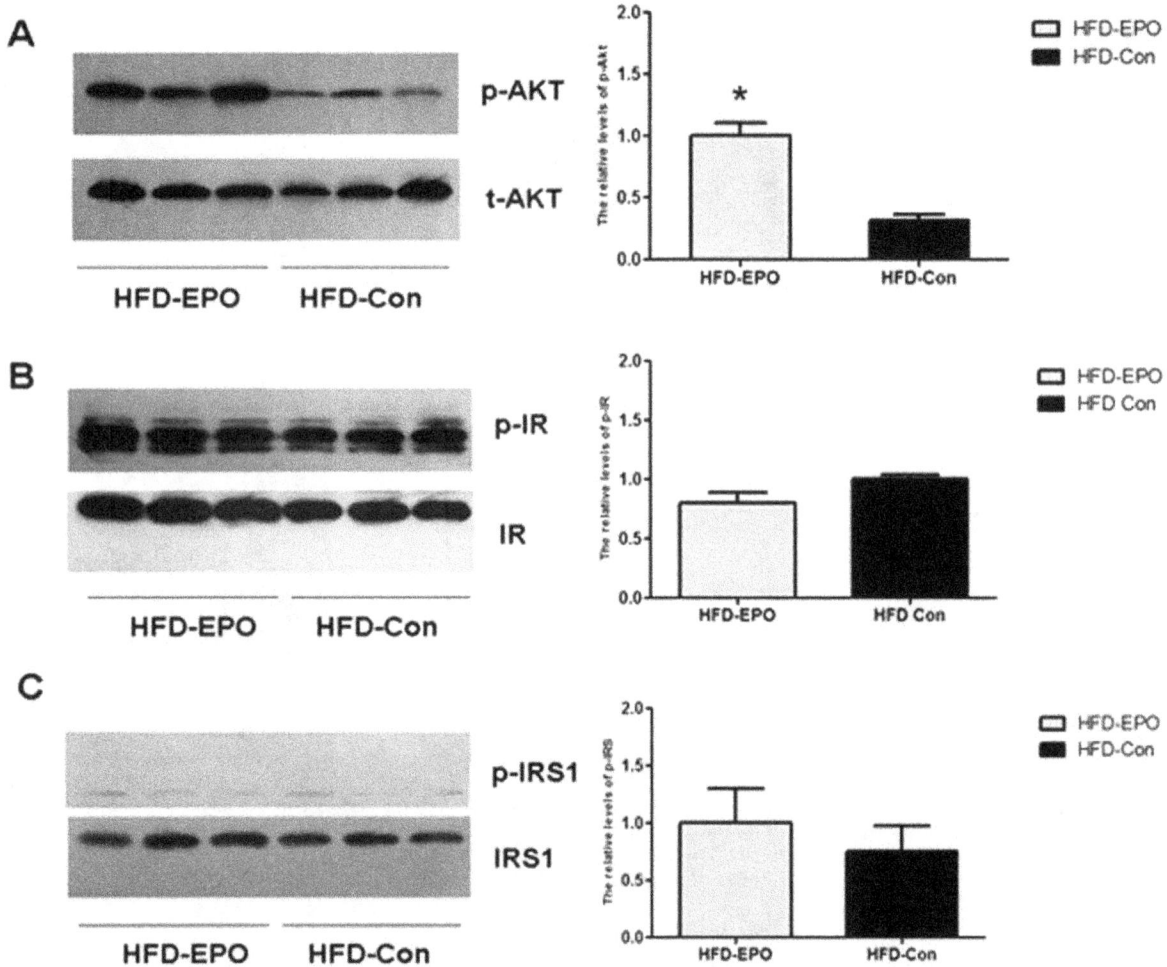

Figure 3. The effect of EPO on the levels of insulin signaling events in the liver. The levels of total Akt, IR and IRS1 and phosphorylated Akt, IR and IRS1 in the livers of individual mice were determined by Western blot assays and the relative levels of Akt, IR and IRS1 phosphorylation were analyzed by densimetric analysis using ImageJ software. Data shown are representative images and expressed as the mean ± SEM of individual groups (n = 6 per group) of mice from three separate experiments. (**A**) Western blot and quantitative analyses of the levels of Akt activation. (**B**) Western blot and quantitative analyses of the levels of IR activation. (**C**) Western blot and quantitative analyses of the levels of IRS1 activation. *P<0.05 vs. the HFD-Con group.

liver by a DNA binding-based ELISA assay. We found that the activity of NF-κB p65 binding to the specific DNA in the livers from the HFD-EPO group of mice was similar to that from the NC group of mice and significantly lower than that from the HFD-Con group of mice (p<0.05, Fig. 6A). Accordingly, these data indicated that EPO treatment significantly mitigated the HFD-enhanced NF-κB activation in the livers of mice.

TLR4 is a transmembrane receptor of free fat acid and pathogens, and can activate the NF-κB pathway. We also characterized the levels of TLR4 expression in the livers from the HFD-fed mice by RT-PCR and Western blot assays. We found that the relative levels of TLR4 mRNA transcripts and proteins in the livers from the HFD-EPO group of mice were significantly reduced, as compared with that in the HFD-Con group of mice (p<0.05, Fig. 6B and C). Notably, TLR4 and other inflammatory cytokines can activate the MAPK pathways, including the JNK, ERK and p38 MAPK. We finally tested the JNK, ERK and p38 MAPK expression and activation in the livers of HFD-fed mice by Western blot assays. We found similar levels of total JNK, ERK and p38 MAPK expression in the livers between the HFD-EPO and HFD-Con groups of mice, suggesting

that EPO treatment did not modulate their expression in the livers of HFD-fed mice (Fig. 6D–F). However, the relative levels of phosphorylated JNK, but not ERK and p38 MAPK, in the livers from the HFD-EPO group of mice were significantly lower than that from the HFD-Con group of mice. Therefore, treatment with EPO significantly mitigated the HFD-up-regulated TLR4 expression and NF-κB and JNK, but not ERK and p38 MAPK, activation in the livers of HFD-fed mice.

Discussion

In the present study, we found that EPO treatment significantly reduced the body weights and improved glucose intolerance in the HFD-fed mice. Furthermore, EPO treatment enhanced the PI3K/Akt phosphorylation and mitigated the HFD-induced PEPCK, G6Pase, TNF-α, IL-6 and TLR4 expression, and NF-κB and JNK activation in the livers of mice. These data suggest that EPO-regulated glucose tolerance may be at least partially mediated by enhancing the insulin-related signaling and inhibiting gluconeogenesis and inflammation-related signaling in the livers of HFD-fed mice.

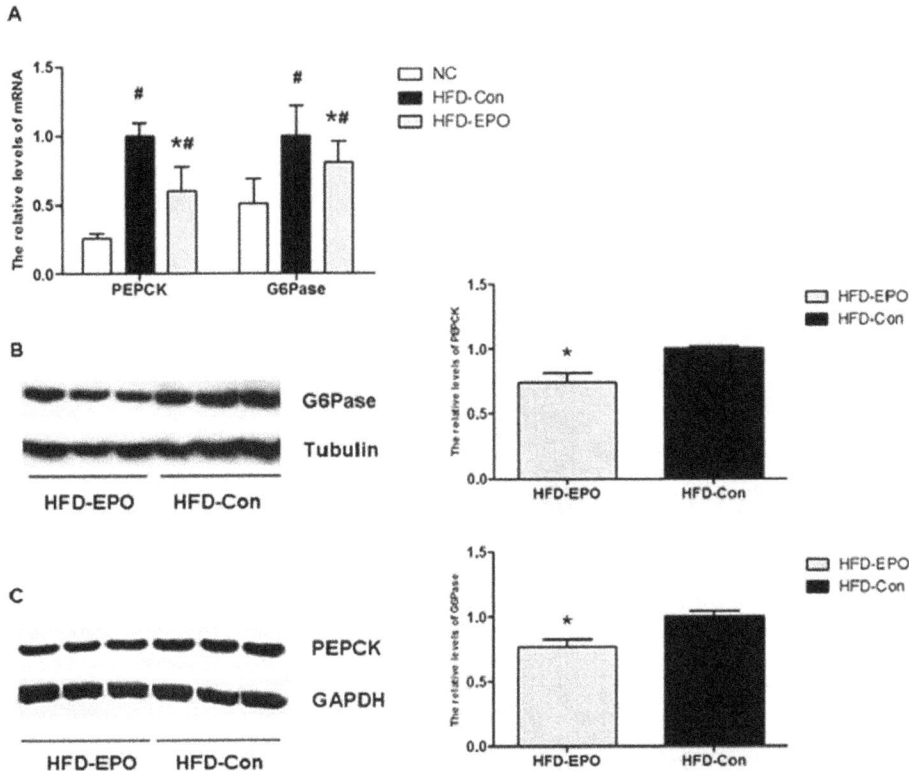

Figure 4. The effect of EPO on the expression of PEPCK and G6Pase in the liver. The relative levels of PEPCK and G6Pase in the livers of individual mice were determined by quantitative RT-PCR and Western blot assays. Data are representative images or expressed as the mean ± SEM of individual group (n = 8 per group) of mice from three separate experiments. (**A**) RT-PCR analysis of the relative levels of PEPCK and G6Pase mRNA transcripts to control GAPDH in the liver. (B) Western blot and quantitative analysis of the relative levels of PEPCK in the liver. (**C**) Western blot and quantitative analysis of the relative levels of G6Pase in the liver. [#]P<0.05 vs. the NC group, *P<0.05 vs. the HFD-Con group.

The PI3K/Akt pathway is a crucial regulator of glucose transportation, glycolysis, protein synthesis, lipogenesis, glycogen synthesis and gluconeogenesis [11,12]. Impairment in the Akt activation is associated with aberrant gluconeogenesis and glucose intolerance while restoration of insulin-induced Akt phosphorylation improves insulin sensitivity and glucose tolerance in the HFD-fed mice [13]. Previous studies have shown that EPO binds to and activates the EPOR, which recruits the p85 subunit of the PI3K through its Src homology 2 (SH2) domain and activates the PI3K and Akt [31,32]. Subsequently, the activated PI3K/Akt cascade regulates the survival and apoptosis as well as other functions in other non-liver organs [15–18]. In the present study, we detected the EPOR mRNA transcription in the liver and found that EPO treatment enhanced the Akt, but not the IR and IRS1, phosphorylation in the livers of HFD-fed mice. These data suggest that EPO may directly activate the PI3K/Akt pathway and overcome the HFD-induced impairment in the insulin-related signaling, leading to the improvement of glucose intolerance in the livers of HFD-fed mice. Our data extended previous findings and indicated that EPO also activated the PI3K/Akt pathway in the livers of HFD-fed mice.

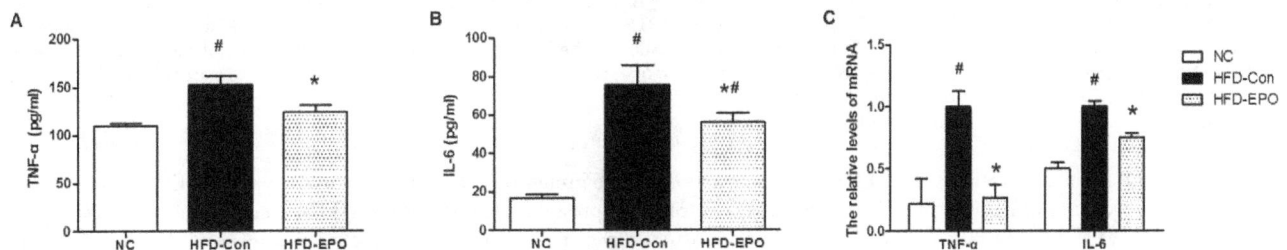

Figure 5. The effect of EPO on inflammatory cytokine expression in mice. At the end of treatment, blood samples were obtained from individual mice and the levels of serum TNF-α and IL-6 were measured by ELISA. In addition, the relative levels of TNF-α and IL-6 mRNA transcripts to control GAPDH were analyzed by quantitative RT-PCR. Data are expressed as the mean ± SEM of the concentrations of serum cytokines or the relative levels of cytokine mRNA transcripts to control GAPDH in each group (n = 8) from three separate experiments. (A) ELISA for the levels of serum TNF-α. (B) ELISA for the levels of serum IL-6. (C) RT-PCR analysis of the relative levels of cytokine mRNA transcripts. [#]P<0.05 vs. the NC group, *P<0.05 vs. the HFD-Con group.

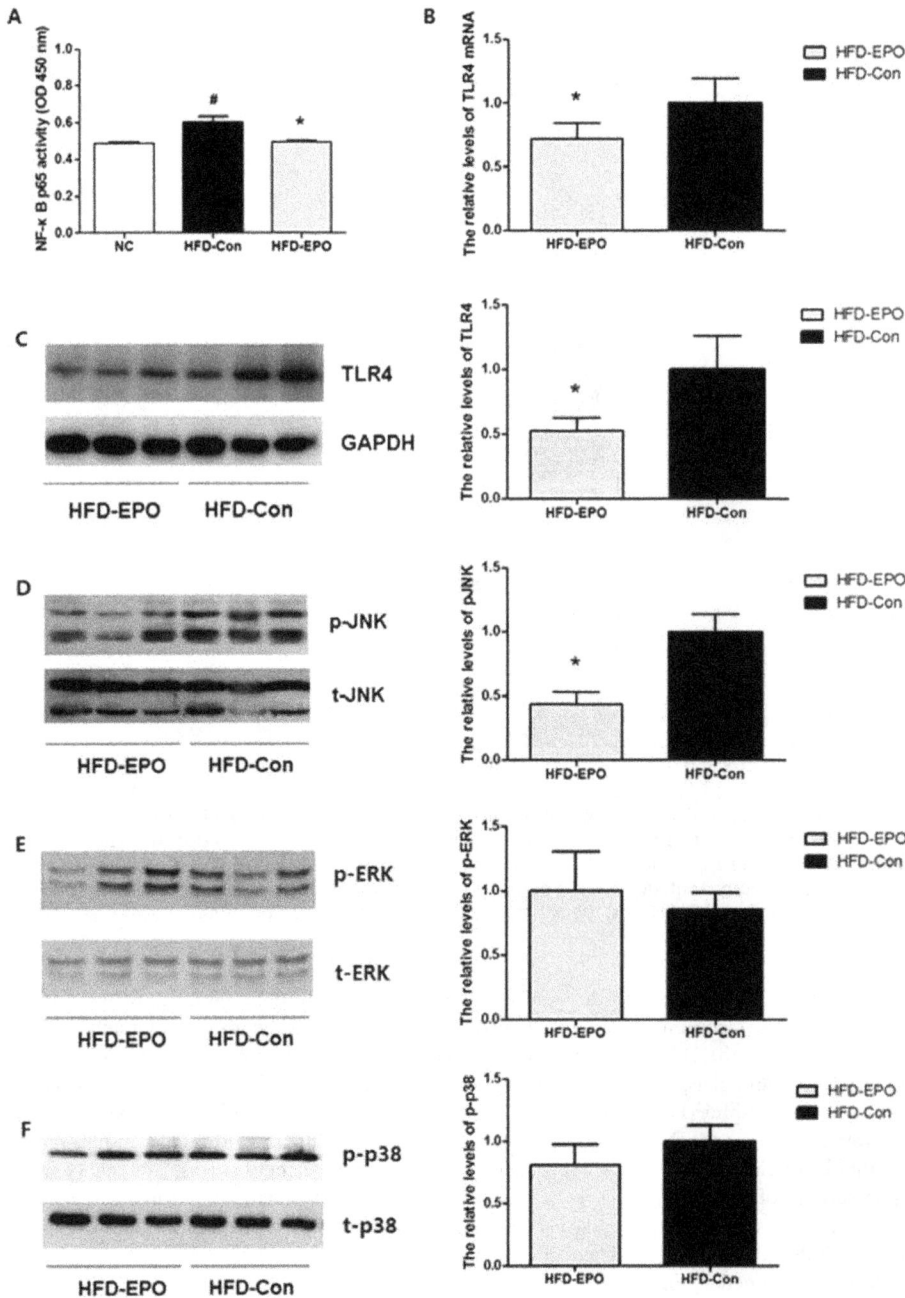

Figure 6. The effect of EPO on the expression of inflammatory signaling events in the liver. The levels of activated NF-κB p65 in the liver were determined by DNA binding-based ELISA (**A**). The relative levels of TLR4 expression were characterized by RT-PCR (**B**) and Western blot assays (**C**). The relative levels of JNK (**D**), ERK (**E**) and p38 MAPK (**F**) phosphorylation in the liver were characterized by Western blot assay and densimetric analysis. Data are representative images or expressed as the mean ± SEM of each group (n=6) of mice from three separate experiments. #P<0.05 vs. the NC group, *P<0.05 vs. the HFD-Con group.

Insulin-related signaling, such as the PI3K/Akt activation, inhibits gluconeogenesis, which is crucial for the maintenance of blood glucose levels and the PEPCK and G6Pase expression, two rate-limiting enzymes that control glucose production [13,14]. We found that EPO treatment mitigated the HFD-up-regulated PEPCK and G6Pase expression in the livers of HFD-fed mice. Interestingly, we detected significantly lower levels of fasting serum insulin in the HFD-EPO group of mice than that in the HFD-Con group of mice. It is possible that EPO directly activates the PI3K/Akt pathway, which overcomes the HFD-induced impairment in

the insulin-related signaling, and inhibits the PEPCK and G6Pase expression, attenuating the HFD-induced gluconeogenesis in the liver and contributing to the improvement of glucose intolerance in HFD-fed mice. Therefore, even after the establishment of insulin resistance, EPO can still activate the PI3K/Akt pathway and inhibit gluconeogenesis, regulating glucose homeostasis.

Chronic low-grade inflammation and pro-inflammatory cytokines, such as TNF-α and IL-6 as well as others, contribute to the development of glucose intolerance and insulin resistance-related metabolic syndrome and T2D [19–21,24]. The TLR4 can activate the NF-κB, JNK, ERK and p38 MAPK pathways, inducing inflammatory cytokine production [22,33]. We found that EPO treatment mitigated the HFD-up-regulated TLR4 expression, NF-κB and JNK activation and TNF-α and IL-6 production in the livers of HFD-fed mice. Our data were consistent with previous findings that impairment in the TLR4-related NF-κB signaling inhibits the HFD-induced inflammation [20,34] and activation of EPOR down-regulates TLR4 expression and NF-κB and JNK activation [26,35–37]. Given that TNF-α and IL-6 as well as the NF-κB activation are crucial for the development of glucose intolerance and insulin resistance [22,24,38], our data support the notion that inhibition of inflammation-related NF-κB activation may be a promising strategy for the intervention of glucose intolerance. Therefore, our novel findings may provide new insights into the regulation of EPO on inflammation-related glucose intolerance.

The insulin-related PI3K activation can activate the downstream ERK pathway and inflammatory cytokines can also activate the ERK and p38 MAPK pathways. However, we did not observe that EPO treatment significantly altered the ERK and p38 MAPK activation in the livers of HFD-fed mice. The unchanged ERK activation may be complicated by up-regulated PI3K activation in the EPO-treated mice and increased levels of pro-inflammatory cytokine production in the HFD-Con group of mice. The unaltered p38 MAPK activation suggests that the EPOR-related JAK/STAT5 signaling may be insufficient in interfering with the inflammation-related p38 MAPK activation in the livers of HFD-fed mice. We are interested in further investigating the cross-talk between the EPOR-related signaling and pro-inflammatory cytokine-mediated JAK/STAT signaling in hepatocytes.

The mitochondrial oxidative phosphorylation in the liver and skeletal muscles is associated with the development of obesity and insulin resistance [39]. A previous study has shown that EPO treatment enhances muscular fat oxidation, improving insulin sensitivity [7]. In this study, we centered on the effect of EPO on glucose tolerance and gluconeogenesis as well as the possible mechanisms in the livers of HFD-fed mice. We found that EPO treatment significantly reduced the body weights in HFD-fed mice and we speculate that EPO treatment may also enhance fat oxidation in the liver, contributing to the improvement of glucose intolerance in the HFD-fed mice. Now, we are investigating how EPO-related signaling regulates hepatic mitochondrial oxidative phosphorylation and lipid metabolism in the HFD-fed mice.

Conclusion

Our data indicated that EPO treatment significantly reduced the body weights and the levels of fasting blood glucose and serum insulin, and improved glucose intolerance in the HFD-fed mice. Furthermore, we found that EPO treatment significantly enhanced the PI3K/Akt activation, but inhibited the PEPCK and G6Pase expression in the livers of HFD-fed mice. In addition, EPO treatment mitigated the HFD-induced TLR4 expression, the NF-κB and JNK activation and TNF-α and IL-6 expression in the livers of HFD-fed mice. Collectively, our data suggest that EPO may activate the Akt pathway and inhibit gluconeogensis and inflammation-related signaling in the liver, leading to the improvement of glucose intolerance in the HFD-fed mice. Hence, our findings may provide new insights into the mechanisms by which EPO regulates glucose tolerance and insulin resistance. Given that EPO has been used in humans, EPO or new EPOR agonists may be valuable for the intervention of glucose intolerance-related metabolic syndrome and T2D.

Acknowledgments

We acknowledge Mr. or Miss. Wenwen Guo, Zhenming Cai, Xiufang Liu and Huan Zhang for their technical assistance.

Author Contributions

Conceived and designed the experiments: RM DLZ YPW. Performed the experiments: RM DHY. Analyzed the data: RM YB. Contributed reagents/materials/analysis tools: RM DLZ YPW. Wrote the paper: RM DLZ.

References

1. Morino K, Neschen S, Bilz S, Sono S, Tsirigotis D, et al. (2008) Muscle-specific IRS-1 Ser->Ala transgenic mice are protected from fat-induced insulin resistance in skeletal muscle. Diabetes 57: 2644–2651.
2. Cani PD, Amar J, Iglesias MA, Poggi M, Knauf C, et al. (2007) Metabolic endotoxemia initiates obesity and insulin resistance. Diabetes 56: 1761–1772.
3. Burger D, Xenocostas A, Feng QP (2009) Molecular basis of cardioprotection by erythropoietin. Curr Mol Pharmacol 2: 56–69.
4. Khedr E, El-Sharkawy M, Abdulwahab S, Eldin EN, Ali M, et al. (2009) Effect of recombinant human erythropoietin on insulin resistance in hemodialysis patients. Hemodial Int 13: 340–346.
5. Tuzcu A, Bahceci M, Yilmaz E, Bahceci S, Tuzcu S (2004) The comparison of insulin sensitivity in non-diabetic hemodialysis patients treated with and without recombinant human erythropoietin. Horm Metab Res 36: 716–720.
6. Katz O, Stuible M, Golishevski N, Lifshitz L, Tremblay ML, et al. (2010) Erythropoietin treatment leads to reduced blood glucose levels and body mass: insights from murine models. J Endocrinol 205: 87–95.
7. Hojman P, Brolin C, Gissel H, Brandt C, Zerahn B, et al. (2009) Erythropoietin over-expression protects against diet-induced obesity in mice through increased fat oxidation in muscles. PLoS One 4: e5894.
8. Teng R, Gavrilova O, Suzuki N, Chanturiya T, Schimel D, et al. (2011) Disrupted erythropoietin signalling promotes obesity and alters hypothalamus proopiomelanocortin production. Nat Commun 2: 520.
9. Saltiel AR, Kahn CR (2001) Insulin signalling and the regulation of glucose and lipid metabolism. Nature 414: 799–806.
10. Cornier MA, Dabelea D, Hernandez TL, Lindstrom RC, Steig AJ, et al. (2008) The metabolic syndrome. Endocr Rev 29: 777–822.
11. Saltiel AR, Pessin JE (2002) Insulin signaling pathways in time and space. Trends Cell Biol 12: 65–71.
12. Taniguchi CM, Emanuelli B, Kahn CR (2006) Critical nodes in signalling pathways: insights into insulin action. Nat Rev Mol Cell Biol 7: 85–96.
13. Whiteman EL, Cho H, Birnbaum MJ (2002) Role of Akt/protein kinase B in metabolism. Trends Endocrinol Metab 13: 444–451.
14. O'Brien RM, Granner DK (1996) Regulation of gene expression by insulin. Physiol Rev 76: 1109–1161.
15. Mudalagiri NR, Mocanu MM, Di Salvo C, Kolvekar S, Hayward M, et al. (2008) Erythropoietin protects the human myocardium against hypoxia/reoxygenation injury via phosphatidylinositol-3 kinase and ERK1/2 activation. Br J Pharmacol 153: 50–56.
16. Cassis P, Gallon L, Benigni A, Mister M, Pezzotta A, et al. (2012) Erythropoietin, but not the correction of anemia alone, protects from chronic kidney allograft injury. Kidney Int 81: 903–918.
17. Cho GW, Koh SH, Kim MH, Yoo AR, Noh MY, et al. (2010) The neuroprotective effect of erythropoietin-transduced human mesenchymal stromal cells in an animal model of ischemic stroke. Brain Res 1353: 1–13.
18. Wang L, Chopp M, Gregg SR, Zhang RL, Teng H, et al. (2008) Neural progenitor cells treated with EPO induce angiogenesis through the production of VEGF. J Cereb Blood Flow Metab 28: 1361–1368.
19. Shoelson SE, Lee J, Goldfine AB (2006) Inflammation and insulin resistance. J Clin Invest 116: 1793–1801.
20. Tsukumo DM, Carvalho-Filho MA, Carvalheira JB, Prada PO, Hirabara SM, et al. (2007) Loss-of-function mutation in Toll-like receptor 4 prevents diet-induced obesity and insulin resistance. Diabetes 56: 1986–1998.
21. Kim JJ, Sears DD (2010) TLR4 and Insulin Resistance. Gastroenterol Res Pract 2010: 212563
22. Arkan MC, Hevener AL, Greten FR, Maeda S, et al. (2005) IKK-beta links inflammation to obesity-induced insulin resistance. Nat Med 11: 191–198.
23. Tanti JF, Jager J (2009) Cellular mechanisms of insulin resistance: role of stress-regulated serine kinases and insulin receptor substrates (IRS) serine phosphorylation. Curr Opin Pharmacol 9: 753–762.
24. Hotamisligil GS (2006) Inflammation and metabolic disorders. Nature 444: 860–867.
25. Ben-Ari Z, Zilbermints V, Pappo O, Avlas O, Sharon E, et al. (2011) Erythropoietin Increases Survival and Attenuates Fulminant Hepatic Failure

Injury Induced by d-Galactosamine/Lipopolysaccharide in Mice. Transplantation 92: 18–24.

26. Hochhauser E, Pappo O, Ribakovsky E, Ravid A, Kurtzwald E, et al. (2008) Recombinant human erythropoietin attenuates hepatic injury induced by ischemia/reperfusion in an isolated mouse liver model. Apoptosis 13: 77–86.

27. Schmeding M, Rademacher S, Boas-Knoop S, Roecken C, Lendeckel U, et al. (2010) rHuEPo reduces ischemia-reperfusion injury and improves survival after transplantation of fatty livers in rats. Transplantation 89: 161–168.

28. Eipel C, Hubschmann U, Abshagen K, Wagner KF, Menger MD, et al. (2012) Erythropoietin as additive of HTK preservation solution in cold ischemia/reperfusion injury of steatotic livers. J Surg Res 173: 171–179.

29. Kleemann R, van Erk M, Verschuren L, van den Hoek AM, Koek M, et al. (2010) Time-resolved and tissue-specific systems analysis of the pathogenesis of insulin resistance. PLoS One 5: e8817.

30. Kleemann R, Gervois PP, Verschuren L, Staels B, Princen HM, et al. (2003) Fibrates down-regulate IL-1-stimulated C-reactive protein gene expression in hepatocytes by reducing nuclear p50-NFkappa B-C/EBP-beta complex formation. Blood 101: 545–551.

31. He TC, Zhuang H, Jiang N, Waterfield MD, Wojchowski DM (1993) Association of the p85 regulatory subunit of phosphatidylinositol 3-kinase with an essential erythropoietin receptor subdomain. Blood 82: 3530–3538.

32. Summers SA, Yin VP, Whiteman EL, Garza LA, Cho H, et al. (1999) Signaling pathways mediating insulin-stimulated glucose transport. Ann N Y Acad Sci 892: 169–186.

33. Hirosumi J, Tuncman G, Chang L, Gorgun CZ, Uysal KT, et al. (2002) A central role for JNK in obesity and insulin resistance. Nature 420: 333–336.

34. Suganami T, Tanimoto-Koyama K, Nishida J, Itoh M, Yuan X, et al. (2007) Role of the Toll-like receptor 4/NF-kappaB pathway in saturated fatty acid-induced inflammatory changes in the interaction between adipocytes and macrophages. Arterioscler Thromb Vasc Biol 27: 84–91.

35. Rodrigues CE, Sanches TR, Volpini RA, Shimizu MH, Kuriki PS, et al. (2012) Effects of continuous erythropoietin receptor activator in sepsis-induced acute kidney injury and multi-organ dysfunction. PLoS One 7: e29893.

36. Pappo O, Ben-Ari Z, Shevtsov E, Avlas O, Gassmann M, et al. (2010) The role of excessive versus acute administration of erythropoietin in attenuating hepatic ischemia-reperfusion injury. Can J Physiol Pharmacol 88: 1130–1137.

37. Nairz M, Schroll A, Moschen AR, Sonnweber T, Theurl M, et al. (2011) Erythropoietin contrastingly affects bacterial infection and experimental colitis by inhibiting nuclear factor-kappaB-inducible immune pathways. Immunity 34: 61–74.

38. Yuan M, Konstantopoulos N, Lee J, Hansen L, Li ZW, et al. (2001) Reversal of obesity- and diet-induced insulin resistance with salicylates or targeted disruption of Ikkbeta. Science 293: 1673–1677.

39. Buchner DA, Yazbek SN, Solinas P, Burrage LC, Morgan MG, et al. (2011) Increased mitochondrial oxidative phosphorylation in the liver is associated with obesity and insulin resistance. Obesity (Silver Spring) 19: 917–924.

15

Improved Glucose Metabolism In Vitro and In Vivo by an Allosteric Monoclonal Antibody that Increases Insulin Receptor Binding Affinity

John A. Corbin[1]*, Vinay Bhaskar[1], Ira D. Goldfine[2], Daniel H. Bedinger[1], Angela Lau[1], Kristen Michelson[1], Lisa M. Gross[1], Betty A. Maddux[2], Hua F. Kuan[1], Catarina Tran[1], Llewelyn Lao[1], Masahisa Handa[1], Susan R. Watson[1], Ajay J. Narasimha[1], Shirley Zhu[1], Raphael Levy[1], Lynn Webster[1], Sujeewa D. Wijesuriya[1], Naichi Liu[1], Xiaorong Wu[1], David Chemla-Vogel[1], Steve R. Lee[1], Steve Wong[1], Diane Wilcock[1], Mark L. White[1]

1 Department of Preclinical Research, XOMA Corporation, Berkeley, California, United States of America, 2 Department of Medicine, University of California San Francisco, San Francisco, California, United States of America

Abstract

Previously we reported studies of XMetA, an agonist antibody to the insulin receptor (INSR). We have now utilized phage display to identify XMetS, a novel monoclonal antibody to the INSR. Biophysical studies demonstrated that XMetS bound to the human and mouse INSR with picomolar affinity. Unlike monoclonal antibody XMetA, XMetS alone had little or no agonist effect on the INSR. However, XMetS was a strong positive allosteric modulator of the INSR that increased the binding affinity for insulin nearly 20-fold. XMetS potentiated insulin-stimulated INSR signaling ~15-fold or greater including; autophosphorylation of the INSR, phosphorylation of Akt, a major enzyme in the metabolic pathway, and phosphorylation of Erk, a major enzyme in the growth pathway. The enhanced signaling effects of XMetS were more pronounced with Akt than with Erk. In cultured cells, XMetS also enhanced insulin-stimulated glucose transport. In contrast to its effects on the INSR, XMetS did not potentiate IGF-1 activation of the IGF-1 receptor. We studied the effect of XMetS treatment in two mouse models of insulin resistance and diabetes. The first was the diet induced obesity mouse, a hyperinsulinemic, insulin resistant animal, and the second was the multi-low dose streptozotocin/high-fat diet mouse, an insulinopenic, insulin resistant animal. In both models, XMetS normalized fasting blood glucose levels and glucose tolerance. In concert with its ability to potentiate insulin action at the INSR, XMetS reduced insulin and C-peptide levels in both mouse models. XMetS improved the response to exogenous insulin without causing hypoglycemia. These data indicate that an allosteric monoclonal antibody can be generated that markedly enhances the binding affinity of insulin to the INSR. These data also suggest that an INSR monoclonal antibody with these characteristics may have the potential to both improve glucose metabolism in insulinopenic type 2 diabetes mellitus and correct compensatory hyperinsulinism in insulin resistant conditions.

Editor: Kathrin Maedler, University of Bremen, Germany

Funding: This research was funded by XOMA Corporation. The funders had a role in study design, data collection and analysis, decision to publish, or preparation of the manuscript.

Competing Interests: All authors except Betty Maddux and Ira Goldfine were employees of XOMA when these studies were carried out.

* E-mail: corbinjohn@gmail.com

Introduction

It has been proposed that receptor antibodies may represent a novel class of therapeutics for regulating glucose metabolism in type 2 diabetes mellitus (T2DM) [1]. The insulin receptor (INSR) is a central node for glycemic control in cells of the major metabolic insulin responsive tissues and therefore, is a key target for antibodies that could either mimic or potentiate insulin action in diabetes [2]. Spontaneously occurring human INSR autoantibodies, and mouse monoclonal antibodies generated to the human INSR have been investigated [3–13]. In humans, autoantibodies to the INSR typically cause severe insulin resistance [6,7,10]. Very rarely, INSR autoantibodies bind to and stimulate the INSR resulting in hypoglycemia [6,8]. In addition, monoclonal antibod-

ies to the INSR produced in mice have been used to characterize this receptor [3–5,14]. Some of these monoclonal antibodies have been shown to mimic insulin action in vitro, but they have not been tested in animal models of diabetes.

Many of the aforementioned antibodies to the INSR inhibit insulin binding to the orthosteric site (insulin binding site). In addition, antibodies that bind to allosteric sites (not the orthosteric site) of receptors can also impact cell signaling [15–17]. Recently, we reported the discovery and characterization of XMetA, an allosteric antibody to the INSR that was a direct agonist [18,19]. XMetA had had no effect on the binding of insulin to the INSR; however it stimulated INSR signaling in cultured cells and reduced hyperglycemia in mouse models of diabetes. In addition to being agonists, allosteric antibodies could also act as positive allosteric modulators of the INSR by enhancing insulin binding affinity and increasing metabolic signaling, without directly activating the INSR. In the present study we describe the discovery and characterization of one such positive allosteric modulator of the INSR, XMetS. In cultured cells, XMetS markedly enhanced insulin binding affinity leading to potentiation of insulin-stimulated INSR signaling resulting in enhanced glucose transport. Moreover, XMetS reduced hyperinsulinemia and hyperglycemia in two mouse models of insulin resistance and diabetes.

Research Design and Methods

XMetS Discovery

The extracellular domain of the human INSR (hINSR) (R&D Systems, MN) was biotinylated (Sulfo-NHS-LC-Biotin, Pierce, Rockford, IL) and incubated with a saturating concentration (10 μM) of human insulin (hINS; Sigma-Aldrich, St. Louis, MO) to complex the INSR with insulin. These complexes were conjugated to streptavidin-coated magnetic beads (Dynabeads® M-280, Invitrogen Dynal AS, Oslo, Norway) to generate the panning reagent. All subsequent steps were carried out in the presence of 10 μM human insulin to maintain biotinylated hINSR that was complexed to hINS (biotin-hINSR/hINS).

Two naïve human antibody phage display libraries (XOMA Corporation, Berkeley, CA) were panned employing standard methods [20,21]. Prior to panning, phage were deselected against unconjugated streptavidin-coated magnetic beads to remove nonspecific phage antibodies. Deselected phage were then incubated with biotin-hINSR/hINS streptavidin beads. hINSR/hINS streptavidin bead-bound phage were eluted and used to infect TG1 bacterial cells (Stratagene, La Jolla, CA). Phage were then rescued with helper phage M13KO7 (New England Biolabs, MA). Individual colonies were picked and grown in 96-well plates, and were then used to generate bacterial periplasmic extracts according to standard methods [20]. The binding properties of monovalent Fab and scFv anti-INSR antibodies from lysates were screened by FACS (fluorescence-activated cell sorting).

For the majority of the subsequent functional studies shown herein, we employed CHO cells transfected with the B isoform of either the human INSR (CHO-hINSR) or mouse INSR (CHO-mINSR). The B isoform of the INSR was employed because it is the predominant isoform of the INSR in adult metabolic insulin responsive tissues [22,23]. As determined by FACS [24], both these human and mouse INSR-transfected cell lines had approximately 250,000 surface receptors per cell compared to untransfected CHO cells (parental CHO cells), which had less than 5,000 surface INSR per cell. For comparative studies of XMetS and insulin binding, CHO cells were also transfected with the A isoform of the hINSR and were selected to have approximately 250,000 surface receptors per cell. Under the conditions employed for the subsequent cellular studies, the surface receptor levels did not change. INSR molar concentrations in the assays were calculated based on the cell surface receptor content, number of cells utilized, and the volume of the reaction. For comparative studies of receptor autophosphorylation, CHO cells transfected with the human insulin-like growth factor-1 receptors (CHO-hIGF-1R) were studied that had approximately 300,000 surface receptors per cell.

Screening studies using both CHO-hINSR and CHO-mINSR cells identified XMetS, an antibody that preferentially bound to the insulin occupied INSR (but not insulin alone), indicating the potential for positive allosteric modulation activity [25]. This clone was reformatted into a fully human divalent IgG2 monoclonal

antibody that was employed in all studies described herein unless indicated otherwise. A monovalent Fab version of XMetS was also generated and tested.

XMetS Binding as Assessed by FACS

For FACS, CHO-hINSR cells (2×10^6/ml) were washed and resuspended in phosphate buffered saline (PBS) with 0.5% fatty acid-free bovine serum albumin and 0.1% sodium azide (FACS buffer; Invitrogen, Carlsbad, CA). Cells were preincubated for 10 minutes at 4°C in the presence of 100 nM human insulin (Sigma-Aldrich). Next, increasing concentrations of XMetS were added to the cell suspension and incubated at 15°C for 120 minutes. Cells were then washed and resuspended in Alexa Fluor® 647-conjugated goat anti-human IgG (1:200; Invitrogen, Carlsbad, CA). The cells were incubated for 30 minutes at 4°C, washed twice and analyzed on a FACScan™ flow cytometer (Becton Dickinson, San Jose, CA).

XMetS and Insulin Binding Assessed by Kinetic Exclusion Assay (KinExA™)

In order to measure the effect of insulin on the binding affinity of XMetS for both isoforms of the hINSR, and the B isoform of the mINSR, we employed equilibrium assays under conditions where there was either no insulin present or where saturating insulin concentrations (>100 nM) were present. XMetS (50 pM) was incubated for 18 hours on a rotator at 5°C in PBS with 0.25% bovine serum albumin and 0.1% sodium azide with increasing concentrations of CHO cells (max 2×10^7/ml) expressing either the hINSR or mINSR. Following this incubation, the viability of all cells was greater than 85% as measured by trypan blue exclusion. Cells were pelleted by centrifugation and the amount of free XMetS remaining in solution was measured by immunofluorescence using a KinExA™ instrument (Sāpidyne Instruments, Boise, Idaho) [26]. Briefly, polymethylmethacrylate (PMMA) beads (Sāpidyne Instruments) were coated with 65 μg/mL goat anti-human-IgG antibody (Jackson Immuno Research, West Grove, PA) and captured human antibody was detected with an anti-human IgG-PE labeled antibody (Jackson Immuno Research) diluted 1:1000. XMetS concentration data were curve-fit using KinExA™ software (standard affinity curve fit model) [27] to yield an estimate of the relative change in XMetS binding affinity as expressed in terms of equilibrium dissociation (K_D) values.

In order to measure the effect of XMetS on the binding affinity of insulin for both isoforms of the hINSR, and the B isoform of the mINSR, we employed equilibrium assays under conditions where there was either no XMetS or where saturating XMetS concentrations (>30 nM) were present. Human insulin (50 pM, Sigma-Aldrich) and either XMetS or an anti-keyhole limpet hemocyanin IgG2 isotype control antibody (>30 nM) were incubated for 18 hours on a rotator at 5°C in PBS with 0.25% bovine serum albumin and 0.1% sodium azide with increasing concentrations of either CHO-hINSR or CHO-mINSR cells. Cells were pelleted by centrifugation and the amount of free insulin in solution was measured by immunofluorescence using a KinExA™ instrument [26]. Briefly, PMMA beads (Sapidyne Instruments) were coated with 65 μg/mL D6C4 anti-insulin monoclonal Ab (Fitzgerald Industries) and captured insulin was detected with 0.15 μg/mL biotin labeled D3E7 anti-insulin monoclonal antibody (Fitzgerald Industries, Acton, MA) mixed with 1 μg/mL streptavidin-phycoerythrin (Jackson Immuno Research). Insulin concentration data were curve-fit using KinExA™ software [27] (standard affinity curve fit model) to yield an estimate of the relative change in insulin binding affinity as expressed in terms of equilibrium dissociation (K_D) values.

The impact of XMetS, on the kinetics of insulin binding to the hINSR was assessed with time course studies under conditions where the XMetS concentration was saturating (>30 nM). Either XMetS or control antibody was preincubated for 30 minutes at 5°C with CHO-hINSR cells expressing the B isoform of the hINSR (2×10^7/ml). Next, human insulin (200 pM) was added and cells were incubated for up to 80 minutes at 5°C. At each time point of the incubation period, an aliquot of cells was pelleted by centrifugation. The concentration of free insulin remaining in the supernatant was measured using an electrochemiluminescent assay (Meso Scale Discovery, Gaithersburg, MD) and bound insulin was calculated. Briefly, MSD (Meso Scale Discovery) plates were coated 10 μg/mL D6C4 anti-insulin monoclonal antibody (Fitzgerald Industries) and captured insulin was detected with 0.3 μg/mL biotin labeled D3E7 anti-insulin monoclonal antibody (Fitzgerald Industries) mixed with 1.3 μg/mL streptavidin-europium (Meso Scale Discovery). Insulin concentration data and equilibrium dissociation (K_D) values determined by the aforementioned equilibrium KinExA™ assays were used to curve-fit the data and calculate the on-rate and off-rate of insulin by employing KinExA™ software (direct kinetics curve fit model).

The Effect of XMetS on Insulin Signaling in Cultured Cells

For studies of receptor autophosphorylation, CHO cells expressing either the hINSR or the hIGF-1R were preincubated in serum-free culture medium with XMetS (33 nM) for 30 minutes at 37°C followed by a 10-minute incubation with increasing concentrations of the cognate ligand (either insulin or IGF-1). Quantitation of tyrosine phosphorylated INSR and IGF-1R were determined by ELISA (Millipore, Billerica, MA) [28]. Receptor autophosphorylation data were curve-fit using GraphPad Prism™ software (sigmoidal dose-response, variable slope) to generate EC_{50} values.

For studies of Akt phosphorylation, CHO cells expressing the hINSR B isoform were preincubated in serum-free culture medium with either XMetS (14 nM for the IgG2 and 140 nM for the Fab) or 70 nM control antibody for 10 minutes at 37°C followed by a 10-minute incubation with increasing concentrations of insulin. Total Akt and Akt phosphorylated at Ser473 were quantified using an electrochemiluminescent assay (Meso Scale Discovery). Akt phosphorylation data were curve-fit using GraphPad Prism™ software (sigmoidal dose-response, variable slope) to generate EC_{50} values.

In order to quantitate the positive allosteric modulatory effects of XMetS on insulin-stimulated Akt activation by the INSR, a Schild analysis was conducted [25,29,30]. CHO cells expressing the hINSR were preincubated in serum-free culture medium with XMetS concentrations ranging from 0–50 nM for 10 minutes at 37°C followed by a 10 minute incubation with increasing concentrations of insulin. Total Akt and Akt phosphorylated at Ser473 were quantified as above, and the data were curve-fit using GraphPad Prism™ software (allosteric EC50 shift) to generate the parameters of INSR allosteric modulation by XMetS.

For studies of Erk1/2 phosphorylation, CHO cells expressing the hINSR B isoform were preincubated in serum-free culture medium with 33 nM XMetS for 10 minutes at 37°C followed by a 10 minute incubation with increasing concentrations of either insulin. Total Erk1/2 and Erk1/2 phosphorylated at Thr202/Tyr204 were measured using an electrochemiluminescent assay (Meso Scale Discovery). Erk1/2 phosphorylation data were curve-fit using GraphPad Prism™ software (sigmoidal dose-response, variable slope) to generate EC_{50} values.

To measure 2-deoxy-glucose uptake, rat L6 muscle cells expressing both hINSR B isoform and human GLUT-4 [31]

were preincubated in serum-free medium for 60 minutes at 37°C with either 33 nM XMetS or control antibody. Next, cells were incubated with increasing concentrations of insulin for 10 minutes. [^{3}H]-2-deoxy-D-glucose was then added for 20 minutes and its uptake measured [14,31]. Glucose uptake data were curve-fit using GraphPad Prism™ software (sigmoidal dose-response, variable slope) to generate EC_{50} values.

MCF-7 human breast cancer cells (ATCC, Manassas, VA) were cultured in Dulbecco's Modified Eagles Medium (DMEM) containing glucose at 4.5 g/L supplemented with 10% FBS and 2 mM glutamine (Invitrogen, Carlsbad, CA) for normal maintenance. For the proliferation assay, cells (1×10^4) were seeded in 96 well white opaque microtiter plates and allowed to reattach. After 24 hrs, cells were washed twice with pre-warmed PBS. They were then incubated in DMEM (without phenol red) containing glucose at 1 g/L supplemented with 0.1% FBS and 2 mM glutamine (Invitrogen, Carlsbad, CA) for another 24 hrs. Next, either 33 nM XMetS or control antibody was added to the cells along with varying concentrations of either insulin, IGF-1 or IGF-2 (Sigma-Aldrich, St. Louis, MO). Cells were incubated at 37°C for 48 hrs and cell proliferation was measured using the CellTiter-Glo® Luminescent Cell Viability Assay (Promega, Madison, WI). Proliferation data were curve-fit using Prism™ software (sigmoidal dose-response) to generate EC_{50} values. Saos-2 osteosarcoma cells (ATCC, Manassas, VA) were treated in a similar manner except that they were incubated for 72 hrs prior to measurement of cell proliferation.

Ethics Statement

Animal experiments were approved by the XOMA Corporation Institutional Animal Care and Use Committee (IACUC) and performed in accordance with IACUC guidelines. All animals were maintained in a pathogen-free environment and allowed free access to food and water.

Mouse Models of Insulin Resistance and Diabetes

In the diet-induced obesity model [32] (18–20 weeks of age), C57BL/6 mice (The Jackson Laboratory, Sacramento, CA) were fed a high fat diet (65 kcal% fat) for 12–14 weeks. Mice were then randomized into two groups ($n = 10$). Mice were treated twice weekly, by intraperitoneal (IP) injection, with either XMetS or the anti-keyhole limpet hemocyanin IgG2 control antibody (10 mg/kg). Age-matched, lean C57BL/6 mice were fed a standard chow diet (Harlan, Indianapolis, IN) and treated twice weekly with the control antibody (10 mg/kg). A glucose tolerance test was performed after one week of antibody administration. For the glucose tolerance test, mice were fasted overnight for 14 hours followed by a glucose challenge (1 g/kg; Mediatech, Manassas, VA) by IP injection. Whole venous blood was obtained from the tail vein at 0, 15, 30, 60 90, and 120 minutes following challenge and evaluated for blood glucose. For all mouse studies, blood glucose was measured using the AlphaTRAK® Blood Glucose Monitoring System (Abbott, Chicago, IL).

In the multi-low dose streptozotocin/high-fat diet model [33], six-week old male ICR mice were fed a 40 kcal% fat, 35 kcal% sucrose diet (Research Diets, New Brunswick, NJ) for 4 weeks. Streptozotocin (Sigma, St. Louis, MO) was injected IP at 40 mg/kg for 5 consecutive days during the third week of high fat diet feeding. After an additional week, mice were randomized into two groups ($n = 8$). They were then treated twice weekly by IP injection with either XMetS or control antibody (10 mg/kg). Non-diabetic ICR mice were fed a standard chow diet (Harlan, Indianapolis, IN) and treated twice weekly with the control antibody (10 mg/kg). Fasting blood glucose was evaluated weekly following a 14-

hour overnight fast. An IP glucose tolerance test (1 g/kg glucose) was performed after 3 weeks of antibody administration, following a 14-hour overnight fast. After five weeks of antibody administration, insulin tolerance tests were carried out following a 4-hour fast by administering insulin (0.75 U/kg; Roche Diagnostics, Indianapolis, IN) intraperitoneally and measuring venous blood for glucose at 0, 30, 60, 90 and 120 minutes after insulin challenge.

At the conclusion of the above studies (multi-low dose streptozotocin/high-fat diet = 6 weeks; diet induced obesity = 4 weeks) mice were sacrificed and terminal plasma was collected by cardiac puncture following a 14-hour overnight fast. Fasting values for plasma glucose, beta-hydroxybutyrate (multi-low dose streptozotocin/high-fat diet only), total cholesterol and HDL cholesterol were measured by standard colorimetric methods (Wako Chemicals, Richmond, VA). Insulin and C-peptide were measured by ELISA (Alpco Diagnostics, Salem NH). Statistical analyses were carried out using a two-tailed student's unpaired t test.

Results

I. Studies in vitro with Cultured Cells

XMetS binds to the INSR. Allosteric modulating antibodies that potentiated the binding of insulin to the INSR were identified by panning naïve human antibody phage display libraries against the recombinant extracellular domain of the INSR which was complexed to insulin. Antibodies that preferentially bound to the INSR in the presence of insulin were then identified. This panning and screening approach was designed to specifically select for positive allosteric modulating antibodies because of the reciprocal relationship between a positive allosteric modulator and the ligand (i.e. the modulator enhances the binding affinity of the ligand, and in turn, the ligand enhances the binding affinity of the modulator) [25]. Using FACS, we qualitatively assessed the binding of XMetS to the INSR B and A isoforms (CHO-hINSR B and CHO-hINSR A cells) in cultured CHO cells expressing high levels of both isoforms. XMetS bound to both INSR isoforms in a similar manner (**Figure 1**). XMetS also bound similarly to the B isoform of the mINSR (data not shown). XMetS did not to parental CHO cells (**Figure 1**).

Quantitative studies defining XMetS as a positive allosteric modulator of the human and mouse INSR. Kinetic exclusion assays (KinExA™) were employed to

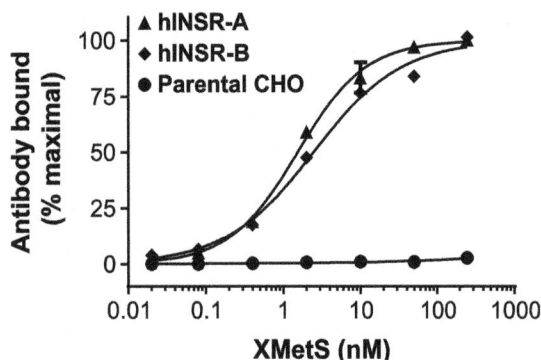

Figure 1. XMetS binds to the A and B isoforms of the INSR with high affinity. CHO cells expressing either the B or A isoform of the hINSR, and parental CHO cells were preincubated for 10 minutes at 4°C in the presence of 100 nM insulin followed by a 120 minute incubation at 15°C with increasing concentrations of XMetS. XMetS binding to the INSR was measured by FACS. Mean of duplicate determinations are shown.

quantitatively assess the reciprocal binding interactions between XMetS and insulin to the hINSR. First, the impact of insulin on the binding affinity of XMetS to the INSR was measured (**Figures 2A and 2B**). XMetS alone bound to CHO-hINSR cells expressing the B isoform of the receptor with an equilibrium dissociation constant (K_D) of 3.0 nM (95% confidence interval (CI): 2.5 to 3.2 nM), but bound only weakly to parental CHO cells (data not shown). XMetS binding affinity was enhanced 16-fold (K_D = 190 pM, 95% CI: 140 to 250 pM) in the presence of insulin (**Figure 2A**). Similar results were obtained with the A isoform of the INSR; XMetS alone bound to CHO-hINSR cells expressing the A isoform of the receptor with an equilibrium dissociation constant (K_D) of 4.0 nM (95% confidence interval (CI): 2.0 to 5.1 nM), and in the presence of insulin XMetS bound with a K_D of 139 pM (95% CI: 50 to 290 pM) (data not shown). The interaction of XMetS with the mINSR was also investigated. XMetS bound to CHO-mINSR cells with a K_D of 520 pM (95% CI: 197 pM to 1.1 nM) in the absence of insulin. As with CHO-hINSR B isoform cells, the binding affinity of XMetS to CHO-mINSR cells increased 16-fold in the presence of insulin (K_D = 33 pM, 95% CI: 10.4 to 66 pM) (**Figure 2B**).

Second, the impact of XMetS on the binding affinity of insulin to the INSR (**Figures 2C and 2D**) was assessed. In the absence of XMetS, insulin bound to CHO-hINSR cells expressing the B isoform of the receptor with a K_D of 270 pM (95% CI: 142 to 434 pM) (**Figure 2C**). In the presence of XMetS, binding of insulin was enhanced 18-fold (K_D of 15 pM, 95% CI: 6 to 23 pM). Similar results were obtained with the A isoform of the INSR; in the absence of XMetS, insulin bound to CHO-hINSR cells expressing the A isoform of the receptor with a K_D of 536 pM (95% CI: 27 to 920 pM), and in the presence of XMetS insulin bound with a K_D of 15 pM, 95% CI: 6 to 23 pM) (data not shown). In the absence of XMetS, insulin bound to CHO-mINSR cells with a K_D of 650 pM) 95% CI: 300 to 930 pM) (**Figure 2D**). In the presence of XMetS, binding of insulin to mINSR was enhanced 11-fold to 57 pM (95% CI: 17 to 124 pM). These data indicated that XMetS was a positive allosteric modulator of both the hINSR and mINSR that markedly enhanced insulin binding affinity. Moreover, the reciprocal nature of the binding interactions between XMetS and insulin further demonstrated that XMetS was a positive allosteric modulator [25] of the INSR. Because XMetS had similar effects on the A and B isoforms of the hINSR, as well as the mINSR, all subsequent in vitro experiments were carried out with the B isoform of the hINSR.

Time course studies were conducted to elucidate the kinetic parameters involved in the enhancement of insulin binding to the INSR by XMetS (**Figure 2E**). XMetS did not significantly alter the observed association rate of insulin binding to the CHO-hINSR cells. Based on the equilibrium K_D parameters determined above and these time course data, the calculated association rates [27] for insulin binding to the INSR in the presence or absence of XMetS were unchanged (8.5×10^5 M^{-1}, sec^{-1}, 95% CI: 4.7×10^5 to 1.4×10^6 M^{-1}, sec^{-1} vs. 9.5×10^5 M^{-1}, sec^{-1}, 95% CI: 6.2×10^5 to 1.4×10^6 M^{-1}, sec^{-1}). In contrast, the calculated dissociation rates in the presence or absence of XMetS were markedly different ($2.2 \pm 1.7 \times 10^{-4}$ sec^{-1}, and $1.4 \pm 0.7 \times 10^{-5}$ sec^{-1} respectively). These data indicate that the positive modulation of insulin affinity by XMetS primarily resulted from a reduction of the dissociation rate between insulin and the INSR.

The effect of XMetS on insulin-mediated INSR autophosphorylation. The binding of insulin to the INSR induces tyrosine autophosphorylation, the major indicator of receptor activation [2]. Similar to its enhancement of insulin

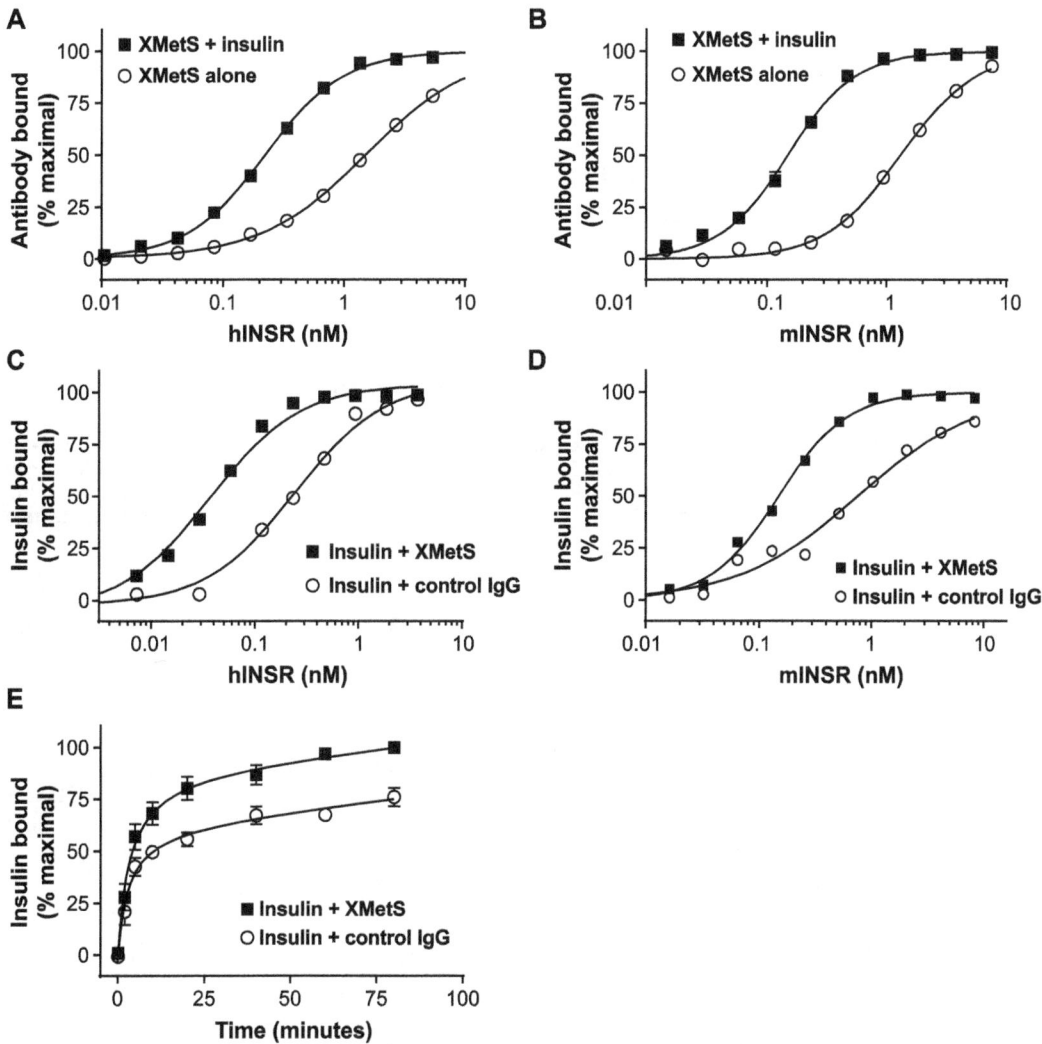

Figure 2. Insulin increases XMetS binding affinity to the INSR and XMetS increases insulin binding affinity to the INSR. A and **B** (*XMetS binding to the INSR*). 50 pM XMetS was incubated with increasing concentrations of either (**A**) CHO-hINSR cells or (**B**) CHO-mINSR for 18 hours at 5°C in the presence and absence of insulin. Free antibody concentrations were quantified by immunofluorescence (KinExA™), and this value was used to calculate bound XMetS. Mean of duplicate determinations are shown. **C** and **D** (*Insulin binding to the INSR*). 50 pM insulin was incubated with increasing concentrations of either (**C**) CHO-hINSR cells or (**D**) CHO-mINSR cells for 18 hours at 5°C in the presence of either XMetS or control antibody. Free insulin was quantified by immunofluorescence (KinExA™) and this value was used to calculate bound insulin. Mean of duplicate determinations are shown. **E**. Human insulin (200 pM) was incubated with CHO-hINSR cells for up to 80 minutes at 5°C with either XMetS or control antibody. At each time point, cells were pelleted by centrifugation. The concentration of free insulin in the supernatant was measured by immunofluorescence and bound insulin was then calculated. Mean ± SD from three separate experiments are shown.

binding affinity, XMetS induced a 14-fold increase in INSR autophosphorylation in response to insulin (**Figure 3A**), indicating that it was a positive allosteric modulator of both insulin binding and INSR activation. The EC_{50} for INSR autophosphorylation in the absence of XMetS was 7.3 nM (95% CI: 5.6 to 8.9 nM), but fell to 0.51 (95% CI: 0.44 to 0.6 nM) in the presence of XMetS. XMetS alone had no direct agonist effect on INSR autophosphorylation. The receptor for IGF-1 (IGF-1R) is closely related to the INSR [34]. In order to examine the receptor specificity of XMetS, we compared the effects of XMetS on IGF-1-mediated activation of the IGF-1R expressed in CHO cells (**Figure 3B**). In contrast to the sensitizing effect of XMetS on insulin stimulation of the INSR, the antibody had no effect on enhancing IGF-1-mediated IGF-1R autophosphorylation.

The effect of XMetS on insulin-mediated Akt and Erk activation in cells expressing the hINSR. Two major

enzymes that are activated via signaling by both isoforms of the INSR are Akt and Erk [2]. Akt is a key mediator of metabolic signaling downstream of the INSR whereas Erk is a key mediator of mitogenic (growth) signaling downstream of the INSR [2]. The influence of XMetS on insulin-mediated Akt and Erk activation in CHO-hINSR cells expressing the B isoform of the INSR was studied. These studies assessed whether the positive modulating effect of XMetS on autophosphorylation of the hINSR B isoform (**Figure 3A**) was associated with enhanced downstream intracellular signaling. XMetS induced a greater than 30-fold increase in the sensitivity of insulin-stimulated Akt phosphorylation as observed by a pronounced left shift in the dose response curve (**Figure 4A and 4B**). The EC_{50} for insulin stimulated pAkt activation in the absence of XMetS was 1.1 nM (95% CI: 0.94 to 1.29 nM) and decreased to 0.027 nM (95% CI: 0.022 to 0.032 nM) in the presence of XMetS (**Figure 4A**). At high

A

B

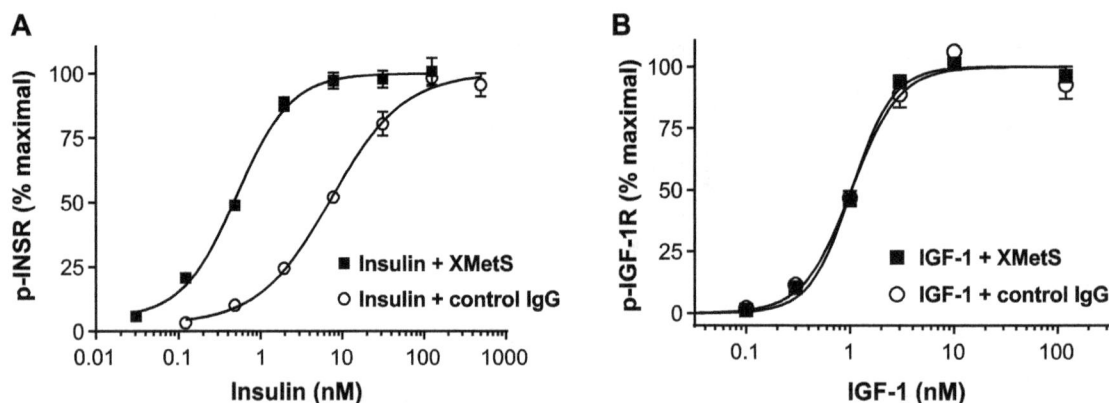

Figure 3. XMetS enhances insulin-dependent INSR autophosphorylation, but does not potentiate IGF-1-dependent IGF-1R autophosphorylation. A. CHO-hINSR cells were preincubated for 30 minutes at 37°C with either XMetS or control antibody, then incubated for 10 minutes with increasing concentrations of insulin. **B.** CHO-IGF-1R cells were preincubated for 30 minutes at 37°C with either XMetS or control antibody, then incubated for 10 minutes with increasing concentrations of IGF-1. Autophosphorylation was measured by ELISA. Mean ± SD from triplicate determinations are shown.

concentrations, XMetS alone, had only a small (~10%) direct agonist effect on this function. These data suggested that the potentiation of insulin-mediated INSR activation by XMetS also translated to an enhancement of downstream signaling. The monovalent Fab version of XMetS induced an 8-fold increase in the sensitivity of insulin-stimulated Akt phosphorylation (**Figure 4A**). The EC_{50} for insulin-stimulated Akt phosphorylation in the presence of the Fab form of XMetS was 0.133 (95% CI: 0.103 to 0.173 nM). These data indicated that the modulatory effects of XMetS were independent of antibody valence.

In order to quantitate the potency of XMetS on INSR modulation, the dose response of insulin-dependent pAkt activation was assessed at XMetS concentrations ranging from 0 to 50 nM (**Figure 4B**). The concentration of XMetS required to induce a half-maximal left shift of insulin-dependent Akt phosphorylation dose response curve occurred at 0.25 nM (95% 0.07 CI: to 0.85 nM) (**Figure 4C**). These dose response data were also fit using a mathematical model of allosteric modulation [25] to determine if the antibody was acting to enhance downstream INSR signaling in addition to enhancing insulin binding and INSR activation by autophosphorylation. The calculated cooperativity factor for potentiation of insulin action on the INSR by XMetS was 37 (log $\alpha\beta = 1.57$, 95% CI: 1.41 to 1.73). This cooperativity factor incorporates both positive modulation of insulin binding affinity (α) and positive modulation of signaling efficacy (β) by XMetS. Using the observed enhancement of insulin affinity by XMetS (α) as determined by KinExA^{TM} analysis (18-fold), the enhancement of insulin signaling efficacy (β) in this system was estimated to be approximately 2-fold [35]. The analysis also yielded an estimate of the affinity of XMetS for the INSR in the absence of insulin of 8.5 nM (log$K_B = 0.93$ nM, 95% CI: 0.67 to 1.2 nM), which is similar to the affinity value as determined by KinExA^{TM} analysis for this interaction. These data indicated therefore, that XMetS acted mainly to enhance insulin binding affinity but also significantly increased the efficacy of insulin signaling through the INSR.

XMetS also potentiated insulin dependent Erk1/2 phosphorylation in CHO cells expressing the hINSR, but to a lesser extent than Akt phosphorylation. The EC_{50} for insulin-stimulated pErk1/2 activation in the absence of XMetS was 26.4 nM (95% CI: 13.8 to 50.5 nM) and decreased to 5.5 nM (95% CI: 3.8 to 8.0 nM) in the presence of XMetS (**Figure 4D**). In contrast to

pAkt activation, XMetS at high concentrations had no direct agonist effect on pErk1/2 phosphorylation.

The effect of XMetS on insulin-mediated glucose uptake and cancer cell proliferation. To determine whether XMetS potentiated insulin-stimulated glucose transport in muscle, a major target tissue for insulin, we employed L6 cultured muscle cells that express both hINSR and GLUT-4 [31]. In these cells, XMetS enhanced insulin-stimulated 2-deoxy-D-glucose (2DG) uptake (**Figure 5A**). The EC_{50} for insulin-stimulated 2DG uptake in the absence of XMetS was 2.7 nM (95% CI: 1.4 to 5.3 nM) and decreased to 0.50 nM (95% CI: 0.26 to 0.97 nM) in the presence of XMetS. XMetS alone had little or no effect on this function. Thus, potentiation of insulin binding to the INSR by XMetS resulted in enhanced metabolic signal activation and enhanced glucose uptake.

In addition to its effects on metabolic functions such as glucose transport, insulin can also stimulate the growth and proliferation of cancer cells, a potential concern when either insulin or insulin analogs are employed for therapeutic purposes [36–38]. Because XMetS enhanced the binding affinity of the INSR for insulin, we studied the effect of XMetS on insulin-stimulated proliferation of MCF-7 human breast cancer cells. In contrast to the observed impact of XMetS on insulin-stimulated glucose transport, XMetS did not influence the EC_{50} of insulin-stimulated proliferation in these cells, relative to control antibody (insulin plus XMetS $EC_{50} = 1.5$ nM, 95% CI: 0.4 to 5.3 nM vs. insulin plus control IgG $EC_{50} = 1.7$ nM, 95% CI: 0.9 to 3.5 nM) (**Figure 5B**). XMetS also did not influence the effect of insulin on the proliferation of Saos-2 human osteosarcoma cells (**Figure 5C**). Moreover, XMetS did not influence the effects of IGF-1 on the proliferation of both cancer cell lines (data not shown).

II. Studies in vivo

In vivo studies with XMetS. To assess whether the observed positive modulation of the INSR by XMetS *in vitro* translated into an improvement in insulin action *in vivo*, we performed studies in both insulin resistant and diabetic mice. We first assessed the effects of XMetS in diet induced obesity mice, a model of obesity and insulin resistance [32]. After four weeks of treatment, fasting glucose levels in the obese mice treated with control antibody were over 240 mg/dL compared to approximately 160 mg/dL in similarly treated lean mice. Fasting glucose levels in obese mice

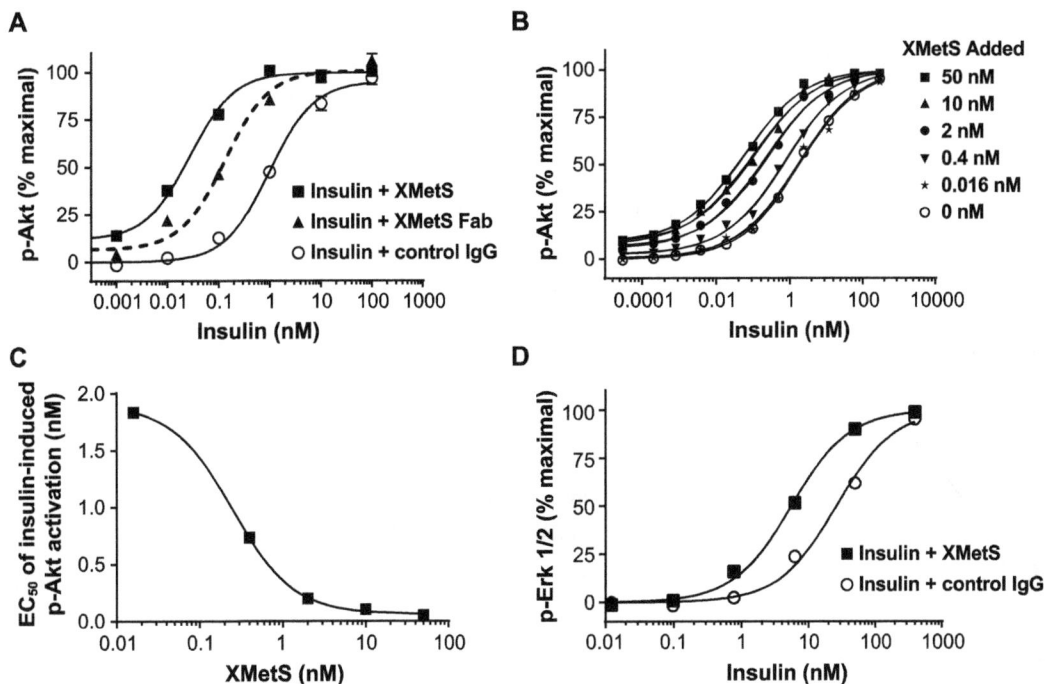

Figure 4. XMetS potentiates insulin-dependent Akt and Erk phosphorylation. A. CHO-hINSR cells were preincubated for 10 minutes at 37°C with either the IgG2 form of XMetS, the Fab form of XMetS, or control antibody followed by a 10 minute incubation with increasing concentrations of insulin. Phosphorylation of Akt was then determined. **B**. CHO-hINSR cells were preincubated for 10 minutes at 37°C with a wide range of XMetS concentrations followed by a 10 minute incubation with increasing concentrations of insulin. Schild analysis [30] of these data was carried out using a curve fit algorithm (Prism, allosteric EC_{50} shift). **C**. EC_{50} values were determined from each curve fit (of the data presented in B) and are plotted as a function of XMetS concentration. **D**. CHO-hINSR cells were preincubated for 10 minutes at 37°C with either XMetS or control antibody followed by a 10 minute incubation with increasing concentrations of insulin and phosphorylation of Erk was then determined. The mean of duplicate determinations are shown.

treated with XMetS for 4 weeks were similar to normal mice treated with control antibody (**Table 1**). Compared to the normal mice, glucose tolerance in obese mice was significantly impaired. Treatment of obese mice with XMetS normalized glucose tolerance (**Figure 6**). In obese mice, fasting insulin levels were twice that of normal mice and fasting C-peptide was also elevated (**Table 1**), reflecting insulin resistance. Treatment of obese mice with XMetS for four weeks lowered both fasting insulin and C-peptide to levels below normal mice. In addition, elevated non-HDL cholesterol levels in obese mice were also significantly improved by XMetS treatment. XMetS treatment did not affect body weight in obese mice, indicating that the improvements in the above parameters elicited by XMetS were not the result of weight reduction (**Table 1**). At no time did any of the mice treated with XMetS manifest symptomatic hypoglycemia.

We next studied the effects of XMetS in the multi-low dose, streptozotocin/high-fat diet mouse model of diabetes that exhibits both insulin resistance and relative insulinopenia [33]. Diabetic mice treated with control antibody exhibited progressive elevations of fasting glucose levels over six weeks (**Figure 7A, Table 2**). Fasting hyperglycemia was markedly improved after one week of XMetS treatment and this effect was maintained for the duration of the study. As in diet induced obesity mice, XMetS did not induce symptomatic hypoglycemia.

To determine whether XMetS improved insulin responsiveness in multi-low dose, streptozotocin/high-fat diet mice, exogenous insulin was administered to mice treated with either XMetS or control antibody. The response to insulin in diabetic mice was significantly compromised relative to that of normal mice, indicating that they were insulin resistant. Treatment of multi-

low dose, streptozotocin/high-fat diet mice with XMetS prevented this insulin resistance (**Figure 7B**). In addition, diabetic mice were glucose intolerant. When these mice were treated with XMetS, they displayed markedly improved glucose tolerance with glucose levels similar to those of normal mice (**Figure 7C**).

After six weeks, multi-low dose, streptozotocin/high-fat diet mice had lost significant body weight relative to normal mice as a result of prolonged insulinopenia; XMetS partially prevented this disease-mediated weight loss (**Table 2**). Both C-peptide and insulin were decreased in XMetS-treated diabetic mice relative to diabetic animals treated with control antibody, reflecting increased insulin sensitivity. Beta-hydroxybutyrate levels were markedly elevated in multi-low dose, streptozotocin/high-fat diet mice and these levels were dramatically reduced when the diabetic mice were treated with XMetS. Elevated total cholesterol and non-HDL cholesterol were also reduced in the diabetic animals by XMetS treatment (**Table 2**).

Discussion

Previously we identified an allosteric anti-INSR antibody, XMetA [18]. We found that XMetA was a direct agonist of the INSR that did not influence insulin binding but activated INSR signaling both in vitro and in vivo. In the present study, we report the identification and characterization of another type of allosteric anti-INSR antibody, XMetS. In contrast to XMetA, XMetS was not a direct agonist of the INSR; rather, XMetS markedly enhanced the affinity of the INSR for insulin. Thus, XMetS was a positive allosteric modulator of the INSR. In accordance with this type of allosteric mechanism we also demonstrated that insulin

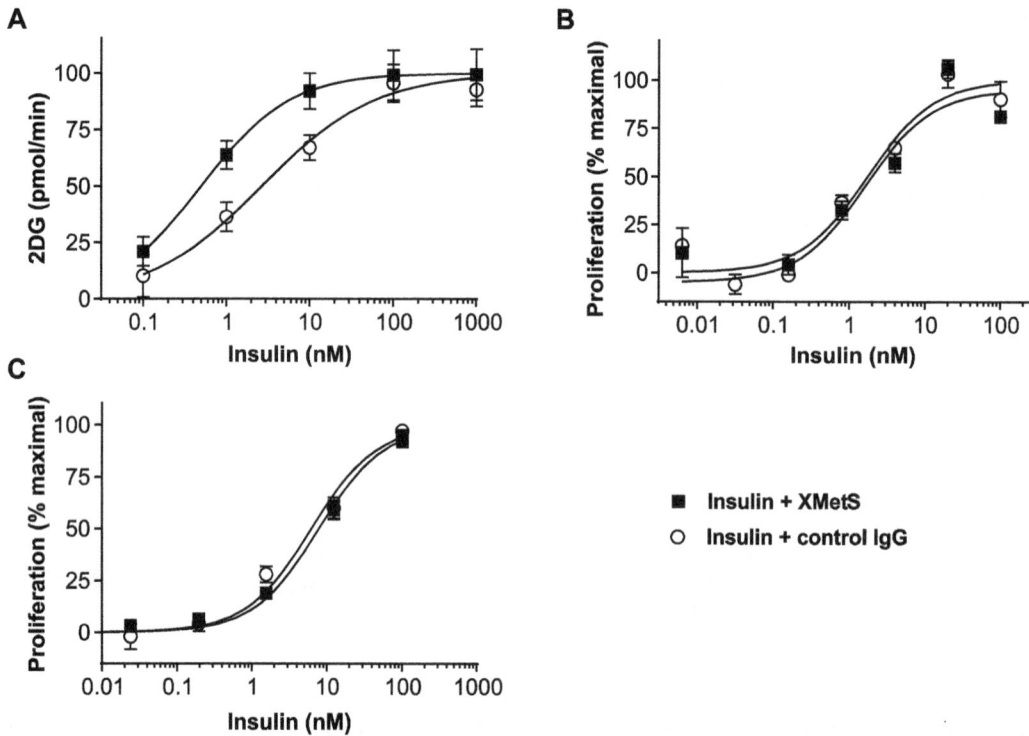

Figure 5. XMetS potentiates insulin-mediated 2-deoxy-D-glucose uptake in L6 muscle cells, but does not enhance the growth of cancer cells. A. L6 cells expressing both isoform B of the hINSR and GLUT-4 were preincubated with either XMetS or control antibody for 60 minutes at 37°C followed by a 10 minute incubation with increasing concentrations of insulin. [^{3}H]-2-deoxy-D-glucose (2DG) was added and uptake was measured after 20 minutes. **B.** MCF-7 human breast cancer cells were incubated for 48 hours at 37°C with increasing concentrations of insulin in the presence of either XMetS or control antibody, and cell proliferation was determined by CellTiter Glo® assay. **C.** Saos-2 human osteosarcoma cells were incubated for 72 hours at 37°C with increasing concentrations of insulin in the presence of either XMetS or control antibody, and cell proliferation was determined by CellTiter Glo® assay. The mean ± SD from triplicate determinations are shown.

reciprocally enhanced the binding affinity of XMetS for the INSR as has been shown for other positive allosteric modulators [25]. XMetS potentiated INSR signaling in cultured cells. Moreover,

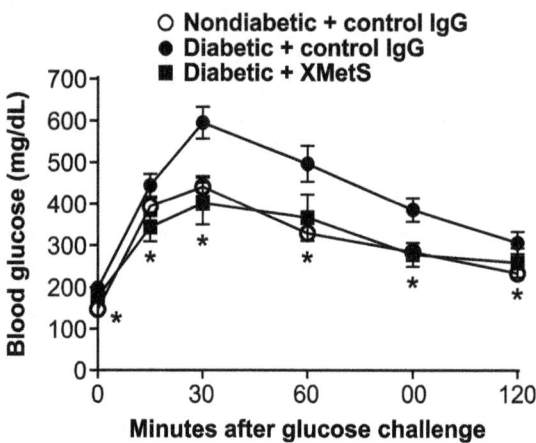

Figure 6. XMetS improves glucose metabolism in diet induced obesity mice. C57BL/6 diet induced obesity mice were treated twice weekly with either control antibody (10 mg/kg) or XMetS (10 mg/kg). Age-matched, lean C57BL/6 mice were treated twice weekly with control antibody (10 mg/kg). After one week of treatment and following a 14-hour overnight fast, a glucose bolus was administered intraperitoneally (1 g/kg) and blood glucose levels were measured for 120 minutes. Mean ± SEM are shown (n = 10 mice/group).

XMetS was active in vivo, improving glucose metabolism in two mouse models of insulin resistance and diabetes.

Others have described monoclonal antibodies to the INSR that were generated using hybridoma technology [4,39,40]. In some instances, antibodies were observed to modestly (2-fold or less) increase insulin binding to the INSR [4]. However, neither the in vitro nor in vivo effects of these antibodies on INSR signaling were extensively characterized.

We find that XMetS markedly enhanced insulin binding affinity in cells expressing either the hINSR or the mINSR. Kinetic analysis indicated that XMetS positively modulated insulin binding affinity by decreasing the dissociation rate of insulin from the INSR without affecting the association rate of insulin. These data suggested that XMetS positively modulated the INSR by stabilizing the ligand bound conformation of the receptor resulting in higher affinity for insulin. Both the monovalent Fab and divalent IgG$_2$ forms of XMetS acted as positive allosteric modulators of the INSR. This observation suggests that the mechanism by which XMetS stabilized the ligand bound form of the INSR does not require intra- or intermolecular crosslinking if the INSR. Hence, the mechanism for XMetS differs from the proposed mechanism by which insulin activates the INSR via intramolecular crosslinking [41]. It will be important to elucidate the details of XMetS INSR modulation on a structural level. However, such an analysis requires knowledge of the full length ligand activated INSR and the conformation changes associated with activation, both of which have not been fully determined [42,43].

Table 1. Metabolic profile of diet induced obesity mice treated with XMetS and controls.

	Non-diabetic+control IgG	Diabetic+control IgG	Diabetic+XMetS
Body Weight (g)	30.1±1.7*	37.0±3.4	36.8±3.1
Glucose (mg/dL)	163±10*	243±12	189±18*
Total cholesterol (mg/dL)	104±9*	136±12	121±20
Non-HDL cholesterol (mg/dL)	33±8*	63±17	46±14*
Insulin (pg/mL)	338±84*	670±395	209±171*
C-peptide (pM)	224±52*	333±117	112±104*

At the end of the 4-week study with diet induced obesity mice, the animals were fasted 14 hours, weighed and plasma was obtained to determine the above parameters. Mice (n = 10/group) were treated with antibody at 10 mg/kg, twice weekly. Values are shown as mean ± SEM. *p<0.05 vs. diabetic+control IgG.

After insulin binds to the INSR it activates receptor autophosphorylation, which leads in turn to activation of downstream signaling. Similar to its effect on insulin binding affinity, XMetS potentiated insulin-dependent INSR autophosphorylation by 14-fold indicating that the enhancement of insulin binding was associated with improved insulin-mediated INSR activation. The effect of XMetS was specific to the INSR as it did not potentiate activation of the IGF-1R by IGF-1.

A key signaling event triggered by INSR activation is the phosphorylation and activation of the intracellular enzyme Akt [2], which leads to cellular glucose uptake. XMetS markedly

enhanced insulin dependent Akt phosphorylation greater than 30-fold in cultured cells expressing the INSR. In accordance with its effect on Akt activation mediated by the INSR, XMetS potentiated insulin-stimulated 2-deoxy-D-glucose uptake in cultured muscle cells expressing the INSR.

In humans, insulin may enhance tumor progression via the INSR, while insulin analogs with INSR dissociation rates slower than insulin may have greater mitogenic activity [44]. XMetS slowed the rate of dissociation of insulin from the INSR. Thus, we studied the effect of XMetS on insulin-stimulated proliferation in MCF-7 breast cancer cells and Saos-2 osteosarcoma cells, two

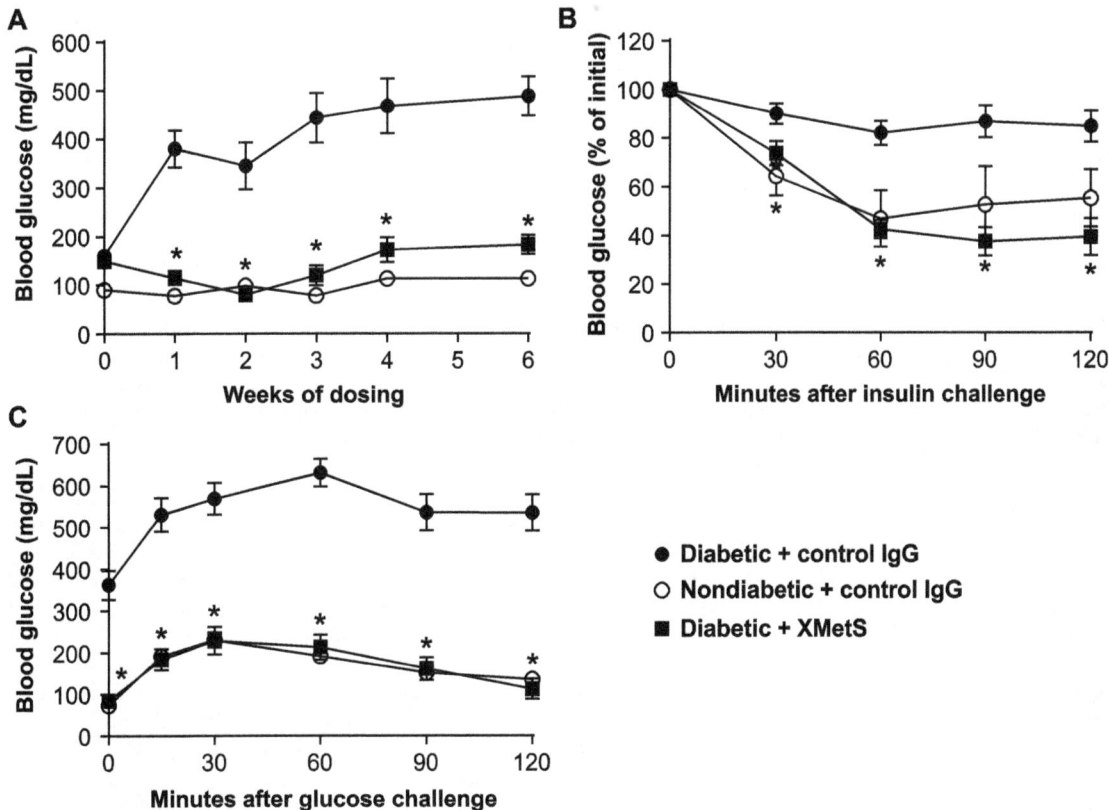

Figure 7. XMetS improves glucose metabolism in multi-low dose, streptozotocin/high-fat diet mice. A–C. ICR multi-low dose, streptozotocin/high-fat diet mice were treated twice weekly with either control antibody (10 mg/kg) or XMetS (10 mg/kg). Age-matched non-diabetic ICR mice were treated twice weekly with control antibody (10 mg/kg). A. Blood glucose levels were obtained weekly for six weeks following a 14-hour fast. B. After five weeks of treatment and following a 4-hour fast, insulin was administered intraperitoneally (0.75 U/kg) and blood glucose levels were obtained for an additional 120 minutes. C. After three weeks of treatment and following a 14-hour fast, a glucose bolus was administered intraperitoneally (1 g/kg) and blood glucose levels were measured for 120 minutes. Mean ± SEM are shown (n = 8 mice/group).

Table 2. Metabolic profile of multi-low dose, streptozotocin/high-fat diet mice treated with XMetS and controls.

	Non-diabetic+control IgG	Diabetic+control IgG	Diabetic+XMetS
Body Weight (g)	42.5±3.1*	35.5±3.2	38.4±2.3*
Beta hydroxybutyrate (mmol/L)	0.26±0.05*	4.79±1.8	1.05±0.61*
Glucose (mg/dL)	113±19*	488±40	183±20*
Total cholesterol (mg/dL)	154±17*	175±29	159±31
Non-HDL cholesterol (mg/dL)	34±10*	101±32	63±21*
Insulin (pg/mL)	1006±332*	336±301	137±51*
C-peptide (pM)	204±69*	142±67	67±63*

At the end of the 6-week study with multi-low dose, streptozotocin/high-fat diet mice, the animals were fasted 14 hours, weighed and plasma was obtained to determine the above parameters. Mice (n = 8/group) were treated with antibody at 10 mg/kg, twice weekly. Values are shown as mean ± SEM. *p<0.05 vs. diabetic+control IgG.

cancer cells lines that are commonly used to determine the mitogenic effects of insulin analogs [37]. We observed that XMetS did not enhance the effect of either insulin or IGF-1 on the proliferation of these cell lines. In the present study we found that the observed potentiation by XMetS on insulin induced Erk activation was less that the potentiation of insulin-stimulated Akt activation by XMetS. Studies have indicated that insulin stimulation of the MAP kinase pathway including enhanced Erk phosphorylation may be associated with mitogenesis [36]. Thus one potential explanation for the lack of effect of XMetS on ligand induced proliferation of cancer cells may be related to the relatively limited effect of XMetS on insulin-dependent Erk activation.

Recently, Vigneri *et. al.* proposed the concept that certain molecules, including monoclonal antibodies, that either activate or modulate metabolic INSR signaling without increasing cell proliferation would be of therapeutic value [38]. We previously reported that XMetA, an INSR agonist antibody, selectively activated metabolic but not mitogenic functions including the proliferation of cancer cells [18]. We now find that XMetS, a positive allosteric modulator of the INSR, also does not agonize or potentiate insulin-mediated cancer cell proliferation. These observations suggest that allosteric antibodies with the unique profiles of either XMetA or XMetS may be of therapeutic value. We therefore studied whether the in vitro ability of XMetS to potentiate the binding of insulin to the INSR and enhance intracellular signaling and glucose transport, were reflected in vivo by enhanced insulin responsiveness and improved glucose metabolism in obese and diabetic animals.

In the diet induced obesity mouse, a model of obese insulin resistance and hyperglycemia, XMetS reduced fasting blood glucose levels and normalized glucose tolerance. Improved glycemic control in these animal models was accompanied by reduced insulin and C-peptide levels, suggesting that XMetS increased insulin sensitivity and lowered the requirement for insulin. This reduction of compensatory hyperinsulinemia caused by XMetS may contribute to the lack of hypoglycemia that was observed in the diseased mice treated with this antibody.

In insulin resistant, insulinopenic multi-low dose, streptozotocin/high-fat diet mice, XMetS also markedly improved fasting hyperglycemia and normalized glucose tolerance. These diabetic mice had a diminished ability to respond to exogenous insulin and were therefore insulin resistant. XMetS restored the ability of insulin to lower glucose levels in these mice, indicating decreased insulin resistance. In concert with this observation, XMetS also lowered insulin and C-peptide values, further indicating that it

improved insulin sensitivity. In addition to its beneficial effects on glucose metabolism, XMetS lowered beta hydroxybutyrate levels in multi-low dose, streptozotocin/high-fat diet mice and improved dyslipidemia as reflected by a reduction of elevated non-HDL cholesterol. XMetS also partially ameliorated the disease related weight loss that was observed in these mice.

An INSR mutant has been described (K460E) [45], that exhibits increased affinity for insulin and induces insulin resistance in humans through a proposed mechanism that involves accelerated INSR degradation [46]. Insulin analogues have also been described that exhibit higher affinity for the INSR with enhanced mitogenic activity (e.g. AspB10) ([47–49]. These effects are the opposite of those for XMetS which increases insulin sensitivity and does not enhance mitogenic activity. Although direct experimental comparisons with XMetS have not been carried out, the present data suggest that the mechanisms by which these INSR and insulin mutants increase the affinity of insulin binding to the INSR are considerably different than the mechanism(s) employed by XMetS. Further studies on insulin processing and INSR trafficking will be required to elucidate these differential effects.

In humans, the natural history of T2DM has been described in multiple populations [50–55]. The insulin resistance of T2DM results in part from obesity and physical inactivity that are now prevalent in many developed and developing countries [56]. Initially, most individuals become insulin resistant due to defects in the INSR signaling pathway [55,57,58]. To compensate, the pancreatic beta cell initially produces and secretes additional insulin in an attempt to maintain euglycemia [51,52,58,59]. However, in many instances compensatory insulin secretion eventually diminishes as a result of beta cell dysfunction leading to uncontrolled hyperglycemia. While current treatments for early T2DM patients may initially provide satisfactory regulation of blood glucose, many patients ultimately require exogenous insulin [51,52,59]. This progression underscores the need for new therapies that may enhance the ability of endogenous insulin to activate the INSR. Such agents could improve glycemic control, prevent compensatory hyperinsulinemia, and possibly delay or obviate the need for exogenous insulin therapy by preserving beta cell function. The studies described herein demonstrate that an allosteric monoclonal antibody to the INSR, XMetS, positively modulates insulin binding to the INSR resulting in improved glucose metabolism both in vitro and in vivo. Importantly, XMetS does not potentiate insulin-stimulated proliferation of cancer cells. Thus, these studies suggest that this type of allosteric monoclonal antibody could have therapeutic utility for the treatment of T2DM.

Acknowledgments

The authors wish to thank Jesse Roth, Patrick J. Scannon and Paul Ruben, for critical reading of the manuscript and helpful comments.

Author Contributions

Conceived and designed the experiments: JAC VB IDG MLW. Performed the experiments: DHB AL KM LMG BAM HFK CT LL MH SRW AJN SZ RL LW SDW NL XW DC SRL SW. Analyzed the data: JAC IDG VB. Wrote the paper: JAC VB IDG DW MLW.

References

1. Ussar S, Vienberg SG, Kahn CR (2011) Receptor antibodies as novel therapeutics for diabetes. Sci Transl Med 3: 113ps147.
2. Taniguchi CM, Emanuelli B, Kahn CR (2006) Critical nodes in signalling pathways: insights into insulin action. Nat Rev Mol Cell Biol 7: 85–96.
3. Goldfine ID, Roth RA (1986) Monoclonal antibodies to the insulin receptor as probes of insulin receptor structure and function. Horiz Biochem Biophys 8: 471–502.
4. Soos MA, Siddle K, Baron MD, Heward JM, Luzio JP, et al. (1986) Monoclonal antibodies reacting with multiple epitopes on the human insulin receptor. Biochem J 235: 199–208.
5. Siddle K, Soos MA, O'Brien RM, Ganderton RH, Taylor R (1987) Monoclonal antibodies as probes of the structure and function of insulin receptors. Biochem Soc Trans 15: 47–51.
6. Lupsa BC, Chong AY, Cochran EK, Soos MA, Semple RK, et al. (2009) Autoimmune forms of hypoglycemia. Medicine (Baltimore) 88: 141–153.
7. Le Marchand-Brustel Y, Gorden P, Flier JS, Kahn CR, Freychet P (1978) Anti-insulin receptor antibodies inhibit insulin binding and stimulate glucose metabolism in skeletal muscle. Diabetologia 14: 311–317.
8. De Pirro R, Roth RA, Rossetti L, Goldfine ID (1984) Characterization of the serum from a patient with insulin resistance and hypoglycemia. Evidence for multiple populations of insulin receptor antibodies with different receptor binding and insulin-mimicking activities. Diabetes 33: 301–304.
9. Arioglu E, Andewelt A, Diabo C, Bell M, Taylor SI, et al. (2002) Clinical course of the syndrome of autoantibodies to the insulin receptor (type B insulin resistance): a 28-year perspective. Medicine (Baltimore) 81: 87–100.
10. Zick Y, Rees-Jones RW, Taylor SI, Gorden P, Roth J (1984) The role of antireceptor antibodies in stimulating phosphorylation of the insulin receptor. J Biol Chem 259: 4396–4400.
11. Kahn CR, Baird K, Filier JS, Jarrett DB (1977) Effects of autoantibodies to the insulin receptor on isolated adipocytes. Studies of insulin binding and insulin action. J Clin Invest 60: 1094–1106.
12. Kahn CR, Baird KL, Jarrett DB, Flier JS (1978) Direct demonstration that receptor crosslinking or aggregation is important in insulin action. Proc Natl Acad Sci U S A 75: 4209–4213.
13. Flier JS, Kahn CR, Roth J, Bar RS (1975) Antibodies that impair insulin receptor binding in an unusual diabetic syndrome with severe insulin resistance. Science 190: 63–65.
14. Brunetti A, Maddux BA, Wong KY, Hofmann C, Whittaker J, et al. (1989) Monoclonal antibodies to the human insulin receptor mimic a spectrum of biological effects in transfected 3T3/HIR fibroblasts without activating receptor kinase. Biochem Biophys Res Commun 165: 212–218.
15. Koschubs T, Dengl S, Durr H, Kaluza K, Georges G, et al. (2012) Allosteric antibody inhibition of human hepsin protease. Biochem J 442: 483–494.
16. Cazorla M, Arrang JM, Premont J (2011) Pharmacological characterization of six trkB antibodies reveals a novel class of functional agents for the study of the BDNF receptor. Br J Pharmacol 162: 947–960.
17. Hino T, Arakawa T, Iwanari H, Yurugi-Kobayashi T, Ikeda-Suno C, et al. (2012) G-protein-coupled receptor inactivation by an allosteric inverse-agonist antibody. Nature 482: 237–240.
18. Bhaskar V, Goldfine ID, Bedinger DH, Lau A, Kuan HF, et al. (2012) A fully human, allosteric monoclonal antibody that activates the insulin receptor and improves glycemic control. Diabetes 61: 1263–1271.
19. Bhaskar V, Lau A, Goldfine ID, Narasimha AJ, Gross LM, et al. (2012) XMetA, an allosteric monoclonal antibody to the insulin receptor, improves glycaemic control in mice with diet-induced obesity. Diabetes Obes Metab.
20. Aitken R (2001) Methods in Molecular Biology. In: O'Brien PM, editor. Antibody phage display: methods and protocols. Totowa, NJ: Humana Press.
21. Barbas CF, Burton DR, Scott JK, Silverman GJ (2001) Phage Display: A Laboratory Manual. Plainview, NY: Cold Spring Harbor Laboratory Press.
22. Seino S, Bell GI (1989) Alternative splicing of human insulin receptor messenger RNA. Biochem Biophys Res Commun 159: 312–316.
23. Moller DE, Yokota A, Caro JF, Flier JS (1989) Tissue-specific expression of two alternatively spliced insulin receptor mRNAs in man. Mol Endocrinol 3: 1263–1269.
24. Zloza A, Sullivan YB, Connick E, Landay AL, Al-Harthi L (2003) CD8+ T cells that express CD4 on their surface (CD4dimCD8bright T cells) recognize an antigen-specific target, are detected in vivo, and can be productively infected by T-tropic HIV. Blood 102: 2156–2164.
25. Christopoulos A, Kenakin T (2002) G protein-coupled receptor allosterism and complexing. Pharmacol Rev 54: 323–374.
26. Rathanaswami P, Babcook J, Gallo M (2008) High-affinity binding measurements of antibodies to cell-surface-expressed antigens. Anal Biochem 373: 52–60.
27. Xie L, Mark Jones R, Glass TR, Navoa R, Wang Y, et al. (2005) Measurement of the functional affinity constant of a monoclonal antibody for cell surface receptors using kinetic exclusion fluorescence immunoassay. J Immunol Methods 304: 1–14.
28. Ryan CJ, Zavodovskaya M, Youngren JF, Campbell M, Diamond M, et al. (2008) Inhibitory effects of nordihydroguaiaretic acid (NDGA) on the IGF-1 receptor and androgen dependent growth of LAPC-4 prostate cancer cells. Prostate 68: 1232–1240.
29. Colquhoun D (2007) Why the Schild method is better than Schild realised. Trends Pharmacol Sci 28: 608–614.
30. Schild HO (1947) pA, a new scale for the measurement of drug antagonism. Br J Pharmacol Chemother 2: 189–206.
31. Maddux BA, See W, Lawrence JC Jr, Goldfine AL, Goldfine ID, et al. (2001) Protection against oxidative stress-induced insulin resistance in rat L6 muscle cells by mircomolar concentrations of alpha-lipoic acid. Diabetes 50: 404–410.
32. Surwit RS, Feinglos MN, Rodin J, Sutherland A, Petro AE, et al. (1995) Differential effects of fat and sucrose on the development of obesity and diabetes in C57BL/6J and A/J mice. Metabolism 44: 645–651.
33. Arulmozhi DK, Kurian R, Bodhankar SL, Veeranjaneyulu A (2008) Metabolic effects of various antidiabetic and hypolipidaemic agents on a high-fat diet and multiple low-dose streptozocin (MLDS) mouse model of diabetes. J Pharm Pharmacol 60: 1167–1173.
34. Frasca F, Pandini G, Sciacca L, Pezzino V, Squatrito S, et al. (2008) The role of insulin receptors and IGF-I receptors in cancer and other diseases. Arch Physiol Biochem 114: 23–37.
35. Conn PJ, Christopoulos A, Lindsley CW (2009) Allosteric modulators of GPCRs: a novel approach for the treatment of CNS disorders. Nat Rev Drug Discov 8: 41–54.
36. Belfiore A, Frasca F, Pandini G, Sciacca L, Vigneri R (2009) Insulin receptor isoforms and insulin receptor/insulin-like growth factor receptor hybrids in physiology and disease. Endocr Rev 30: 586–623.
37. Sciacca L, Le Moli R, Vigneri R (2012) Insulin analogs and cancer. Front Endocrinol (Lausanne) 3: 21.
38. Vigneri R, Squatrito S, Frittitta L (2012) Selective insulin receptor modulators (SIRM): a new class of antidiabetes drugs? Diabetes 61: 984–985.
39. Morgan DO, Roth RA (1986) Mapping surface structures of the human insulin receptor with monoclonal antibodies: localization of main immunogenic regions to the receptor kinase domain. Biochemistry 25: 1364–1371.
40. Forsayeth JR, Caro JF, Sinha MK, Maddux BA, Goldfine ID (1987) Monoclonal antibodies to the human insulin receptor that activate glucose transport but not insulin receptor kinase activity. Proc Natl Acad Sci U S A 84: 3448–3451.
41. De Meyts P, Whittaker J (2002) Structural biology of insulin and IGF1 receptors: implications for drug design. Nat Rev Drug Discov 1: 769–783.
42. Smith BJ, Huang K, Kong G, Chan SJ, Nakagawa S, et al. (2010) Structural resolution of a tandem hormone-binding element in the insulin receptor and its implications for design of peptide agonists. Proc Natl Acad Sci U S A 107: 6771–6776.
43. Menting JG, Whittaker J, Margetts MB, Whittaker LJ, Kong GK, et al. (2013) How insulin engages its primary binding site on the insulin receptor. Nature 493: 241–245.
44. Kurtzhals P, Schaffer L, Sorensen A, Kristensen C, Jonassen I, et al. (2000) Correlations of receptor binding and metabolic and mitogenic potencies of insulin analogs designed for clinical use. Diabetes 49: 999–1005.
45. Kadowaki T, Bevins CL, Cama A, Ojamaa K, Marcus-Samuels B, et al. (1988) Two mutant alleles of the insulin receptor gene in a patient with extreme insulin resistance. Science 240: 787–790.
46. Taylor SI, Kadowaki T, Kadowaki H, Accili D, Cama A, et al. (1990) Mutations in insulin-receptor gene in insulin-resistant patients. Diabetes Care 13: 257–279.
47. Drejer K, Kruse V, Larsen UD, Hougaard P, Bjorn S, et al. (1991) Receptor binding and tyrosine kinase activation by insulin analogues with extreme affinities studied in human hepatoma HepG2 cells. Diabetes 40: 1488–1495.
48. Hansen BF, Danielsen GM, Drejer K, Sorensen AR, Wiberg FC, et al. (1996) Sustained signalling from the insulin receptor after stimulation with insulin analogues exhibiting increased mitogenic potency. Biochem J 315 (Pt 1): 271–279.
49. Authier F, Di Guglielmo GM, Danielsen GM, Bergeron JJ (1998) Uptake and metabolic fate of [HisA8,HisB4,GluB10,HisB27]insulin in rat liver in vivo. Biochem J 332 (Pt 2): 421–430.
50. Lyssenko V, Almgren P, Anevski D, Perfekt R, Lahti K, et al. (2005) Predictors of and longitudinal changes in insulin sensitivity and secretion preceding onset of type 2 diabetes. Diabetes 54: 166–174.

51. Martin BC, Warram JH, Krolewski AS, Bergman RN, Soeldner JS, et al. (1992) Role of glucose and insulin resistance in development of type 2 diabetes mellitus: results of a 25-year follow-up study. Lancet 340: 925–929.

52. Chen YD, Jeng CY, Hollenbeck CB, Wu MS, Reaven GM (1988) Relationship between plasma glucose and insulin concentration, glucose production, and glucose disposal in normal subjects and patients with non-insulin-dependent diabetes. J Clin Invest 82: 21–25.

53. Warram JH, Martin BC, Krolewski AS, Soeldner JS, Kahn CR (1990) Slow glucose removal rate and hyperinsulinemia precede the development of type II diabetes in the offspring of diabetic parents. Ann Intern Med 113: 909–915.

54. Lillioja S, Mott DM, Spraul M, Ferraro R, Foley JE, et al. (1993) Insulin resistance and insulin secretory dysfunction as precursors of non-insulin-dependent diabetes mellitus. Prospective studies of Pima Indians. N Engl J Med 329: 1988–1992.

55. Defronzo RA (2009) Banting Lecture. From the triumvirate to the ominous octet: a new paradigm for the treatment of type 2 diabetes mellitus. Diabetes 58: 773–795.

56. (2011) National Diabetes Fact Sheet. CDC.

57. Kolterman OG, Gray RS, Griffin J, Burstein P, Insel J, et al. (1981) Receptor and postreceptor defects contribute to the insulin resistance in noninsulin-dependent diabetes mellitus. J Clin Invest 68: 957–969.

58. Reaven GM (1988) Banting lecture 1988. Role of insulin resistance in human disease. Diabetes 37: 1595–1607.

59. Reaven GM, Olefsky JM (1978) The role of insulin resistance in the pathogenesis of diabetes mellitus. Adv Metab Disord 9: 313–331.

16

Association between Serum Leptin Concentrations and Insulin Resistance

Hui Zuo[1,2]*, Zumin Shi[3], Baojun Yuan[1], Yue Dai[1], Gaolin Wu[1], Akhtar Hussain[2]

1 Department of Nutrition and Food Hygiene, Jiangsu Provincial Center for Disease Control and Prevention, Nanjing, China, **2** Department of Community Medicine, Institute of Health and Society, Faculty of Medicine, University of Oslo, Oslo, Norway, **3** Discipline of Medicine, University of Adelaide, Adelaide, Australia

Abstract

Background: Insulin resistance contributes to the cardio-metabolic risk. The effect of leptin in obese and overweight population on insulin resistance was seldom reported.

Methods: A total of 1234 subjects (572 men and 662 women) aged ≥18 y was sampled by the procedure. Adiposity measures included BMI, waist circumference, hip circumference, WHR, upper arm circumference, triceps skinfold and body fat percentage. Serum leptin concentrations were measured by an ELISA method. The homeostasis model (HOMA-IR) was applied to estimate insulin resistance.

Results: In men, BMI was the variable which was most strongly correlated with leptin, whereas triceps skinfold was most sensitive for women. More importantly, serum leptin levels among insulin resistant subjects were almost double compared to the subjects who had normal insulin sensitivity at the same level of adiposity in both men and women, after controlling for potential confounders. In addition, HOMA-IR increased significantly across leptin quintiles after adjustment for age, BMI, total energy intake, physical activity and smoking status in both men and women (p for trend <0.0001).

Conclusions: There was a significant association between HOMA-IR and serum leptin concentrations in Chinese men and women, independently of adiposity levels. This may suggest that serum leptin concentration is an important predictor of insulin resistance and other metabolic risks irrespective of obesity levels. Furthermore, leptin levels may be used to identify the cardio-metabolic risk in obese and overweight population.

Editor: Rocio I. Pereira, University of Colorado Denver, United States of America

Funding: This work was funded by the Norwegian Research Council, Norway. The funders had no role in study design, data collection and analysis, decision to publish, or preparation of the manuscript.

Competing Interests: The authors have declared that no competing interests exist.

* E-mail: huizuo97@gmail.com

Introduction

Obesity is now a global epidemic [1,2]. It is one of the most significant causes of ill-health worldwide [3–5]. Anti-adiposity efforts to reverse the increasing trend are somewhat disappointing. However, all overweight or obese people do not have the same risk of developing insulin resistance, resulting in adiposity-related health risks such as type 2 diabetes, metabolic syndrome and cardiovascular diseases.

Leptin, an adipose tissue-derived hormone, activates researchers' interest with a new insight since its discovery [6,7]. It plays an important role in the pathophysiology of obesity [5]. Leptin acts centrally to decrease food intake and modulate glucose and fat metabolism [8].

Circulating leptin level was found to be proportional to adipose tissue mass, and body fat percentage was possibly the best adiposity-related predictor of serum leptin concentrations in human, which may be due to leptin resistance [9,10]. However, it is not always easily accessible to directly measure the percentage of body fat, especially in epidemiological studies [11,12]. In the studies on the association between leptin and indirect measures of adiposity, the most frequently used measures were body mass index (BMI) and waist circumference [13–16]. Very few studies [17,18] reported information about surrogate dimension of other variables such as waist-to-hip ratio (WHR), arm circumference or triceps skinfold in relation to leptin. Also, it is unknown the proxy performance of body fat percentage estimated using prediction equation.

Although most surveys indicated a positive relationship of leptin and insulin resistance in their populations [16,19,20], others showed inconsistent results [14,21,22]. However, data on the effect of leptin in obese and overweight population on insulin resistance are scarce, other than one study focusing in diabetic women [14]. Furthermore, it remains unclear whether ethnic difference affects such association in addition to lifestyle factors such as smoking [13,23].

Therefore, we have investigated the role of leptin in insulin resistance at different levels of obesity controlling for potential confounding factors including lifestyle and diet in a Chinese population.

Table 1. Descriptive statistics of demographic, anthropometric and biochemical parameters in 1234 participants, stratified by sex.

	Men	Women	P value
n	572	662	
Age (years)	50.4±0.6	48.6±0.6	0.031
Anthropometric measures[a]			
BMI (kg/m²)	23.4±0.2	23.5±0.1	0.607
Waist circumference (cm)	83.6±0.4	79.2±0.4	<0.0001
Hip circumference (cm)	94.5±0.4	93.9±0.4	0.228
WHR	0.88±0.003	0.84±0.003	<0.0001
Upper arm circumference (cm)	27.5±0.1	26.5±0.1	<0.0001
Triceps skinfold (mm)	17.3±0.3	23.9±0.3	<0.0001
BF (%)	24.1±0.2	35.1±0.1	<0.0001
Total energy intake (kcal/d)[a]	2661±45	2242±42	<0.0001
Physical activity (MET-h/week)[a]	168.3±4.9	159.6±4.4	0.191
Smoking (%)	51.9	2.3	<0.0001
Biochemical parameters[a]			
Fasting glucose (mmol/L)	5.20±0.05	5.20±0.05	0.936
Fasting insulin (uU/ml)	5.47±0.21	6.58±0.19	<0.0001
HOMA-IR[b]	0.92±0.03	1.20±0.03	<0.0001
Leptin (ng/ml)[b]	1.45±0.05	8.32±0.05	<0.0001

BMI, body mass index; WHR, waist-to-hip ratio; BF (%), body fat percentage; HOMA-IR, homeostasis model assessment of insulin resistance.
Data are means ± SEM, unless otherwise indicated.
[a]Adjusted for age.
[b]Geometric means ± SEM.

Methods and Subjects

Study Design

Data used in this study were derived from the 2006 wave of the China Health and Nutrition Survey (CHNS) in Jiangsu Province. The CHNS study is a nationwide ongoing open cohort in China, started from 1989. More detailed information was described elsewhere [24]. Jiangsu was the only province that collected blood samples in that project in the 2006 wave. Therefore the study consisted of face-to-face questionnaire interviews, physical examinations, and laboratory analysis in Jiangsu. The study sample was drawn from six areas (two cities: Suzhou and Yangzhou; four counties: Shuyang, Taixing, Haimen, and Jinhu) following a multistage random cluster process. Socioeconomic status in these areas was a primary consideration. Further, 4 villages and townships in each county and 4 urban and suburban neighborhoods in each city were selected randomly. In total, 16 villages and townships within the counties and 8 urban and suburban neighborhoods within the cities were selected, respectively.

Subjects

The study sample consisted of 572 men and 662 women aged ≥18 y from those household sampled by the procedure. Excluded were persons who had an age <18 y (n = 81), who had previously diagnosed diabetes (n = 48), who had any of missing anthropometric or leptin data (n = 59). The study was approved by the Review Board of Jiangsu Provincial Center for Disease Control and Prevention. All participants provided written consent. The

subjects were compensated for their participation. The response rate was 91.3%.

Adiposity Measures

Anthropometric data were measured by trained health workers following standard protocols. Weight in light clothing and without shoes was measured to the nearest 0.1 kg and height was measured to the nearest 0.1 cm. BMI was calculated as weight (kg)/height squared (m²). It was categorized as normal weight (BMI<24), overweight (BMI≥24 to <28), obese (BMI≥28) according to the Chinese standard [25]. Waist circumference was measured to the nearest 0.1 cm with an inelastic tape at the mid-way between the lowest rib and the iliac crest with the subject standing at the end of gentle expiration. Central obesity was defined as WC≥90 cm in men and ≥80 cm in women according to the International Diabetes Federation criteria [26]. Hip circumference was measured with the same tape to the nearest 0.1 cm at the maximum circumference over the buttocks. Upper arm circumference was measured to the nearest 0.1 cm with the left arm hanging relaxed. The measurement was taken midway between the tip of the acromion and olecranon process. Triceps skinfold was measured to the nearest mm in triplicate with a Lange skinfold caliper (Beta Technology Ltd, Cambridge, Maryland) having a pressure of 10 g/mm² of contact surface area. The measurement was taken over the triceps muscle at the midpoint of the left posterior upper arm. Body fat percentage (BF %) was estimated using ethnic specific prediction equations: $BF\% = 1.04*BMI - 10.9*sex +0.1*age +5.7$ [where BMI = body mass index (kg/m2); sex: females = 0, males = 1; and age in years] for Chinese [27].

Biochemical Analysis

Blood was collected by venipuncture from participants after overnight fasting. The fasting status was verbally confirmed by subjects before the blood sampling. All blood samples were collected in three vacuum tubes and processed within three hours. All specimens were then shipped to the Jiangsu Provincial Center for Disease Control and Prevention and were stored at −70°C for later laboratory testing. Fasting glucose was assessed by an enzymology method using OLYMPUS Chemistry Analyzer AU400 (Mishima Olympus CO., LTD, Shizuoka-ken, Japan). Insulin was measured by ELISA Kit (Millipore Corporation, Billerica, MA, USA). The homeostasis model assessment for insulin resistance (HOMA-IR) score was calculated as fasting insulin (mU/L) * fasting glucose (mmol/L)/22.5 [28]. Its highest quartile was used to define insulin resistance. Serum leptin concentrations were measured using Linco Human Leptin ELISA Kit (Linco Research, St. Charles, MO, USA), the sensitivity of which was 0.5 ng/ml – 100 ng/ml. The average intra- and inter-assay coefficients of variation were 4.7% and 7.2%, respectively.

Diet, Physical Activity and Smoking Status Assessment

A semi-quantitative food frequency questionnaire (FFQ) [29] was used to collect dietary intake information. The questionnaire has been validated and compared with weighted food records and reported to be a useful method for the collection of individual food consumption information in face-to-face interviews, especially in studying the relationship between diet, nutrition and chronic diseases [29]. Participants were asked to recall their usual frequency and quantity of intakes of 33 food groups and beverages during the previous year with a series of detailed questions. Strict quality control procedures were took to minimize potential recall bias during the survey, which included well training of the survey workers, the use of food models, and so on. Intake of each food item was calculated by multiplying the reported frequency of the

Table 2. Correlation analysis of serum leptin concentrations with different adiposity measures in men and women.

	Men (n = 572)			Women (n = 662)		
	Unadjusted	Model 1	Model 2	Unadjusted	Model 1	Model 2
BMI (kg/m2)	0.665***	–	0.521***	0.489***	–	0.372***
Waist circumference (cm)	0.637***	0.287***	0.483***	0.385***	0.119**	0.307***
Hip circumference (cm)	0.550***	0.198***	0.379***	0.352***	0.088*	0.280***
WHR	0.342***	0.129**	0.240***	0.196***	0.061	0.151**
Upper arm circumference (cm)	0.549***	0.196***	0.382***	0.422***	0.163***	0.399***
Triceps skinfold (mm)	0.481***	0.289**	0.392***	0.525***	0.350***	0.449***
BF (%)	0.615***	–	0.521***	0.410***	–	0.372***

Model 1, adjusted for age and BMI.
Model 2, adjusted for age, total energy intake (quintile), physical activity (quintile), smoking status (yes/no) and HOMA-IR (quintile).
Analysis was performed on log-transformed leptin concentration due to non-normality distribution.
*p<0.05,
**p<0.01,
***p<0.0001.

food by estimated portion size of the food per time. It was then converted into g/day for further analysis. Total energy intake was computed by using the Chinese Food Composition Table [30]. Physical activities including domestic, occupational, transportation and leisure-time physical activity were assessed in terms of metabolic equivalent (MET)-hours-per-week to account for both intensity and time spent on activities. The level of physical activity was the product of time spent in each activity multiplied by specific MET values based on the "Compendium of Physical Activities" [31]. Domestic physical activity was defined as activities such as food shopping for the family, food preparation and cooking, washing and ironing clothes and house cleaning. Occupational physical activity was defined as activities such as light-intensity (e.g., office work, counter salesperson, lab technician, etc.), moderate-intensity (e.g., driver, electrician) and vigorous-intensity physical activity (e.g., farmer, athlete, dancer, steel worker, construction worker). Transportation physical activity was defined by various transportation methods such as on foot, by bicycle, by bus/subway or by car/taxi/motorcycle. Leisure-time physical activity included martial arts, gymnastics/dancing/acrobatics, track and field (running, etc.)/swimming, soccer/basketball/tennis, badminton/volleyball and other (ping pong, Tai Chi, etc.). Current smoking status was classified as dichotomous variables (yes/no).

Statistical Analysis

Distribution of leptin and HOMA-IR were highly skewed to the right, so geometric means and natural logs are presented in the analysis. Continuous variables were presented as means ± SEM. Means of serum leptin concentrations and HOMA-IR were generated and compared between the groups using the analysis of covariance (ANCOVA) procedure, adjusting for potential confounders. Pearson correlation coefficients were used to examine the association between serum leptin concentrations and different adiposity measures in men and women. The linear trend of adjusted geometric means of HOMA-IR across leptin quintiles was tested to assess the association between HOMA-IR and serum leptin concentrations in men and women after adjustment for age, BMI, total energy intake, physical activity and smoking status. Statistical analyses were performed separately for men and women, due to significant sex difference in serum leptin concentrations.

In addition, we generated predictive models for serum leptin concentrations and HOMA-IR, respectively, by using multivariate regression analysis. The candidate independent variables were gender, age, BMI, waist circumference, WHR, hip circumference, upper arm circumference, triceps skinfold, total energy intake, physical activity, smoking, insulin and HOMA-IR for serum leptin concentrations. The candidate independent variables were the same as above except substituting insulin and HOMA-IR to leptin for the prediction of HOMA-IR. Multivariate analyses excluded persons with missing values for any factor included in the model. Diagnostic measures including multicollinearity and interaction were examined in the predictive model. Interaction was performed by introducing production term into the model.

Stepwise procedure and adjusted R^2 selection method were used for choosing optimal predictors. We also report the model R^2 as a measure of the proportion of the variance in the values of dependent variable explained by the multivariate regression model. Only interaction terms were eligible in the model if it was significant, and had good predictive power (a larger model R^2) and no multicollinearity. The values of p<0.05 were considered statistically significant. All analyses were conducted using the SAS (version 8.1, SAS Institute, Cary, NC).

Results

Among 1234 study participants in our study, 416 (33.7%) were overweight and 118 (9.6%) were obese according to the Chinese criteria. Descriptive statistics of demographic, anthropometric and biochemical parameters for men and women are shown in Table 1. Women were a bit younger than men in general. There was no difference of BMI, hip circumference, physical activity and fasting glucose level between men and women. Men had higher waist circumference, WHR, upper arm circumference and a higher intake of total energy than women (p<0.0001). In contrast, triceps skinfold, body fat percentage, fasting insulin, HOMA-IR and leptin levels were significantly higher in women (p<0.0001). Smokers accounted for 51.9% in men and only 2.3% in women.

Table 2 reports the correlation coefficients for men and women between serum leptin concentrations with different adiposity measures. Prior to adjustments, all adiposity parameters were significantly correlated with serum leptin concentrations (p<0.0001). In men, BMI had the strongest correlation with

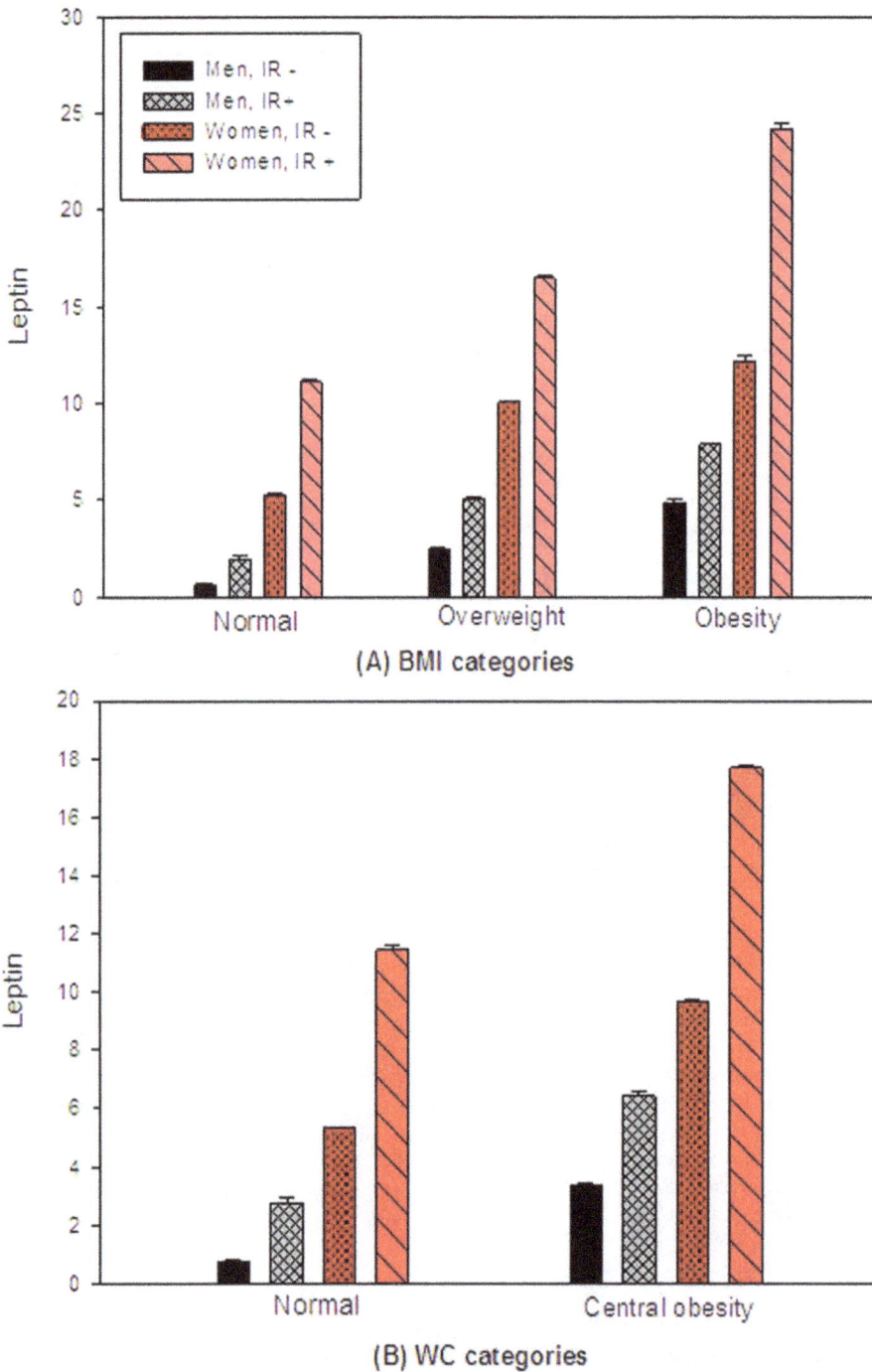

Figure 1. Serum leptin levels between participants with and without insulin resistance across different categories of adiposity in men and women, after adjustment for age, total energy intake (quintile), physical activity (quintile) and smoking status (yes/no). (Data are geometric means and SEM; Insulin resistance was defined as HOMA-IR >1.67 in men and >1.88 in women; P<0.001 between IR - and IR+groups at the same categories in men and women except P = 0.052 between two groups in obese women).

leptin, followed by waist circumference and BF (%). In women, the counterpart was triceps skinfold, followed by BMI and upper arm circumference. After controlling for age and BMI, all the variables except WHR in women remained significant. After further adjustment for age, total energy intake, physical activity, smoking status and HOMA-IR, the strong positive correlations still kept significant for all the variables in both men and women. In addition, serum leptin concentrations were more correlated with

adiposity measures in women aged ≥52 y compared to those aged <52 y by stratified analysis (data not shown).

Figure 1 presents serum leptin levels between participants with and without* insulin resistance across different categories of adiposity in men and women. After controlling for potential confounders, we found that participants with insulin resistance had significantly higher leptin levels compared to those without the condition, at all levels of adiposity, measured by BMI or waist

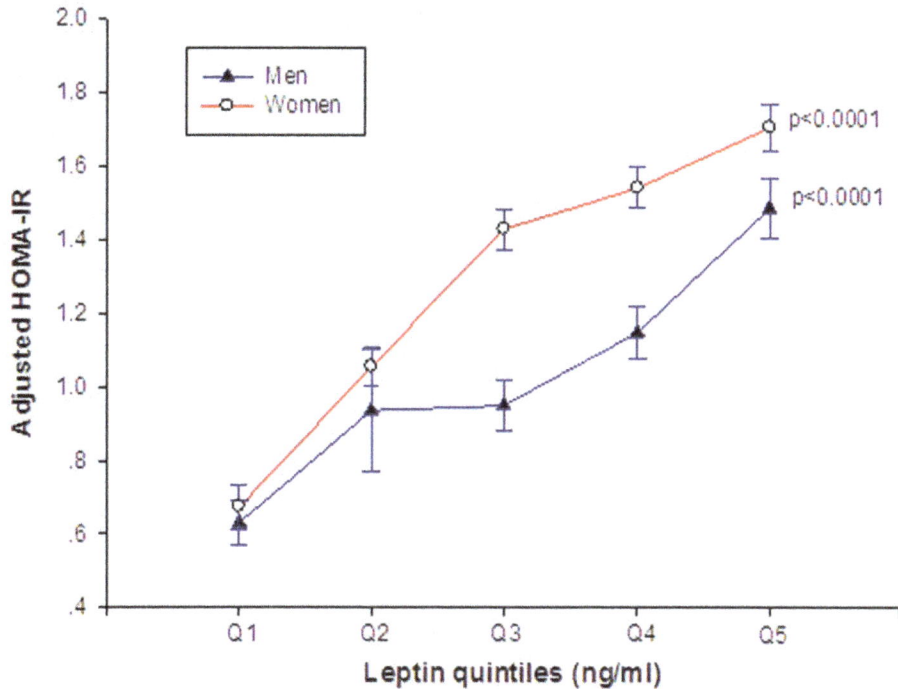

Figure 2. The association between HOMA-IR and serum leptin concentrations in men and women after adjustment for age, BMI, total energy intake (quintile), physical activity (quintile) and smoking status (yes/no). Geometric means ± SEM.

circumference. The leptin level was almost double among the insulin resistance group compared to those without the condition.

Table 3. Multivariate regression analysis standardized ß coefficients (SE) for leptin concentration in Chinese adults in the 2006 CHNS study, Jiangsu.

	Model 1[a]			Model 2[b]		
	ß	SE	P value	ß	SE	P value
Gender	–	–	–	−0.404	0.073	<0.0001
Age (years)	–	–	–	−0.079	0.002	<0.0001
BMI (kg/m^2)	0.330	0.009	<0.0001	0.135	0.012	<0.0001
Waist circumference (cm)	0.314	0.003	<0.0001	0.161	0.004	<0.0001
Triceps skinfold (mm)	0.317	0.004	<0.0001	0.218	0.004	<0.0001
Total energy intake (kcal/d, quintile)	–	–	–	−0.081	0.023	0.0001
Physical activity (MET-h/week, quintile)	–	–	–	−0.076	0.020	<0.0001
Smoking (yes/no)	–	–	–	−0.185	0.130	<0.0001
HOMA-IR	–	–	–	0.274	0.040	<0.0001
Energy*smoking	–	–	–	0.138	0.044	0.0003

Analysis was performed on log-transformed leptin concentration and HOMA-IR due to non-normality distribution.
[a]Model 1, BMI, waist circumference and triceps skinfold were put into the model separately, only information on the three adiposity measures was shown.
[b]Model 2, all independent variables in the table were put into the model simultaneously; Gender (0 women, 1 men); Smoking (0 no, 1 yes); Energy*smoking, interaction term between total energy intake (kcal/d, quintile) and smoking (yes/no); Model $R^2 = 0.69$.

As shown in Figure 2, HOMA-IR increased significantly across leptin quintiles after adjustment for age, BMI, total energy intake, physical activity and smoking status in both men and women (p for trend<0.0001).

The serum leptin concentration was predicted by gender, age, BMI, waist circumference, triceps skinfold, total energy intake, physical activity, smoking, HOMA-IR and interaction term between total energy intake and smoking. Gender and HOMA-IR and triceps skinfold were the major determinants. All these independent variables explained 69% of the variance of leptin concentrations in the regression model. Moreover, in order to avoid potential over-adjustment, BMI, waist circumference and triceps skinfold were separately analyzed in model 1. We observed that all the ß coefficients of them were larger than 0.3 (Table 3).

Discussion

Our study demonstrated that leptin was independently associated with all measures of adiposity. Furthermore, our data suggest that among the overweight/obese population those with insulin resistance had a significant higher level of leptin concentration compared to those overweight/obese who were not insulin resistant even after controlling for a number of potential confounding factors. There was a gender difference in the association of various levels of adiposity measures with leptin. In men, BMI had the strongest association with leptin. While in women, it was triceps skinfold.

Diverse adiposity measures available in our study allowed us to compare the strength of the association with leptin. Despite of disparities existed, all adiposity measures were significantly correlated with serum leptin concentrations in both men and women. Overall, we found BMI, universally used as proxy indicator of general obesity, had a satisfactory performance to correlate with leptin, especially in men. Also, we found triceps skinfold was most strongly correlated with leptin in women. Our results are in agreement with two studies, one from US [17] and one from China [18]. Gender and age differences in the estimation of the strength of association with leptin may be explained by the effect of sex hormones [4]. In addition, the proxy performance of body fat percentage (BF %) calculated using prediction equation [27] was reported for the first time by our study.

Although a large number of studies have reported the association between HOMA-IR and serum leptin concentrations. Their interrelationship independent of adiposity level was not largely addressed. Most studies found a significant and independent association between HOMA-IR and leptin in their populations [16,19,20], which was confirmed by the present study. However, some studies reported inconsistent results [14,21,32].

Of note, we found that serum leptin levels among insulin resistant subjects were almost double compared to those subjects who were not insulin resistant at the same level of adiposity in both men and women. Our results are consistent with a study specifically focusing on diabetic women [14]. This finding may provide an insight into the explanation why the metabolic risk was different among persons with same degree of adiposity.

Regression analyses showed that lifestyles such as dietary energy intake, physical activity and smoking were all inversely associated with leptin, which is in line with previous studies [13,23,33]. Possible explanation for smoking is that nicotine might indirectly reduce leptin secretion via enhanced plasma catecholamine concentration [23]. The inverse association between physical activity and leptin concentrations may be explained by several mechanisms: leptin is proposed to activate the melanocortin-4 receptor in the arcuate nucleus and then influence physical activity; physical activity may also regulate the leptin level directly through reducing its synthesis or by improved insulin sensitivity [33].

In addition, results of prediction model building further confirmed that HOMA-IR and leptin were important determinants and predictors of each other. Letpin may play an independent role in developing insulin resistance and other metabolic risks. However, the casual relationship in this study cannot be identified owing to its design. Another limitation of the study is possible residual confounding due to indirect methods to estimate adiposity. However, the striking rise of overweight and obesity epidemic in the world requires special attention. Understanding the pathophysiological role of leptin and insulin resistance may help address the problem.

In summary, the association between leptin and insulin resistance was demonstrated irrespective of obesity levels. Further, significant higher level of leptin was found in insulin resistant subjects compared to the subjects without the condition at the same level of obesity in both gender. This finding may provide an insight into the explanation why the metabolic risk was different among persons with same degree of adiposity and may help identify the people at risk for diabetes and/or cardiovascular diseases across adiposity level and thereby an important contribution in clinical and preventive measures.

Acknowledgments

We are sincerely grateful to the CHNS project initiated by the Carolina Population Center at the University of North Carolina at Chapel Hill and the National Institute of Nutrition and Food Safety at the China CDC. Also, we thank all of the study participants and their families, and the entire study team for their valuable contributions.

Author Contributions

Conceived and designed the experiments: HZ ZS AH. Performed the experiments: HZ ZS BY YD GW. Analyzed the data: HZ. Contributed reagents/materials/analysis tools: HZ. Wrote the paper: HZ.

References

1. Caballero B (2007) The Global Epidemic of Obesity: An Overview. Epidemiologic Reviews 29: 1–5.
2. Laddu D, Dow C, Hingle M, Thomson C, Going S (2011) A Review of Evidence-Based Strategies to Treat Obesity in Adults. Nutrition in Clinical Practice 26: 512–525.
3. Haslam DW, James WPT (2005) Obesity. The Lancet 366: 1197–1209.
4. Meyer MR, Clegg DJ, Prossnitz ER, Barton M (2011) Obesity, insulin resistance and diabetes: sex differences and role of oestrogen receptors. Acta Physiologica 203: 259–269.
5. Mantzoros CS (1999) The role of leptin in human obesity and disease: a review of current evidence. Ann Intern Med 130: 671–680.
6. Zhang YY, Proenca R, Maffei M, Barone M, Leopold L, et al. (1994) Positional cloning of the mouse obese gene and its human homologue. Nature 372: 425–432.
7. Halaas JL, Gajiwala KS, Maffei M, Cohen SL, Chait BT, et al. (1995) Weight-Reducing Effects of the Plasma Protein Encoded by the Obese Gene. Science 269: 543–546.
8. Lapidus L, Bengtsson C, Larsson B, Pennert K, Rybo E, et al. (1984) Distribution of adipose tissue and risk of cardiovascular disease and death: a 12 year follow up of participants in the population study of women in Gothenburg, Sweden. British Medical Journal 289: 1257–1261.
9. Mahabir S, Baer D, Johnson LL, Roth M, Campbell W, et al. (2007) Body Mass Index, percent body fat, and regional body fat distribution in relation to leptin concentrations in healthy, non-smoking postmenopausal women in a feeding study. Nutr J 6: 3.
10. Considine RV, Sinha MK, Heiman ML, Kriauciunas A, Stephens TW, et al. (1996) Serum immunoreactive leptin concentrations in normal-weight and obese humans. New England Journal of Medicine 334: 292–295.
11. Mally K, Trentmann J, Heller M, Dittmar M (2011) Reliability and accuracy of segmental bioelectrical impedance analysis for assessing muscle and fat mass in older Europeans: a comparison with dual-energy X-ray absorptiometry. European Journal of Applied Physiology 111: 1879–1887.
12. Haapala I, Hirvonen A, Niskanen L, Uusitupa M, Kroger H, et al. (2002) Anthropometry, bioelectrical impedance and dual-energy X-ray absorptiometry in the assessment of body composition in elderly Finnish women. Clinical Physiology and Functional Imaging 22: 383–391.

13. Ruige JB, Dekker JM, Blum WF, Stehouwer CD, Nijpels G, et al. (1999) Leptin and variables of body adiposity, energy balance, and insulin resistance in a population-based study. The Hoorn Study. Diabetes Care 22: 1097–1104.
14. Nakhjavani M, Esteghamati A, Tarafdari AM, Nikzamir A, Ashraf H, et al. (2011) Association of plasma leptin levels and insulin resistance in diabetic women: a cross-sectional analysis in an Iranian population with different results in men and women. Gynecological Endocrinology 27: 14–19.
15. Monti V, Carlson JJ, Hunt SC, Adams TD (2006) Relationship of Ghrelin and Leptin Hormones with Body Mass Index and Waist Circumference in a Random Sample of Adults. Journal of the American Dietetic Association 106: 822–828.
16. Mente A, Razak F, Blankenberg S, Vuksan V, Davis AD, et al. (2010) Ethnic Variation in Adiponectin and Leptin Levels and Their Association With Adiposity and Insulin Resistance. Diabetes Care 33: 1629–1634.
17. Ruhl CE, Everhart JE (2001) Leptin concentrations in the United States: relations with demographic and anthropometric measures. American Journal of Clinical Nutrition 74: 295–301.
18. Hu FB, Chen C, Wang B, Stampfer MJ, Xu X (2001) Leptin concentrations in relation to overall adiposity, fat distribution, and blood pressure in a rural Chinese population. International Journal of Obesity 25: 121–125.
19. Esteghamati A, Khalilzadeh O, Anvari M, Rashidi A, Mokhtari M, et al. (2009) Association of Serum Leptin Levels With Homeostasis Model Assessment-Estimated Insulin Resistance and Metabolic Syndrome: The Key Role of Central Obesity. Metabolic Syndrome and Related Disorders 7: 447–452.
20. Huang KC, Lin RCY, Kormas N, Lee LT, Chen CY, et al. (2004) Plasma leptin is associated with insulin resistance independent of age, body mass index, fat mass, lipids, and pubertal development in nondiabetic adolescents. International Journal of Obesity 28: 470–475.
21. Panahloo A, MohamedAli V, Pinkney J, Goodrick S, Coppack S, et al. (1997) Relationships between plasma leptin and insulin concentrations, but not insulin resistance, in non-insulin dependent diabetes mellitus. Diabetes 46: 1340–1340.
22. Ceddia RB, Koistinen HA, Zierath JR, Sweeney G (2002) Analysis of paradoxical observations on the association between leptin and insulin resistance. FASEB J 16: 1163–1176.
23. Reseland JE, Mundal HH, Hollung K, Haugen F, Zahid N, et al. (2005) Cigarette smoking may reduce plasma leptin concentration via catecholamines. Prostaglandins Leukot Essent Fatty Acids 73: 43–49.

24. Popkin BM, Du S, Zhai F, Zhang B (2010) Cohort Profile: The China Health and Nutrition Survey-monitoring and understanding socio-economic and health change in China, 1989–2011. International Journal of Epidemiology 39: 1435–1440.

25. Bei-Fan Z (2002) Predictive values of body mass index and waist circumference for risk factors of certain related diseases in Chinese adults: study on optimal cut-off points of body mass index and waist circumference in Chinese adults. Asia Pac J Clin Nutr 11 Suppl 8: S685–693.

26. Alberti KGMM, Zimmet P, Shaw J (2005) The metabolic syndrome–a new worldwide definition. The Lancet 366: 1059–1062.

27. Deurenberg-Yap M, Schmidt G, van Staveren WA, Deurenberg P (2000) The paradox of low body mass index and high body fat percentage among Chinese, Malays and Indians in Singapore. International Journal of Obesity 24: 1011–1017.

28. Matthews DR, Hosker JP, Rudenski AS, Naylor BA, Treacher DF, et al. (1985) Homeostasis model assessment: insulin resistance and beta-cell function from fasting plasma glucose and insulin concentrations in man. Diabetologia 28: 412–419.

29. Zhao W, Hasegawa K, Chen J (2006) The use of food-frequency questionnaires for various purposes in China. Public Health Nutrition 5: 829–833.

30. Yang Y (2005) Chinese Food Composition Table 2004. Beijing: Peking University Medical Press. 351 p.

31. Zuo H, Shi Z, Yuan B, Dai Y, Hu G, et al. (2012) Interaction between physical activity and sleep duration in relation to insulin resistance among non-diabetic Chinese adults. BMC Public Health 12: 247.

32. Wang Z, Zhuo Q, Fu P, Piao J, Tian Y, et al. (2010) Are the associations of plasma leptin and adiponectin with type 2 diabetes independent of obesity in older Chinese adults? Diabetes/Metabolism Research and Reviews 26: 109–114.

33. Esteghamati A, Khalilzadeh O, Ashraf H, Zandieh A, Morteza A, et al. (2010) Physical activity is correlated with serum leptin independent of obesity: results of the national surveillance of risk factors of noncommunicable diseases in Iran (SuRFNCD-2007). Metabolism 59: 1730–1735.

17

Effects of Selective and Non-Selective Glucocorticoid Receptor II Antagonists on Rapid-Onset Diabetes in Young Rats

Jacqueline L. Beaudry[1], Emily C. Dunford[1], Trevor Teich[1], Dessi Zaharieva[1], Hazel Hunt[2], Joseph K. Belanoff[2], Michael C. Riddell[1]*

1 School of Kinesiology and Health Science, Faculty of Health, Muscle Health Research Center and Physical Activity and Chronic Disease Unit, York University, Toronto, Ontario, Canada, 2 Corcept Therapeutics, Menlo Park, California, United States of America

Abstract

The blockade of glucocorticoid (GC) action through antagonism of the glucocorticoid receptor II (GRII) has been used to minimize the undesirable effects of chronically elevated GC levels. Mifepristone (RU486) is known to competitively block GRII action, but not exclusively, as it antagonizes the progesterone receptor. A number of new selective GRII antagonists have been developed, but limited testing has been completed in animal models of overt type 2 diabetes mellitus. Therefore, two selective GRII antagonists (C113176 and C108297) were tested to determine their effects in our model of GC-induced rapid-onset diabetes (ROD). Male Sprague-Dawley rats ($\sim$ six weeks of age) were placed on a high-fat diet (60%), surgically implanted with pellets containing corticosterone (CORT) or wax (control) and divided into five treatment groups. Each group was treated with either a GRII antagonist or vehicle for 14 days after surgery: CORT pellets (400 mg/rat) + antagonists (80 mg/kg/day); CORT pellets + drug vehicle; and wax pellets (control) + drug vehicle. After 10 days of CORT treatment, body mass gain was increased with RU486 (by $\sim$20% from baseline) and maintained with C113176 administration, whereas rats given C108297 had similar body mass loss ($\sim$15%) to ROD animals. Fasting glycemia was elevated in the ROD animals ($>$20 mM), normalized completely in animals treated with RU486 (6.2 ± 0.1 mM, $p<0.05$) and improved in animals treated with C108297 and C113176 (14.0 ± 1.6 and 8.8 ± 1.6 mM, $p<0.05$ respectively). Glucose intolerance was normalized with RU486 treatment, whereas acute insulin response was improved with RU486 and C113176 treatment. Also, peripheral insulin resistance was attenuated with C113176 treatment along with improved levels of β-cell function while C108297 antagonism only provided modest improvements. In summary, C113176 is an effective agent that minimized some GC-induced detrimental metabolic effects and may provide an alternative to the effective, but non-selective, GRII antagonist RU486.

Editor: Jan Peter Tuckermann, University of Ulm, Germany

Funding: This study was funded by Corcept Theraputics and the Natural Sciences and Engineering Research Council of Canada (NSERC) grant to MCR. JLB is a recipient of an NSERC-Canadian Graduate Scholarship Doctoral Award. The funders had no role in data collection or analysis. The funders did help to prepare the manuscript for submission.

Competing Interests: HH and JB are employees of Corcept Theraputics, which develops glucocorticoid receptor ligands for clinical use. Corcept Theraputics provided the antagonists for this study and financed part of the experiments.

* E-mail: mriddell@yorku.ca

Introduction

Glucocorticoids (GCs) are naturally occurring steroid-derived hormones that are essential for healthy whole-body metabolism and adaptation to stressful environments. The hypothalamic-pituitary-adrenal (HPA) axis is the main regulator of GC secretion (cortisol in humans and corticosterone in rodents), operating normally in a diurnal rhythm and in response to stressors to increase GC release [1]. GCs act as ligands and bind to receptors including GC receptors II (GRII) that are found ubiquitously throughout the body. The mineralocorticoid receptor (MR) also binds GCs with high affinity [2], but expression of this receptor is lower than GRII in most tissues except for in the hippocampus, kidneys, adipose tissue and heart [3] and plays a larger role in non-stressful conditions. Once the GRII is occupied by a ligand, the complex translocates to the nucleus where it acts as a transcription factor to activate or repress the expression of genes necessary for cell proliferation, inflammation, immune development, reproduction [4] and energy homeostasis [5,6].

Acute elevations in GCs are important for many biological functions; however, chronically high levels of GCs, such as those observed in patients suffering from Cushing's syndrome [7], result in unwanted metabolic disturbances such as attenuated lean tissue growth [8], increased whole body insulin resistance [9], elevated fasting glucose levels [10] and increased risk for type 2 diabetes mellitus (T2DM) development [11–13]. Currently, there are a large number of rodent [14–16] and human [17,18] studies suggesting that the rise in circulating and/or cellular levels of GCs is connected with diabetes onset. At the cellular level, the pre-receptor enzyme, 11β-hydroxysteroid dehydrogenase type 1 (11β-HSD1) is responsible for conversion of inactive GCs into active GCs. This activity increases GC concentrations leading to the progression of tissue specific metabolic dysfunction [19] and, if left untreated, T2DM development [20]. GRII antagonists have become an active area of interest as they may eliminate unwanted metabolic effects of elevated GCs.

Mifepristone (RU486) is a non-selective GRII antagonist that competitively blocks the GRII, the progesterone receptor (PR), but not the MR [21]. This receptor antagonist has recently gained FDA approval (Korlym[TM], 2012) for the treatment of patients with hypercortisolemia or Cushing's syndrome with established hyperglycemia, since it has been shown clinically to improve glucose tolerance in these patients [22–24]. However, RU486 treatment requires consistent patient monitoring as it can result in various side effects such as endometrial hypertrophy, hypokalemia, and aborted pregnancy [21,25]. Currently, more specific antagonists selective for the GRII are being developed in the hope of eliminating the progesterone blocking properties of RU486 administration. A few studies of selective GRII antagonists have been conducted in rodent models [26–28]. In these studies, selective GRII antagonists have been shown to play a role in the attenuation of detrimental GRII-dependent pathways in the brain [26], whole-body steady state glucose metabolism [27], and body mass gain [28]. However, no studies in this field have been conducted to investigate the role of selective GRII antagonists in a model of elevated GCs indicative of Cushing's syndrome and diabetes development.

Recently, we have developed a rodent model of rapid-onset diabetes (ROD) that involves the administration of increased levels of GCs by a slow release corticosterone pellet in combination with a high-fat diet (HFD) in young male Sprague-Dawley rats [29,30]. We are interested in the effects of GRII antagonists on ROD and hypothesized that this therapeutic treatment will help to prevent ROD development. In this present study, we tested two selective GRII antagonists, C113176 and C108297, in comparison to the non-selective GRII antagonist, RU486, in our established rodent model of ROD. We show that a new selective GRII antagonist, C113176, has beneficial effects in our model of ROD, attenuating the pathophysiological outcomes of elevated GCs and high-fat feeding, including perturbed body composition, elevated fasting glucose concentrations, insulin resistance and reduced insulin release by pancreatic β-cells.

Materials and Methods

This study was carried out in accordance with the recommendations of the Canadian Council for Animal Care guidelines and was approved by the York University Animal Care Committee (Protocol # 2010-15(R2)). All surgical procedures were performed under isoflurane anaesthesia, and all efforts were made to minimize animal suffering.

Rodent Treatment and Experimental Design

Three sets of 20 male Sprague Dawley rats (Charles River Laboratories, 225–250 g, six weeks post-weaned) were individually housed (lights on 12 h: lights off 12 h cycle) after one week of acclimatization to the rodent facilities. Upon surgery day (day 0), each rat received a subcutaneous implantation of either corticosterone (CORT) pellets (4×100 mg; Sigma, Canada, Cat # C2505) or wax (control) pellets, as previously described [29]. Immediately following surgery all rats were given *ad libitum* access to a high-fat diet (HFD), 60% of the total calories from fat and 5.1 kcal per gram of pellet (D12492, Research diets); this diet was maintained to the end of the experimental protocol. Rats recovered in sterile cages for two days and were then separated into five groups while being maintained on a HFD and were

assigned either vehicle or GRII antagonist treatment (RU486, C113176 and C108297) at a dose of 80 mg/kg/day. These antagonists have been partially characterized with respect to binding efficiencies to GR, MR, PR, androgen receptor (AR), and estrogen receptor (ER) in human HepG2 and Rat H4 cells (Table 1). The compounds RU486, C113176 and C108297 have been shown to readily distribute into liver, adipose tissue, and brain tissue and to have similar pharmacokinetic profiles (Communications with Corcept Therapeutics). The antagonist dose was chosen based on doses used in earlier studies [27]. The following treatment groups were created; wax+ vehicle gavage controls (controls), CORT+vehicle (ROD), CORT+RU486 (RU486), CORT+C108297 (C108297), CORT+C113176 (C113176). All antagonists were first dissolved in DMSO which was further dissolved in a vehicle consisting of 0.5% HPMC + 0.1% Tween 80 by approximately 30 seconds of sonication. ROD animals who were given only vehicle received 10% DMSO + vehicle instead of an antagonist compound. Antagonists and vehicles were administered with a syringe and oral gavage tube (Instech, Plymouth, PA USA, Cat # FTP-18-75) twice daily, approximately 10 hours apart. Body mass and food intake were measured and recorded daily for each rodent using an electronic scale (Mettler Toledo, Canada) and any changes in the rodents' health were noted and monitored.

Blood Sampling

Plasma CORT levels were sampled on the morning of the 7th and 14th day after pellet implantation at approximately 0800 h, using the animal's saphenous vein. Blood samples were collected in lithium-heparin coated microvette capillary tubes (Sarstedt, Des Grandes Prairies, Montreal, Québec, Canada, Cat # 16.443.100) and centrifuged at 12,000 rpm for 5 minutes so that the plasma could be collected into polyethylene tubes and stored at −80°C until further analysis. These samples were later analyzed for CORT levels using a radioimmunoassay kit (MP Biomedical, OH, USA).

Fed whole blood glucose concentrations were measured on day seven using a handheld glucometer (Bayer, Contour, NY, USA). On day 11, animals were fasted overnight (16 hours) and on day 12, animals were administered an oral glucose tolerance test (OGTT, 1.5 g/kg body mass). An insulin tolerance test (ITT) was administered on day 16 after an overnight fast by intraperitoneal

Table 1. Binding affinities (Ki) and TAT activity assay data for RU486, C108297 and C113176 to GR, MR, PR, AR, and ER in hepatocytes.

	Compounds		
	RU486	C108297	C113176
GR	0.09 nM	0.28 nM	0.26 nM
MR	5.5 μM	0% @ 10 μM	20% @ 10 μM
PR	1 nM	26% @ 10 μM	0% @ 10 μM
AR	15 nM	12% @ 10 μM	2% @ 10 μM
ER	392 nM	3% @ 10 μM	37% @ 10 μM
Human HepG2	3 nM	25 nM	11 nM
Rat H4	2 nM	14 nM	4 nM

Note: The Ki in human HepG2 and rat H4 cells were calculated based on the IC50 data from TAT assay using dexamethasone treatment. Data provided by Corcept Therapeutics Incorporated.

(i.p.) insulin injection, (as described in [29,30]). For these tests, all blood glucose concentrations were also measured with a handheld glucometer and blood samples drawn from saphenous vein were collected in microvette tubes (Sarstedt). The animals' plasma was subsequently analyzed for insulin (Crystal Chem, IL, USA, Cat # 90060) using the high-range assay method and for non-esterified fatty acids (NEFA) levels (HR Series NEFA-HR, Wako Chemicals). Glucose area under the curve (AUC) and insulin AUC was measured relative to each individual's fasting insulin levels (i.e. each groups baseline) to assess the groups' responsiveness to oral glucose challenge. The acute insulin response (AIR) to oral glucose challenge was determined by the difference between basal (fasting) insulin levels and insulin levels 15 minutes following an oral glucose gavage (as described in [30,31]). This measurement represents the ability of the pancreatic β-cells to respond to exogenous glucose load. The glucose AUC measured during the ITT was determined by the net inverse relationship between the individual fasting and 30-minute blood glucose post insulin injection.

Homeostatic Model Assessment for Insulin Resistance (HOMA-IR) was calculated as previously reported in [29] and is based on the following equation: Glucose (mM)×Insulin (μ units·L)/22.5 [32]. This calculation represents basal glucose and insulin action on peripheral tissues, and primarily reflects the relationship between hepatic glucose output and insulin secretion [33]. Homeostatic Model Assessment for β-cells (HOMA-β) was calculated based on the following equation: 20×Insulin (μ units·L)/Glucose (mM)-3.5 [32]. This measurement represents basal pancreatic β-cell function in response to basal glucose levels.

For technical and experimental reasons, the day of termination ranged from 2–5 days after the ITT to allow for subsequent tissue collection. Trunk blood was collected for further analysis. Tissues collected from animals euthanized via decapitation were as follows: liver, heart, epididymal fat pads, and skeletal muscles such as epitrochlearis, soleus, gastrocnemius and tibialis anterior.

Histology

Liver and skeletal muscle tissue from euthanized animals were snap frozen, cryosectioned (10 μm thick) and stained with Oil Red O for neutral lipid content as previously described [34]. Muscle and liver sections were fixed with 3.7% formaldehyde for 1 h at room temperature while an Oil Red O solution composed of 0.5 g Oil Red O powder (Sigma-Aldrich, Canada) and 100 ml of 60% triethyl phosphate (Sigma-Aldrich, Canada) was mixed and filtered. Following fixation in 3.7% formaldehyde, slides were immersed in filtered Oil Red O solution for 30 minutes at room temperature. Slides immediately underwent five washes with ddH2O, were allowed to dry for 10 minutes and were sealed with Permount (Sigma-Aldrich, Canada). Skeletal muscle and liver images were acquired at 10× and 20× magnifications respectively using a Nikon Eclipse 90i microscope (Nikon, Canada) and Q-imaging MicroPublisher 3.3 RTV camera with Q-capture Software. Intensity of Oil Red O staining of IMCL droplets on serial sections of the tibialis anterior was assessed with Adobe Photoshop CS6, converted to greyscale and reported as the average optical density (60 fibers were counted per muscle section). The greyscale is evaluated on a range of 0 (completely black) to 255 (completely white).

Western Blotting

We quantified protein expression for key determinants of adipose tissue metabolism including CD36, adipose tissue triglyceride lipase (ATGL), hormone sensitive lipase (HSL) and 11β-HSD1. Western blot analysis was carried out according to previously published work [30,35]. In brief, 50 μgs of protein lysate from epididymal fat protein was run on a 10% (CD36, ATGL, HSL) or 12% (11β-HSD1) SDS-page gel and proteins were transferred to a PVDF membrane (Bio-Rad, Canada). Membranes were blocked in 10% powdered milk and Tris-buffered saline with Tween 20 at room temperature for 1 hour. Membranes were then incubated overnight at 4°C with their respective primary antibodies (CD36, 1:1000, ab133625, Abcam, Toronto, ON; ATGL, 1:500, sc-50223, Santa Cruz Biotechnology, Dallas, TX; HSL, 1:1000, sc-25843, Santa Cruz Biotechnology; 11β-HSD1, 1:1000, Cat#10004303, Cayman Chemical Company, Ann Arbor, MI;). The following morning the membranes were washed with TBST and incubated with anti-mouse (1:10000, Cat#ab6789, Abcam) or anti-rabbit (1:10000, Cat#ab6721, Abcam) secondary antibodies for 1 hour at room temperature. Membranes were then washed and imaged. Images were detected on a Kodak In vivo FX Pro imager and molecular imaging software (Carestream Image MI SE, version S.0.2.3.0, Rochester, New York) was used to quantify protein content. To minimize reprobing due similar molecular weights, α-tubulin (1:40000, ab7291, Abcam) was used as a loading control for 11β-HSD1 and HSL, and β-actin (1:20000, ab6276, Abcam) was used for CD36 and ATGL.

Glucose Stimulated Insulin Secretion (GSIS)

Islet isolations and *ex vivo* glucose challenges were carried out as previously reported [30]. Collagenase pancreas digestion was followed by Histopaque-1077 (H8889, Sigma, Canada) pellet suspension followed by re-suspension in KREB's buffer. Islets were handpicked and cultured in filtered RPMI buffer (Wisent) overnight (24 h) at 37°C, 5% CO2. Islets were separated into a 12-well culture plate (6–10 islets/well in 3 batches) and given a 30-minute pre-incubation period as previously described [30]. Islets were given fresh KREB's buffer with 2.8 mM glucose + 0.1% BSA for 1 hour at 37°C, 5% CO2. Media was changed to KREB's buffer with 16.7 mM glucose + 0.1% BSA for 1 hour at 37°C, 5% CO2. Immediately following each incubation period, media was collected, centrifuged and stored at −20°C for further analysis. Insulin was measured using a radioimmunoassay kit (Millipore, Billerica, MA, USA).

Statistical Analysis

All data are represented as a mean ± standard error (SE), with a criterion of p<0.05 and were assessed using one-way ANOVAs as a means of statistical significance. All individual differences were evaluated using Tukey's post-hoc test unless otherwise stated as a student's t-test (Statistica 6.0 software and Prism Graph Pad version 5.1). Results from post-hoc analyses were denoted on each figure bar using letters. If bars do not share the same letters then mean values were found to be statistically significant between treatment groups. If bars share the same letter then mean values were found to not be statistically significant from each other.

Results

Body Mass

GC antagonist treatment commenced on day 2 of pellet treatment and body mass was measured every day relative to day 0 (pre-surgery) for 10 days. Animals weighed ~300–325 g prior to pellet surgery (Figure 1 shows the fold changes in mass over the 10 day period). ROD treatment resulted in ~15% body mass loss relative to pre-surgery mass and ~50% body mass difference compared to control animals 10 days after CORT treatment. In comparison, RU486 treatment increased body mass gain relative to ROD treated animals by day 4. Body mass continued to rise during the treatment period and ultimately resulted in ~20% mass gain over the 10 day period. It is suspected that because of the initial mass lost from day 0 to 2, RU486 treatment did not fully reverse body mass loss in CORT treated animals when compared to controls (final mass on day ten: 352.7±5.9 g, vs. 397.6±6.1 g, in the RU486 treated animals and control animals respectively, p<0.05, Figure 1B). C113176 treatment recovered body mass to pre-surgery levels by day 8 (mass on day 10, 317.6±3.8 g), whereas C108297 treatment resulted in an overall mass loss of ~15% (mass on day 10, 259.3±4.4 g), similar to the ROD animals (mass on day 10, 266.5±3.1 g, Figure 1B).

Corticosterone and Food Intake

Normally, circulating CORT concentrations follow a diurnal pattern in rodents and fluctuate from high levels in early evening hours (i.e. peak, ~2000 h) to low levels in early morning hours (i.e. basal, ~0800 h). In this study, blood was sampled on day 7 and on

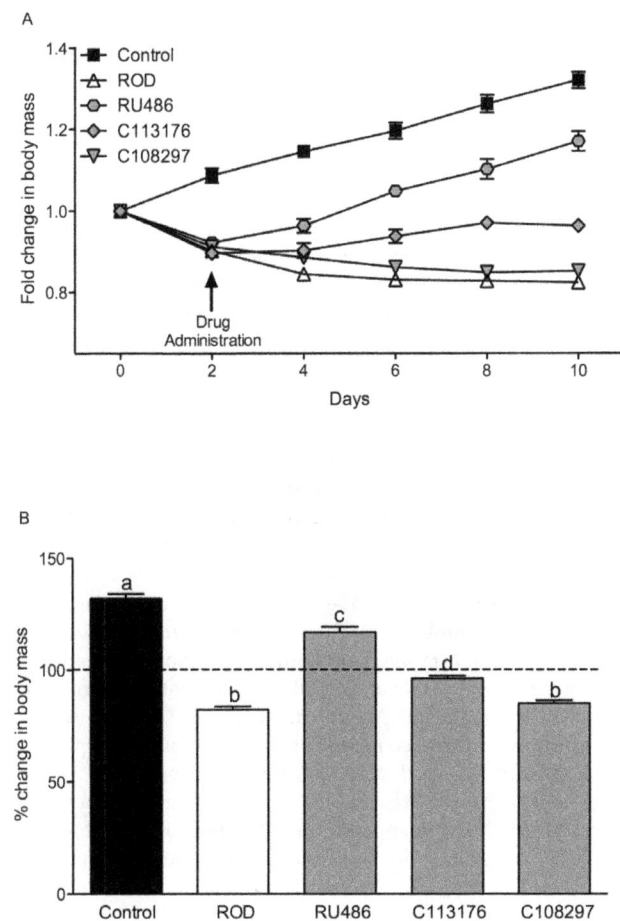

Figure 1. C113176 treatment maintains body mass while RU486 increases body mass with ROD treatment. Animal body mass (g) were recorded every two days for 10 days as a measure of fold change from day 0, pellet surgery (A). Animal body mass on day 10 was measured as a percent change of body mass from day 0 (B). The dotted line (100%) represents no change in body mass from day 0. Arrow indicates that 2 days after pellet surgeries respective antagonists or vehicle were administered at 80 mg/kg/day to each treatment group. Bars that do not share similar letters denote statistical significance, p<0.05, one-way ANOVA using Tukey's post-hoc test. n=7-10. All values are means ± SE.

day 14 at ~0800 h to determine basal CORT levels. Control animals had normal basal CORT levels on day 7 and day 14, values that were about 3-4-fold lower than all other treatment groups that received CORT pellets (p<0.05, Table 2). CORT pellet groups treated with ROD, RU486, C113176 and C108297 all had similar basal CORT levels at day 7 and 14 (p>0.05, i.e. not significant, Table 2).

Food intake was measured on day 10 of pellet treatment. ROD treated animals had an increase in absolute food intake compared to controls (p>0.05, Table 2). RU486 treated animals had the highest absolute food intake compared to all other groups (p<0.05, Table 2). Animals that were treated with C113176 or C108297 had similar absolute food intake to control animals (Table 2). Daily total kilocalorie intake relative to body mass was elevated in all CORT treated animals compared to controls (p<0.05); however, relative food intake was highest in ROD animals compared to all groups (p<0.05). Relative food intake was similar between RU486, C113176 and C108297 groups. Therefore, antagonist treatment lowered relative food intake compared to ROD animals but did not normalize food intake compared to the controls.

Hormone and Blood Analyses

Fed blood glucose concentrations were elevated in ROD animals compared to controls (p<0.05, Table 3). RU486 normalized fed blood glucose levels whereas C113176 and C108297 treated animals had similar levels compared to ROD treated animals (Table 3). All animals were fasted on the night of day 11 for ~16 h. Fasting blood glucose concentrations, measured the following day, were highest in ROD animals by ~4-fold compared to controls (p<0.05, Table 3). RU486 treatment normalized fasted glucose levels compared to controls, while C113176 treatment resulted in improved but not complete normalization of fasting blood glucose concentrations (Table 3). C108297 treated animals had significantly lower fasting blood glucose levels compared to ROD animals; however, they had fasting blood glucose levels that were also higher than controls and RU486 treated rats (p<0.05, Table 3). ROD, RU486, C113176 and C108297 treated rats had higher fasting insulin concentrations compared to controls (p<0.05, Table 3). However, RU486 treatment resulted in lower fasting insulin levels compared to ROD animals, or rats treated with C113176 or C108297 (p<0.05). Fasting NEFAs were measured on day 12, as high levels of free fatty acids are associated with an increased risk of diabetes [36]. ROD, C113176 and C108297 treated rats demonstrated ~2-fold increase in fasting NEFAs compared to controls (p<0.05, Table 3). In contrast, RU486 normalized fasting NEFA concentrations to levels found in control animals.

Glucose Tolerance and Insulin Response

An OGTT was performed on all animals on day 12 after an overnight fast to determine glucose tolerance and insulin response to exogenous glucose challenge (Figure 2A). The ROD group had the highest glucose concentrations throughout the OGTT challenge (Figure 2A) with a glucose AUC ~2-fold higher than controls (p<0.05, Figure 2A'). RU486 treatment normalized glucose tolerance, with results similar to those observed in the control group. C113176 treatment resulted in lower glucose levels compared to the ROD group (Figure 2A), but glucose AUC values in the animals treated with C113176 were still ~2-fold higher than those observed in the control group (p<0.05, Figure 2A'). Treatment with C108297 also lowered glucose levels compared to the ROD treated group, but glucose AUC was still ~2-fold higher than in control animals. All fasting and glucose-stimulated

Table 2. Corticosterone concentrations, absolute and relative food intake.

	Control		ROD		RU486		C113176		C108297	
	Day 7	Day 14	Day 7	Day 14	Day 7	Day 14	Day 7	Day 14	Day 7	Day 14
Corticosterone (ng/ml)	169 ± 50^a	61 ± 30^a	623 ± 38^b	537 ± 41^b	611 ± 61^b	401 ± 65^b	711 ± 63^{bc}	637 ± 58^b	442 ± 61^b	344 ± 60^b
	Day 10		Day 10		Day 10		Day 10		Day 10	
Food Intake (g)	20.9 ± 0.6^a		$24.0\pm1.2^{b*}$		26.3 ± 1.0^b		21.1 ± 1.3^a		20.3 ± 1.6^a	
Food Intake (kcal/g/BM)	0.23 ± 0.4^a		0.46 ± 0.02^b		0.40 ± 0.01^c		0.40 ± 0.02^c		0.40 ± 0.03^c	

Note: BM = Body Mass. Different letters denote statistical significance, $p < 0.05$, $n = 6$–10. The * indicates that a significant difference was performed by a student's unpaired t-test. All values are mean $\pm$ SE.

insulin levels were elevated in ROD treated animals compared to controls ($p < 0.05$, Figure 2B). Insulin AUC was measured during the OGTT to determine *in vivo* insulin response to exogenous glucose. ROD, C113176 and C108297 treated animals had a similar AUC compared to control animals and interestingly, RU486 treatment resulted in a ~3-fold increase in insulin AUC compared to controls ($p < 0.05$, Figure 2B'). Acute insulin response (AIR) was measured to determine insulin response at 15 minutes post oral glucose gavage. ROD animals had reduced AIR compared to all other groups ($p < 0.05$, Figure 2C). RU486 treatment resulted in ~3-fold increase in AIR compared to the values in the control group ($p < 0.05$), and C113176 treatment resulted in similar AIR levels to those observed with RU486 treatment, with higher AIR compared to animals in the control group (Figure 2C). Animals treated with C108297 showed no differences compared to control animals or ROD treated animals ($p > 0.05$).

Insulin Sensitivity, Insulin Resistance and β-Cell Function

To determine peripheral insulin sensitivity, primarily through skeletal muscle insulin action, an insulin tolerance test (ITT) was performed on all treatment groups. All of the values were plotted as a percent change from each individual's fasting blood glucose level (Figure 3A), since baseline glucose levels differed among the groups. Inverted glucose AUC was calculated as an index of insulin sensitivity (Figure 3A'). The ROD group had the lowest insulin sensitivity (Figure 3A'), while all three antagonists resulted in normalized insulin sensitivity when compared to controls (Figure 3A'). To determine insulin resistance as measured primarily by liver insulin action, the HOMA-IR index was used. ROD animals were ~40 and 30-fold more insulin resistant than control animals and RU486 treated groups, respectively ($p < 0.05$, Figure 3B). RU486 treated animals were more insulin resistant than control animals (by~2-fold). However, they were less insulin

resistant than the ROD and the selective GRII antagonist treated groups. C113176 and C108297 treated animals showed attenuated increases in insulin resistance when compared to ROD animals. However, these treatment groups remained more insulin resistant than control animals and RU486 treated animals ($p < 0.05$, Figure 3B). The HOMA-β index was used to determine β-cell function; higher values indicate elevated β-cell response to basal glucose concentrations. No differences were found between ROD animals and control treated animals. Both RU486 and C113176 treatments improved β-cell function by ~5-fold compared to all other groups ($p < 0.05$, Figure 3C). C108297 treatment did not significantly impact the HOMA-β index. It is important to note that HOMA-β represents basal β-cell function and although ROD animals did not show differences between the controls they do have impaired β-cell response to glucose (Figure 2C), and they clearly do not provide adequate insulin levels to reverse hyperglycemia in either the fasted or fed state.

Body Composition

Relative visceral fat mass was represented by the measured amount of isolated epididymal fat pad mass divided by body mass. All treatment groups had increased relative visceral fat mass compared to the control group ($p < 0.05$, Table 4). No differences in fat mass were found between the groups treated with the antagonists. Liver mass was also increased in all treatment groups compared to controls ($p < 0.05$) except for animals treated with RU486, in which liver mass was normalized (Table 4). Heart mass was increased with ROD and C108297 treatment and normalized with RU486 treatment. Animals treated with C113176 showed slight improvements compared to control animals ($p < 0.05$, Table 4). It is known that CORT treatment specifically impairs white muscle growth [37]. As expected, ROD animals had lower epitrochlearis mass compared to all other treatment groups ($p < 0.05$). All groups that were administered an antagonist did

Table 3. Fed and fasting glucose, insulin, and non-esterified fatty acids (NEFAs) levels on day 12.

	Control	ROD	RU486	C113176	C108297
Fed Blood Glucose (mM)	6.6 ± 0.2^a	20.6 ± 1.4^b	9.5 ± 1.3^a	20.7 ± 1.3^b	23.6 ± 2.3^b
Fasted Blood Glucose (mM)	4.8 ± 0.2^a	21.0 ± 0.6^b	6.2 ± 0.1^{ac}	8.8 ± 1.6^c	14.0 ± 1.6^d
Fasted Insulin (ng/ml)	0.85 ± 0.16^a	6.75 ± 0.58^b	3.64 ± 0.15^c	6.46 ± 1.04^b	5.22 ± 0.73^b
Fasted NEFAs(mM)	0.45 ± 0.03^a	1.08 ± 0.07^b	0.49 ± 0.05^a	1.10 ± 0.15^b	1.06 ± 0.12^b

Note: Different letters denote statistical significance, $p < 0.05$, $n = 6$–10. All values are means $\pm$ SE.

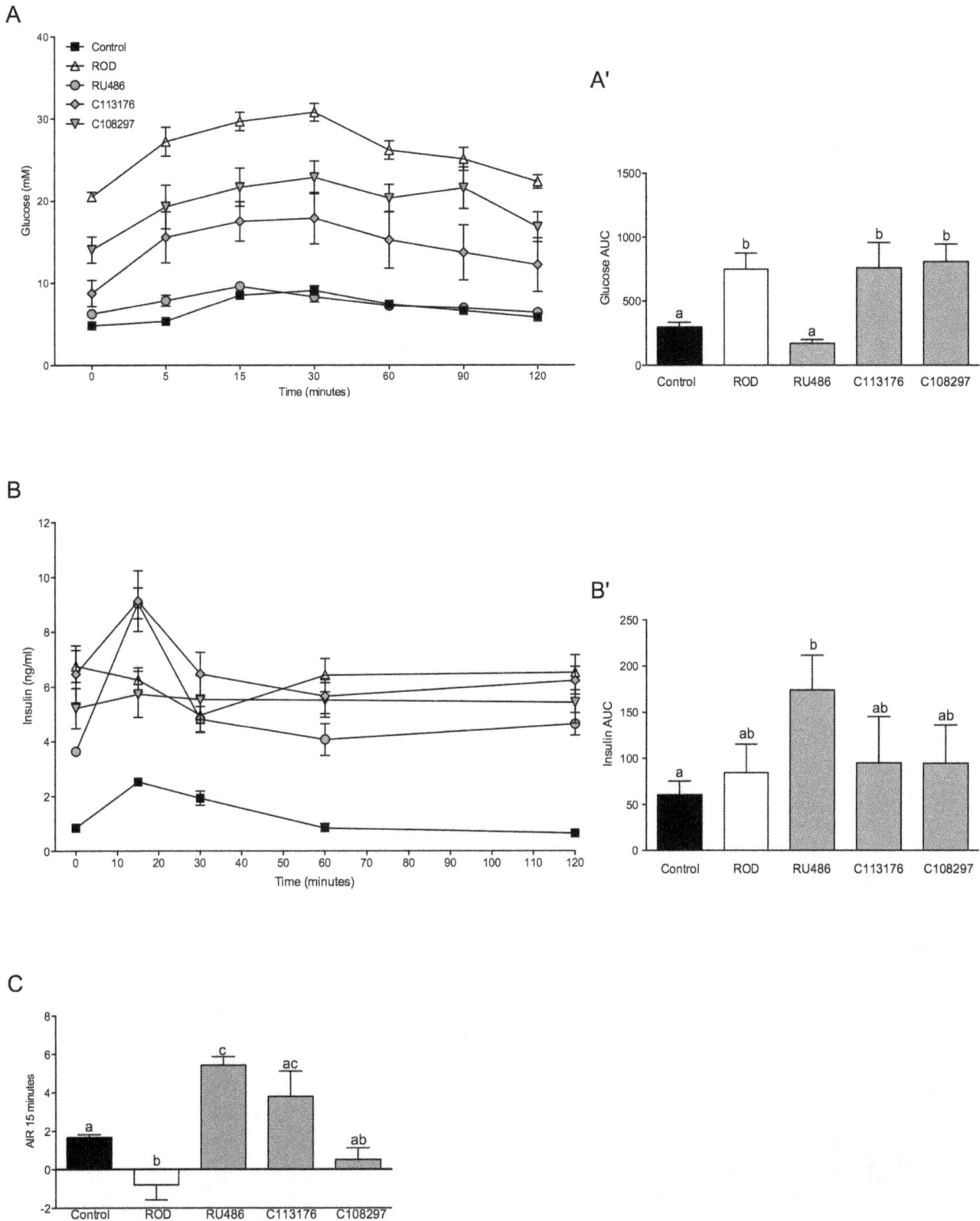

Figure 2. Glucose intolerance and acute insulin response (AIR) is improved with RU486 and C113176 treatment. Fasting (basal, 0 minutes) and stimulated blood glucose levels (mM) were measured at 5, 15, 30, 60, 90 and 120 minutes post oral glucose gavage (A). Glucose area under the curve (AUC) was calculated based on fasting blood glucose of individual animals (A'). Fasting (basal, 0 minutes) and glucose-stimulated insulin levels (ng/ml) were measured at 15, 30, 60, and 120 minutes post oral glucose gavage (B). Insulin area under the curve (AUC) was calculated based on fasting individual insulin levels within each group (B'). To measure insulin capacity acute insulin response (AIR) was measured by the difference in insulin levels between fasting insulin and 15 minutes post glucose gavage (C). Negative values represent a decrease in insulin response, indicating impairment in insulin secretion. Bars that do not share similar letters denote statistical significance, $p < 0.05$, one-way ANOVA using Tukey's post-hoc. A student's unpaired t-test was performed between controls and ROD, C108297 and C113176 groups (C). $n = 7–10$. All values are means $\pm$ SE.

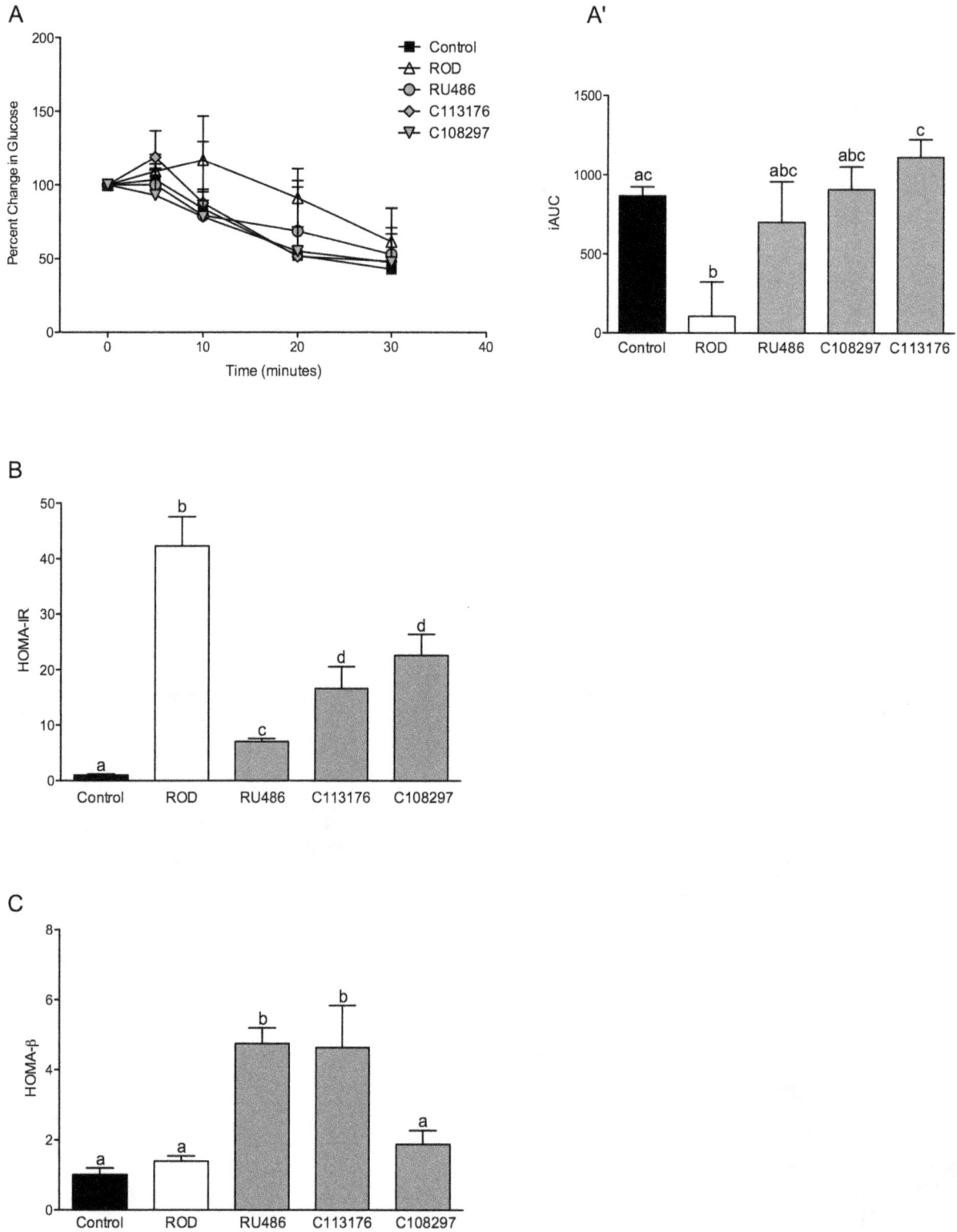

Figure 3. Peripheral insulin sensitivity and β-cell function is enhanced with RU486 and C113176 administration. Percent change of blood glucose levels (mM) relative to individual fasting blood glucose at 5, 10, 20 and 30 minutes post insulin i.p. injection using a handheld glucometer (A). The glucose AUC was measured by the net inverse glucose AUC during the ITT (A'). HOMA-IR index was used to measure whole-body insulin resistance (B). HOMA-β index was used to measure pancreatic β-cell function (C). Bars that do not share similar letters denote statistical significance, $p < 0.05$ one-way ANOVA using Tukey's post-hoc test. n = 7–10. All values are means ± SE.

not show changes in muscle mass relative to the animals in the control group (Table 4). The soleus muscle primarily consists of red, slow twitch muscle fibers and has been previously shown to increase with ROD treatment [29], although the mechanisms for this change remain unknown. ROD animals demonstrated an increase in soleus muscle mass (p<0.05, Table 4) whereas RU486 treated animals only had a slight trend towards an increase in soleus muscle mass compared to control animals (p>0.05, Table 4). There were no differences between tibialis anterior muscle mass among the various treatment groups (Table 4).

Fat Accumulation in Muscle and Liver

Oil Red O staining of liver and tibialis anterior muscle sections was used to quantify fat accumulation in all treatment groups. ROD treatment increased red stain in muscle tissue and appearance of lipid droplets in liver tissue compared to controls (Figure 4). RU486 was the only antagonist that promoted normalized lipid accumulation in both the liver and type IIa muscle fibers relative to controls animals (115.76±10.12 vs. 127.3±4.74, arbitrary units). The animals treated with the selective antagonists (C113176 and C108297) had similar ectopic lipid accumulation compared to ROD treated animals (144.52±3.17, 144.9±2.62, and 142.58±7.44 vs. 141.58±2.98, n = 3–4 per group).

Protein Content in Visceral Fat

At the tissue level, inactive GCs become activated by the action of the pre-receptor enzyme 11β-HSD1, which acts to convert inactive GCs into active GCs. Recent studies have shown that inhibition of 11β-HSD1 activity helps to reverse metabolic pathological conditions such as T2DM [38]. ROD treatment resulted in ~4-fold increase in 11β-HSD1 content in epididymal fat compared to controls (p<0.05, Figure 5). RU486, but not C113176 nor C108293, treatment normalized levels of 11β-HSD1 content in epididymal fat (p<0.05). CD36 is a protein known to regulate fatty acid uptake into the adipose tissue [39]. ROD treatment increased CD36 protein content by ~3-fold (p<0.05) but no changes were found in protein content amongst the groups treated with the antagonists (Figure 5B). ATGL and HSL are well known markers of lipolysis that modulate the release of fatty acids from triglyceride storage [35]. ROD, RU486, C113176 and C108297 treated groups, all had increased ATGL protein content compared to controls (all p<0.05), and no differences were found between the antagonist treated groups (Figure 5C). Finally, ROD and all other antagonist treated groups tended to have higher HSL protein levels relative to controls, but these difference from control failed to reach statistical significance (all p>0.05, Figure 5D).

GSIS (Glucose Stimulated Insulin Secretion)

Pancreatic islets were isolated from all animals and insulin secretion was stimulated by an exogenous glucose challenge. ROD treatment resulted in an elevation in GSIS in both low (2.8 mM) and high (16.7 mM) glucose media concentrations compared to controls (p<0.05, Figure 6). RU486 and C113176 normalized GSIS in low and high glucose media concentrations compared to controls. C108297 treatment resulted in similar levels as ROD treatment that had higher GSIS in high glucose media compared to control animals (p<0.05) with similar levels of GSIS compared to ROD treated islets.

Discussion

This study is the first to investigate the effectiveness of selective and non-selective GRII antagonists in a rodent model of ROD induced by GCs and HFD. We show that of the tested compounds, C113176 treatment is the more effective selective GRII antagonist as it attenuates elevated fasting glucose, reinstates β-cell function, and improves insulin resistance. The other selective antagonist tested in this study, C108297, also provides modest attenuation in hyperglycemia and peripheral insulin resistance and no changes to insulin response *in vivo* or β-cell function in this ROD model despite increased *ex vivo* β-cell response. However, by comparison, the non-selective antagonist RU486 demonstrated superior effectiveness in this animal model of hyperglucocorticoidemia/diabetes, completely normalizing all abnormal features of growth and metabolism. Nonetheless, the new selective antagonist C113176 may be of some therapeutic advantage for treatment of the metabolic features of hyperglucocorticoidemia/diabetes since it does not bind to the progesterone receptor.

Elevated GCs induce a severe state of hypercatabolism that can lead to drastic metabolic complications, such as muscle wasting, low bone density and inhibited structural growth [7]. GCs can also act in an anabolic fashion, promoting increased food intake and body fat deposition, especially in the abdominal region, thereby increasing an individual's risk for the development of diabetes [7]. We have previously reported that ROD treatment decreases overall body mass (~50%) but increases visceral adiposity compared to control animals [29]. In the present study, we show that RU486 treatment reverses body mass loss caused by ROD treatment, increasing body mass gain by ~20% compared to pre-surgery mass (Fig. 1A and B). Previous results show that RU486 and C108297 treatment lower body mass gain in C57BL/6J mice consuming a HFD and given access to 11% sucrose for 4 weeks [27]. An obese phenotype is also alleviated with RU486 [28,40–42] and C108297 [42] in other rodent and human models of

Table 4. Anthropometric data for epididymal fat pad, liver, heart, epitrochlearis, soleus and tibialis anterior mass (g/kg of body mass).

	Control	ROD	RU486	C113176	C108297
Epididymal Fat Pad (g/kg)	15.9±0.7[a]	25.0±1.7[b]	26.3±0.7[b]	26.4±1.6[b]	23.3±1.5[b]
Liver (g/kg)	38.3±1.1[a]	74.0±3.5[b]	43.1±2.8[a]	62.8±4.5[b]	73.4±4.8[b]
Heart (g/kg)	2.6±0.1[a]	4.1±0.2[b]	2.9±0.1[a]	3.6±0.1[c]	4.0±0.1[bc]
Epitrochlearis (g/kg)	0.13±0.01[a]	0.09±0.01[b]	0.13±0.01[a]	0.11±0.01[ab]	0.14±0.02[a]
Soleus (g/kg)	0.34±0.01[a]	0.45±0.03[b]	0.38±0.02[ab]	0.41±0.02[b]	0.44±0.02[b]
Tibialis Anterior (g/kg)	1.61±0.05[a]	1.51±0.08[a]	1.54±0.04[a]	1.88±0.06[a]	1.55±0.07[a]

Note: Different letters denote statistical significance, p<0.05, n = 6–10. All values are means ± SE.

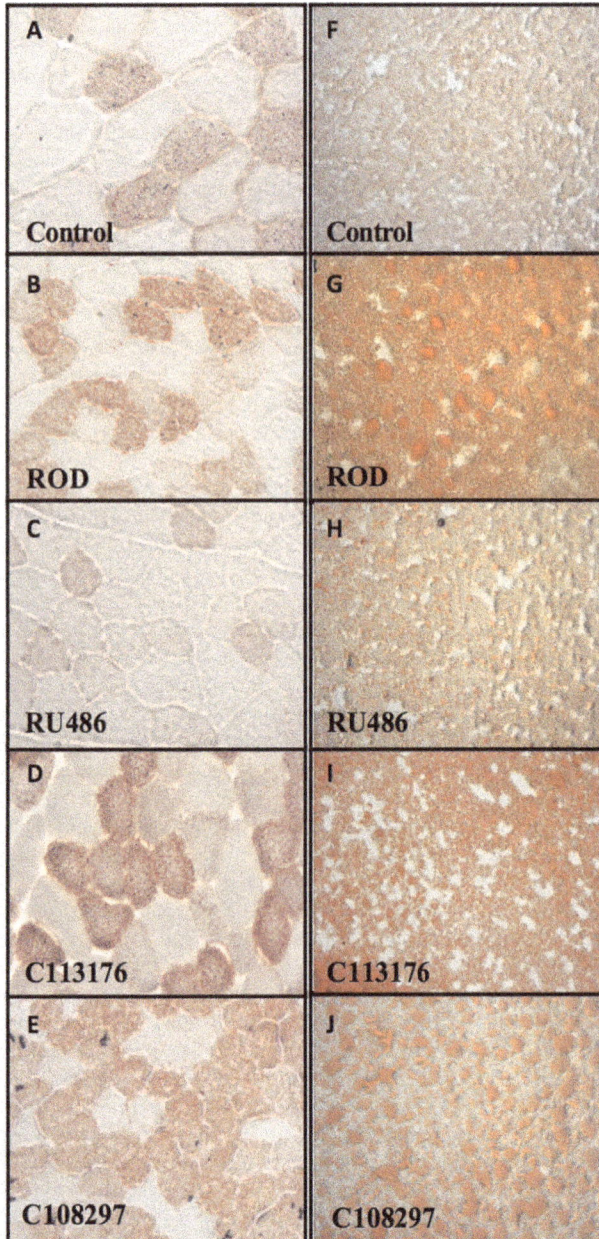

Figure 4. Fat accumulation is normalized with RU486 in skeletal muscle and liver cross sections. To determine fat content in skeletal muscle, tibialis anterior muscle was dissected and stained with a neutral lipid stain (Oil Red O) (A–E). Cross sections of liver were also stained with Oil Red O to measure lipid content (F–J).

disease. However, to our knowledge, C113176 administration in animals with elevated GCs who are consuming a high fat diet has never before been reported. We demonstrate in this study that C113176 antagonism restores pre-surgery body mass at day 8 of treatment and animals continue to maintain a healthy body mass until the termination of the study. In contrast, C108297 treatment promoted mass loss similar to that observed in untreated ROD animals, a finding that could be considered detrimental in this particular animal model of severe cachexia. In other studies, C108297 has been shown to decrease mass gain in C57BL/6J mice [27] as well as in rats treated with olanzapine, an anti-psychotic medication associated with weight gain in rodents and

humans [42]. Body composition analysis was not reported in these studies to determine if the drug influenced lean or fat mass or both. Therefore, C113176 antagonism might be an appropriate treatment for body mass management in humans with Cushing's syndrome because C108297 did not prevent body mass loss.

RU486 has been used to effectively treat metabolic disturbances and hypertension in patients with Cushing's syndrome [24]. It is readily absorbed, has a half-life up to 48 hours, and has a greater binding affinity to GRII than GC agonists such as dexamethasone (3 to 4 times) and cortisol itself (18 times) [43–45]. The potent blockade of the GRII with RU486 administration interrupts GC negative feedback to the HPA axis, which could have an effect on corticosterone levels. In our study, there were no differences in CORT AM levels between ROD and antagonist treated animals (Table 2). This finding is not surprising as our model of ROD administers exogenous GCs via CORT pellets at a level that already inhibits HPA axis negative feedback and reduces adrenal GC production [29]. It can therefore be concluded that the results of the antagonists on whole-body metabolism are not due to differences in CORT levels as these were unchanged by the antagonists. It is known that increased levels of stress hormones not only promote hyperphagia [29], but also influence food choice decisions towards higher caloric foods [46]. In this study, ROD treatment resulted in increased relative food intake compared to control animals and the GRII antagonist treated groups. Our study confirms that relative food intake is lower with the administration of GRII antagonists, as has been reported for RU486 treatment in rodents on a HFD [47] and in humans with Cushing's syndrome [24,40]. In addition, RU486 treatment in obese fa/fa rats with increased levels of circulating GCs, results in lower food intake [48] while no alterations in feeding are found in lean rats given the antagonist [49]. Moreover, studies investigating the effects of selective GRII antagonists on weight gain show no differences in food intake in healthy rodents despite decreases in body mass gain [28]. Taken together, these results suggest that GRII antagonism helps limit hyperphagia in Cushing's syndrome and in diabetic animals.

RU486 administration improves glycemic control and insulin sensitivity in rodents given HFD for 4 weeks [27] and lowers glycated hemoglobin levels in patients with Cushing's syndrome who often exhibit poor glycemic control [24]. In our study, we show that RU486 administration results in normalized glycemic control, and that C113176 lowers fasting glucose better than C108297, but does not improve glucose tolerance compared to ROD treated animals (Figure 2A and A'). Moreover, RU486 results in higher insulin AUC during oral glucose challenge suggesting an elevated insulin response to exogenous glucose, whereas the selective GRII antagonists show no effect on insulin secretion (Figure 2B'). Both RU486 and C113176 treatment resulted in higher AIRs to oral glucose challenge compared to the other treatment groups thereby suggesting that enhanced β-cell function occurs with GRII antagonism (Figure 2C). Animals treated with C108297 tended to have lower AIR compared to controls, suggesting poor β-cell sensitivity to exogenous glucose, similar to the effects seen in ROD animals. In accordance with these findings, we recently have shown that ROD treatment results in impaired islet glucose responsiveness in vivo and ex vivo, which likely exacerbates the poor glucose control caused by reduced insulin sensitivity [30]. Importantly, this present study suggests that the non-selective GRII antagonist RU486 reverses defective insulin responsiveness in vivo, which may help to explain normal glucose control in these treated animals. In addition, β-cell function in vivo, as assessed by HOMA-β, is improved with both RU486 and C113176 treatment but not with C108297 treatment

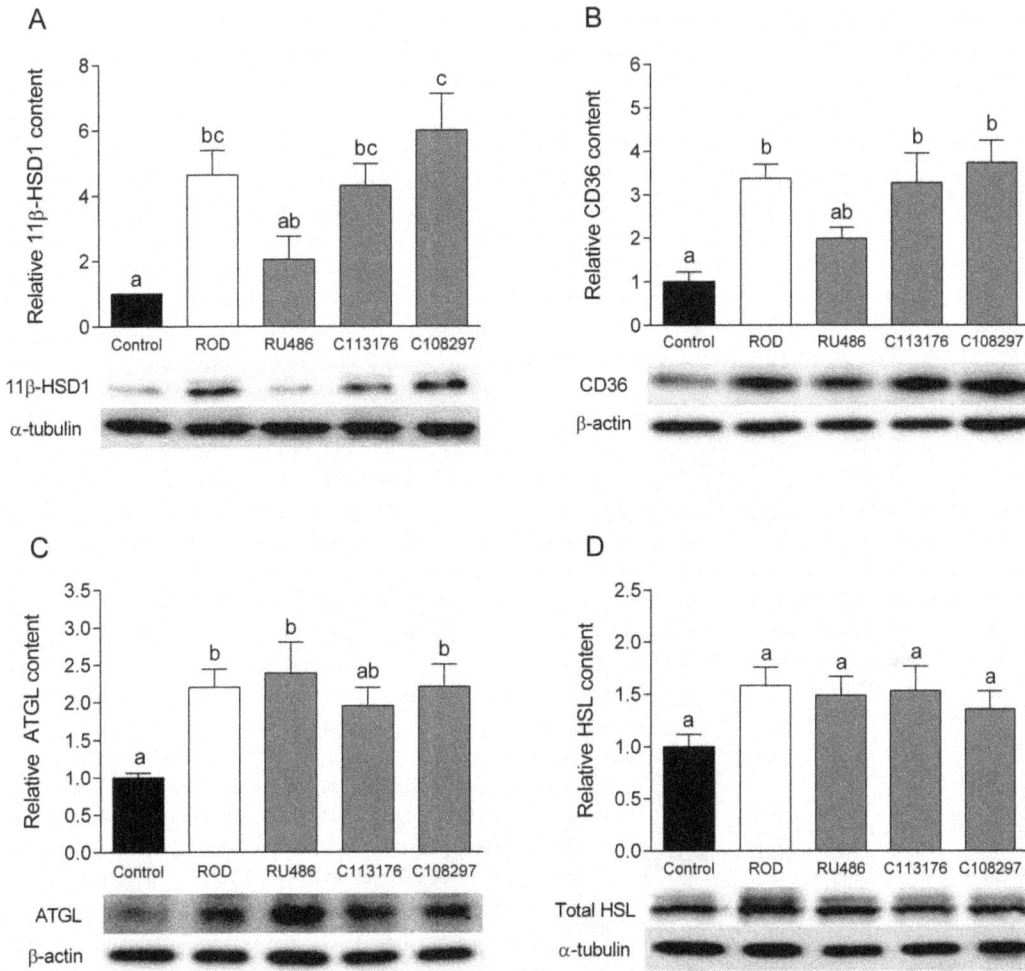

Figure 5. 11β-HSD1 content in visceral fat is attenuated with RU486 treatment but not with C113176 or C108297 treatment. No changes were found in lipolytic protein levels with treatment of antagonists. 11β-HSD1 content was measured in epididymal fat pads to represent visceral adipose tissue and expressed relative to α-tubulin content (A). CD36 protein levels were measured from epididymal fat pads (B) as well as adipose triglyceride lipase (ATGL) (C) and hormone-sensitive lipase (HSL) (D) protein levels as markers of lipolytic adipose tissue activity and expressed relative to loading control. Bars that do not share similar letters denote statistical significance, p<0.05 one-way ANOVA using Tukey's post-hoc test. n = 5–6. All values are means ± SE.

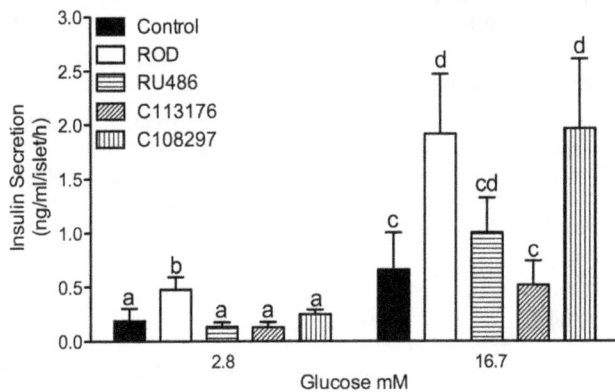

Figure 6. Glucose stimulated insulin secretion (GSIS) was normalized with RU486 and C113176 treatment. GSIS in isolated islets was measured in low (2.8 mM) and high (16.7 mM) glucose media for 1-hour incubations expressed as ng/ml/islet/hour. Bars that do not share similar letters denote statistical significance, p<0.05 one-way ANOVA using student's unpaired t-test. n = 3–7. All values are means ± SE.

(Figure 3C). Moreover, dynamic insulin responses to glucose challenge also appear enhanced by RU486 (Figures 2B′ and C). There are very few studies to date that investigate the effects of RU486 on β-cell function *in vivo* and to the best of our knowledge this study is the first to report on β-cell function *in vivo* with selective GRII antagonism. As such, it is possible to suggest that improvements to β-cell function *in vivo* are through exclusive inhibition of GRII as seen with C113176 administration. However, more investigations are required to fully understand the mechanisms of action with selective GRII antagonism.

Elevated GCs in rodents induce peripheral tissue abnormalities that affect liver and skeletal muscle insulin sensitivity/signalling, thereby promoting hyperglycemia [39,50,51]. In our study, we show that RU486, C113176 and C108297 normalize whole body insulin sensitivity (Figure 3A and A′) although C108297 was the only group that was statistically significant from the ROD group. The blockade of the GRII with RU486 helps to reduce peripheral insulin resistance in individuals with mild GC excess [52]. Our study confirms that insulin resistance, as measured by HOMA-IR was normalized with RU486 while attenuated with C113176 and

C108297 administration (Figure 3B). Liver and skeletal muscle lipid accumulation is elevated in ROD treated animals, ultimately contributing to peripheral insulin resistance [29,39]. Interestingly, only RU486 administration lowered both skeletal muscle and liver fat content compared to the ROD animals, with the other selective GRII antagonists having no noticeable effect (Figure 4). Therefore, more studies are required to investigate the mechanisms of action, especially with C113176 administration, on improving insulin resistance.

Patients with Cushing's syndrome have an increased risk of obesity, which heightens their risk (60–80%) of developing diabetes as the disease progresses [13]. Recent research shows that administration of RU486 results in normal body mass gain in rodents and in healthy men [40,41]. In addition, selective GRII antagonists such as C112716 and C113083 have been shown to help reverse olanzapine-induced mass gain in rats [28]. In our study we found that none of the GRII antagonists normalized the visceral adiposity that is readily observable in ROD treated animals (Table 4). We propose that it is likely that GRII antagonism inhibits GC-induced lipolysis [53,54] or off-target non-genomic effects that may indirectly increase GC tissue action [55], thereby promoting visceral adiposity. Moreover, increased 11β-HSD1 activity in adipose tissue has been linked to obese and/or insulin resistant individuals [56]. Our ROD model demonstrates increased 11β-HSD1 content in visceral fat compared to controls. RU486 attenuates 11β-HSD1 content (Figure 5), contradicting the idea that an increase in GC activity results in more visceral adiposity as RU486 treated animals had similar visceral adiposity to the ROD treated animals. Therefore, we propose that the increase in visceral adiposity with RU486 is due to the anti-lipolytic effects of increased insulin levels as all ROD treated groups had a higher level of insulin than controls (Table 4). Insulin is an anabolic hormone that down-regulates non-genomic actions of GCs (lipolysis) [54,57], thereby promoting increased adiposity. In support of this, we found that ROD treatment increases lipolytic enzyme protein content in visceral fat depots and none of the antagonists appeared to normalize these increases (Figure 5 B–D). Together these data suggest that although GRII antagonism does not lower visceral adiposity it may decrease lipolytic GC action in the adipose tissue of RU486 treated rats, in part indicating a lesser risk of developing adiposity-induced abnormalities.

Previously we have shown that ROD treatment results in increased islet 11β-HSD1 content as well as elevated GSIS in isolated islets [30]. RU486 administration to insulin secreting cells *in vitro* reverses β-cell dysfunction through improvements in insulin biosynthesis, release and content [58] as well as β-cell [Ca2+]i response to glucose [59]. Our study confirms these results as we show that RU486 and C113176 normalize GSIS compared to controls whereas C108297 has similar GSIS compared to ROD animals (Figure 6). This is the first study to report the effects of selective GRII antagonists on *ex vivo* islet GSIS. We observe that

C113176 is an effective antagonist on GC action in the islet and it normalizes GSIS whereas C108297 does not demonstrate the same result. More studies are required *in vitro* to replicate and further investigate the mechanisms of C113176 action on GSIS.

It is evident that GCs play a critical role in regulating whole body physiology [60] and reducing their action, if concentrations are too elevated, can help eliminate some unwanted effects. Although RU486 binds to the GRII with high affinity (0.3 nM) it also binds with high affinity to the progesterone receptor, resulting in endometrial wall thickening causing early disruption to pregnancy in females (reviewed in, [21]). Therefore, selective GRII antagonists have a major advantage over non-selective antagonists and presently there is a significant effort underway to find replacements for non-selective GRII blockers [61]. More experiments need to be completed before the best antagonist is identified but in our study we consistently see that one compound, C113176, attenuate diabetes symptoms. The advantage of C113176 is that it binds to the GRII with excellent affinity (0.28 nM) and does not bind significantly to ER, AR, PR or MR (Table 1). It has been found to be more potent than C108297 in functional TAT (tyrosine amino transferase) *in vitro* assays that measure inhibition of dexamethasone-induced activity in HepG2 cells and ratH4 cells (Corcept Therapeutics Inc.). For example, in HepG2 cells, the Ki values for C108297 and C113176 are 25 and 11 nM, and in rat H4 cells, the Ki values are 14 and 4 nM, respectively (Table 1). Compounds such as C108297 are described as having some beneficial effects in inhibiting GC action. However, C108297 does not completely reverse adverse GC effects in our ROD model. Perhaps, as previously described [26], this antagonist may actually work as a partial agonist, which could account for some of the results presented.

This study describes the various metabolic and morphologic outcomes of administering selective and non-selective GRII antagonists to our rodent model of ROD. We show that in comparison to RU486, C113176 provides therapeutic advantages over C108297 in ROD animals. C113176 helps to attenuate fasting hyperglycemia, insulin resistance and improves AIR, and pancreatic β-cell response. It may be a reasonable alternative medication to help patients suffering from Cushing's syndrome and other diseases associated with elevated GCs. Although C113176 did not completely normalize all complications of diabetes, it did provide clear benefits without any observable adverse effects. Thus, C113176 may be a good alternative to the non-selective GRII antagonist RU486.

Author Contributions

Conceived and designed the experiments: JLB ECD HH MCR. Performed the experiments: JLB ECD DPZ TT. Analyzed the data: JLB ECD DPZ TT HH JB MCR. Contributed reagents/materials/analysis tools: HH JB MCR. Wrote the paper: JLB ECD MCR. Edited the manuscript: JLB ECD DPZ TT HH JB MCR.

References

1. Funder JW (1997) Glucocorticoid and mineralocorticoid receptors: Biology and clinical relevance. Annu Rev Med 48: 231–240.
2. De Kloet ER, Vreugdenhil E, Oitzl MS, Joels M (1998) Brain corticosteroid receptor balance in health and disease. Endocr Rev 19: 269–301.
3. Zhou J, Cidlowski JA (2005) The human glucocorticoid receptor: One gene, multiple proteins and diverse responses. Steroids 70: 407–417.
4. Rhen T, Cidlowski JA (2005) Antiinflammatory action of glucocorticoids–new mechanisms for old drugs. N Engl J Med 353: 1711–1723.
5. Andrews RC, Walker BR (1999) Glucocorticoids and insulin resistance: Old hormones, new targets. Clin Sci (Lond) 96: 513–523.
6. McMahon M, Gerich J, Rizza R (1988) Effects of glucocorticoids on carbohydrate metabolism. Diabetes Metab Rev 4: 17–30.
7. Shibli-Rahhal A, Van Beek M, Schlechte JA (2006) Cushing's syndrome. Clin Dermatol 24: 260–265.
8. Kelly HW, Sternberg AL, Lescher R, Fuhlbrigge AL, Williams P, et al. (2012) Effect of inhaled glucocorticoids in childhood on adult height. N Engl J Med 367: 904–912.
9. Schacke H, Docke WD, Asadullah K (2002) Mechanisms involved in the side effects of glucocorticoids. Pharmacol Ther 96: 23–43.
10. Nielsen MF, Caumo A, Chandramouli V, Schumann WC, Cobelli C, et al. (2004) Impaired basal glucose effectiveness but unaltered fasting glucose release and gluconeogenesis during short-term hypercortisolemia in healthy subjects. Am J Physiol Endocrinol Metab 286: E102–10.

11. Hoes JN, van der Goes MC, van Raalte DH, van der Zijl NJ, den Uyl D, et al. (2011) Glucose tolerance, insulin sensitivity and beta-cell function in patients with rheumatoid arthritis treated with or without low-to-medium dose glucocorticoids. Ann Rheum Dis 70: 1887–1894.

12. Lansang MC, Hustak LK (2011) Glucocorticoid-induced diabetes and adrenal suppression: How to detect and manage them. Cleve Clin J Med 78: 748–756.

13. Simmons LR, Molyneaux L, Yue DK, Chua EL (2012) Steroid-induced diabetes: Is it just unmasking of type 2 diabetes? ISRN Endocrinol 2012: 910905.

14. Chan O, Inouye K, Riddell MC, Vranic M, Matthews SG (2003) Diabetes and the hypothalamo-pituitary-adrenal (HPA) axis. Minerva Endocrinol 28: 87–102.

15. Matthews LC, Hanley NA (2011) The stress of starvation: Glucocorticoid restraint of beta cell development. Diabetologia 54: 223–226.

16. Wang Y, Nakagawa Y, Liu L, Wang W, Ren X, et al. (2011) Tissue-specific dysregulation of hexose-6-phosphate dehydrogenase and glucose-6-phosphate transporter production in db/db mice as a model of type 2 diabetes. Diabetologia 54: 440–450.

17. Anagnostis P, Athyros VG, Tziomalos K, Karagiannis A, Mikhailidis DP (2009) Clinical review: The pathogenetic role of cortisol in the metabolic syndrome: A hypothesis. J Clin Endocrinol Metab 94: 2692–2701.

18. Rosmond R (2005) Role of stress in the pathogenesis of the metabolic syndrome. Psychoneuroendocrinology 30: 1–10.

19. Stewart PM (1996) 11 beta-hydroxysteroid dehydrogenase: Implications for clinical medicine. Clin Endocrinol (Oxf) 44: 493–499.

20. Bujalska IJ, Draper N, Michailidou Z, Tomlinson JW, White PC, et al. (2005) Hexose-6-phosphate dehydrogenase confers oxo-reductase activity upon 11 beta-hydroxysteroid dehydrogenase type 1. J Mol Endocrinol 34: 675–684.

21. Johanssen S, Allolio B (2007) Mifepristone (RU 486) in cushing's syndrome. Eur J Endocrinol 157: 561–569.

22. Belavic JM (2013) Drug updates and approvals: 2012 in review. Nurse Pract 38: 24–42.

23. [Anonymous]. (2012) Mifepristone (korlym) for cushing's syndrome. Med Lett Drugs Ther 54: 46–47.

24. Fleseriu M, Biller BM, Findling JW, Molitch ME, Schteingart DE, et al. (2012) Mifepristone, a glucocorticoid receptor antagonist, produces clinical and metabolic benefits in patients with cushing's syndrome. J Clin Endocrinol Metab 97: 2039–2049.

25. Goldberg JR, Plescia MG, Anastasio GD (1998) Mifepristone (RU 486): Current knowledge and future prospects. Arch Fam Med 7: 219–222.

26. Zalachoras I, Houtman R, Atucha E, Devos R, Tijssen AM, et al. (2013) Differential targeting of brain stress circuits with a selective glucocorticoid receptor modulator. Proc Natl Acad Sci 110:7910–7915.

27. Asagami T, Belanoff JK, Azuma J, Blasey CM, Clark RD, et al. (2011) Selective glucocorticoid receptor (GR-II) antagonist reduces body weight gain in mice. J Nutr Metab 2011: 235389. 10.1155/2011/235389.

28. Belanoff JK, Blasey CM, Clark RD, Roe RL (2011) Selective glucocorticoid receptor (type II) antagonists prevent weight gain caused by olanzapine in rats. Eur J Pharmacol 655: 117–120.

29. Shpilberg Y, Beaudry JL, D'Souza A, Campbell JE, Peckett A, et al. (2012) A rodent model of rapid-onset diabetes induced by glucocorticoids and high-fat feeding. Dis Model Mech. doi:10.1242/dmm.008912

30. Beaudry JL, D'Souza A, Teich T, Tsushima R, Riddell MC (2013) Exogenous glucocorticoids and a high-fat diet cause severe hyperglycemia and hyperinsulinemia and limit islet glucose responsiveness in young male sprague-dawley rats. Endocrinology 154: 3197–3208.

31. Holness MJ, Smith ND, Greenwood GK, Sugden MC (2005) Interactive influences of peroxisome proliferator-activated receptor alpha activation and glucocorticoids on pancreatic beta cell compensation in insulin resistance induced by dietary saturated fat in the rat. Diabetologia 48: 2062–2068.

32. Wallace TM, Levy JC, Matthews DR (2004) Use and abuse of HOMA modeling. Diabetes Care 27: 1487–1495.

33. Hoffman RP (2008) Indices of insulin action calculated from fasting glucose and insulin reflect hepatic, not peripheral, insulin sensitivity in african-american and caucasian adolescents. Pediatr Diabetes 9: 57–61.

34. Koopman R, Schaart G, Hesselink MK (2001) Optimisation of oil red O staining permits combination with immunofluorescence and automated quantification of lipids. Histochem Cell Biol 116: 63–68.

35. Campbell JE, Peckett AJ, D'souza AM, Hawke TJ, Riddell MC (2011) Adipogenic and lipolytic effects of chronic glucocorticoid exposure. Am J Physiol Cell Physiol 300: C198–209.

36. Taskinen MR (2003) Diabetic dyslipidaemia: From basic research to clinical practice. Diabetologia 46: 733–749.

37. Roy RR, Gardiner PF, Simpson DR, Edgerton VR (1983) Glucocorticoid-induced atrophy in different fibre types of selected rat jaw and hind-limb muscles. Arch Oral Biol 28: 639–643.

38. Chrousos GP (2004) Is 11beta-hydroxysteroid dehydrogenase type 1 a good therapeutic target for blockade of glucocorticoid actions? Proc Natl Acad Sci U S A 101: 6329–6330.

39. D'souza AM, Beaudry JL, Szigiato AA, Trumble SJ, Snook LA, et al. (2012) Consumption of a high-fat diet rapidly exacerbates the development of fatty liver disease that occurs with chronically elevated glucocorticoids. Am J Physiol Gastrointest Liver Physiol 302: G850–863.

40. Gross C, Blasey CM, Roe RL, Allen K, Block TS, et al. (2009) Mifepristone treatment of olanzapine-induced weight gain in healthy men. Adv Ther 26: 959–969.

41. Beebe KL, Block T, Debattista C, Blasey C, Belanoff JK (2006) The efficacy of mifepristone in the reduction and prevention of olanzapine-induced weight gain in rats. Behav Brain Res 171: 225–229.

42. Belanoff JK, Blasey CM, Clark RD, Roe RL (2010) Selective glucocorticoid receptor (type II) antagonist prevents and reverses olanzapine-induced weight gain. Diabetes Obes Metab 12: 545–547.

43. Bourgeois S, Pfahl M, Baulieu EE (1984) DNA binding properties of glucocorticosteroid receptors bound to the steroid antagonist RU-486. EMBO J 3: 751–755.

44. Heikinheimo O, Kontula K, Croxatto H, Spitz I, Luukkainen T, et al. (1987) Plasma concentrations and receptor binding of RU 486 and its metabolites in humans. J Steroid Biochem 26: 279–284.

45. Sartor O, Cutler GB Jr (1996) Mifepristone: Treatment of cushing's syndrome. Clin Obstet Gynecol 39: 506–510.

46. Dallman MF (2003) Fast glucocorticoid feedback favors 'the munchies'. Trends Endocrinol Metab 14: 394–396.

47. Okada S, York DA, Bray GA (1992) Mifepristone (RU 486), a blocker of type II glucocorticoid and progestin receptors, reverses a dietary form of obesity. Am J Physiol 262: R1106–10.

48. Langley SC, York DA (1990) Effects of antiglucocorticoid RU 486 on development of obesity in obese fa/fa zucker rats. Am J Physiol 259: R539–44.

49. Taylor AI, Frizzell N, McKillop AM, Flatt PR, Gault VA (2009) Effect of RU486 on hepatic and adipocyte gene expression improves diabetes control in obesity-type 2 diabetes. Horm Metab Res 41: 899–904.

50. Friedman JE, Yun JS, Patel YM, McGrane MM, Hanson RW (1993) Glucocorticoids regulate the induction of phosphoenolpyruvate carboxykinase (GTP) gene transcription during diabetes. J Biol Chem 268: 12952–12957.

51. Vander Kooi BT, Onuma H, Oeser JK, Svitek CA, Allen SR, et al. (2005) The glucose-6-phosphatase catalytic subunit gene promoter contains both positive and negative glucocorticoid response elements. Mol Endocrinol 19: 3001–3022.

52. Debono M, Chadarevian R, Eastell R, Ross RJ, Newell-Price J (2013) Mifepristone reduces insulin resistance in patient volunteers with adrenal incidentalomas that secrete low levels of cortisol: A pilot study. PLoS One 8: e60984. doi:10.1371/journal.pone.0060984

53. Haller J, Mikics E, Makara GB (2008) The effects of non-genomic glucocorticoid mechanisms on bodily functions and the central neural system. A critical evaluation of findings. Front Neuroendocrinol 29: 273–291.

54. Peckett AJ, Wright DC, Riddell MC (2011) The effects of glucocorticoids on adipose tissue lipid metabolism. Metabolism 60: 1500–1510.

55. Spiga F, Harrison LR, Wood SA, Atkinson HC, MacSweeney CP, et al. (2007) Effect of the glucocorticoid receptor antagonist org 34850 on basal and stress-induced corticosterone secretion. J Neuroendocrinol 19: 891–900.

56. Deschoolmeester J, Palming J, Persson T, Pereira MJ, Wallerstedt E, et al. (2013) Differences between men and women in the regulation of adipose 11beta-HSD1 and in its association with adiposity and insulin resistance. Diabetes Obes Metab 15:1056–60.

57. Dallman MF, la Fleur SE, Pecoraro NC, Gomez F, Houshyar H, et al. (2004) Minireview: Glucocorticoids-food intake, abdominal obesity, and wealthy nations in 2004. Endocrinology 145: 2633–2638.

58. Linssen MM, van Raalte DH, Toonen EJ, Alkema W, van der Zon GC, et al. (2011) Prednisolone-induced beta cell dysfunction is associated with impaired endoplasmic reticulum homeostasis in INS-1E cells. Cell Signal 23: 1708–1715.

59. Koizumi M, Yada T (2008) Sub-chronic stimulation of glucocorticoid receptor impairs and mineralocorticoid receptor protects cytosolic Ca2+ responses to glucose in pancreatic beta-cells. J Endocrinol 197: 221–229.

60. van Raalte DH, Ouwens DM, Diamant M (2009) Novel insights into glucocorticoid-mediated diabetogenic effects: Towards expansion of therapeutic options? Eur J Clin Invest 39: 81–93.

61. Mohler ML, He Y, Wu Z, Hong SS, Miller DD (2007) Non-steroidal glucocorticoid receptor antagonists: The race to replace RU-486 for anti-glucocorticoid therapy. Expert Opin Ther Pat 17: 59–81.

18

The rs225017 Polymorphism in the 3′UTR of the Human *DIO2* Gene is Associated with Increased Insulin Resistance

Leonardo B. Leiria, José M. Dora, Simone M. Wajner, Aline A. F. Estivalet, Daisy Crispim*, Ana Luiza Maia

Thyroid Section, Endocrine Division, Hospital de Clínicas de Porto Alegre, Universidade Federal do Rio Grande do Sul, Porto Alegre, RS, Brazil

Abstract

The Thr92Ala (rs225014) polymorphism in the type 2 deiodinase (*DIO2*) gene has been associated with insulin resistance (IR) and decreased enzyme activity in human tissues but kinetic studies failed to detect changes in the mutant enzyme, suggesting that this variant might be a marker of abnormal *DIO2* expression. Thus, we aimed to investigate whether other *DIO2* polymorphisms, individually or in combination with the Thr92Ala, may contribute to IR. The entire coding-region of *DIO2* gene was sequenced in 12 patients with type 2 diabetes mellitus (T2DM). Potentially informative variants were evaluated in 1077 T2DM patients and 516 nondiabetic subjects. IR was evaluated using the homeostasis model assessment (HOMA-IR) index. *DIO2* gene sequencing revealed no new mutation but 5 previously described single nucleotide polymorphisms (SNPs). We observed that all T2DM patients displaying high HOMA-IR index (n = 6) were homozygous for the rs225017 (T/A) polymorphism. Further analysis showed that the median fasting plasma insulin and HOMA-IR of T2DM patients carrying the T/T genotype were higher than in patients carrying the A allele (P = 0.013 and P = 0.002, respectively). These associations were magnified in the presence of the Ala92Ala genotype of the Thr92Ala polymorphism. Moreover, the rs225017 and the Thr92Ala polymorphisms were in partial linkage disequilibrium ($|D'| = 0.811$; $r^2 = 0.365$). In conclusion, the rs225017 polymorphism is associated with greater IR in T2DM and it seems to interact with the Thr92Ala polymorphism in the modulation of IR.

Editor: Qingyang Huang, Central China Normal University, China

Funding: This study was supported by grants from Conselho Nacional de Desenvolvimento Científico e Tecnológico (CNPq), Coordenação de Aperfeiçoamento de Pessoal de Nivel Superior (CAPES) and Fundo de Incentivo a Pesquisa (FIPE), Brazil. The funders had no role in study design, data collection and analysis, decision to publish, or preparation of the manuscript.

Competing Interests: The authors have declared that no competing interests exist.

* Email: dcmoreira@hcpa.ufrgs.br

Introduction

Thyroid hormones are critical to the development, growth and metabolism of virtually all tissues [1,2]. The iodothyronine deiodinases types 1 (D1), 2 (D2) and 3 (D3) are selenoenzymes of the oxidoreductase family which catalyze iodine removal from the outer (D1 and D2) or inner (D1 and D3) ring of thyroid hormones. While D1 and D2 convert T4 to the metabolically active hormone T3, D3 inactivates both T4 and T3 [2]. In humans, D2 is the most important deiodinase for intracellular T3 generation in target tissues [1,2] and, together with D1, contributes for 80% of peripheral T3 [3]. The gene that encodes D2 (*DIO2*) is expressed in the thyroid, pituitary, brain, heart, placenta, skeletal muscle and adipocytes [4,5,6,7,8,9]. D2 activity is tightly regulated at transcriptional, post-transcriptional and post-translational levels [10,11], which thereby supports the hypothesis that this enzyme plays an important homeostatic role in metabolism.

Type 2 diabetes mellitus (T2DM) is a heterogeneous group of disorders usually characterized by varying degrees of insulin insufficiency and insulin resistance (IR), which result in increased blood glucose concentrations. Ultimately, IR results either from inappropriately increased hepatic gluconeogenesis or decreased glucose disposal rate in tissues such as skeletal muscle, adipose tissue and liver [12].

Glucose homeostasis may be affected by thyroid status [13,14]. Thyroid hormone affects insulin action in skeletal muscle and adipose tissue in part by upregulating the expression of the glucose transporter 4 (GLUT4) and, therefore, increasing glucose uptake [15,16]. An increase in both hepatic endogenous glucose disposal and insulin mediated-glucose uptake is observed in patients with hyperthyroidism when compared with euthyroid subjects [17,18,19]. In contrast, studies showed that, in hypothyroidism, there is a decrease in both glucose disposal [19] and insulin mediated-glucose uptake in muscle, and also an impaired ability of insulin to stimulate glucose disposal related to insulinaemia [19,20]. In animal models, experimental induction or spontaneous forms of thyroid dysfunction are also associated with impaired glucose tolerance [20]. Mice with targeted disruption of the *dio2* gene have higher insulin levels during glucose tolerance tests and reduced glucose uptake during insulin tolerance tests, consistent with the occurrence of IR [21]. According to these findings, it is plausible to postulate that a lower intracellular D2-generated T3 in skeletal muscle might create a state of relative intracellular hypothyroidism, decreasing the expression of genes involved in energy use, such as GLUT4, and thus resulting in increased IR.

Previous studies have demonstrated that polymorphisms in the *DIO2* gene might interfere in the phenotypic expression of D2 [7,22]. The *DIO2* single-nucleotide polymorphism (SNP), in which a threonine (Thr) changes to alanine (Ala) at codon 92 (Thr92Ala, rs225014, A/G), was associated with IR in obese white women and with a 20% lower glucose disposal rate in white non-diabetic women [23]. The Ala92Ala genotype was also associated with a more pronounced IR in patients with T2DM and the frequency of this variant allele was found to be increased in some ethnic groups, such as Pima Indians and Mexican-Americans, who have a higher prevalence of IR [23]. Even though some studies have failed to demonstrate an association between the Thr92Ala polymorphism and glycemic traits or T2DM [24,25,26], the association between this polymorphism and T2DM is supported by data reported in a recent systematic review and meta-analysis [27]. However, the mechanism by which this occurs is still not clear. Decreased D2 activity has been observed in human tissue biopsy samples [7,27] but studies failed to identify any changes in the *ex vivo* biochemical properties of the mutant enzyme [7,28], suggesting that this variant might be only a marker for abnormal *DIO2* expression. Here, we aimed to determine whether other SNPs in the *DIO2* gene, individually or in combination with the Thr92Ala polymorphism, contribute to the IR phenotype.

Materials and Methods

Ethics statement

The information obtained during the study did not affect the patients' diagnosis or treatment. The protocol was approved by the Committee on Research Ethics from Hospital de Clínicas de Porto Alegre, and all subjects signed an informed consent term. Clinical investigation was conducted according to the principles expressed in the Declaration of Helsinki.

Study population

In the first phase of this study, we used direct automated sequencing of the *DIO2* gene to search for SNPs in 12 T2DM patients with different degrees of IR. These 12 patients were selected from two subgroups in our T2DM population: 6 patients with a low HOMA-IR index (ranging from 0.32 to 1.3) and 6 patients with a high HOMA-IR index (6.2–23.4). The results generated by sequencing the *DIO2* gene in T2DM patients were compared with the sequences of the human *DIO2* gene available in GenBank (http://www.ncbi.nlm.nih.gov/genbank/).

In the second phase of the study, allele and genotype frequencies of a potentially informative *DIO2* variants found by sequencing were compared between 1077 patients with T2DM and 516 nondiabetic subjects. The criteria used to select the variant for further analysis were: 1) the polymorphism was not known to be a neutral variation; 2) it involved change between chemically different amino acids or was localized at regulatory regions, such as the promoter or 3'- untranslated region (3'UTR); 3) its frequency was not low (minor allele frequency less than 5% in the literature or GenBank); and 4) the frequency of the variant was different in the groups under analysis (in this case, low and high HOMA-IR groups) [29,30]. Additionally, haplotypes constructed from the combination of this polymorphism with the Thr92Ala polymorphism were analyzed regarding their effect on IR in T2DM patients.

The 1077 patients with T2DM were selected from a multicenter study that started recruiting patients in southern Brazil in 2002 and whose purpose was to investigate risk factors for T2DM and

its complications. Initially, it included 4 tertiary-teaching hospitals in the Brazilian state of Rio Grande do Sul, namely Grupo Hospitalar Conceição, Hospital São Vicente de Paula, Hospital Universitário de Rio Grande and Hospital de Clínicas de Porto Alegre. The detailed description of that study can be found elsewhere [31]. The group of subjects without diabetes was composed of 516 healthy volunteers who came to Hospital de Clínicas de Porto Alegre to donate blood.

Clinical and anthropometric profiles and laboratory analyses

A standard questionnaire was used to collect information from all patients about age, age at T2DM diagnosis and drug treatment. All patients with T2DM were white. The ethnic group was defined on the basis of self-classification and subjective classification (skin color, nose and lip shapes, hair texture and family history).

All T2DM patients underwent physical and laboratory evaluations. They were weighed (barefoot and wearing light outdoor clothing) and had their height measured. Body mass index (BMI) was calculated as weight (kg) divided by height squared (m^2). Blood pressure (BP) was measured twice, in the sitting position, with a 5-min rest between measurements, using a mercury sphygmomanometer (Korotkoff phases I and V). The mean of the two measurements was used to record systolic and diastolic BP. Arterial hypertension was defined as BP≥140/90 mmHg or use of antihypertensive drugs regardless of BP at the time of assessment.

Serum samples for laboratory tests were collected after a 12-h fast from all patients with T2DM. Glucose levels were determined by a glucose oxidase method; creatinine by the Jaffé reaction; glycated haemoglobin (A1C) by an ion-exchange HPLC procedure (Merck-Hitachi L-9100 glycated haemoglobin analyzer, Merck, Darmstadt, Germany; reference range: 2.7–6.0%); and total plasma cholesterol, HDL-cholesterol, and triglycerides, by enzymatic methods. LDL-cholesterol was calculated using the Friedewald equation. Serum insulin was measured by radioassay (Elecsys Systems 1010/2010/modular analytics E170, Roche Diagnostics, Indianapolis, IN). Insulin sensitivity was estimated by the HOMA-IR index [fasting insulin (milliunits per millilitre) x fasting glucose (millimoles per litre)/22.5] [32]. The mean HOMA-IR index of control subjects in our laboratory was 1.84±1.02 [33].

Molecular analysis

DNA was extracted from peripheral blood leukocytes by a standardized salting-out procedure. A search for variants of the *DIO2* gene was performed in 12 patients with T2DM by direct sequencing of all exons, partial intron sequences (500 bp of exon-intron junctions), and 5'UTR and 3'UTR sequences (1000 bp each, including the selenocysteine insertion sequence element - ESECIS - in the 3'UTR). Screening of this limited number of individuals may fail to detect some rarer polymorphisms; however, this number seems to be adequate to identify representative variants which are sufficiently polymorphic to warrant association studies. Direct sequencing in an automated ABI 3100 *Avant Genetic Analyzer* (Life Technologies, Foster City, CA, USA) was performed using ABI Prism Big Dye Terminator Cycle Sequence Ready reaction kit (Life Technologies) according to the manufacturers' recommendations, and using primers described in **Table S1**.

Potentially informative variants identified through the sequencing of the *DIO2* gene were selected for subsequent genotyping in all patients with T2DM and nondiabetic subjects. These SNPs, together with the rs225014 (Thr92Ala) polymorphism, were determined using primers and probes contained in Human

Custom TaqMan Genotyping Assays 40x (Assays-By-Design Service, Life Technologies). Sequences of primers and probes used for genotyping are shown in **Table S1**. Reactions were conducted in 96-well plates, at a total reaction volume of 5 μL and using 2 ng of genomic DNA, TaqMan Genotyping Master Mix 1x (Life Technologies), and Custom TaqMan Genotyping Assay 1x (Life Technologies). Plates were then placed in a real-time PCR thermal cycler (7500 Fast Real-Time PCR System, Life Technologies) and heated for 10 minutes at 95°C, followed by 45 cycles of 95°C for 15 seconds and 62°C for 1 minute. Fluorescence data files of each plate were analyzed using automated allele-calling software (SDS 2.1, Life Technologies).

Statistical analyses

Results are expressed as mean ± SD, % or median (minimum-maximum values). Allelic frequencies were determined by gene counting, and departures from the Hardy-Weinberg equilibrium (HWE) were investigated using chi-squared test. Linkage disequilibrium (LD) between the candidate polymorphism and the Thr92Ala polymorphism was examined using Lewontin's D′ |D′| and r^2 measures [34,35]. Haplotypes constructed from the combination of these *DIO2* polymorphisms and their frequencies were inferred using the Phase 2.1 program, which uses a Bayesian statistical method [35,36]. We also used this program to compare the distributions of *DIO2* haplotypes between patients with T2DM and nondiabetic subjects by permutation analyses of 1,000 random replicates [35].

Clinical and laboratory characteristics were compared using ANOVA, unpaired Student *t* test or chi-squared test, as appropriate. Variables with a skewed distribution were logarithmically transformed before analyses. To check if the candidate polymorphism was independently associated with T2DM, a multiple logistic regression analysis was performed with T2DM as the dependent variable and age, sex, and the possible informative polymorphism as independent variables. A linear regression analysis was performed to evaluate the independent association between the candidate polymorphism and IR parameters after adjusting for covariates (age, sex, BMI and use of T2DM medication). Haplotype interaction between the candidate polymorphism and the Thr92Ala polymorphism in modulating fasting insulin and HOMA-IR index was tested by general linear model univariate analyses (GLM), after adjusting for covariates (age, sex, BMI and use of T2DM medication). In these interaction analyses, each of the polymorphisms was modeled as a dichotomous variable.

All analyses were performed using the SPSS 18.0 (SPSS, Chicago, IL, USA). The level of statistical significance was set at P less than 0.05. Power calculations for the case-control study were done using the software PEPI, version 4.0, and showed that this study has a power of approximately 80% at a significance level of 0.05 to detect an OR of 1.35 or higher (for a 40% frequency of the minor allele).

Results

DIO2 screening and identification of candidate polymorphisms for association with insulin resistance

An interim study comprising samples of 12 patients with T2DM was used to search for polymorphisms in the *DIO2* gene. This first phase study identified 448 amplicons (data not shown). Although no new mutation was detected in the data set, 5 previously described SNPs were identified (**Figure 1**). These SNPs included two polymorphisms in the 5′ flanking region (rs199598135,

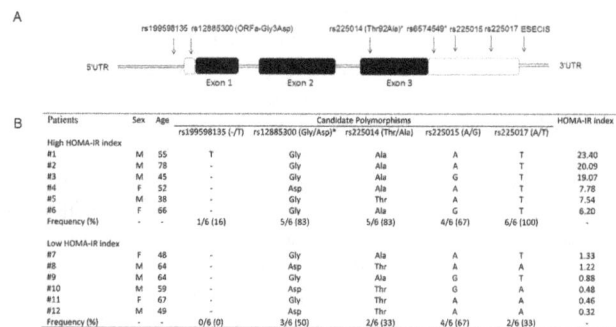

Figure 1. Candidate polymorphisms identified by sequencing of the *DIO2* gene. A. The vertical arrows show the five candidate variants in human *DIO2* gene identified through sequencing. Black boxes are coding regions. *polymorphisms associated with T2DM/IR/fasting insulin. ESECIS, Selenocysteine Insertion Sequence Element; 3′UTR = 3′-untranslated region. **B.** The characteristics of the 12 patients with T2DM selected for the screening of the *DIO2* gene. These patients had extreme HOMA-IR indexes and were selected from two subgroups according low or high HOMA-IR values.

rs12885300), one polymorphism in exon 3 (rs225014 - Thr92Ala), and two in the 3′UTR (rs225015, rs225017).

The characteristics of the 12 patients with T2DM selected for the screening of the *DIO2* gene, as well as the occurrence of the 5 *DIO2* polymorphisms identified in these patients are shown in **Figure 1**. We observed that the T/T genotype of the rs225017 (A/T) polymorphism was more frequent in patients with a high HOMA-IR index (6 in 6) than in patients with a low HOMA-IR index (2 in 6). Moreover, the relative frequency of this polymorphism for white subjects in GenBank was 0.36 whereas in our sample was 0.66 (P = 0.129). This polymorphism also fills the criteria for selecting an informative polymorphism (see Material and Methods Section) and was then selected for further analysis in an association study. The Thr92Ala polymorphism also fulfilled the above criteria; however, this polymorphism was already reported in our sample population as being associated with both T2DM risk [27] and increased IR and insulin levels [37]. Thus, in the present study, we aimed to evaluate whether haplotypes constructed from the combination of Thr92Ala polymorphism with the rs225017 polymorphism are associated with IR in T2DM patients.

The rs225017 variant and T2DM development in a case-control study

The baseline characteristics of the 1077 patients with T2DM and the 516 nondiabetic subjects included in the study were as follows: mean age was 59.2±10.1 years *vs.* 46.2±10.3 years (P< 0.001), and males comprised 47% and 63% of the sample (P< 0.001).

The T allele frequency of the rs225017 polymorphism did not differ significantly between patients with T2DM and nondiabetic subjects (0.51 *vs.* 0.48, P=0.196). In addition, genotypes frequencies of this polymorphism were similar between T2DM patients and nondiabetic subjects (25.9% A/A, 47.2% A/T, 26.9% T/T vs. 28.5% A/A, 46.9% A/T, 24.6% T/T; P=0.452). These findings did not change after logistic regression analysis adjusting for age and sex (OR=1.15, 95% CI=0.86–1.55; P=0.354). Genotype frequencies of the rs225017 polymorphism were in HWE in patients with T2DM and nondiabetic subjects (P>0.05).

Table 1. Clinical and laboratory characteristics of patients with T2DM broken down according to *DIO2* rs225017 (T/A) polymorphism.

| | Total (n = 1077) | Genotypes | | |
		A/A or A/T (n = 798)	T/T (n = 279)	P
Age (Years)	59.2±10.1	59.6±9.8	58.2±10.3	0.051
Duration of diabetes (Years)	11.7±8.8	12.1±9.0	10.5±7.9	0.009
Sex (% males)	47.0	49.0	42.0	0.038
BMI (kg/m²)	28.9±4.9	28.8±4.8	29.3±5.3	0.117
Total cholesterol (mmol/l)	5.4±1.2	5.4±1.2	5.5±1.2	0.419
Systolic BP (mm Hg)	141.9±23.2	141.9±23.7	141.8±21.8	0.953
Diastolic BP (mm Hg)	85.0±12.8	84.8±12.7	85.6±13.1	0.823
HDL cholesterol (mmol/l)	1.17±0.3	1.17±0.3	1.16±0,3	0.753
LDL cholesterol (mmol/l)	1.29±1.1	1.29±1.1	1.31±1.1	0.533
Serum creatinine (μmol/l)[a]	102.8 (35.4–937)	81.4 (26.5–937)	79.6 (35.4–540)	0.127
Triglycerides (mmol/l)[a]	2.00 (0.3–13.2)	2.00 (0.3–13.2)	1.99 (0.5–8.7)	0.821
Fasting plasma glucose (mmol/l)	9.4 (2.9–21.9)	9.3 (2.9–21.9)	9.8 (3.3–20.5)	0.144
SU/Met/SU + Met (%)	32.5/38.5/16.5	31.1/36.0/14.3	34.8/45.9/22.9	0.249/0.027/0.015
A1C (%)	7.2±2.0	7.1±2.0	7.3±1.8	0.343
Fasting insulin (UI/ml)[a,b]	13.9 (1–46.1)	10.6 (1–44.9)	15.7 (3.2–46.1)	0.005
HOMA–IR index[a,b]	3.8 (0.3–20.1)	3.5 (0.3–19.5)	5.2 (0.6–20.1)	0.005

Data are mean ± SD, median (minimum - maximum values) or %. A1C, glycated haemoglobin; BMI, body mass index; HOMA-IR, homeostasis model assessment - insulin resistance; Met, metformin; SU, sulfonylureas; WHR, waist-to-hip ratio; P values were estimated by χ^2 or ANOVA, as appropriate.
[a]Variables which were logarithmically transformed before analyses.
[b]For comparisons of fasting insulin levels and HOMA-IR index among rs225017 genotypes, we analyzed only 227 individuals (162 individuals harboring the A/A or A/T genotypes and 65 individuals harboring the T/T genotype).

The rs225017 DIO2 polymorphism is associated with insulin resistance in patients with T2DM

Table 1 summarizes the clinical and laboratory characteristics of patients with T2DM grouped according to the different genotypes of the rs225017 polymorphism. Assuming a recessive model of inheritance, patients with A/A or A/T genotypes were grouped and compared with patients carrying the T/T genotype. T2DM duration (P = 0.009), sex proportion (P = 0.038) and use of metformin alone (P = 0.027) or metformin + sulfonylurea (P = 0.015) for treatment of T2DM were differentially distributed between patients with the T/T genotype and A allele carriers. It is worth mentioning that none of the variables showed in **Table 1** attained statistical significance when assuming dominant (A/A *vs.* A/T-T/T) or additive (A/A *vs.* T/T) models of inheritance (data not shown).

A subgroup of 227 patients with T2DM who were not receiving insulin was further analyzed for IR measurements. This subgroup was representative of the whole sample: mean age was 59.3±9.3 years (P = 0.803 for the comparison with the whole sample), mean T2DM duration was 11.2±8.2 years (P = 0.580), mean A1C was 7.3±1.7% (P = 0.12), and mean BMI was 28.9±4.7 kg/m² (P = 0.89). Males comprised 45.3% (n = 103) of the sample (P = 0.45).

In this subgroup of patients, median fasting plasma insulin levels were higher in patients with the T/T genotype than in patients carrying the A allele [15.71 (3.2–46.1) *vs.* 10.57 (1–44.9), P = 0.005], whereas fasting plasma glucose levels did not differ significantly between groups (P = 0.144). Moreover, T/T genotype patients showed a higher HOMA-IR index than patients carrying the A allele [5.20 (0.6–20.1) *vs.* 3.50 (0.3–19.5), P = 0.005]. Because insulin sensitivity is known to be affected by multiple

independent factors, multiple linear regression analyses were performed with HOMA-IR index ($\log_{10}$ HOMA-IR) or insulin level ($\log_{10}$ fasting insulin) as dependent variables. The T/T genotype of the rs225017 polymorphism remained significantly associated with HOMA-IR [standardized coefficient B for T/T genotype $= -0.366$, 95% CI $(-0.654--0.078)$; P = 0.013] and insulin levels [standardized coefficient B for T/T genotype $= -0.268$, 95% CI $(-0.441--0.096)$; P = 0.002], after adjusting for age, sex, BMI and use of medication for T2DM (mainly metformin or sulfonylureas).

Association of the DIO2 rs225017 and Thr92Ala variants with insulin resistance

We used a Bayesian statistical method to estimate the frequencies of different haplotypes produced by the combination of the rs225017 and Thr92Ala polymorphisms in patients with T2DM. The first letter of the haplotypes refers to the Thr92Ala polymorphism, and the second, to the rs225017 polymorphism. The wild type haplotype (Thr/A) was observed in 49.0% of the sample, the Thr/T haplotype was observed in 18.0%, the Ala/A haplotype in 4.0%, and the Ala/T haplotype (double mutated) in 29.0% of the sample.

Taking these results into account, we tested whether any haplotype constituted by the rs225017 and Thr92Ala polymorphisms might affect fasting plasma insulin levels or HOMA-IR index differently as compared with the effect of each polymorphism analyzed separately. To test this hypothesis, we performed GLM analyses using fasting insulin levels or the HOMA-IR index as the dependent variable, and age, sex, BMI, use of medication for T2DM and the polymorphic combinations of the two *DIO2* variants as independent variables. These interaction analyses are

Table 2. Interaction analyses between the *DIO2* rs225017 (T/A) and rs225014 (Thr92Ala) polymorphisms according to fasting plasma insulin and HOMA-IR index.

| | rs225017 | | | | | | |
| | A/X | | | T/T | | | |
Thr92Ala	Thr/X (n=138)	Ala/Ala (n=14)	P^a	Thr/X (n=35)	Ala/Ala (n=30)	P^a	F; P^b
Age (years)	59.7±9.9	57.2±10.5	0.177	58.2±10.6	58.1±10.0	0.941	-
Sex (% males)	49.0	42.0	0.439	39.0	49.0	0.417	-
BMI (kg/m²)	28.8±4.9	28.6±4.5	0.865	29.4±5.5	29.3±5.1	0.959	-
SU/Met/SU + Met (%)	31.3/35.6/14.0	28.6/50.0/14.0	0.830/0.270/0.997	35.3/51.5/22.0	34.3/40.3/24.0	0.907/0.196/0.803	-
Fasting insulin (UI/ml)^{c,d}	10.8 (1-44.9)	8.6 (4.0-39.0)	0.794	11.9 (4.5-44.6)	16.8 (3.2-46.1)	0.011	11.072; 0.001
HOMA-IR index^{c,e}	3.5 (0.3-19.5)	2.8 (1.6-13.6)	0.916	3.9 (0.6-13.5)	6.1 (0.9-20.1)	0.034	4.740; 0.010

Data are mean ± SD, median (minimum - maximum values) or %. BMI, body mass index; HOMA-IR, homeostasis model assessment - insulin resistance; Met, metformin; SU, sulfonylureas.
^{a}Data were analyzed using the Student t test or χ^2, as appropriate.
^{b}F and P values obtained from the general linear model-interaction analyses, after adjusting for age, sex, BMI and use of medication for T2DM.
^{c}Variables which were logarithmically transformed before analyses.
^{d}Adjusted R squared for fasting plasma insulin =0.135.
^{e}Adjusted R squared for HOMA-IR =0.111.

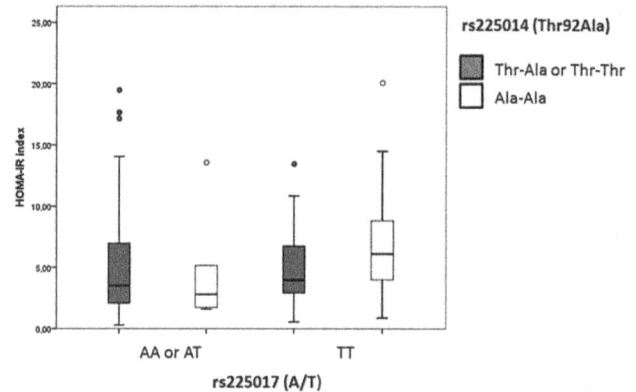

Figure 2. Possible interaction between rs225017 and Thr92Ala variants in modulation of insulin resistance. HOMA-IR indexes in T2DM patients according to different genotypes of *DIO2* rs225017 (A/T) and rs225014 (Thr92Ala) polymorphisms. Results are expressed as median (percentiles 25% and 75%). Circles represent outlier values. Interaction P value =0.010, adjusted for age, sex, BMI, and use of medication for T2DM.

shown in **Table 2**. Patients carrying the Ala/Ala – T/T haplotype showed higher fasting insulin values than patients with other genotype combinations, adjusting for covariables (F = 11.072, P = 0.001). Likewise, patients carrying the Ala/Ala – T/T haplotype showed a higher HOMA-IR index than patients with other genotype combinations (F = 4.740; P = 0.010) (**Figure 2**).

To determine whether the rs225017 (A/T) and rs225014 (Thr92Ala) polymorphisms were in LD in T2DM patients, we used Lewontin's $|D'|$ and r^2 measures. The analysis showed that the rs225017 polymorphism was in partial LD with the rs225014 polymorphism ($|D'| = 0.811$; $r^2 = 0.365$). These results were confirmed in the HAPMAP Project (http://hapmap.ncbi.nlm.nih.gov/).

Discussion

Insulin resistance is a heterogeneous disorder influenced by multiple environmental and genetic factors [38,39,40]. Previous studies indicate that the Thr92Ala polymorphism in the *DIO2* gene is involved in IR pathogenesis [7,23,37]. Even though the Ala/Ala genotype was associated with lower D2 activity in thyroid biopsy samples, *in vitro* studies did not show any change in the biochemical properties of the mutated enzyme, suggesting that this SNP might be only a polymorphic marker [7]. Therefore, here we searched for other informative SNPs in the *DIO2* gene which might be associated with IR or T2DM. We report a new *DIO2* polymorphism associated with increased IR in T2DM patients. Homozygosis for the allele T of the rs225017 (A/T) polymorphism was associated with IR in patients with T2DM, whereas patients carrying a combination of the T/T genotype of the rs225017 polymorphism and the Ala/Ala genotype of the Thr92Ala polymorphism showed an increased HOMA-IR index as compared with patients with other genotype combinations, suggesting that they might interact in the modulation of IR.

The rs205017 (A/T) polymorphism is located at the 3'UTR of the *DIO2* gene. In selenoenzymes, the 3'UTR contains the selenocysteine insertion sequence (SECIS), which is very important for looping formation in the mechanism of cis-acting mRNA structure of selenocysteine insertion [41,42]. The 3'UTR is also the main site for ligation of microRNAs (miRNAs) that can function as translational repressors or triggers of transcript degradation by partially pairing to this region in target mRNAs [43]. Currently, it is universally recognized that miRNAs are major regulators of gene expression and key controllers of several biologic and pathologic processes, as such those involved in the T2DM pathogenesis [44]. Hence, it is reasonable to speculate that the rs205017 polymorphism could be involved in a ligation site for a given miRNA, decreasing the *DIO2* expression. Therefore, we used the TargetScan software to look for potential miRNA targets in the *DIO2* gene [45]. Six predicted interaction regions with miRNA families were found in the *DIO2* sequence: miR-9, miR-29abcd, miR-30abcdef, miR-193, miR-203 and miR-216a. Interestingly, miR-9, miR-29 and miR-30 seem to have a role in insulin resistance [44,46]. Although the rs225017 SNP is not located at any of these miRNA regions, it is close to some of them and, therefore, we could not rule out a potential effect of this SNP on *DIO2* gene expression. Alternatively, it could be obstructing the mechanism of selenocysteine insertion and, thereby, reducing the amount of D2 available for the activation of T3. In this context, polymorphic D2, generated from the Ala/T haplotype sequence, might generate less T3 in skeletal muscle and adipocytes, which, consequently, may create a local state of intracellular hypothyroidism, decreasing the expression of genes involved in metabolism, such as GLUT4, and leading to IR.

Recently, the *DIO2* rs6574549 polymorphism, also located at the 3'UTR, was associated with elevated fasting insulin levels and higher insulin action, but not with T2DM in Pima Indians [47]. This polymorphism may also be a candidate for the functional variant associated with IR. The rs6574549 polymorphism is in strong LD with the Thr92Ala [47] and rs205017 [48] polymorphisms (LD>0.8; HAPMAP Project, http://hapmap.ncbi.nlm.nih.gov/). Therefore, further studies are necessary to determine: 1) which polymorphism is the functional variant interacting with the Thr92Ala polymorphism in the modulation of IR; 2) whether there is another functional polymorphism in the *DIO2* gene yet to be identified; and 3) whether these polymorphisms have combined effects on D2 function. The results presented here add to the understanding of the molecular interactions controlling IR and might partially explain the association with the Thr92Ala polymorphism.

Some factors unrelated to the rs205017 and Thr92Ala polymorphisms may have interfered with the findings of the present study. First, medications for T2DM treatment may have played a role because some are known to affect insulin sensitivity.

However, we minimized such possibility by excluding insulin-treated patients from the group of 227 patients analyzed for IR. Furthermore, the rs205017 variant and the Ala/Ala-T/T haplotype remained independently associated with the HOMA-IR index and plasma insulin levels after adjusting for medications for T2DM, including metformin and sulfonylurea. In addition, none of the patients were using thiazolidinediones, agents that change insulin sensitivity. Second, IR was assessed by calculation of the HOMA-IR index rather than by the reference method, the euglycaemic-hyperinsulinemic clamp [32,49,50]. Although the HOMA-IR index is only an approximate estimate of IR, it is simple to calculate and shows a good correlation with the reference method [32,49]; therefore, it is a good approach for cohort and epidemiological studies [50]. Third, we cannot rule out the possibility of stratification bias in our sample, although we studied only self-defined white subjects and thus reduced the risk of false positive or false negative associations due to this bias. In addition, the 227 patients with T2DM analyzed for IR were representative of the whole sample (n = 1077) with respect to age, T2DM duration, A1c, sex, BMI and presence of arterial hypertension. The frequencies of the rs205017 and Thr92Ala polymorphisms were also similar between these 227 patients and the whole T2DM sample (data not shown). Fourth, screening only 12 patients with T2DM for the occurrence of *DIO2* polymorphisms might have failed to detect rare polymorphisms [49]; however, this number was enough to detect most representative variants, which are sufficiently polymorphic to warrant association studies. Finally, our results might represent a type 1 error, but the scientific plausibility of the reported association provides evidence against it.

In summary, the *DIO2* rs225017 (A/T) polymorphism is a new polymorphism associated with IR in white patients with T2DM, and it seems to interact with the Thr92Ala polymorphism in the modulation of this characteristic. Further studies are needed to evaluate the functional and epidemiological importance of the rs205017 polymorphism in IR and T2DM.

Author Contributions

Conceived and designed the experiments: LBL AAFE DC ALM. Performed the experiments: LBL AAFE SMW. Analyzed the data: LBL JMD SMW AAFE DC ALM. Contributed reagents/materials/analysis tools: DC ALM. Wrote the paper: LBL DC ALM.

References

1. Yen PM (2001) Physiological and molecular basis of thyroid hormone action. Physiol Rev 81: 1097–1142.
2. Maia AL, Goemann IM, Meyer EL, Wajner SM (2011) Deiodinases: the balance of thyroid hormone: type 1 iodothyronine deiodinase in human physiology and disease. J Endocrinol 209: 283–297.
3. Maia AL, Kim BW, Huang SA, Harney JW, Larsen PR (2005) Type 2 iodothyronine deiodinase is the major source of plasma T3 in euthyroid humans. J Clin Invest 115: 2524–2533.
4. Croteau W, Davey JC, Galton VA, St Germain DL (1996) Cloning of the mammalian type II iodothyronine deiodinase. A selenoprotein differentially expressed and regulated in human and rat brain and other tissues. J Clin Invest 98: 405–417.
5. Itagaki Y, Yoshida K, Ikeda H, Kaise K, Kaise N, et al. (1990) Thyroxine 5'-deiodinase in human anterior pituitary tumors. J Clin Endocrinol Metab 71: 340–344.
6. Salvatore D, Tu H, Harney JW, Larsen PR (1996) Type 2 iodothyronine deiodinase is highly expressed in human thyroid. J Clin Invest 98: 962–968.
7. Canani LH, Capp C, Dora JM, Meyer EL, Wagner MS, et al. (2005) The type 2 deiodinase A/G (Thr92Ala) polymorphism is associated with decreased enzyme velocity and increased insulin resistance in patients with type 2 diabetes mellitus. J Clin Endocrinol Metab 90: 3472–3478.
8. Grozovsky R, Ribich S, Rosene ML, Mulcahey MA, Huang SA, et al. (2009) Type 2 deiodinase expression is induced by peroxisomal proliferator-activated receptor-gamma agonists in skeletal myocytes. Endocrinology 150: 1976–1983.
9. Heemstra KA, Soeters MR, Fliers E, Serlie MJ, Burggraaf J, et al. (2009) Type 2 iodothyronine deiodinase in skeletal muscle: effects of hypothyroidism and fasting. J Clin Endocrinol Metab 94: 2144–2150.
10. Steinsapir J, Bianco AC, Buettner C, Harney J, Larsen PR (2000) Substrate-induced down-regulation of human type 2 deiodinase (hD2) is mediated through proteasomal degradation and requires interaction with the enzyme's active center. Endocrinology 141: 1127–1135.
11. Gereben B, Goncalves C, Harney JW, Larsen PR, Bianco AC (2000) Selective proteolysis of human type 2 deiodinase: a novel ubiquitin-proteasomal mediated mechanism for regulation of hormone activation. Mol Endocrinol 14: 1697–1708.
12. Frojdo S, Vidal H, Pirola L (2009) Alterations of insulin signaling in type 2 diabetes: a review of the current evidence from humans. Biochim Biophys Acta 1792: 83–92.

13. Chidakel A, Mentuccia D, Celi FS (2005) Peripheral metabolism of thyroid hormone and glucose homeostasis. Thyroid 15: 899–903.
14. Kim SR, Tull ES, Talbott EO, Vogt MT, Kuller LH (2002) A hypothesis of synergism: the interrelationship of T3 and insulin to disturbances in metabolic homeostasis. Med Hypotheses 59: 660–666.
15. Weinstein SP, O'Boyle E, Haber RS (1994) Thyroid hormone increases basal and insulin-stimulated glucose transport in skeletal muscle. The role of GLUT4 glucose transporter expression. Diabetes 43: 1185–1189.
16. Torrance CJ, Devente JE, Jones JP, Dohm GL (1997) Effects of thyroid hormone on GLUT4 glucose transporter gene expression and NIDDM in rats. Endocrinology 138: 1204–1214.
17. Dimitriadis G, Baker B, Marsh H, Mandarino L, Rizza R, et al. (1985) Effect of thyroid hormone excess on action, secretion, and metabolism of insulin in humans. Am J Physiol 248: E593–601.
18. Dimitriadis G, Maratou E, Alevizaki M, Boutati E, Psara K, et al. (2005) Thyroid hormone excess increases basal and insulin-stimulated recruitment of GLUT3 glucose transporters on cell surface. Horm Metab Res 37: 15–20.
19. Rochon C, Tauveron I, Dejax C, Benoit P, Capitan P, et al. (2003) Response of glucose disposal to hyperinsulinaemia in human hypothyroidism and hyperthyroidism. Clin Sci (Lond) 104: 7–15.
20. Dubaniewicz A, Kaciuba-Uscilko H, Nazar K, Budohoski L (1989) Sensitivity of the soleus muscle to insulin in resting and exercising rats with experimental hypo- and hyper-thyroidism. Biochem J 263: 243–247.
21. Marsili A, Aguayo-Mazzucato C, Chen T, Kumar A, Chung M, et al. (2011) Mice with a targeted deletion of the type 2 deiodinase are insulin resistant and susceptible to diet induced obesity. PLoS One 6: e20832.
22. Coppotelli G, Summers A, Chidakel A, Ross JM, Celi FS (2006) Functional characterization of the 258 A/G (D2-ORFa-Gly3Asp) human type-2 deiodinase polymorphism: a naturally occurring variant increases the enzymatic activity by removing a putative repressor site in the 5′ UTR of the gene. Thyroid 16: 625–632.
23. Mentuccia D, Proietti-Pannunzi L, Tanner K, Bacci V, Pollin TI, et al. (2002) Association between a novel variant of the human type 2 deiodinase gene Thr92Ala and insulin resistance: evidence of interaction with the Trp64Arg variant of the beta-3-adrenergic receptor. Diabetes 51: 880–883.
24. Maia AL, Dupuis J, Manning A, Liu C, Meigs JB, et al. (2007) The type 2 deiodinase (DIO2) A/G polymorphism is not associated with glycemic traits: the Framingham Heart Study. Thyroid 17: 199–202.
25. Mentuccia D, Thomas MJ, Coppotelli G, Reinhart LJ, Mitchell BD, et al. (2005) The Thr92Ala deiodinase type 2 (DIO2) variant is not associated with type 2 diabetes or indices of insulin resistance in the old order of Amish. Thyroid 15: 1223–1227.
26. Grarup N, Andersen MK, Andreasen CH, Albrechtsen A, Borch-Johnsen K, et al. (2007) Studies of the common DIO2 Thr92Ala polymorphism and metabolic phenotypes in 7342 Danish white subjects. J Clin Endocrinol Metab 92: 363–366.
27. Dora JM, Machado WE, Rheinheimer J, Crispim D, Maia AL (2010) Association of the type 2 deiodinase Thr92Ala polymorphism with type 2 diabetes: case-control study and meta-analysis. Eur J Endocrinol 163: 427–434.
28. Peeters RP, van Toor H, Klootwijk W, de Rijke YB, Kuiper GG, et al. (2003) Polymorphisms in thyroid hormone pathway genes are associated with plasma TSH and iodothyronine levels in healthy subjects. J Clin Endocrinol Metab 88: 2880–2888.
29. Adams DR, Sincan M, Fuentes Fajardo K, Mullikin JC, Pierson TM, et al. (2011) Analysis of DNA sequence variants detected by high-throughput sequencing. Hum Mutat 33: 599–608.
30. Cooper DN, Chen JM, Ball EV, Howells K, Mort M, et al. (2010) Genes, mutations, and human inherited disease at the dawn of the age of personalized genomics. Hum Mutat 31: 631–655.
31. Canani LH, Costa LA, Crispim D, Goncalves Dos Santos K, Roisenberg I, et al. (2005) The presence of allele D of angiotensin-converting enzyme polymorphism is associated with diabetic nephropathy in patients with less than 10 years duration of Type 2 diabetes. Diabet Med 22: 1167–1172.
32. Bonora E, Targher G, Alberiche M, Bonadonna RC, Saggiani F, et al. (2000) Homeostasis model assessment closely mirrors the glucose clamp technique in the assessment of insulin sensitivity: studies in subjects with various degrees of glucose tolerance and insulin sensitivity. Diabetes Care 23: 57–63.
33. Seligman BG, Biolo A, Polanczyk CA, Gross JL, Clausell N (2000) Increased plasma levels of endothelin 1 and von Willebrand factor in patients with type 2 diabetes and dyslipidemia. Diabetes Care 23: 1395–1400.
34. Hedrick PW (1987) Gametic disequilibrium measures: proceed with caution. Genetics 117: 331–341.
35. Barrett JC, Fry B, Maller J, Daly MJ (2005) Haploview: analysis and visualization of LD and haplotype maps. Bioinformatics 21: 263–265.
36. Stephens M, Smith NJ, Donnelly P (2001) A new statistical method for haplotype reconstruction from population data. Am J Hum Genet 68: 978–989.
37. Estivalet AA, Leiria LB, Dora JM, Rheinheimer J, Boucas AP, et al. (2010) D2 Thr92Ala and PPARgamma2 Pro12Ala polymorphisms interact in the modulation of insulin resistance in type 2 diabetic patients. Obesity (Silver Spring) 19: 825–832.
38. Irvin MR, Wineinger NE, Rice TK, Pajewski NM, Kabagambe EK, et al. (2011) Genome-wide detection of allele specific copy number variation associated with insulin resistance in African Americans from the HyperGEN study. PLoS One 6: e24052.
39. North KE, Williams K, Williams JT, Best LG, Lee ET, et al. (2003) Evidence for genetic factors underlying the insulin resistance syndrome in american indians. Obes Res 11: 1444–1448.
40. North KE, Almasy L, Goring HH, Cole SA, Diego VP, et al. (2005) Linkage analysis of factors underlying insulin resistance: Strong Heart Family Study. Obes Res 13: 1877–1884.
41. Mix H, Lobanov AV, Gladyshev VN (2007) SECIS elements in the coding regions of selenoprotein transcripts are functional in higher eukaryotes. Nucleic Acids Res 35: 414–423.
42. Ryan K, Bauer DL (2008) Finishing touches: post-translational modification of protein factors involved in mammalian pre-mRNA 3′ end formation. Int J Biochem Cell Biol 40: 2384–2396.
43. Ambros V (2004) The functions of animal microRNAs. Nature 431: 350–355.
44. Guay C, Regazzi R (2013) Circulating microRNAs as novel biomarkers for diabetes mellitus. Nat Rev Endocrinol 9: 513–521.
45. Lewis BP, Burge CB, Bartel DP (2005) Conserved seed pairing, often flanked by adenosines, indicates that thousands of human genes are microRNA targets. Cell 120: 15–20.
46. Guay C, Roggli E, Nesca V, Jacovetti C, Regazzi R (2011) Diabetes mellitus, a microRNA-related disease? Transl Res 157: 253–264.
47. Nair S, Muller YL, Ortega E, Kobes S, Bogardus C, et al. (2012) Association analyses of variants in the DIO2 gene with early-onset type 2 diabetes mellitus in Pima Indians. Thyroid 22: 80–87.
48. Altshuler DM, Gibbs RA, Peltonen L, Altshuler DM, Gibbs RA, et al. (2010) Integrating common and rare genetic variation in diverse human populations. Nature 467: 52–58.
49. Emoto M, Nishizawa Y, Maekawa K, Hiura Y, Kanda H, et al. (1999) Homeostasis model assessment as a clinical index of insulin resistance in type 2 diabetic patients treated with sulfonylureas. Diabetes Care 22: 818–822.
50. Wallace TM, Levy JC, Matthews DR (2004) Use and abuse of HOMA modeling. Diabetes Care 27: 1487–1495.

19

CDKAL1-Related Single Nucleotide Polymorphisms are Associated with Insulin Resistance

Mathias Rask-Andersen[1]*[9], Gaëtan Philippot[1][9], George Moschonis[2], George Dedoussis[2], Yannis Manios[2], Claude Marcus[3], Robert Fredriksson[1], Helgi B. Schiöth[1]

1 Department of Neuroscience, Functional Pharmacology, Uppsala University, BMC, Uppsala, Sweden, **2** Department of Nutrition and Dietetics, Harokopio University, Athens, Greece, **3** Department for Clinical Science, Intervention and Technology, Karolinska Institutet, Division of Pediatrics, National Childhood Obesity Centre, Stockholm, Sweden

Abstract

Five novel loci recently found to be associated with body mass in two GWAS of East Asian populations were evaluated in two cohorts of Swedish and Greek children and adolescents. These loci are located within, or in the proximity of: CDKAL1, PCSK1, GP2, PAX6 and KLF9. No association with body mass has previously been reported for these loci in GWAS performed on European populations. The single nucleotide polymorphisms (SNPs) with the strongest association at each loci in the East Asian GWAS were genotyped in two cohorts, one obesity case control cohort of Swedish children and adolescents consisting of 496 cases and 520 controls and one cross-sectional cohort of 2293 nine-to-thirteen year old Greek children and adolescents. SNPs were surveyed for association with body mass and other phenotypic traits commonly associated with obesity, including adipose tissue distribution, insulin resistance and daily caloric intake. No association with body mass was found in either cohort. However, among the Greek children, association with insulin resistance could be observed for the two CDKAL1-related SNPs: rs9356744 ($\beta = 0.018$, p = 0.014) and rs2206734 ($\beta = 0.024$, p = 0.001). CDKAL1-related variants have previously been associated with type 2 diabetes and insulin response. This study reports association of CDKAL1-related SNPs with insulin resistance, a clinical marker related to type 2 diabetes in a cross-sectional cohort of Greek children and adolescents of European descent.

Editor: Lin Chen, The University of Chicago, United States of America

Funding: The study was supported by the Swedish Research Council, the Brain Research Foundation, Novo Nordisk Foundation, Engkvist and the Åhlens Foundation. The funders had no role in study design, data collection and analysis, decision to publish, or preparation of the manuscript.

Competing Interests: The authors have declared that no competing interests exist.

* E-mail: Mathias.Rask-Andersen@neuro.uu.se

Introduction

The worldwide obesity epidemic is a major public health concern associated with increased morbidity and mortality [1]. Obesity shows comorbidity with e.g. type 2 diabetes mellitus (T2DM), cardiovascular disease, hypertension and certain types of cancer [2–4]. However, the exact mechanisms behind the development of obesity are not fully understood. Even though recent lifestyle changes have likely triggered the increased prevalence of obesity, a genetic predisposition has been indicated to substantially contribute to the etiology of this condition [5–7]. As of today, at least 32 obesity-associated loci have been identified in by the GIANT-consortium [8–9]. These findings come from meta-analyses of genome-wide association studies (GWAS) and are predominantly based on subjects of European ancestry.

Recently, two GWAS identified five novel loci associated with BMI in East Asians [10–11] that have, as of yet, not been associated with body mass in European cohorts. The loci were located in or near the CDKAL1, PCSK1, GP2, PAX6 and KLF9 genes. The aim of this study was to determine if these SNPs were associated with BMI also in Europeans. We therefore analyzed the strongest associated SNPs reported in the two GWAS performed on East Asian populations: rs9356744, rs2206734, rs652722, rs11142387, rs261967 and rs12597579 for associations with obesity and body mass in a case control cohort for obesity consisting of 1016 Swedish children and adolescents recruited in the Stockholm area, as well as in a cross-sectional national cohort of 2293 Greek children and adolescents recruited from schools. Phenotypic traits commonly associated with BMI were also surveyed, including adipose tissue distribution (hip- and waist circumference and thickness of skinfolds), homeostasis model assessment of insulin resistance (HOMA-IR) and daily caloric intake [12].

Methods

Ethics statement: Healthy Growth Study, Greek children and adolescents

An extended letter and a consent form were provided to each parent having a child in one of the primary schools explaining the aims of the study. Parents who agreed to participate in the study had to sign the consent form and provide their contact details. The study was approved by the Greek Ministry of Education and the

Ethical Committee of Harokopio, University of Athens, Athens, Greece.

Ethics statement: Case control study for obesity, Swedish children and adolescents

The study was approved by the Regional Committee of Ethics, Stockholm. All subjects, or their legal guardians, gave their written informed consent.

Healthy Growth Study, Greek children and adolescents

The Healthy Growth Study, a large scale cross-sectional epidemiological study, was initiated in May 2007. The survey population consisted of 2657 school children aged 9–13 years attending the fifth and sixth grade of primary school (Table 1), as previously described [13–15]. Standard procedures and equipment were used to measure body weight and height in all study participants. Body weight without shoes in the minimal amount of clothing possible was measured using a Seca digital scale Model 770 (Seca Alpha, Hamburg, Germany), to the nearest 10 g. Height was measured to the nearest 0.1 cm, in standing position without shoes, shoulders in a relaxed position, arms hanging freely and head aligned in Frankfurt plane, using a commercial stadiometer (Leicester Height Measure, Invicta Plastics Ltd, Oadby, UK). BMI z-score was calculated relative to the International Obesity Task Force (IOTF) definitions [16]. Blood samples were obtained for screening tests after a 12 h overnight fast. Plasma separation of blood was performed by centrifugation (3000 rpm for 15 min). Serum insulin concentrations were measured using a chemiluminescence immunoassay (Kyowa Medex Ltd, Minami-Ishiki, Japan). Insulin resistance (IR) was calculated through the homeostasis model assessment (Equation 1) [17].

$$HOMA-IR = \frac{Glucose\left(\frac{mmol}{l}\right) \times Insulin\left(\mu\frac{U}{ml}\right)}{22.5} \quad \text{(Equation 1)}$$

DNA for genotyping was available for 2293 individuals (1154 males and 1132 females). Waist and hip circumference was measured at standing position using non-elastic tape (Hoechstmass, Sulzback, Germany) to the nearest 0.1 cm. Measurements were taken around the trunk, at the umbilicus midway between the lower rib margin and the iliac crest. Thickness of four skinfolds (triceps, biceps, subscapular and suprailiac) were measured to the nearest 0.1 mm with a Large skinfold caliper (Cambridge, Maryland). Triceps and biceps skinfold thickness was measured on the right arm hanging freely at the side of the body, with the

skinfold being picked up 1 cm below the midpoint mark over the triceps and biceps. Subscapular skinfold thickness was measured in standing position, arms hanging in a relaxed position after identifying the inferior angle of the scapula. The skinfold was picked up 1 cm below the subscapular mark. Suprailiac skinfold thickness was measured above the iliac crest along the axis of the anterior line. Pubertal maturation (Tanner Stage) was determined by four well-trained pediatricians. Breast development in girls and genital development in boys was examined according to the pubertal maturation classification (Tanner Stage 1 to 5) [18]. The study was approved by the Greek Ministry of Education and the Ethical Committee of Harokopio University, Athens, Greece.

Case control study for obesity, Swedish children and adolescents

The cohort of Swedish children was comprised of 1016 children and adolescents in two groups, as described previously [13,15]. One group consisted of 496 obese children (236 boys and 260 girls) registered at the National Childhood Obesity centre at Karolinska University Hospital, Huddinge, Sweden. The second group consisted of 520 healthy adolescents with normal weight (253 boys and 267 girls) recruited from 17 upper secondary schools in the Stockholm area, Sweden (Table 1). Body weight and height were measured to the nearest 0.1 kg and 1 cm, respectively. BMI z-score was calculated according to the International Obesity Task Force (IOTF) definitions [16]. A BMI z-score >2 is commonly utilized as a cutoff for defining obesity. In the obese group, patients with T2DM were excluded. Subjects in the control group that were overweight, obese or had metabolic diseases were also excluded.

SNP genotyping

Genotyping of gene variants was carried out using the predesigned Taqman single-nucleotide polymorphism genotyping assay (Applied Biosystems, Foster city, USA) and an ABI7900 genetic analyzer with SDS 2.2 software at the Uppsala Genome Center (http://www.genpat.uu.se/node462).

Statistical analysis

All statistical analyses were made using PLINK (http://pngu. mgh.harvard.edu/purcell/plink) [19]. Quantitative skewed variables were log transformed if needed to meet the assumptions of parametric statistics. Deviation from Hardy-Weinberg equilibrium was tested for using the Pearson's χ^2- test. Association between genotypes and phenotypes in the Greek cohort were analyzed with linear regression, assuming an additive model. All analyses in the Greek cohort were adjusted for age, gender and pubertal development (Tanner stage). Analyses of secondary phenotypic traits were also adjusted for BMI z-score. The Swedish cohort was analyzed using logistic regression and was adjusted for age and

Table 1. Descriptive characteristics of the cohorts of Greek and Swedish children and adolescents.

	N (boys/girl)	Age (years)	Body weight (kg)	Length (m)	BMI z-score	HOMA-IR	Daily caloric intake (kcal/day)
Greek cohort							
	2293 (1154/1132)	11.2±0.7	45.3±11.1	1.49±7.8	0.84±1.27	2.381±1.720	1785±552.4
Swedish cohort							
Controls	520 (253/267)	17.0±0.9	63.5±10.1	1.73±0.09	$-3.0\times10^{-4}\pm0.8$		
Cases	496 (236/260)	12.8±3.2	92.9±29.1	1.59±0.16	3.35±1.65		

gender. Results are presented as odds ratios (OR) with 95% confidence interval (CI). We applied the False Discovery Rate by Benjamini and Hochberg [20] to correct for multiple testing. Associations were considered significant if the adjusted p value <0.05.

Power calculation

Power calculation for the Swedish and Greek cohorts were performed in CaTS power calculator (http://www.sph.umich.edu/csg/abecasis/CaTS/) and Quanto (http://hydra.usc.edu/gxe/) utilizing effect sizes reported in the previous GWAS [10–11] as well as child and adolescent obesity prevalence of 4.3% [21]. We estimate a 20–40% power, depending on effect size and allele frequency, to observe effects on BMI for the studied SNPs of medium to high allele frequency (CDKAL1-, KLF9-, PCSK1- and PAX9-related SNPs) in the cohort of Greek children and adolescents. Our power was lower (~10%) for detecting association of the GP2-related SNP rs12597579 with body mass due to the low frequency of this SNP (7%). In the case control cohort of Swedish obese children and adolescents, we estimate a 40–70% power to detect associations of the medium to high frequency SNPs with obesity, depending on allele frequency. Again, the low frequency of rs12597579 leads to a lower power for this SNP at about 18%.

Results

Genotyping was performed on 2293 subjects in the Greek cohort and 1016 subjects in the Swedish cohort. The call rate was between 98.5–99.7%. No deviation from Hardy-Weinberg equilibrium was observed. In our analysis we were unable to observe any effect of the studied SNPs on body mass in the cohort of Greek children and adolescents (Table S1). We were also unable to observe any association with obesity in the case control study of Swedish children and adolescents (Table S2). Analyses of waist-to-hip ratio and skinfold thickness also failed to reveal any association with the studied SNPs (Table S3).

Association of CDKAL1-related SNPs rs9356744 and rs2206734 with insulin resistance

Linear regression revealed associations between HOMA-IR and two SNPs within the CDKAL1 gene: rs9356744 and rs2206734 ($\beta = 0.018$, adjusted $p = 0.042$ and $\beta = 0.024$, adjusted $p = 0.025$ respectively) in models adjusted for age, gender, body mass and pubertal development (Table 2).

Association of rs652722 with daily caloric intake

Linear regression revealed association between rs652722 and daily caloric intake among the Greek children. The minor allele of rs652722, near the PAX6 gene was associated with lower daily caloric intake ($\beta = -0.010$, nominal $p = 0.020$) in models adjusted for age, gender, body mass and pubertal development. However, this association was not significant after correcting for multiple testing (Table 3).

Discussion

The strongest associated SNPs at five loci associated with BMI in East Asians [10–11] were evaluated for association with BMI and related traits in two cohorts of children of European ancestry: one cross-sectional cohort of Greek children and one case-control study of obese Swedish children and adolescents. The effects on body mass observed in East Asian populations could not be replicated in our studies indicating heterogenic effects of these loci across European and East Asian populations. These results are in line with reports from the GIANT consortium [22]. Despite reporting some directionally consistent effects as the East Asian GWAS, the effects of variants at these loci were not powerful enough to reach the criteria for statistical significance in the analysis by the GIANT consortium. It must be highlighted that our study utilized cohorts of children, which could indicate that genetic effects of variations at these loci have a higher penetrance in adults, as the two GWAS on East Asians primarily performed their studies on adult populations [10–11]. Statistical power is also a potential limiting factor due to the relatively small sizes of our cohorts. In the case of the GP2-related SNP rs12597579, this may be further compounded by the low frequency of its minor allele (minor allele frequency approximately 5–7%).

However, the SNPs within the T2DM associated gene CDKAL1, rs9356744 and rs2206734, were observed to be associated with HOMA-IR ($\beta = 0.02$, adjusted $p = 0.042$ and $\beta = 0.025$, adjusted $p = 0.025$, respectively) in linear regression models co-varied for body mass, age, gender and pubertal development (Table 2). HOMA-IR is an estimate of IR which describes the interplay between plasma glucose and insulin release from the pancreatic islets. It is determined through measurements of fasting insulin and plasma glucose [17,23]. An elevated IR, a cut-off value 2.60 is commonly used, denotes an insufficiency of insulin-mediated glucose uptake and is one of the central features of T2DM and also one of the key features of the metabolic syndrome [24–25]. A study in U.S subjects found obese children and adolescents (12–19 years old) to have a higher IR compared to normal weight children and adolescents (4.93 vs. 2.30) [26].

Table 2. Association of SNPs with HOMA-IR in the Greek cohort.

SNP	Gene	genotypic distribution	HWE	MAF (%)	n	HOMA-IR β	p-value	FDR
rs261967	PCSK1	CC/CA/AA (444/1083/749)	0.15	43.3	1973	0.0027	0.69	0.99
rs9356744	CDKAL1	CC/CT/TT (229/997/1054)	0.81	31.9	1977	0.018	**0.014***	**0.042***
rs2206734	CDKAL1	TT/TC/CC (114/773/1393)	0.62	22.0	1976	0.024	**0.0041****	**0.025***
rs11142387	KLF9	AA/AC/CC (470/1174/636)	0.10	46.4	1976	−0.10	0.99	0.99
rs652722	PAX6	TT/TC/CC (157/858/1265)	0.48	25.7	1976	0.0012	0.88	0.99
rs12597579	GP2	TT/TC/CC (13/291/1973)	0.52	7.00	1973	−0.024	0.08	0.16

β - regression coefficient. MAF – minor allele frequency. HWE – Hardy Weinberg equilibrium deviation test presented as p-value. *p<0.05, **p<0.005.
Linear regression was used to analyze association with phenotypic traits. Models were adjusted for BMI z-score, gender, age and pubertal development (tanner stage).

Table 3. Analysis of association of rs652722 with daily caloric intake in the Greek cohort.

SNP	Gene	Genotypic distribution	MAF (%)	n	Daily caloric intake β	p-value	FDR
rs261967	PCSK1	CC/CA/AA (229/997/1054)	43.3	2250	−0.0017	0.65	0.76
rs9356744	CDKAL1	CC/CT/TT (229/997/1054)	31.9	2254	0.0044	0.29	0.58
rs2206734	CDKAL1	TT/TC/CC (114/773/1393)	22.0	2254	0.0060	0.19	0.57
rs11142387	KLF9	AA/AC/CC (470/1174/636)	46.4	2254	−0.0025	0.53	0.76
rs652722	PAX6	TT/TC/CC (157/858/1265)	25.7	2254	−0.010	**0.02***	0.12
rs12597579	GP2	TT/TC/CC (13/291/1973)	7.00	2251	−0.0023	0.76	0.76

β - regression coefficient. MAF – minor allele frequency. HWE – Hardy Weinberg equilibrium deviation test presented as p-value. *p<0.05.
Linear regression was used to analyze association with phenotypic traits. Models were adjusted for BMI z-score, gender, age and pubertal development (tanner stage).

Insulin resistance has also been suggested as a prognostic marker for development of T2DM although causality has not been firmly established [27–28].

The directionalities of the effects of rs2206734 and rs9356744 on BMI observed in East Asians [10–11] are opposite compared to the effects on insulin resistance observed by us. However, our findings are in line with those of Okada et al. who also reported the T allele of rs2206734, which was associated with lower BMI in a cohort of East Asians, to be associated with an increased risk of T2DM [10]. Our findings are also in line with several studies showing associations of CDKAL1-related genetic variants with T2DM [29–30]. CDKAL1 encodes a methylthiotransferase that modifies tRNA to enhance the translational accuracy of the pro-insulin transcript [31]. A study with knockout mice indicated the involvement of CDKAL1 in exocytosis of first phase insulin in β-cells [32].

A trend towards associations with body mass and IR were observed for the GP2-related SNP rs12597579 ($\beta = -0.024$, nominal p = 0.079). The low minor allele frequency of this SNP unfortunately limits the statistical power of our analysis. Replication in larger cohorts may clarify potential effects of this locus on body mass and IR. GP2 is an interesting candidate gene at this locus due to its high expression in the pancreas. Rs12597579 is located ~65 kb downstream from the GP2 gene on chromosome 16. GP2 is highly expressed in the pancreas and especially within the islets of Langerhans [33–34]. Specifically, the GP2 protein is expressed in the secretory granules of acinar-cells and is the most abundant protein in the pancreatic secretory granule membrane, accounting for 35% of total membrane protein [35–36]. More recently, GP2 has been shown to be present in the microfold (M) cells of the follicle-associated epithelium (FAE) of intestinal Peyer's patches [37]. There is evidence of a potential autoantigen function of GP2 for pancreatic autoantibody (PAB), which is involved in Crohn's disease [38], but the full function of the GP2 gene is yet to be elucidated. Due to the high, close to exclusive, expression of GP2 in the islets of Langerhans, according to the gene atlas of the mouse and human protein encoding transcripts [39], accessed via BioGPS.org, evaluation of genetic variants in or near this gene could be highly relevant to diabetes research.

Some indication of association of rs652722 with a lower caloric intake was observed at nominal p-values, but not when correcting for multiple testing. According to the SCAN database [40] this SNP is in linkage disequilibrium with several other SNPs that influence genes potentially important for body weight regulation [11]. The PAX6 gene is located in the closest proximity of this locus and is expressed in all endocrine cells, e.g. ghrelin cells,

during development [41]. After development, the expression of PAX6 is necessary in the control of, among several other hormones, glucagon and insulin [42–43]. Homozygous PAX6 deleted mice showed symptoms of diabetes and severe weight loss [44], which points to a possible connection between PAX6-associated SNPs and metabolic function.

In summary, we observe associations between SNPs identified to be associated to body mass in two recently published GWAS performed in East Asian subjects with phenotypic traits associated with T2DM, in two cohorts of children and adolescents of European descent. In a cohort of Greek children and adolescents, CDKAL1-related SNPs rs9356744 and rs9356734 were observed to be associated with IR. The results provide candidate genetic markers for IR, which may be of great importance in both research and clinical practice.

Supporting Information

Table S1 Association of SNPs with BMI z-score in the Greek cohort. Linear regression was used to analyze association with BMI z-score. Models were adjusted for gender, age and pubertal development (tanner stage).

Table S2 Logistic regression was used to analyze association of SNPs with obesity in the cohort of Swedish children and adolescents. Models were adjusted for gender and age.

Table S3 Association of SNPs with adipose tissue distributions in the Greek cohort. Linear regression was used to analyze association with phenotypic traits. Models were adjusted for BMI z-score, gender, age and pubertal development (tanner stage).

Acknowledgments

Genotyping was performed by the SNP&SEQ Technology Platform in Uppsala, which is supported by Uppsala University, Uppsala University Hospital, Science for Life Laboratory - Uppsala and the Swedish Research Council (Contracts 80576801 and 70374401). We thank the Healthy Growth Study Group for their contribution in this study. The Healthy Growth Study Group consists of (1) Harokopio University Research Team/Department of Nutrition and Dietetics: Yannis Manios (Coordinator), George Moschonis (Project manager), Katerina P Skenderi, Evangelia Grammatikaki, Odysseas Androutsos, Sofia Tanagra, Alexandra Koumpitski, Paraskevi-Eirini Siatitsa, Anastasia Vandorou, Aikaterini-Efstathia

Kyriakou, Vasiliki Dede, Maria Kantilafti, Aliki-Eleni Farmaki, Aikaterini Siopi, Sofia Micheli, Louiza Damianidi, Panagiota Margiola, Despoina Gakni, Vasiliki Iatridi, Christina Mavrogianni, Kelaidi Michailidou, Aggeliki Giannopoulou, Efstathoula Argyri, Konstantina Maragkopoulou, Maria Spyridonos, Eirini Tsikalaki, Panagiotis Kliasios, Anthi Naoumi, Konstantinos Koutsikas, Katerina Kondaki, Epistimi Aggelou, Zoi Krommyda, Charitini Aga, Manolis Birbilis, Ioanna Kosteria, Amalia Zlatintsi, Elpida Voutsadaki, Eleni-Zouboulia Papadopoulou, Zoi Papazi, Maria Papadogiorgakaki, Fanouria Chlouveraki, Maria Lyberi, Nora Karatsikaki-Vlami, Eva Dionysopoulou and Efstratia Daskalou. (2) Aristotle University of Thessaloniki/School of Physical Education and Sports Sciences: Vassilis Mougios, Anatoli Petridou, Konstantinos Papaioannou, Georgios Tsalis, Ananis Karagkiozidis, Konstantinos Bougioukas, Afroditi Sakellaropoulou and Georgia Skouli. (3) University of Athens/Medical School: George P Chrousos, Maria Drakopoulou and Evangelia Charmandari.

Author Contributions

Conceived and designed the experiments: MRA HBS RF. Performed the experiments: HBS RF MRA GP. Analyzed the data: GP MRA. Contributed reagents/materials/analysis tools: GM GD YM CM. Wrote the paper: GP MRA.

References

1. Flegal KM, Graubard BI, Williamson DF, Gail MH (2007) Cause-specific excess deaths associated with underweight, overweight, and obesity. Jama 298: 2028–2037.
2. Kelly T, Yang W, Chen CS, Reynolds K, He J (2008) Global burden of obesity in 2005 and projections to 2030. Int J Obes (Lond) 32: 1431–1437.
3. Bogardus C (2009) Missing heritability and GWAS utility. Obesity (Silver Spring) 17(2): 209–10.
4. Lopez AD, Mathers CD, Ezzati M, Jamison DT, Murray CJ (2006) Global and regional burden of disease and risk factors, 2001: systematic analysis of population health data. Lancet 367: 1747–1757.
5. Maes HH, Neale MC, Eaves LJ (1997) Genetic and environmental factors in relative body weight and human adiposity. Behav Genet 27: 325–351.
6. Stunkard AJ, Foch TT, Hrubec Z (1986) A twin study of human obesity. Jama 256: 51–54.
7. Fontaine KR, Redden DT, Wang C, Westfall AO, Allison DB (2003) Years of life lost due to obesity. Jama 289: 187–193.
8. Speliotes EK, Willer CJ, Berndt SI, Monda KL, Thorleifsson G, et al. (2010) Association analyses of 249,796 individuals reveal 18 new loci associated with body mass index. Nat Genet 42: 937–948.
9. Willer CJ, Speliotes EK, Loos RJ, Li S, Lindgren CM, et al. (2009) Six new loci associated with body mass index highlight a neuronal influence on body weight regulation. Nat Genet 41: 25–34.
10. Okada Y, Kubo M, Ohmiya H, Takahashi A, Kumasaka N, et al. (2012) Common variants at CDKAL1 and KLF9 are associated with body mass index in east Asian populations. Nat Genet: 44(3): 302–6.
11. Wen W, Cho YS, Zheng W, Dorajoo R, Kato N, et al. (2012) Meta-analysis identifies common variants associated with body mass index in east Asians. Nat Genet 44(3): 307–11.
12. Shiwaku K, Anuurad E, Enkhmaa B, Nogi A, Kitajima K, et al. (2004) Overweight Japanese with body mass indexes of 23.0–24.9 have higher risks for obesity-associated disorders: a comparison of Japanese and Mongolians. Int J Obes Relat Metab Disord 28: 152–158.
13. Rask-Andersen M, Jacobsson JA, Moschonis G, Ek AE, Chrousos GP, et al. (2012) The MAP2K5-linked SNP rs2241423 is associated with BMI and obesity in two cohorts of Swedish and Greek children. BMC Med Genet 13: 36.
14. Moschonis G, Tanagra S, Vandorou A, Kyriakou AE, Dede V, et al. (2010) Social, economic and demographic correlates of overweight and obesity in primary-school children: preliminary data from the Healthy Growth Study. Public Health Nutr:1693–700.
15. Jacobsson JA, Rask-Andersen M, Riserus U, Moschonis G, Koumpitski A, et al. (2012) Genetic variants near the MGAT1 gene are associated with body weight, BMI and fatty acid metabolism among adults and children. Int J Obes (Lond) 36(1):119–29.
16. Cole TJ (2000) Commentary: Beware regression to the mean. Bmj 321: 281.
17. Matthews DR, Hosker JP, Rudenski AS, Naylor BA, Treacher DF, et al. (1985) Homeostasis model assessment: insulin resistance and beta-cell function from fasting plasma glucose and insulin concentrations in man. Diabetologia 28: 412–419.
18. Tanner JM (1955) Growth at Adolescence. Oxford: Blackwell Scientific.
19. Purcell S, Neale B, Todd-Brown K, Thomas L, Ferreira MA, et al. (2007) PLINK: a tool set for whole-genome association and population-based linkage analyses. Am J Hum Genet ()81(3): 559–75.
20. Benjamini Y, Hochberg Y (1995) Controlling the False Discovery Rate: a Practical and Powerful Approach to Multiple Testing Journal of the Royal Statistical Society Series B (Methodological) 57: 289–300.
21. Neovius M, Janson A, Rossner S (2006) Prevalence of obesity in Sweden. Obes Rev 7: 1–3.
22. Speliotes EK, Willer CJ, Berndt SI, Monda KL, Thorleifsson G, et al. (2010) Association analyses of 249,796 individuals reveal 18 new loci associated with body mass index. Nat Genet: 937–48.
23. Qu HQ, Li Q, Rentfro AR, Fisher-Hoch SP, McCormick JB (2011) The definition of insulin resistance using HOMA-IR for Americans of Mexican descent using machine learning. PLoS One 6(6): e21041.
24. Ascaso JF, Pardo S, Real JT, Lorente RI, Priego A, et al. (2003) Diagnosing insulin resistance by simple quantitative methods in subjects with normal glucose metabolism. Diabetes Care 26: 3320–3325.
25. Dumas M-E, Kinross J, Nicholson JK (2013) Metabolic Phenotyping and Systems Biology Approaches to Understanding Metabolic Syndrome and Fatty Liver Disease. Gastroenterology 146: 46–62.
26. Lee JM, Okumura MJ, Davis MM, Herman WH, Gurney JG (2006) Prevalence and determinants of insulin resistance among U.S. adolescents: a population-based study. Diabetes Care 29: 2427–32.
27. Nijpels G (1998) Determinants for the progression from impaired glucose tolerance to non-insulin-dependent diabetes mellitus. Eur J Clin Invest 2: 8–13.
28. Ten S, Maclaren N (2004) Insulin resistance syndrome in children. J Clin Endocrinol Metab 89(6): 2526–39.
29. Steinthorsdottir V, Thorleifsson G, Reynisdottir I, Benediktsson R, Jonsdottir T, et al. (2007) A variant in CDKAL1 influences insulin response and risk of type 2 diabetes. Nat Genet 39(6):770–5.
30. Unoki H, Takahashi A, Kawaguchi T, Hara K, Horikoshi M, et al. (2008) SNPs in KCNQ1 are associated with susceptibility to type 2 diabetes in East Asian and European populations. Nat Genet 40:1098–1102.
31. Brambillasca S, Altkrueger A, Colombo SF, Friederich A, Eickelmann P, et al. (2012) CDK5 regulatory subunit-associated protein 1-like 1 (CDKAL1) is a tail-anchored protein in the endoplasmic reticulum (ER) of insulinoma cells. J Biol Chem 287(50):41808–19.
32. Ohara-Imaizumi M, Yoshida M, Aoyagi K, Saito T, Okamura T, et al. (2010) Deletion of CDKAL1 affects mitochondrial ATP generation and first-phase insulin exocytosis. PLoS One 5(12):e15553.
33. Fukuoka S, Freedman SD, Scheele GA (1991) A single gene encodes membrane-bound and free forms of GP-2, the major glycoprotein in pancreatic secretory (zymogen) granule membranes. Proc Natl Acad Sci U S A 88: 2898–2902.
34. Hoops TC, Rindler MJ (1991) Isolation of the cDNA encoding glycoprotein-2 (GP-2), the major zymogen granule membrane protein. Homology to uromodulin/Tamm-Horsfall protein. J Biol Chem 266: 4257–4263.
35. Ronzio RA, Kronquist KE, Lewis DS, MacDonald RJ, Mohrlok SH, et al. (1978) Glycoprotein synthesis in the adult rat pancreas. IV. Subcellular distribution of membrane glycoproteins. Biochim Biophys Acta 508: 65–84.
36. Yu S, Lowe A (2009) The pancreatic zymogen granule membrane protein, GP2, binds Escherichia coli type 1 Fimbriae. BMC Gastroenterology 9: 58.
37. Hase K, Kawano K, Nochi T, Pontes GS, Fukuda S, et al. (2009) Uptake through glycoprotein 2 of FimH(+) bacteria by M cells initiates mucosal immune response. Nature 462(7270): 226–30.
38. Roggenbuck D, Hausdorf G, Martinez-Gamboa L, Reinhold D, Buttner T, et al. (2009) Identification of GP2, the major zymogen granule membrane glycoprotein, as the autoantigen of pancreatic antibodies in Crohn's disease. Gut 58(12):1620–8.
39. Su AI, Wiltshire T, Batalov S, Lapp H, Ching KA, et al. (2004) A gene atlas of the mouse and human protein-encoding transcriptomes. Proc Natl Acad Sci U S A 101: 6062–67.
40. Gamazon ER, Zhang W, Konkashbaev A, Duan S, Kistner EO, et al. (2010) SCAN: SNP and copy number annotation. Bioinformatics 26(2):259–62.
41. Heller RS, Stoffers DA, Liu A, Schedl A, Crenshaw EB 3rd, et al. (2004) The role of Brn4/Pou3f4 and Pax6 in forming the pancreatic glucagon cell identity. Dev Biol 268: 123–134.
42. Sander M, Neubuser A, Kalamaras J, Ee HC, Martin GR, et al. (1997) Genetic analysis reveals that PAX6 is required for normal transcription of pancreatic hormone genes and islet development. Genes Dev 11: 1662–73.
43. Gosmain Y, Marthinet E, Cheyssac C, Guerardel A, Mamin A, et al. (2010) Pax6 controls the expression of critical genes involved in pancreatic {alpha} cell differentiation and function. J Biol Chem 285(43):33381–93.
44. Hart AW, Mella S, Mendrychowski J, van Heyningen V, Kleinjan DA (2013) The developmental regulator Pax6 is essential for maintenance of islet cell function in the adult mouse pancreas. PLoS One 8(1):e54173.

20

Comparison of Liver Fat Indices for the Diagnosis of Hepatic Steatosis and Insulin Resistance

Sabine Kahl[1,2], **Klaus Straßburger**[1], **Bettina Nowotny**[1,2], **Roshan Livingstone**[1], **Birgit Klüppelholz**[3], **Kathrin Keßel**[1], **Jong-Hee Hwang**[1], **Guido Giani**[3], **Barbara Hoffmann**[4], **Giovanni Pacini**[5], **Amalia Gastaldelli**[6], **Michael Roden**[1,2,7]*

1 Institute for Clinical Diabetology, German Diabetes Center at Heinrich-Heine University, Düsseldorf, Germany, 2 Department of Endocrinology and Diabetology, Heinrich-Heine University Düsseldorf, Düsseldorf, Germany, 3 Institute for Biometrics and Epidemiology, German Diabetes Center at Heinrich-Heine University, Düsseldorf, Germany, 4 IUF – Leibniz Research Institute for Environmental Medicine, Düsseldorf, Germany, 5 National Research Council, Institute of Biomedical Engineering, Metabolic Unit, Padova, Italy, 6 National Research Council, Institute of Clinical Physiology, Pisa, Italy, 7 German Center for Diabetes Research, Partner Düsseldorf, Germany

Abstract

Context: Hepatic steatosis, defined as increased hepatocellular lipid content (HCL), associates with visceral obesity and glucose intolerance. As exact HCL quantification by ^{1}H-magnetic resonance spectroscopy (^{1}H-MRS) is not generally available, various clinical indices are increasingly used to predict steatosis.

Objective: The purpose of this study was to test the accuracy of NAFLD liver fat score (NAFLD-LFS), hepatic steatosis index (HSI) and fatty liver index (FLI) against ^{1}H-MRS and their relationships with insulin sensitivity and secretion.

Design, Setting and Participants: Ninety-two non-diabetic, predominantly non-obese humans underwent clinical examination, ^{1}H-MRS and an oral glucose tolerance test (OGTT) to calculate insulin sensitivity and β-cell function. Accuracy of indices was assessed from the area under the receiver operating characteristic curve (AROC).

Results: Median HCL was 2.49% (0.62;4.23) and correlated with parameters of glycemia across all subjects. NAFLD-LFS, FLI and HSI yielded AROCs of 0.70, 0.72, and 0.79, respectively, and related positively to HCL, insulin resistance, fasting and post-load β-cell function normalized for insulin resistance. Upon adjustment for age, sex and HCL, regression analysis revealed that NAFLD-LFS, FLI and HSI still independently associated with both insulin sensitivity and β-cell function.

Conclusion: The tested indices offer modest efficacy to detect steatosis and cannot substitute for fat quantification by ^{1}H-MRS. However, all indices might serve as surrogate parameters for liver fat content and also as rough clinical estimates of abnormal insulin sensitivity and secretion. Further validation in larger collectives such as epidemiological studies is needed.

Editor: Michael Müller, University of East Anglia, United Kingdom

Funding: This project was conducted in the context of the pretest studies of the German National Cohort (www.nationale-kohorte.de). These were funded by the Federal Ministry of Education and Research (BMBF), Förderkennzeichen 01ER1001A-I and supported by the participating universities, institutes of the Leibniz Association, the European Foundation for the Study of Diabetes (EFSD Clinical Research Grant in the Field of Diabetes 2010), the German Diabetes Association, the Schmutzler-Stiftung, the ICEMED Helmholtz-Alliance and the German Center for Diabetes Research (DZD e.V.). The study design of the National Cohort, basis for our study, was done by the German national cohort epidemiologic planning committee and project management team, and approved by Prof. Dr. Karl-Heinz Jöckel, chairman of the scientific board of the German National Cohort. The funders had no role in study design, data collection and analysis, decision to publish, or preparation of the manuscript.

Competing Interests: Unrelated to this study, M. R. has financial relationships with Boehringer Ingelheim Pharma, Eli Lilly, Novartis Pharma GmbH, Novo Nordisk, Sanofi-Aventis Deutschland GmbH and Takeda Pharma Ges. mbH, Austria. B. N. had travel costs paid by Sanofi-Aventis Deutschland GmbH. There are no patents, products in development or marketed products to declare.

* E-mail: michael.roden@ddz.uni-duesseldorf.de

Introduction

Hepatic steatosis is the most frequent liver disease in Western countries, closely associates with insulin resistance, visceral obesity, dyslipidemia and type 2 diabetes (T2DM) and is now classified among non-alcoholic fatty liver diseases (NAFLD) in the absence of excessive alcohol intake [1]. The gold standard for diagnosis of NAFLD is the liver biopsy, which is only justified in severe liver disease [2]. ^{1}H-magnetic resonance spectroscopy (^{1}H-MRS) allows for non-invasive quantification of hepatocellular lipid (HCL) content and for exact diagnosis of steatosis [2], while ultrasound and computed tomography provide rather semi-quantitative estimates [3].

As these techniques are time-consuming, expensive and often unavailable in daily routine, more simple tests have been developed based on routine laboratory and anthropometric parameters. The fatty liver index (FLI) [4], the hepatic steatosis index (HSI) [5] and the NAFLD liver fat score (NAFLD-LFS) [6] yielded satisfying results in their respective collectives, when validated against ultrasound (FLI, HSI) or ^{1}H-MRS (NAFLD-LFS). However, despite the association of steatosis with impaired glucose tolerance [7], FLI and HSI seem to perform less well in insulin resistant states such as T2DM [8].

We aimed to test (i) the diagnostic accuracy of these three indices by comparison with exact quantification of HCL by ^{1}H-MRS and (ii) the relationships with insulin sensitivity and secretion in a non-diabetic, predominantly non-obese collective of white origin in which median liver fat content is supposed to be low and therefore diagnosis of steatosis appears more challenging. Of note, the FLI has been originally developed to detect steatosis, whereas HSI and NAFLD-LFS have been developed to detect NAFLD. To account for these differences, we also analyzed a subgroup of our collective with low-risk alcohol consumption [9].

Study Population and Methods

Study design

This study was performed in the context of the German National Cohort feasibility studies. The protocol is in line with the 1975 Declaration of Helsinki and was approved by the Bavarian Medical Association and the ethical board of Heinrich-Heine University Düsseldorf. All subjects gave their written informed consent to participate.

Overall, from July to October 2011, 148 residents of the Düsseldorf area, aged 22 to 70 years, were recruited from a random sample of the general population. 100 persons agreed to participate in additional clinical examination, blood sampling after 10 hours of fasting, a 2-hours oral glucose tolerance test (OGTT), liver ^{1}H-MRS and whole-body MR imaging (MRI). Persons with non-white origin, T2DM and/or with hepatitis B and C were excluded from analysis, because these conditions are known to specifically affect HCL [10] so that 92 subjects remained for further analyses.

Clinical examination

All participants underwent a structured interview including assessment of mean daily alcohol intake during 7 days using estimated ethanol contents of beverages (beer 5%, wine 12%, shots 40%). The World Health Organization definition was applied for low-risk alcohol (LRA) consumption [9].

Body weight was measured to the nearest 0.1 kg using a calibrated weighting scale (SECA 285; SECA, Hamburg, Germany). Body height and waist circumference (waist) were measured according to standard procedures. Values of systolic (SBP) and diastolic blood pressure (DBP) were measured thrice after 5 min rest in sitting position using a validated automatic device (OMRON HEM 705 IT, OMRON, Mannheim, Germany) and means of the last two measurements were used for analysis.

Oral glucose tolerance test (OGTT)

A 75 g-OGTT (Accu-Chek Dextro O.G-T., Roche, Basel, Switzerland) was performed after at least 10 hrs overnight fasting. Blood samples were drawn at −5, 30, 60 and 120 min of OGTT and dysglycemia was categorized according to international criteria [11].

Laboratory measurements

Alanine aminotransferase (ALT), aspartate aminotransferase (AST), γ-glutamyl transpeptidase (γ-GT) and HDL-cholesterol (HDL-C) were measured on a Cobas MODULAR analyzer (Roche, Basel, Switzerland). Triglycerides (TG) were measured on a Hitachi 912 analyzer (Roche, Basel, Switzerland). Blood glucose was measured from venous whole blood samples using an EPOS

Analyzer 5060 (Eppendorf, Hamburg, Germany). Insulin was determined by microparticle enzyme immunoassay (MEIA) on an AXSYM analyzer (Abbot, Abbot Park, USA), C-peptide (CP) was measured chemiluminimetrically (Immulite1000, Siemens, Erlangen, Germany).

^{1}H-MRS and MRI

All measurements were performed using a 3-T MR scanner (Philips achieva, X-series, Eindhoven, Netherlands). For ^{1}H-MRS, a stimulated echo acquisition mode (STEAM) sequence (repetition time of 4 s, echo time of 10 ms) was performed on a volume of $3 \times 3 \times 2$ cm^3 in the liver. Spectra was collected without water suppression from 32 acquisitions and analyzed using the NUTS software package (Acorn NMR Inc, Livermore, CA, USA). HCL was quantified and corrected for T2 relaxation times with specific weighting for lipids as previously reported [12,13]. Steatosis was defined as HCL values ≥5.56% [14]. Whole body MRI was performed to quantify liver volume (HVOL), total (AT$_{tot}$), subcutaneous (SAT) and visceral (VAT) abdominal adipose tissue using transverse multi-slice turbo-spin echo sequences [15].

Indices of hepatic steatosis
NAFLD liver fat score (NAFLD-LFS) [6].

$$NAFLD - LFS = -2.89 + 1.18 * MS(yes = 1/no = 0)$$
$$+ 0.45 * T2DM(yes = 2/no = 0) + 0.15 * I_0$$
$$+ 0.04 * AST - 0.94 * AST/ALT;$$

with I_0 (μU/ml) representing fasting insulin and AST, fasting AST levels (U/l). Values ≤−0.640 rule out, while values >−0.640 rule in NAFLD. Metabolic syndrome (MS) was defined according to the criteria of the International Diabetes Federation [16].

Hepatic steatosis index (HSI) [5].

$$HSI = 8 * ALT/AST + BMI + 2, if\ DM; +2, if\ female;$$

with values <30 ruling out and values >36 ruling in steatosis.

Fatty liver index (FLI) [4].

$$FLI = logistic(0.953 * ln(TG) + 0.139 * BMI$$
$$+ 0.718 * ln(\gamma GT) + 0.053 * waist - 15.745) * 100;$$

where logistic(x) = $1/(1+e^{-x})$ denotes the logistic function and ln the natural logarithm. Values <30 rule out and values ≥60 rules in steatosis.

Index of percentage HCL
NAFLD-LFS_cont [6].

$NAFLD - LFS\_cont(liver\ fat\%) =$

$10^{(-0.805 + 0.282*MS(yes=1/no=0) + 0.078*T2DM(yes=2/no=0) + 0.525*log(I0 + 0.521log(AST0) - 0.454*log(AST0/ALT))}$

log denotes the decadic logarithm.

Measures of insulin sensitivity and secretion

QUICKI. For fasting conditions, we applied the quantitative insulin sensitivity check index (QUICKI) calculated as $1/[\log(G_0) + \log(I_0)]$, where G_0 and I_0 are fasting glucose and insulin [17].

OGIS. Dynamic insulin sensitivity was assessed with the oral glucose insulin sensitivity index (OGIS), derived from a complex

Table 1. Participants' characteristics.

	No steatosis	Steatosis	No steatosis +LRA	Steatosis +LRA
N (m/f)	75 (29/46)	17 (7/10)	54 (25/29)	11 (6/5)
Age (years)	57.1±12.2	59.9±8.5	56.8±13.1	59.7±9.0
Alcohol (g/d)	18.1±16.1	26.1±18.8	11.1±9.7	18.1±12.9
BMI (kg/m²)	25.3±4.1	28.2±2.8**	25.2±4.1	27.8±2.3§
Waist (cm)	87.1±12.4	94.6±8.5*	87.0±12.3	94.7±6.6§§
SBP (mmHg)	121.6±15.6	128.1±10.3	122.5±14.3	129.5±6.7§
DBP (mmHg)	72.54±8.7	79.3±8.0**	71.9±7.6	80.1±8.9§§
TG (mg/dl)	78 [60;117]	109[84;153]*	79[56;110]	125[87;153]§
HDL-C (mg/dl)	68.3±17.8	58.1±12.7*	67.3±18.2	55.7±12.7§
AST (U/L)	24[21;28]	25[22;32]	24[21;28]	23[21;31]
ALT (U/L)	18[14;25]	26[17;46]**	18[13;24]	26[17;29]§
ãGT (U/L)	20[14;30]	30[20;35]	21[14;30]	30[20;35]
MS (n)	6	4	3	2
G_0 (mg/dl)	75.7±8.3	77.6±10.7	75.5±7.9	77.2±9.5
G_{120} (mg/dl)	89.7±21.5	96.7±26.0	89.7±21.3	92.6±27.7
I_0 (µU/ml)	6[5;9]	8[6;13]*	6[5;9]	8[6;12]§
I_{120} (µU/ml)	37[24;57]	64[38;119]***	33 [23;57]	67[38;102]§
Hep_Extr (%)	69[62;74]	60[57;66]**	69[62;73]	59[56;66]§§
HCL (%)	1.3[0.4;3.4]	13.6[8.3;22.3]	1.1[0.4;2.9]	11.8[8.3;20.1]
HVOL (L)	1.6[1.4;1.8]	1.8[1.8;1.9]**	1.6[1.4;1.8]	1.8[1.7;1.9]§
AT_{tot} (L)	22[18;29]	29[27;32]***	22[18;27]	28[24;32]§
VAT (L)	2.9[1.7;4.4]	4.3[3.3;6.5]**	3.1[1.6;4.4]	4.6[3.3;6.5]§§§
SAT (L)	5.5[4.4;8.1]	7.4[6.6;9.4]	5.4[4.4;7.4]	7.4[5.6;9.4]

Normally distributed data given as mean±standard deviation; Log-normally distributed data as median [25%quartile;75%quartile];
*p<0.05;
**p<0.01 for steatosis vs no steatosis;
§p<0.05;
§§p<0.01,
§§§p<0.001 for steatosis vs no steatosis in LRA.

mathematical model, which represents total glucose disposal or whole body insulin sensitivity [18].

ISIcomp. The Matsuda's index (ISIcomp) was used as another measure of dynamic insulin sensitivity and calculated as $= 10000/\sqrt{(G_0 \times I_0 \times G_m \times I_m)}$, where G_m and I_m are mean glucose and insulin concentrations during OGTT [19].

Fasting β-cell function. During fasting, β-cell function was calculated as CP_0/G_0.

Insulinogenic indices (IGI). During glucose loading, the insulinogenic index was calculated as IGI_Ins $= (I_{30} - I_0)/(G_{30} - G_0)$, where I_{30} and G_{30} are insulin and glucose concentrations at 30 min of OGTT [20,21].

IGI_Ins reflects the appearance of insulin in the peripheral circulation.

For more precise assessing of β-cell (pancreatic, pre-hepatic) function, C-peptide levels were used to calculate the IGI_CP as $(CP_{30} - CP_0)/(G_{30} - G_0)$, where CP_0 and CP_{30} are C-peptide concentrations at fasting and 30 min of OGTT [21].

Disposition Index (DI). The DI is given as product of insulin sensitivity (OGIS) with post-hepatic insulin release function (IGI_Ins$_{tot}$) [22,23].

Adaptation Index (AI). The AI is the product of insulin sensitivity (OGIS) with β-cell function (IGI_CP$_{tot}$) [24,25].

Hepatic insulin extraction. Hepatic insulin extraction was approximated by a function of $1-(AUC_{Ins}/AUC_{CP})$ [26].

Statistical Analyses

The diagnostic performance of the indices was tested by the area under the receiver operating characteristic curve (AROC) [27]. Confidence bounds for comparison between AROC's were done as described [28]. The Clopper-Pearson method [29] was used to calculate exact confidence bounds for sensitivity (Se) and specificity (Sp) at different cut-off limits. The Youden index was calculated as sum of Se and Sp-1 [30].

Variables with skewed distribution were ln-transformed before correlation and regression analyses. Moreover, the logit transformation (logit(x) = ln(x/(1-x)) was applied to the FLI index, divided by 100, to obtain a corresponding linear (approximately normally distributed) index given by

$$FLI_l = 0.953 * ln(TG) + 0.139 * BMI$$
$$+ 0.718 * ln(\gamma GT) + 0.053 * waist - 15.745.$$

This linear index has identical characteristics (ROC, Se, Sp) as the original index and was only used for regression analysis, for all other analyses we applied the original index.

P-values from two-sided tests less than 5% were considered to indicate statistically significant differences. For comparing two

Table 2. Correlation (R) of HCL and indices with insulin sensitivity, β-cell function, liver volume and visceral adipose tissue.

Variable		HCL_ln	NAFLD-LFS	HSI	FLI
Liver fat, volume and fat distribution					
HCL_ln	All	1	0.42***	0.46***	0.50***
	LRA	1	0.26*	0.37**	0.43***
HVOL_ln	All	0.36***	0.38***	0.45***	0.52***
	LRA	0.30*	0.32*	0.39**	0.48***
VAT_ln	All	0.52***	0.52***	0.58***	0.78***
	LRA	0.47***	0.39**	0.54***	0.76***
Insulin sensitivity					
ISIcomp_ln	All	−0.46***	−0.71***	−0.53***	−0.62***
	LRA	−0.34**	−0.56***	−0.48***	−0.59***
OGIS	All	−0.46***	−0.51***	−0.50***	−0.62***
	LRA	−0.39**	−0.27*	−0.43***	−0.55***
QUICKI	All	−0.38***	−0.68***	−0.42***	−0.55***
	LRA	−0.24*	−0.62***	−0.35**	−0.46***
β-cell function					
DI_ln	All	0.36***	0.57***	0.48***	0.47***
	LRA	0.24	0.46***	0.45***	0.47***
B-cell func_ln	All	0.28**	0.57***	0.47***	0.57***
	LRA	0.10	0.46***	0.45***	0.54***
AI	All	0.22*	0.35***	0.33**	0.34***
	LRA	0.14	0.25*	0.29*	0.29*
IGI_CP_ln	All	0.11	0.05	0.02	−0.02
	LRA	0.08	0.06	0.00	−0.03
IGI_Ins_ln	All	0.22*	0.26*	0.19	0.16
	LRA	0.15	0.25*	0.14	0.11
Hep _Extr_ln	All	−0.34***	−0.55***	−0.42***	−0.39***
	LRA	−0.24	−0.46***	−0.42***	−0.39***

*, p<0.05;
**, p<0.01;
***, p<0.001;
B-cell func, B-cell function.

concentration-time curves, we tested specific time points with a Bonferroni-adjusted multiple t-test controlling the family-wise error rate at level 5%. All analyses were performed with SAS for Windows Version 9.2 (SAS Institute, Cary, North Carolina, USA).

Results

Clinical characteristics

Persons with steatosis had higher BMI, waist, DBP, TG, ALT, fasting and 2-hour insulin but lower HDL-C *(Table 1)*. Those with steatosis and low risk alcohol consumption (LRA) also had higher SBP. There were no differences between the respective subgroups with or without LRA.

HCL ranged from 0.03 to 39.01% (median 2.49%; interquartile range (0.62;4.23)) across the whole group (Figure S1 A) and from 0.05 to 30.34% (1.47% (0.60;4.02)) in the LRA subgroup. In the whole group, NAFLD-LFS, HSI and FLI ranged from −4.10 to 2.20, 23.87 to 51.52 and 1.61 to 91.44 with means of −1.81±1.09, 33.71±5.15 and 33.46±26.68, respectively (Figure

S1 B,C,D). NAFLD-LFS, HSI and FLI had comparable values in LRA subjects. All indices differed between persons with and without steatosis of the whole group (NAFLD-LFS: p<0.05; HSI: p<0.001; FLI: p<0.01) and LRA subgroups (p<0.01; p<0.01; p<0.05). All indices correlated with HCL and HVOL in the whole and LRA group. HCL and indices also related to AT_{tot}, SAT and VAT in the whole and LRA group, except for NAFLD-LFS, which did not correlate with AT_{tot} and SAT (Table 2, for AT_{tot} and SAT data not shown).

Diagnostic performance of indices

Across all persons, AROC's were 0.70(95% confidence interval [0.53;0.87]) for NAFLD-LFS, 0.79[0.68;0.90] for HSI, and 0.72[0.59;0.85] for FLI (Figure 1A). In the LRA subgroup, AROC's were 0.75[0.57;0.92], 0.80[0.68;0.92], and 0.75[0.63;0.88], respectively. AROC's did not differ from each other in the whole and LRA group.

Raising the threshold for diagnosing steatosis by HCL above 5.56% improved AROC's for all indices in the whole group (Figure 1B) and in LRA subjects (data not shown). However, AROC of FLI did not further improve at a threshold of 7%.

Applying the originally published cut-off values for each index, which rule in or out steatosis, yielded different diagnostic performance. NAFLD-LFS provided low Se (0.35[0.14;0.62]), but high Sp (0.91[0.82;0.96]). In contrast, HSI had maximal Se (1.00[0.81;1.00]) at the lower cut-off and acceptable Sp (0.75[0.63;0.84]) at the upper cut-off value. FLI had comparable Se (0.76[0.50;0.93]) and Sp (0.83[0.72;0.90]). Analysis of the LRA subgroup revealed similar results (data not shown). We also calculated positive (PPV) and negative predictive values (NPV) of the three indices, with NAFLD-LFS, HSI and FLI having a PPV of 0.46[0.19; 0.75], 0.25[0.16; 0.37] and 0.31[0.18; 0.47]. NPV for NAFLD-LFS, HSI and FLI were 0.86[0.76; 0.93], 0.88[0.77; 0.94] and 0.84[0.73; 0.91], respectively.

To determine optimal cut-off values for each index in our sample, we identified those values that maximize Youden's index. In the whole sample, the optimal cut-off values were −1.02 for NAFLD-LFS yielding a Se of 0.59[0.33; 0.82] and Sp of 0.89[0.80; 0.95], 35.0 for HSI (Se 0.76[0.50; 0.93]; Sp 0.70[0.59; 0.81]), and 29.2 for FLI (Se 0.82[0.56; 0.96]; Sp 0.61[0.49; 0.72]). In the LRA subgroup, the values were −1.12 for NAFLD-LFS (Se 0.64[0.31; 0.89]; Sp 0.87[0.75; 0.95]), 34.0 for HSI (Se 0.91[0.59; 1.0]; Sp 0.67[0.53; 0.79]) and 29.2 for FLI (0.91[0.59; 1.0];0.67[0.53; 0.79]).

After optimization of cut-off values, PPV were 0.56[0.31;0.79] for NAFLD-LFS, 0.37[0.21;0.55] for HSI and 0.33[0.19;0.49] for FLI. NPV were 0.91[0.81;0.96] for NAFLD-LFS, 0.93[0.83;0.98] for HSI and 0.94[0.83;0.99] for FLI. For the LRA subgroup, values were 0.77[0.48;0.95] (PPV) and 0.92[0.81;0.98] (NPV) for NAFLD-LFS, 0.55[0.35;0.74] (PPV) and 0.97[0.86;1.0] (NPV) for HSI, and 0.55[0.35;0.74] (PPV) and 0.97[0.86;1.0] (NPV) for FLI.

Finally, we examined whether specific indices can predict percentage of HCL by applying the previously proposed NAFLD-LFS_cont index using the identical parameters as NAFLD-LFS [6]. NAFLD-LFS_cont correlated with HCL across all (r=0.42, p<0.001) and LRA persons (r=0.27, p<0.05) (Figure 1C). However, the differences between observed and predicted ln-transformed HCL values (residuals) ranged from −3.9 to 2.5 (Figure 1D). Translated to the original scale, this means that the ratio of observed and predicted liver fat ranges from 0.02 to 12.2.

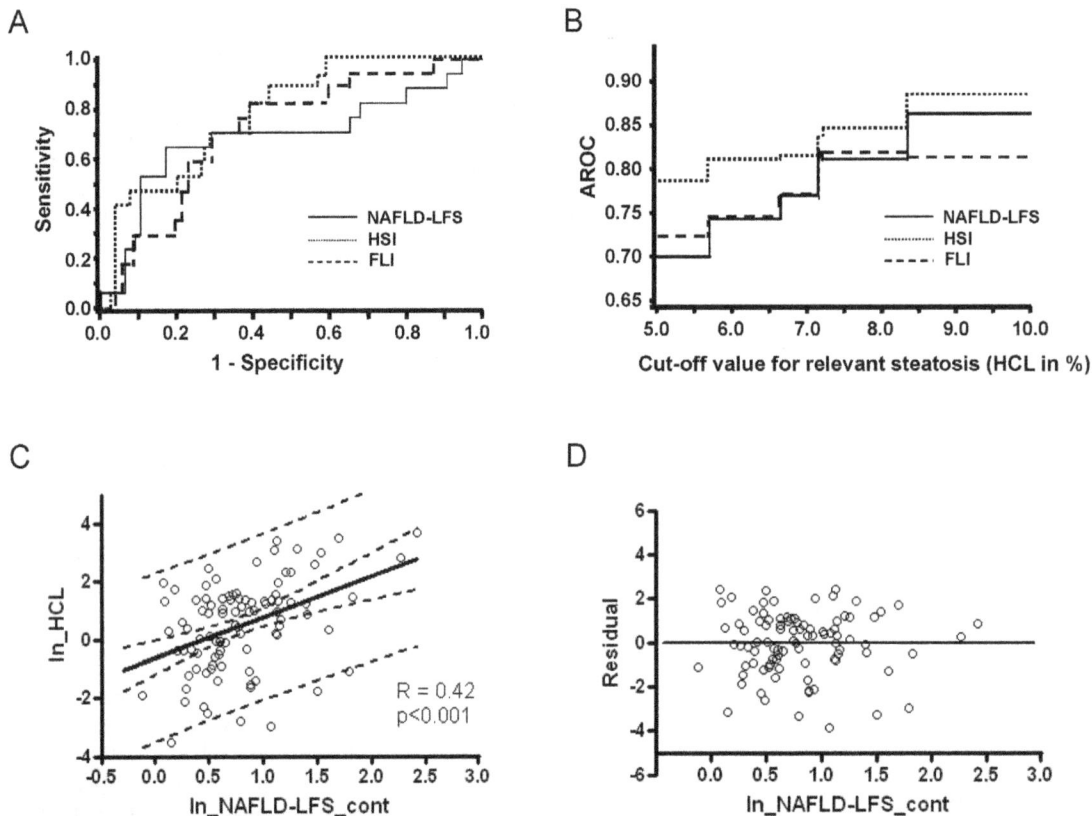

Figure 1. Performance of indices (all subjects). (A) ROC curves of NAFLD-LFS (black line), HSI (dotted line) and FLI (dashed line) (B) AROC's of NAFLD-LFS (black line), HSI (dotted line) and FLI (dashed line) for different HCL cut-offs defining steatosis (C) Correlation of HCL with NAFLD-LFS_cont. Black line, linear regression curve; inner broken lines, 95% confidence limits; outer broken lines, 95% prediction limits (D) Evaluation of goodness of fit by plotting residuals against HCL calculated by NAFLD-LFS_cont.

Correlation of HCL and indices with glycemia, insulin sensitivity and β-cell function

Subjects with steatosis had similar blood glucose, but higher insulin and C-peptide during OGTT than those without steatosis (Figure 2 A,B). In LRA subjects, presumably due to low sample size, differences in insulin and C-peptide levels were less prominent (Figure 2 C,D).

HCL correlated inversely with fasting (QUICKI) and dynamic insulin sensitivity (OGIS, ISIcomp) and positively with fasting β-cell function and post-load insulin release (DI, AI, IGI_Ins) in all, but not in LRA subjects (table 2).

Also, the indices inversely and strongly correlated with QUICKI, OGIS and ISIcomp (table 2). Even after adjustment for age, sex, and HCL (model-1, table 3) and for LRA (model-2, table 3), FLI, NAFLD-LFS and HSI still related to all parameters of insulin sensitivity.

In all and LRA subjects, indices correlated with fasting β-cell function, DI and AI. Only NAFLD-LFS related to IGI_INS (p<0.05) (table 2). Applying model-1 on all subjects, correlations between indices and fasting β-cell function, DI and AI were still present. Also, applying model-2, correlations remained (table 3). LRA subjects showed comparable results with model-1, only HSI did not correlate with AI and NAFLD-LFS was not associated with OGIS (data not shown).

Hepatic insulin extraction differed between subjects with and without FL (table 1) and related to HCL and indices in all (p<0.001), but not in LRA subjects (p = 0.06). However, all indices

correlated with hepatic insulin extraction in all and LRA subjects (table 2).

Discussion

In this non-diabetic, predominantly non-obese collective from the general population NAFLD-LFS, HSI and FLI offer a diagnostic efficacy of 70–80% with lower sensitivities and specificities compared with their original description. Interestingly, this study shows additional features of these indices as predictors of insulin resistance and - to less extent - insulin secretion.

Several factors might contribute to the lower than expected diagnostic efficacy of the indices, including selection and characteristics of the study populations (inclusion criteria, risk factor prevalence) as well as measurement technique [27]. In contrast to the populations from which the indices were derived, our study consists of a sample of non-diabetic, predominantly non-obese white persons from the general population. For NAFLD-LFS, the Finnish collective comprises persons without and with T2DM recruited on a 3-to-1 basis for metabolic studies [6]. HSI was derived from data of a Korean cross-sectional case-control study [5]. Finally, FLI however, was developed from data of the Dionysos Nutrition & Liver study, which included residents of Campogalliano in Italy [4,31], providing a real sampling of general population without particular bias in selection, but development of FLI was based on equally matched persons with and without suspected liver disease (SLD). Comparing these collectives shows marked differences in prevalence of risk factors.

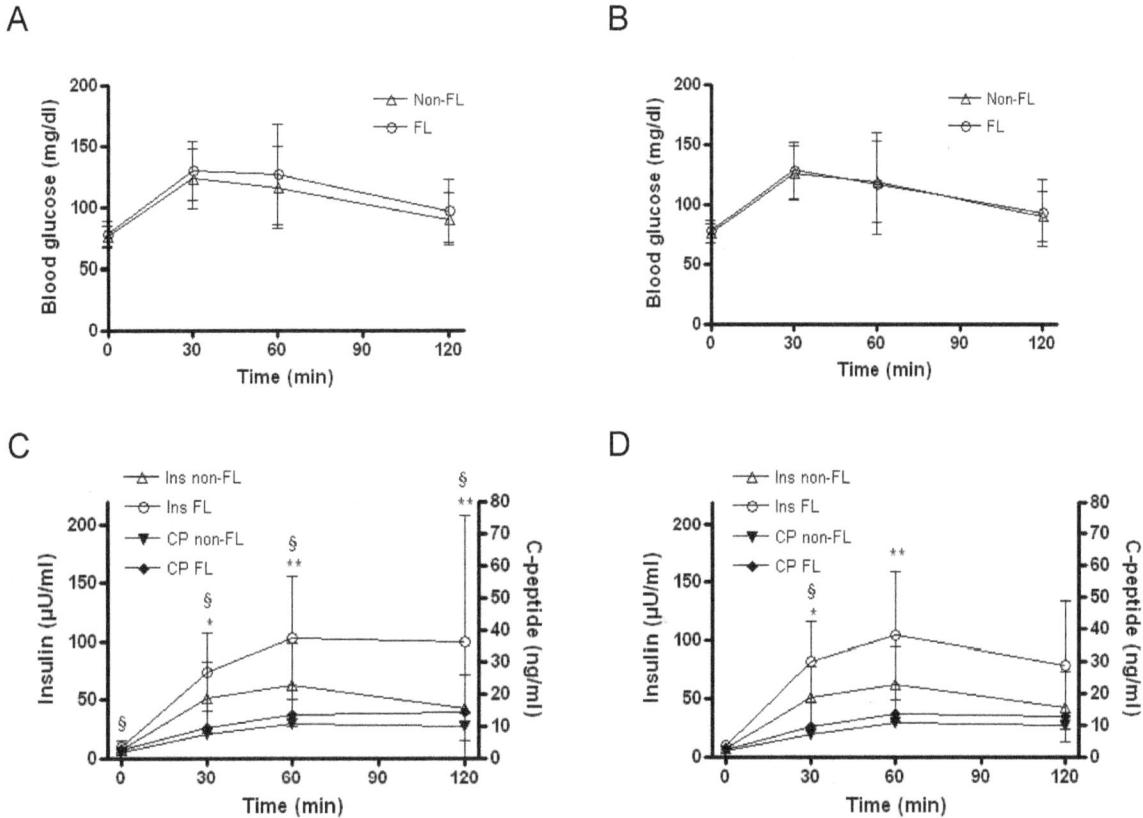

Figure 2. OGTT in subjects with and without steatosis. Plasma glucose (all: A, LRA: B), insulin and C-peptide (all: C, LRA: D) during OGTT in subjects without (non-FL) (insulin: open triangles, C-peptide: black triangles) and with steatosis (FL) (insulin: open circles, C-peptide: black squares). *, $p<0.05$; **, $p<0.01$ for insulin; §, $p<0.05$ for C-peptide.

The NAFLD-LFS collective presents with already increased risk for metabolic diseases such as T2DM due to greater BMI, BP, TG and transaminases [6]. The HSI collective comprised exclusively Asians, who develop NAFLD at lower BMI with 3.5fold greater prevalence in males, both of which differing from whites [32]. Remarkably, both BMI and sex are variables of the HSI. The FLI collective comprised a white sample of the general population, but cases of SLD were matched with cases without SLD and therefore prevalence of the metabolic syndrome and T2DM might not be the same as in the general population [31].

The sensitivity of ultrasound to detect steatosis is about 91% in patients with HCL ≥30% [33], but only 64% for HCL <30%, indicating that ultrasound misses cases of mild steatosis. Thus, HSI and FLI, which have been validated against ultrasound, may have been rather designed to reliably identify patients with medium to severe fatty liver disease than those with mild steatosis. Testing the accuracy of FLI in a smaller group of women with previous gestational diabetes revealed a strong correlation with HCL measured by ^{1}H-MRS [34], whereas FLI and HSI performed less well in patients with T2DM [8]. We found reasonable AROCs for FLI and HSI, but lower diagnostic performance for NAFLD-LFS in our collective. The latter might be due to the lower mean HCL compared to the validation study of NAFLD-LFS [6]. NAFLD-LFS_cont was derived from the NAFLD-LFS collective and developed exclusively to predict percent HCL [6]. The present study showed that the residuals, i.e. the differences between observed and predicted HCL using this specific index, were in most cases as high as the value of HCL contents. This indicates that NAFLD-LFS_cont is not suitable for prediction of HCL at

least in non-diabetic collectives with lower prevalence of steatosis. Thus, these scores offer overall modest performance in the clinical setting– even after optimizing cut-off values for our collective. In detail, sensitivity and specificity differ among the three indices between 0.59 and 0.82 for Se and 0.61 and 0.89 for Sp, respectively. This means that up to 41% of the investigated individuals may be classified as patients without FL, although having FL (false-negative rate) and up to 39% of the individuals may be grouped as FL positive, although having no FL (false-positive rate). These data do not support their use as screening tools, at least for populations with similar characteristics as in the present study with such non-obese persons. Additionally, the positive predictive values indicate that in case of a positive test result, the probability that the patient really has FL is only between 33 and 56%. It might be also critical to adjust cut-offs for FL indices for the tested cohort. Nevertheless, the acceptable correlation between fatty liver indices and exact quantification of HCL suggests that these indices might be appropriate surrogate parameters of liver fat content in large epidemiological studies. It is well accepted that hepatic steatosis associates with insulin resistance and hyperinsulinemia even in lean glucose-tolerant subjects [7]. Likewise, FLI correlates with insulin resistance and T2DM incidence [7,34,35]. Although NAFLD-LFS also predicted T2DM in a French cohort [36], its relationship with insulin resistance has not been assessed. To our knowledge, HSI has also not been analyzed with regard to insulin sensitivity and secretion. Here we clearly show that all three indices, strongly and inversely correlate with measures of insulin sensitivity.

Table 3. Association of indices with insulin sensitivity and β-cell function after adjustment for age, sex, HCL and LRA.

			Model-1 Age,Sex,HCL		Model-2 Age,Sex,HCL,LRA	
		Dependent	Estimate (β)	Partial correlation	Estimate (β)	Partial correlation
NAFLD-LFS	All	OGIS	−22.3***	−0.38	−22.9***	−0.39
HSI			−4.1**	−0.35	−4.3***	−0.35
FLI$_I$			−20.4***	−0.46	−21.1***	−0.46
NAFLD-LFS		QUICKI	−0.03***	−0.62	−0.03***	−0.64
HSI			−0.003**	−0.32	−0.003**	−0.33
FLI$_I$			−0.02***	−0.45	−0.02***	−0.46
NAFLD-LFS		ISIcomp_ln	−0.31***	−0.64	−0.33***	−0.66
HSI			−0.04***	−0.41	−0.04***	−0.42
FLI$_I$			−0.19***	−0.51	−0.20***	−0.52
NAFLD-LFS		Disposition Index_ln	0.22***	0.52	0.23***	0.55
HSI			0.03***	0.38	0.04***	0.40
FLI$_I$			0.13***	0.41	0.14***	0.43
NAFLD-LFS		Adaptation Index	0.04***	0.34	0.04***	0.36
HSI			0.006*	0.24	0.006*	0.24
FLI$_I$			0.03**	0.32	0.03**	0.33
NAFLD-LFS		B-cell func_ln	0.21***	0.53	0.19***	0.53
HSI			0.03***	0.40	0.03***	0.40
FLI$_I$			0.16***	0.56	0.16***	0.56

*, $p < 0.05$;
**, $p < 0.01$;
***, $p < 0.001$;
B-cell func, B-cell function.

Of note, less is known on an association between HCL and β-cell function. While HCL and fasting insulin may correlate [37], data on its relationship with dynamic/OGTT postload β-cell function in collectives with normal and impaired glucose tolerance was contradictory [38,39]. Here, we confirm that HCL relates to various parameters of β-cell function except IGI in all, but not in LRA subjects, and extend this finding to the three indices. The indices only failed to associate with IGI_Ins and IGI_CP, which might result from the pre-described rather low performance of IGI in small- to medium-sized collectives [21].

The novelty of the present study resides in the direct comparison of different indices with HCL measurement by ^{1}H-MRS in a single study population of non-diabetic, predominantly non-obese whites and the finding that - while not specific for prediction of hepatic steatosis - they at least partly reflect glucose homeostasis. On the other hand, this study has also certain limitations. First, this study has a rather small sample size and a collective with low mean HCL contents and prevalence of steatosis. This should not influence Se and Sp of the indices [27] and increases the relevance of these results for general screening of steatosis. However, the predominance of persons with low HCL contents might contribute to the wide confidence intervals for sensitivity and the low positive predictive values thereby under-estimating the value of the indices. The small sample size may also add to the wide confidence intervals for AROCs of the tested indices. Moreover, when comparing AROCs of the different indices, we did not find significant differences in performances, but we cannot fully exclude that there might be differences in performance we cannot detect with our collective. Thus, further validation of these indices should be performed in larger cohorts.

Second, participants with significant consumption of alcohol were not omitted from the analysis of the whole collective, as the relative contribution of ethanol intake to the pathogenesis of NAFLD is still uncertain [4]. In their regression models, Bedogni et al. even report no association between ethanol intake and steatosis [4]. Recent data suggest that - despite the potential interactions between alcohol drinking and liver injury - moderate alcohol intake may have paradoxical, favorable and gender-dependent effects also in the liver [40,41]. However, as heavy drinking is known for its deleterious effects on the liver, we set maximum acceptable alcohol intake to 40 g/d for men and 20 g/d for women, which is below the levels set for heavy drinking (>60 g/d for men and >40 g/d for women), for analyses of the LRA subgroup. Of note, all analyses were also performed in this LRA subgroup, which gave similar results as reported for the whole group.

In conclusion, the tested fatty liver indices offer modest efficacy to detect steatosis and cannot substitute for exact fat quantification by ^{1}H-MRS. However, they might serve as surrogate parameters for liver fat content and also as rough clinical estimates of abnormal insulin sensitivity and secretion. Further validation in larger collectives such as epidemiological studies is needed.

Acknowledgments

We thank Peter Nowotny for technical assistance.

Author Contributions

Conceived and designed the experiments: MR SK BN KS BK RL JHH. Performed the experiments: SK BN RL KK BK. Analyzed the data: SK KS RL JHH GG BH GP AG MR. Contributed reagents/materials/ analysis tools: KS JHH GP. Wrote the paper: SK KS RL JHH GG GP MR. Revision of article: SK KS BN RL BK KK JHH GG BH GP AG MR. Final approval: SK KS BN RL BK KK JHH GG BH GP AG MR.

References

1. Roden M (2006) Mechanisms of Disease: hepatic steatosis in type 2 diabetes-pathogenesis and clinical relevance. Nat Clin Pract Endocrinol Metab 2: 335–348.
2. Barsic N, Lerotic I, Smircic-Duvnjak L, Tomasic V, Duvnjak M (2012) Overview and developments in noninvasive diagnosis of nonalcoholic fatty liver disease. World J Gastroenterol 18: 3945–3954.
3. Webb M, Yeshua H, Zelber-Sagi S, Santo E, Brazowski E, et al. (2009) Diagnostic value of a computerized hepatorenal index for sonographic quantification of liver steatosis. AJR Am J Roentgenol 192: 909–914.
4. Bedogni G, Bellentani S, Miglioli L, Masutti F, Passalacqua M, et al. (2006) The Fatty Liver Index: a simple and accurate predictor of hepatic steatosis in the general population. BMC Gastroenterol 6: 33.
5. Lee JH, Kim D, Kim HJ, Lee CH, Yang JI, et al. (2010) Hepatic steatosis index: a simple screening tool reflecting nonalcoholic fatty liver disease. Dig Liver Dis 42: 503–508.
6. Kotronen A, Peltonen M, Hakkarainen A, Sevastianova K, Bergholm R, et al. (2009) Prediction of non-alcoholic fatty liver disease and liver fat using metabolic and genetic factors. Gastroenterology 137: 865–872.
7. Gastaldelli A, Kozakova M, Hojlund K, Flyvbjerg A, Favuzzi A, et al. (2009) Fatty liver is associated with insulin resistance, risk of coronary heart disease, and early atherosclerosis in a large European population. Hepatology 49: 1537–1544.
8. Guiu B, Crevisy-Girod E, Binquet C, Duvillard L, Masson D, et al. (2012) Prediction for steatosis in type-2 diabetes: clinico-biological markers versus 1H-MR spectroscopy. Eur Radiol 22: 855–863
9. Rehm J, Room R, Monteiro M, Gmel G, Graham K, et al. (2004) Alcohol use. In: Ezzati M, Lopez A, Rodgers A, Murray CJL, eds. Comparative Quantification of Health Risks: Global and regional burden of disease due to selected major risk factors. Geneva, World Health Organization. pp 959–1108.
10. Poynard T, Ratziu V, Naveau S, Thabut D, Charlotte F, et al. (2005) The diagnostic value of biomarkers (SteatoTest) for the prediction of liver steatosis. Comp Hepatol 4: 10.
11. American Diabetes Association (2006) Diagnosis and classification of diabetes mellitus. Diabetes Care 29 Suppl 1: S43–S48.
12. Krssak M, Hofer H, Wrba F, Meyerspeer M, Brehm A, et al. (2010) Non-invasive assessment of hepatic fat accumulation in chronic hepatitis C by 1H magnetic resonance spectroscopy. Eur J Radiol 74: e60–e66.
13. Hamilton G, Yokoo T, Bydder M, Cruite I, Schroeder ME, et al. (2011) In vivo characterization of the liver fat (1)H MR spectrum. NMR Biomed 24: 784–790.
14. Szczepaniak LS, Nurenberg P, Leonard D, Browning JD, Reingold JS, et al. (2005) Magnetic resonance spectroscopy to measure hepatic triglyceride content: prevalence of hepatic steatosis in the general population. Am J Physiol Endocrinol Metab 288: E462–E468.
15. Machann J, Thamer C, Stefan N, Schwenzer NF, Kantartzis K, et al. (2010) Follow-up whole-body assessment of adipose tissue compartments during a lifestyle intervention in a large cohort at increased risk for type 2 diabetes. Radiology 257: 353–363.
16. Alberti KG, Zimmet P, Shaw J (2005) The metabolic syndrome–a new worldwide definition. Lancet 366: 1059–1062.
17. Katz A, Nambi SS, Mather K, Baron AD, Follmann DA, et al. (2000) Quantitative insulin sensitivity check index: a simple, accurate method for assessing insulin sensitivity in humans. J Clin Endocrinol Metab 85: 2402–2410.
18. Mari A, Pacini G, Murphy E, Ludvik B, Nolan JJ (2001) A model-based method for assessing insulin sensitivity from the oral glucose tolerance test. Diabetes Care 24: 539–548.
19. Matsuda M, DeFronzo RA (1999) Insulin sensitivity indices obtained from oral glucose tolerance testing: comparison with the euglycemic insulin clamp. Diabetes Care 22: 1462–1470.
20. Phillips DI, Clark PM, Hales CN, Osmond C (1994) Understanding oral glucose tolerance: comparison of glucose or insulin measurements during the oral glucose tolerance test with specific measurements of insulin resistance and insulin secretion. Diabet Med 11: 286–292.
21. Tura A, Kautzky-Willer A, Pacini G (2006) Insulinogenic indices from insulin and C-peptide: comparison of beta-cell function from OGTT and IVGTT. Diabetes Res Clin Pract 72: 298–301.
22. Kahn SE, Prigeon RL, McCulloch DK, Boyko EJ, Bergman RN, et al. (1993) Quantification of the relationship between insulin sensitivity and beta-cell function in human subjects. Evidence for a hyperbolic function. Diabetes 42: 1663–1672.
23. Szendroedi J, Frossard M, Klein N, Bieglmayer C, Wagner O, et al. (2012) Lipid-induced insulin resistance is not mediated by impaired transcapillary transport of insulin and glucose in humans. Diabetes 61: 3176–3180.
24. Ahren B, Pacini G (1997) Impaired adaptation of first-phase insulin secretion in postmenopausal women with glucose intolerance. Am J Physiol 273: E701–E707.
25. Anderwald C, Pfeiler G, Nowotny P, Anderwald-Stadler M, Krebs M, et al. (2008) Glucose turnover and intima media thickness of internal carotid artery in type 2 diabetes offspring. Eur J Clin Invest 38: 227–237.
26. Stadler M, Anderwald C, Karer T, Tura A, Kastenbauer T, et al. (2006) Increased plasma amylin in type 1 diabetic patients after kidney and pancreas transplantation: A sign of impaired beta-cell function? Diabetes Care 29: 1031–1038.
27. Cook NR (2007) Use and misuse of the receiver operating characteristic curve in risk prediction. Circulation 115: 928–935.
28. DeLong ER, DeLong DM, Clarke-Pearson DL (1988) Comparing the areas under two or more correlated receiver operating characteristic curves: a nonparametric approach. Biometrics 44: 837–845.
29. Clopper CJ, Pearson ES (1934) The use of confidence or fiducial limits illustrated in the case of the binominal. Biometrika 26: 404–413.
30. Youden WJ (1950) Index for rating diagnostic tests. Cancer 3: 32–35.
31. Bedogni G, Miglioli L, Masutti F, Tiribelli C, Marchesini G, et al. (2005) Prevalence of and risk factors for nonalcoholic fatty liver disease: the Dionysos nutrition and liver study. Hepatology 42: 44–52.
32. Weston SR, Leyden W, Murphy R, Bass NM, Bell BP, et al. (2005) Racial and ethnic distribution of nonalcoholic fatty liver in persons with newly diagnosed chronic liver disease. Hepatology 41: 372–379.
33. Palmentieri B, de Sio I, La Mura V, Masarone M, Vecchione R, et al. (2006) The role of bright liver echo pattern on ultrasound B-mode examination in the diagnosis of liver steatosis. Dig Liver Dis 38: 485–489.
34. Bozkurt L, Gobl CS, Tura A, Chmelik M, Prikoszovich T, et al. (2012) Fatty liver index predicts further metabolic deteriorations in women with previous gestational diabetes. PLoS One 7: e32710.
35. Calori G, Lattuada G, Ragogna F, Garancini MP, Crosignani P, et al. (2011) Fatty liver index and mortality: the Cremona study in the 15th year of follow-up. Hepatology 54: 145–152.
36. Balkau B, Lange C, Vol S, Fumeron F, Bonnet F (2010) Nine-year incident diabetes is predicted by fatty liver indices: the French D.E.S.I.R. study. BMC Gastroenterol 10: 56.
37. Perseghin G, Caumo A, Lattuada G, DeCobelli F, Esposito A, et al. (2007) Augmented fasting beta-cell secretion, and not only insulin resistance, is a feature of non-diabetic individuals with fatty liver. Diabetes 56, suppl.1: pA677.
38. Tushuizen ME, Bunck MC, Pouwels PJ, Bontemps S, Mari A, et al. (2008) Lack of association of liver fat with model parameters of beta-cell function in men with impaired glucose tolerance and type 2 diabetes. Eur J Endocrinol 159: 251–257.
39. Rijkelijkhuizen JM, Doesburg T, Girman CJ, Mari A, Rhodes T, et al. (2009) Hepatic fat is not associated with beta-cell function or postprandial free fatty acid response. Metabolism 58: 196–203.
40. Suzuki A, Angulo P, St Sauver J, Muto A, Okada T, et al. (2007) Light to moderate alcohol consumption is associated with lower frequency of hyper-transaminasemia. Am J Gastroenterol 102: 1912–1919.
41. Moriya A, Iwasaki Y, Ohguchi S, Kayashima E, Mitsumune T, et al. (2011) Alcohol consumption appears to protect against non-alcoholic fatty liver disease. Aliment Pharmacol Ther 33: 378–388.

21

Serum 25-Hydroxyvitamin D and Insulin Resistance in Apparently Healthy Adolescents

Dong Phil Choi[1,4], Sun Min Oh[2], Ju-Mi Lee[2], Hye Min Cho[2], Won Joon Lee[2], Bo-Mi Song[1], Yumie Rhee[3], Hyeon Chang Kim[2,4]*

1 Department of Public Health, Graduate School of Yonsei University, Seoul, Korea, **2** Department of Preventive Medicine, Yonsei University College of Medicine, Seoul, Korea, **3** Department of Internal Medicine, Yonsei University College of Medicine, Seoul, Korea, **4** Cardiovascular and Metabolic Diseases Etiology Research Center, Yonsei University College of Medicine, Seoul, Korea

Abstract

Purpose: Vitamin D deficiency is a common condition that is associated with diabetes and insulin resistance. However, the association between vitamin D and insulin resistance has not been fully studied, especially in the general adolescent population. Therefore, we assessed the association between serum 25-hydroxyvitamin D [25(OH)D] level and insulin resistance among apparently healthy Korean adolescents.

Methods: A total of 260 (135 male and 125 female) adolescents in a rural high school were assessed for serum 25(OH)D, fasting plasma glucose, and insulin. All of the participants were aged 15 to 16 years old, and without known hypertension or diabetes. Serum 25(OH)D was analyzed both as a continuous and categorical variable in association with insulin resistance. Insulin resistance was estimated by homeostasis model assessment (HOMA-IR). Increased insulin resistance was operationally defined as a HOMA-IR value higher than the sex-specific 75th percentile.

Results: In male adolescents, every 10 ng/ml decrease in 25(OH)D level was associated with a 0.25 unit increase in HOMA-IR (p = 0.003) after adjusting for age and BMI. Compared to those in the highest quartile, male adolescents in the lowest 25(OH)D quartile were at significantly higher risk for insulin resistance: unadjusted odds ratio 4.06 (95% CI, 1.26 to 13.07); age and BMI adjusted odds ratio 3.59 (95% CI, 1.03 to 12.57). However, 25(OH)D level, either in continuous or categorical measure, was not significantly associated with insulin resistance among female adolescents.

Conclusions: This study suggests that serum 25(OH)D level may be inversely associated with insulin resistance in healthy male adolescents.

Editor: Joseph Devaney, Children's National Medical Center, Washington, United States of America

Funding: This research was supported by Basic Science Research Program through the National Research Foundation of Korea (NRF) grant funded by the Ministry of Education, Science and Technology (MEST) (No. 2010-0007860) and by a faculty research grant of Yonsei University College of Medicine for 2010 (6-2010-0164). The funders had no role in study design, data collection and analysis, decision to publish, or preparation of the manuscript.

Competing Interests: The authors have declared that no competing interests exist.

* Email: hckim@yuhs.ac

Introduction

Vitamin D is an important fat-soluble vitamin that functions in calcium and phosphorus homeostasis and affects bone mineralization. Functions of vitamin D are not limited to skeletal effects, and a non-skeletal action under active investigation is the role of vitamin D in insulin or glucose metabolism [1]. Vitamin D status may play a functional role in glucose homeostasis as *in vitro* and *in vivo* studies have provided biological evidence of its effects on insulin secretion and insulin sensitivity [2–6]. Several epidemiological studies have reported associations between low vitamin D status, as indicated by circulating serum 25-hydroxyvitamin D [25(OH)D], and the risk of type 2 diabetes [7–10], although others have not found such an association [11,12]. A study of the Third National Health and Nutrition Examination Survey (NHANES III) showed an inverse association between serum 25(OH)D level, insulin resistance, and diabetes in non-Hispanic whites and Mexican Americans, but not in non-Hispanic blacks [13]. Serum

25(OH)D level was inversely associated with insulin resistance in a study of Chinese individuals [14], but was not associated with insulin resistance or beta cell function in a study of the Canadian Cree [12].

An association between hypovitaminosis D and insulin resistance has also been reported in overweight or obese adolescents [15–19], but the association was not observed in the general adolescent population [20]. The association between vitamin D and insulin resistance has not been fully explored, especially in healthy adolescents. Therefore, we investigated the association between serum 25(OH)D level and insulin resistance among apparently healthy Korean adolescents.

Materials and Methods

Study population

We conducted a cross-sectional analysis of baseline data collected for an adolescent cohort study. All first-year students of

Table 1. Participants characteristics.

Variable	Total (n = 260)	Male (n = 135)	Female (n = 125)	p-value
Mean ± SD				
Age, year	15.9±0.3	15.9±0.3	15.9±0.3	0.274
Body mass index, kg/m²	21.7±2.9	22.2±3.2	21.2±2.5	0.011
Systolic blood pressure, mmHg	103.4±11.5	109.4±10.8	96.8±8.4	<.001
Diastolic blood pressure, mmHg	57.9±5.9	58.4±6.1	57.4±5.8	0.204
Total cholesterol, mg/dl	156.9±27.2	150.0±26.6	164.5±26.0	<.001
HDL cholesterol, mg/dl	45.6±8.8	43.1±7.7	48.3±9.1	<.001
Triglycerides, mg/dl	83.1±30.3	85.6±30.7	80.4±29.8	0.066
Aspartate aminotransferase, IU/l	20.4±5.7	21.9±7.1	18.7±2.9	<.001
Alanine aminotransferase, IU/l	15.9±9.2	18.5±11.8	13.0±3.2	<.001
Fasting glucose, mg/dl	84.5±6.2	86.0±6.3	82.9±5.8	<.001
Fasting insulin, uIU/mL	8.54±3.12	8.67±3.44	8.42±2.76	0.995
HOMA-IR, mg/dl/mL/uIU	1.79±0.71	1.86±0.79	1.73±0.61	0.314
25(OH)D, ng/ml	15.8±7.2	17.0±6.9	14.4±7.3	<.001
Number (%)				
Smoking (≥100 cigarettes)	13 (5.0)	12 (8.8)	1 (0.8)	0.546
Drinking (≥1 time/month)	16 (6.1)	10 (7.4)	6 (4.8)	0.160
Regular exercise (≥1 time/week)	219 (83.9)	120 (88.2)	99 (79.2)	0.003

Abbreviations: HDL, high-density lipoprotein; HOMA-IR, homeostasis model assessment insulin resistance.

a high school in a rural community in South Korea were invited to participate in the cohort study. Among the total 283 first-year students, 268 students agreed to participate in the study between May 30 and June 22, 2011. After exclusion of seven individuals who were missing serum 25(OH)D measurements and one individual with diagnosed hypertension, 260 students were included for this analysis. All participants were aged between 15 and 16 years (mean age 15.9 years) and had not been previously diagnosed with diabetes mellitus. Written informed consent was obtained from each participant and his/her parent or guardian. Informed consent forms were distributed to eligible students at least one week prior to the examination, so the participating students and their parents had enough time to understand the purpose and process of the study. On the day of examination, research staff checked whether each consent form was completed and signed by the student as well as his/her parent or guardian. The study protocol and consent procedure was approved by the Institutional Review Board of Severance Hospital at Yonsei University College of Medicine (Approval No. 4-20100169).

Measurements

Health-related lifestyle, personal and family medical history were evaluated with self-report questionnaires. Smokers were defined as participants who smoked more than 100 cigarettes in their lifetime. Drinkers were defined as participants who consume alcoholic beverage at least once a month over the last year. Regular exercise was defined as physical activity on a regular basis (at least once a week for 30 minutes at moderate intensity) regardless of indoor or outdoor exercise. Anthropometric measures, performed using the same devices throughout this study, were taken by a trained examiner. Standing height was measured to the nearest 0.1 cm on a stadiometer, and body weight was measured to the nearest 0.1 kg on a digital scale (Seca 763; SECA, Hamburg, Germany) while wearing the school uniform.

Body mass index (BMI) was calculated as weight in kg divided by squared height in meters (kg/m²). Waist circumference (WC) was measured to the nearest 0.1 cm at the level of the superior iliac crest at the end of a normal expiration. Resting blood pressure and pulse rate were measured with an oscillometric device (Dinamap 1846 SX/P; USA). Participants were seated in the examination room for at least five minutes before blood pressure measurement, and then an appropriately sized cuff was applied snugly around the right upper arm at heart level. Cuff size was chosen for each subject according to mid-arm circumference. Two readings at five minute intervals were obtained and averaged to determine systolic blood pressure (SBP) and diastolic blood pressure (DBP) for each individual. When the two readings differed by ≥10 mmHg, additional readings were obtained after five minutes, and the last two readings were averaged.

An overnight fasting blood sample was collected after at least an 8-hour fast. Serum concentrations of total cholesterol, triglycerides, high-density lipoprotein (HDL) cholesterol, aspartate aminotransferase (AST), and alanine aminotransferase (ALT) were measured by enzymatic methods with an autoanalyzer (7600 Autoanalyzer, Hitachi, Tokyo, Japan). Serum 25(OH)D was measured by radioimmunoassay (BioSource, Nivelles, Belgium) with inter-/intra-assay coefficient of variations (CVs) of 5.2% and 3.3%, respectively, and a reference range of 7.6 to 75.0 ng/ml. Fasting plasma glucose (FPG) level was measured by the glucose hexokinase method. Fasting plasma insulin level was measured by the radio immunometric method. Insulin resistance was assessed by homeostatic model assessment (HOMA-IR), calculated as the product of the fasting insulin level (uIU/mL) and the fasting glucose level (mg/dL), divided by 405.

Statistical analyses

All statistical analyses were performed separately for males and females, because there were significant sex-differences in serum

Table 2. Correlations between serum 25(OH)D and metabolic characteristics.

	BMI	SBP	DBP	TC	HDLC	Triglyceride	Glucose	Insulin	HOMA-IR	25(OH)D
BMI	-	0.412***	0.062	0.000	-0.218*	0.240**	0.087	0.330***	0.301***	0.028
SBP	0.362***	-	0.468***	0.073	0.010	0.045	0.063	0.143	0.123	0.040
DBP	0.077	0.610***	-	-0.059	0.021	0.020	-0.116	0.120	0.084	0.038
TC	0.156	0.025	-0.060	-	0.353***	0.226**	0.077	0.033	0.049	-0.213*
HDLC	0.046	-0.019	-0.051	0.370***	-	-0.329***	0.065	-0.098	-0.085	0.016
Triglyceride	0.004	0.061	0.039	0.241**	-0.276**	-	0.053	0.147	0.152	-0.148
Glucose	0.100	0.036	0.084	-0.040	0.176*	0.046	-	0.233**	0.410***	-0.153
Insulin	0.302***	0.226*	-0.001	-0.018	-0.102	0.150	0.191*	-	0.975***	-0.256**
HOMA-IR	0.286***	0.210*	-0.002	-0.035	-0.047	0.130	0.400***	0.966***	-	-0.263**
25(OH)D	0.059	-0.024	0.090	-0.022	0.063	-0.101	0.028	-0.049	-0.049	-

Abbreviations: BMI, body mass index; SBP, systolic blood pressure; DBP, diastolic blood pressure; TC, total cholesterol; HDLC, high-density lipoprotein cholesterol; HOMA-IR, homeostasis model assessment insulin resistance. Males, above the diagona.; Females, under the diagonal. * $p < 0.05$; ** $p < 0.01$; *** $p < 0.001$.

25(OH)D levels and a significant interaction ($p = 0.019$) between sex and 25(OH)D on HOMA-IR levels. Differences between groups in quantitative variables were evaluated by student's t-test, x^2-test, or Wilcoxon rank sum test. Spearman correlation and linear regression analyses were used to examine the relationship between variables. Both categorical (quartile groups) and continuous measures of 25(OH)D were analyzed in association with fasting glucose, insulin, and HOMA-IR levels, with and without adjustment for age and sex. Multiple logistic regression models were also used to evaluate the odds ratio and 95% confidence interval for increased insulin resistance (defined as HOMA-IR ≥ 75 percentile) for quartile groups of serum 25(OH)D as well as for 10 ng/ml decrease of 25(OH)D. In order to assess the independent association between serum 25(OH)D, two adjusted models were employed; first for age and BMI, then for cigarette smoking, alcohol consumption, and regular exercise. All analyses were 2-tailed and performed using SAS system version 9.2 (SAS Institute, Cary, NC, USA).

Results

The characteristics of the study participants are given by sex and in total. Male participants had significantly higher BMI, SBP, AST, ALT, FPG, and 25(OH)D, but significantly lower HDL cholesterol level than female participants. None of the adolescents had fasting glucose higher than 110 mg/dl. Thirteen adolescents (5.0%) were current smokers, 16 (6.1%) consumed alcoholic drinks at least once a month, and 219 (83.9%) exercised on a regular basis (Table 1). Although the participants were recruited from a single high school, their anthropometric distributions and serum 25(OH)D levels were similar to those in the 2007 Korean National Growth Charts and the 2009 Korean National Health and Nutrition Examination Survey. Mean height was 172.8/160.7 cm (male/female) in this study, and the corresponding value from the growth charts was 173.3/160.7 cm. Mean body weight was 66.4/55.5 kg (male/female) in this study and 65.8/54.1 kg in the growth charts. Mean serum 25(OH)D level was 17.0/14.4 ng/ml (male/female) in this study and 17.2/16.4 ng/ml in the Korean National Health and Nutrition Examination Survey [21,22].

Table 2 shows correlations between serum 25(OH)D and other metabolic variables. Serum 25(OH)D level was inversely correlated with total cholesterol ($r = -0.213$, $p = 0.013$), fasting insulin ($r = -0.256$, $p = 0.003$), and HOMA-IR ($r = -0.263$, $p = 0.002$) in males, but not in females. Figure 1 shows clear sex differences in the linear relationship of serum 25(OH)D with fasting glucose, insulin, and insulin resistance. Serum 25(OH)D level was significantly and inversely associated with fasting insulin and HOMA-IR only in male adolescents.

Table 3 shows fasting plasma glucose, insulin, and HOMA-IR levels according to serum 25(OH)D. Male adolescents in the lowest 25(OH)D quartile, when compared to those in the highest quartile, had significantly higher fasting glucose ($p = 0.039$), fasting insulin ($p = 0.012$), and HOMA-IR ($p = 0.008$) levels, even after adjustment for age and BMI. There were also increasing trends in fasting glucose (adjusted p for trend $= 0.060$), fasting insulin (adjusted p for trend $= 0.009$), and HOMA-IR (adjusted p for trend $= 0.007$) according to the decrease of 25(OH)D. When the 25(OH)D level was analyzed as a continuous variable, every 10 ng/ml lower level was associated with a 1.44 mg/dl increase in fasting glucose, 1.02 uIU/mL increase in fasting insulin, and 0.25 unit increase in HOMA-IR among male adolescents. However, in female adolescents, serum 25(OH)D level was not associated with fasting glucose, insulin, or insulin resistance.

Males

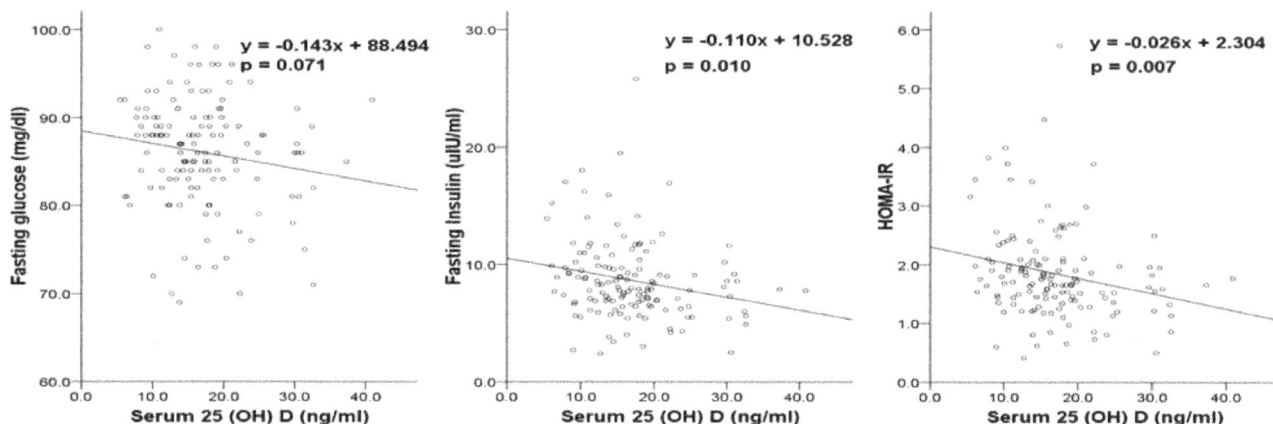

Females

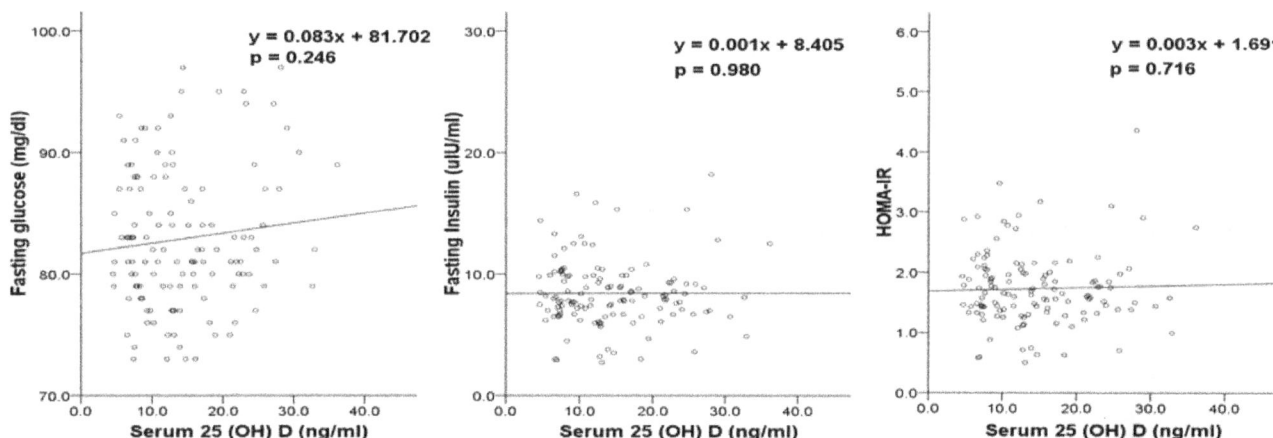

Figure 1. Association between serum 25(OH)D level and glucose metabolism. Upper panels scatter plots with fitted regression lines for 25(OH)D versus fasting glucose, fasting insulin, and HOMA-IR, respectively in males. Lower panels are corresponding scatter plots with fitted regression lines in females. P-values are for the regression coefficients.

Table 4 presents the association between serum 25(OH)D level and increased insulin resistance, which was defined as a HOMA-IR value higher than the 75th percentile. In male adolescents, the lowest 25(OH)D quartile was significantly associated with increased insulin resistance, and this association was consistent when unadjusted (odds ratio 4.06; 95% confidence interval 1.26 to 13.07), adjusted for age and body mass index (odds ratio 3.59; 95% CI 1.03 to 12.57), and adjusted for age, body mass index, smoking, drinking, and regular exercise (odds ratio 3.54; 95% CI 1.01 to 12.41). Continuous measure of 25(OH)D level was also significantly and inversely associated with insulin resistance among male participants. However, this association was not observed among female participants.

Discussion

We observed a significant inverse association between serum 25(OH)D level and insulin resistance in apparently healthy male adolescents, but not in female adolescents. To our knowledge, this is the first study demonstrating an association between a lower serum 25(OH)D level and increased insulin resistance in healthy Asian adolescents. Moreover, our study population has a narrow

age range (15 to 16 years), is relatively lean (mean body mass index 21.7 kg/m^2), and free of metabolic disorders. These characteristics minimized the possible influences of aging, obesity, and comorbidity in the relationship between vitamin D status and insulin resistance. Most of previous studies on the association between vitamin D and insulin resistance were performed in adult populations [23–27]. A few observational studies and clinical trials reported inverse associations between serum 25(OH)D and insulin resistance among overweight or obese adolescents [16–19]. On the other hand, no association between serum 25(OH)D and insulin resistance was observed among high school students in Turkey [20]. A recent study reported a sigmoid-shaped association between vitamin D and insulin resistance [27]. The inverse association between 25(OH)D and insulin resistance was observed only at serum 25(OH)D range from 16 to 36 ng/ml, but not at 25(OH)D values higher than 36 ng/ml or lower than 16 ng/ml [27]. However, in our data, we could not observe such a sigmoid-shaped association, probably because of small sample size or narrow age distribution.

Our participants had relatively low serum 25(OH)D levels. Mean serum 25(OH)D was 15.8 ng/ml, while mean serum 25(OH)D level was reported as 24 ng/ml among U.S. adolescents

Table 3. Serum 25(OH)D levels and fasting plasma glucose, insulin, and insulin resistance.

Serum 25(OH)D, ng/ml	Glucose, mg/dl			Insulin, uIU/ml			HOMA-IR		
	Means ± SE	Difference*	p	Means ± SE	Difference*	p	Means ± SE	Difference*	p
Males									
4th quartile (19.6 to 40.9, n=34)	84.53±1.13	Reference		7.67±0.48	Reference		1.62±0.11	Reference	
3rd quartile (15.9 to 19.3, n=34)	86.26±1.14	1.72	0.265	8.76±0.67	0.71	0.305	1.88±0.15	0.17	0.282
2nd quartile (12.3 to 15.8, n=33)	85.61±1.13	1.27	0.414	8.40±0.58	1.18	0.090	1.79±0.13	0.27	0.091
1st quartile (5.4 to 12.2, n=34)	87.71±0.92	3.25	0.039	9.83±0.59	1.77	0.012	2.14±0.14	0.43	0.008
Continuous measure (per 10 ng/ml decrease)		1.44	0.071		1.02	0.004		0.25	0.003
Females									
4th quartile (18.9 to 36.1, n=32)	84.13±1.11	Reference		8.54±0.51	Reference		1.79±0.12	Reference	
3rd quartile (12.9 to 18.5, n=33)	81.55±0.99	−2.57	0.075	7.53±0.45	−0.86	0.176	1.52±0.09	−0.24	0.094
2nd quartile (8.4 to 12.8, n=29)	82.79±1.08	−1.51	0.311	9.15±0.54	0.63	0.338	1.88±0.12	0.09	0.535
1st quartile (4.5 to 8.3, n=31)	83.16±0.91	−0.74	0.611	8.55±0.46	0.09	0.611	1.76±0.10	−0.01	0.967
Continuous measure (per 10 ng/ml decrease)		−0.86	0.231		0.02	0.953		−0.02	0.752

Abbreviations: HOMA-IR, homeostasis model assessment insulin resistance.
*Adjusted for age and body mass index.

Table 4. Serum 25(OH)D level and the risk of increased insulin resistance.

Serum 25(OH)D, ng/ml	No. (%) of increased insulin resistance*	Odds ratio (95% confidence interval) for increased insulin resistance*					
		Unadjusted		Adjusted for age and BMI		Multiple adjusted**	
Males							
4th quartile (19.6 to 40.9, n=34)	5 (14.7)	1.00		1.00		1.00	
3rd quartile (15.9 to 19.3, n=34)	9 (26.5)	2.09	(0.62 to 7.05)	1.80	(0.50 to 6.52)	1.87	(0.51 to 6.84)
2nd quartile (12.3 to 15.8, n=33)	6 (18.2)	1.29	(0.35 to 4.72)	1.45	(0.37 to 5.64)	1.35	(0.34 to 5.34)
1st quartile (5.4 to 12.2, n=34)	14 (41.2)	4.06	(1.26 to 13.07)	3.59	(1.03 to 12.57)	3.54	(1.01 to 12.41)
Continuous measure (per 10 ng/ml decrease)		2.37	(1.17 to 4.79)	2.29	(1.09 to 4.82)	2.22	(1.04 to 4.74)
Females							
4th quartile (18.9 to 36.1, n=32)	7 (21.9)	1.00		1.00		1.00	
3rd quartile (12.9 to 18.5, n=33)	5 (15.2)	0.64	(0.18 to 2.27)	0.62	(0.17 to 2.32)	0.58	(0.15 to 2.19)
2nd quartile (8.4 to 12.8, n=29)	9 (31.0)	1.61	(0.51 to 5.07)	1.52	(0.46 to 5.01)	1.66	(0.48 to 5.70)
1st quartile (4.5 to 8.3, n=31)	11 (35.5)	1.96	(0.64 to 6.00)	2.34	(0.73 to 7.50)	1.76	(0.53 to 5.83)
Continuous measure (per 10 ng/ml decrease)		1.19	(0.67 to 2.10)	1.24	(0.69 to 2.25)	1.15	(0.63 to 2.10)

Abbreviations: BMI, body mass index.

* Defined as homeostasis model assessment insulin resistance ≥ 75 percentile value (males, 2.09; females, 1.99).

**Adjusted for age, body mass index, smoking, drinking, and regular exercise.

aged 12 to 19 years [28]. Korean high school students devote large amounts of time to studying, and many attend supplemental after-school instruction [29], thus they may not receive sufficient sunlight exposure for adequate cutaneous production of vitamin D. However, we did not collect data on the amount of sunlight exposure. Health effects of insufficient outdoor activity and sunlight exposure need to be further investigated among Korean adolescents. In this study, serum 25(OH)D level was associated with insulin resistance in males, but not in females. This finding suggests that female adolescents, even with vitamin D insufficiency, maintain their insulin sensitivity. The developmental and hormonal differences may explain, at least in part, the sex difference in the associations between serum 25(OH)D level and insulin resistance. Hormonal status during puberty, especially for female adolescents, might affect glucose metabolism. The increase in growth hormone during puberty may contribute to insulin sensitivity via the growth hormone's effect on increasing lipolysis and free fatty acid concentration [30,31]. In addition, a rise in estrogen level in females may suppress secretion of glucose and protect the pancreatic insulin response to glucose [32]. The relationship between vitamin D status and insulin resistance needs to be further investigated across different sex and age groups.

Several limitations of our study should be acknowledged. First, this is a cross-sectional study, thus the causal inference might be limited. Second, we measured serum 25(OH)D level at a single point, and therefore did not assess seasonal variation. However, therefore seasonal variation is unlikely to distort the relationship between 25(OH)D and insulin resistance, because the health examination was performed over a relatively short period. Third, we could not assess the effects of vitamin D supplements. Our study population consisted of healthy high school students, and none of them reported intake of vitamin D supplements. However, we could not exclude the possible intake of a multivitamin formula including vitamin D. Fourth, objective data on sun exposure and time spent outdoors were not available. Thus, we could not investigate the effects of sunlight on the relationship between vitamin D status and insulin resistance. Finally, the study was conducted at a single high school and included one ethnic group, so the study findings cannot be generalized to other adolescent populations.

In conclusion, this study suggests that lower serum 25(OH)D levels may be associated with increased insulin resistance among healthy male adolescents. Sex differences in the association between serum 25(OH)D and insulin resistance need to be further investigated.

Acknowledgments

We are particularly grateful to all adolescents, their parents and the school staff who provided us valuable cooperation.

Author Contributions

Conceived and designed the experiments: DPC HCK. Performed the experiments: DPC SMO JML HMC WJL BS. Analyzed the data: DPC. Contributed reagents/materials/analysis tools: DPC YR HCK. Wrote the paper: DPC.

References

1. Muszkat P, Camargo MB, Griz LH, Lazaretti-Castro M (2010) Evidence-based non-skeletal actions of vitamin D. Arq Bras Endocrinol Metabol 54: 110–117.
2. Johnson JA, Grande JP, Roche PC, Kumar R (1994) Immunohistochemical localization of the 1,25(OH)2D3 receptor and calbindin D28k in human and rat pancreas. Am J Physiol 267: E356–360.
3. Simpson RU, Thomas GA, Arnold AJ (1985) Identification of 1,25-dihydroxyvitamin D3 receptors and activities in muscle. J Biol Chem 260: 8882–8891.
4. Bland R, Markovic D, Hills CE, Hughes SV, Chan SL, et al. (2004) Expression of 25-hydroxyvitamin D3-1alpha-hydroxylase in pancreatic islets. J Steroid Biochem Mol Biol 89–90: 121–125.
5. Maestro B, Campion J, Davila N, Calle C (2000) Stimulation by 1,25-dihydroxyvitamin D3 of insulin receptor expression and insulin responsiveness for glucose transport in U-937 human promonocytic cells. Endocr J 47: 383–391.
6. Alvarez JA, Ashraf A (2010) Role of vitamin d in insulin secretion and insulin sensitivity for glucose homeostasis. Int J Endocrinol 2010: 351385.
7. Isaia G, Giorgino R, Adami S (2001) High prevalence of hypovitaminosis D in female type 2 diabetic population. Diabetes Care 24: 1496.
8. Mattila C, Knekt P, Mannisto S, Rissanen H, Laaksonen MA, et al. (2007) Serum 25-hydroxyvitamin D concentration and subsequent risk of type 2 diabetes. Diabetes Care 30: 2569–2570.
9. Knekt P, Laaksonen M, Mattila C, Harkanen T, Marniemi J, et al. (2008) Serum vitamin D and subsequent occurrence of type 2 diabetes. Epidemiology 19: 666–671.
10. Grimnes G, Emaus N, Joakimsen RM, Figenschau Y, Jenssen T, et al. (2010) Baseline serum 25-hydroxyvitamin D concentrations in the Tromso Study 1994-95 and risk of developing type 2 diabetes mellitus during 11 years of follow-up. Diabet Med 27: 1107–1115.
11. Gulseth HL, Gjelstad IM, Tierney AC, Lovegrove JA, Defoort C, et al. (2010) Serum vitamin D concentration does not predict insulin action or secretion in European subjects with the metabolic syndrome. Diabetes Care 33: 923–925.
12. Del Gobbo LC, Song Y, Dannenbaum DA, Dewailly E, Egeland GM (2011) Serum 25-hydroxyvitamin D is not associated with insulin resistance or beta cell function in Canadian Cree. J Nutr 141: 290–295.
13. Scragg R, Sowers M, Bell C (2004) Serum 25-hydroxyvitamin D, diabetes, and ethnicity in the Third National Health and Nutrition Examination Survey. Diabetes Care 27: 2813–2818.
14. Lu L, Yu Z, Pan A, Hu FB, Franco OH, et al. (2009) Plasma 25-hydroxyvitamin D concentration and metabolic syndrome among middle-aged and elderly Chinese individuals. Diabetes Care 32: 1278–1283.

15. Alemzadeh R, Kichler J, Babar G, Calhoun M (2008) Hypovitaminosis D in obese children and adolescents: relationship with adiposity, insulin sensitivity, ethnicity, and season. Metabolism 57: 183–191.
16. Belenchia AM, Tosh AK, Hillman LS, Peterson CA (2013) Correcting vitamin D insufficiency improves insulin sensitivity in obese adolescents: a randomized controlled trial. Am J Clin Nutr 97: 774–781.
17. Kelishadi R, Salek S, Salek M, Hashemipour M, Movahedian M (2014) Effects of vitamin D supplementation on insulin resistance and cardiometabolic risk factors in children with metabolic syndrome: a triple-masked controlled trial. J Pediatr (Rio J) 90: 28–34.
18. Olson ML, Maalouf NM, Oden JD, White PC, Hutchison MR (2012) Vitamin D deficiency in obese children and its relationship to glucose homeostasis. J Clin Endocrinol Metab 97: 279–285.
19. Kelly A, Brooks LJ, Dougherty S, Carlow DC, Zemel BS (2011) A cross-sectional study of vitamin D and insulin resistance in children. Arch Dis Child 96: 447–452.
20. Erdonmez D, Hatun S, Cizmecioglu FM, Keser A (2011) No relationship between vitamin D status and insulin resistance in a group of high school students. J Clin Res Pediatr Endocrinol 3: 198–201.
21. Lee CG, Moon JS, Choi J-M, Nam CM, Lee SY, et al. (2008) Normative blood pressure references for Korean children and adolescents. Korean J Pediatr 51: 33–41.
22. (2009) Korean National Health and Nutrition Examination Survey Report. Ministry of Health and Welfare.
23. Zhao G, Ford ES, Li C (2010) Associations of serum concentrations of 25-hydroxyvitamin D and parathyroid hormone with surrogate markers of insulin resistance among U.S. adults without physician-diagnosed diabetes: NHANES, 2003-2006. Diabetes Care 33: 344–347.
24. Liu E, Meigs JB, Pittas AG, McKeown NM, Economos CD, et al. (2009) Plasma 25-hydroxyvitamin d is associated with markers of the insulin resistant phenotype in nondiabetic adults. J Nutr 139: 329–334.
25. Kayaniyil S, Vieth R, Retnakaran R, Knight JA, Qi Y, et al. (2010) Association of vitamin D with insulin resistance and beta-cell dysfunction in subjects at risk for type 2 diabetes. Diabetes Care 33: 1379–1381.
26. Chiu KC, Chu A, Go VL, Saad MF (2004) Hypovitaminosis D is associated with insulin resistance and beta cell dysfunction. Am J Clin Nutr 79: 820–825.
27. Heaney RP, French CB, Nguyen S, Ferreira M, Baggerly LL, et al. (2013) A novel approach localizes the association of vitamin D status with insulin resistance to one region of the 25-hydroxyvitamin D continuum. Adv Nutr 4: 303–310.

28. Ginde AA, Liu MC, Camargo CA Jr (2009) Demographic differences and trends of vitamin D insufficiency in the US population, 1988-2004. Arch Intern Med 169: 626–632.

29. Lee M (2003) Korean adolescents' "examination hell" and their use of free time. New Dir Child Adolesc Dev: 9–21.

30. Moran A, Jacobs DR Jr, Steinberger J, Steffen LM, Pankow JS, et al. (2008) Changes in insulin resistance and cardiovascular risk during adolescence: establishment of differential risk in males and females. Circulation 117: 2361–2368.

31. Hoffman RP, Vicini P, Sivitz WI, Cobelli C (2000) Pubertal adolescent male-female differences in insulin sensitivity and glucose effectiveness determined by the one compartment minimal model. Pediatr Res 48: 384–388.

32. Godsland IF (2005) Oestrogens and insulin secretion. Diabetologia 48: 2213–2220.

22

Metabolic Signatures of Cultured Human Adipocytes from Metabolically Healthy versus Unhealthy Obese Individuals

Anja Böhm[1,2,3,4]*, Anna Halama[1], Tobias Meile[5], Marty Zdichavsky[5], Rainer Lehmann[2,3,4], Cora Weigert[1,2,3,4], Andreas Fritsche[2,3,4], Norbert Stefan[2,3,4], Alfred Königsrainer[5], Hans-Ulrich Häring[1,2,3,4], Martin Hrabě de Angelis[1,3,6], Jerzy Adamski[1,3,6], Harald Staiger[1,2,3,4]

1 Helmholtz Zentrum München, German Research Center for Environmental Health, Institute of Experimental Genetics, Genome Analysis Center, Neuherberg, Germany, 2 Department of Internal Medicine IV, Division of Endocrinology, Diabetology, Angiology, Nephrology, and Clinical Chemistry, University Hospital, Eberhard Karls University, Tübingen, Germany, 3 German Center for Diabetes Research, Neuherberg, Germany, 4 Institute for Diabetes Research and Metabolic Diseases of the Helmholtz Center München at the Eberhard Karls University of Tübingen, Tübingen, Germany, 5 Department of General, Visceral and Transplant Surgery, University Hospital, Eberhard Karls University, Tübingen, Germany, 6 Chair of Experimental Genetics, Technical University München, Freising-Weihenstephan, Germany

Abstract

Background and Aims: Among obese subjects, metabolically healthy and unhealthy obesity (MHO/MUHO) can be differentiated: the latter is characterized by whole-body insulin resistance, hepatic steatosis, and subclinical inflammation. Aim of this study was, to identify adipocyte-specific metabolic signatures and functional biomarkers for MHO versus MUHO.

Methods: 10 insulin-resistant (IR) vs. 10 insulin-sensitive (IS) non-diabetic morbidly obese (BMI >40 kg/m^2) Caucasians were matched for gender, age, BMI, and percentage of body fat. From subcutaneous fat biopsies, primary preadipocytes were isolated and differentiated to adipocytes in vitro. About 280 metabolites were investigated by a targeted metabolomic approach intracellularly, extracellularly, and in plasma.

Results/Interpretation: Among others, aspartate was reduced intracellularly to one third (p = 0.0039) in IR adipocytes, pointing to a relative depletion of citric acid cycle metabolites or reduced aspartate uptake in MUHO. Other amino acids, already known to correlate with diabetes and/or obesity, were identified to differ between MUHO's and MHO's adipocytes, namely glutamine, histidine, and spermidine. Most species of phosphatidylcholines (PCs) were lower in MUHO's extracellular milieu, though simultaneously elevated intracellularly, e.g., PC aa C32:3, pointing to increased PC synthesis and/or reduced PC release. Furthermore, altered arachidonic acid (AA) metabolism was found: 15(S)-HETE (15-hydroxy-eicosatetraenoic acid; 0 vs. 120pM; p = 0.0014), AA (1.5-fold; p = 0.0055) and docosahexaenoic acid (DHA, C22:6; 2-fold; p = 0.0033) were higher in MUHO. This emphasizes a direct contribution of adipocytes to local adipose tissue inflammation. Elevated DHA, as an inhibitor of prostaglandin synthesis, might be a hint for counter-regulatory mechanisms in MUHO.

Conclusion/Interpretation: We identified adipocyte-inherent metabolic alterations discriminating between MHO and MUHO.

Editor: Marta Letizia Hribal, University of Catanzaro Magna Graecia, Italy

Funding: This study was supported in part by a grant (01GI0925) from the German Federal Ministry of Education and Research (BMBF) to the German Center for Diabetes Research (DZD e.V.). Norbert Stefan is currently funded by a Heisenberg-Professorship from the German Research Foundation (STE 1096/3-1). The funders had no role in study design, data collection and analysis, decision to publish, or preparation of the manuscript.

Competing Interests: The authors have declared that no competing interests exist.

* E-mail: anja.boehm@med.uni-tuebingen.de

Introduction

Diabetes and obesity have developed to a worldwide problem of mankind, with immense financial and personal burden. The underlying pathomechanisms are not well understood, the prevention strategies are insufficient. Development of the metabolic syndrome demands the interplay of multiple organs, e.g., fat, liver, muscle, gut, and brain. Among these, the liver and in particular adipose tissue play a meaningful impact [1,2]. Continuously, more and more adipokines are found to play a role in atherosclerosis, endothelial dysfunction, metabolic syndrome and diabetes.

In the obese state, several subphenotypes exist, e.g., metabolically healthy and unhealthy obesity (MHO/MUHO) [3,4]; the latter includes whole-body insulin resistance, hepatic steatosis, and subclinical inflammation. Insulin resistance precedes type 2 diabetes for years, but the sequelae exert adverse effects from the beginning [5,6]. There are several metabolomic studies searching for biomarkers of insulin resistance, obesity and glucose intolerance [7–16], but none of them are dealing with adipocyte-

Table 1. Participants' clinical characteristics.

	IS	IR	p	p1	p2
N (women/men)	6/4	6/4	-	-	-
Age (y)	45±9	38±13	0.1	-	-
BMI (kg/m^2)	52.5±8.9	51.1±6.9	0.7	1.0	-
Body fat (%)	48.0±12.1[a]	50.2±11.6	0.7	0.5	-
Lean Body Mass (kg)	76±8	74±8	0.8	0.4	0.2
AUC$_{Glucose\ 0-120}$ (mmol/L)	16.5±2.3	18.1±3.0	0.2	0.0268	0.0256
Glucose$_0$ (mmol/L)	5.5±0.1	5.7±0.2	0.6	0.2	0.2
Glucose$_{120}$ (mmol/L)	7.3±1.3	7.5±	0.9	0.3	0.2
Insulin$_0$ (pmol/L)	111.5±30.1	265.2±12.6	<0.0001	0.0002	<0.0001
Insulin$_{120}$ (pMol/L)	468.8±227	1519.5±689.4	0.0003	0.0003	0.0003
HbA1c (%; mmol/mol)	5.6±0.4; 38±4.4[a]	6.0±0.3; 42±3.3[a]	0.0194	0.0304	0.0244
ISI OGTT ($\cdot 10^6$ Lkg^{-1}min^{-1})	7.04±2.25	2.55±0.64	<0.0001	<0.0001	<0.0001
Metabolic Syndrome (%)#	60	78	0.4	0.2	0.2
Waist circumference (cm)	135±5	133±5	0.9	0.8	0.8
Adipo-IR index	80±27	172±104	0.0017	0.0049	0.0004
RR$_{sys}$ (mmHg)	123±17	131±13	0.2	0.2	0.2
RR$_{dia}$ (mmHg)	80±12	84±9	0.3	0.2	0.2
Free fatty acids (µmol/L)	723±182[a]	651±207	0.4	0.7	0.8
Triglycerides (mg/dL)	154±85	177±90[a]	0.6	0.5	0.6
Total cholesterol (mg/dL)	216±55	198±35	0.5	1.0	1.0
HDL cholesterol (mg/dL)	53±14[a]	41±5[a]	0.0312	0.1	0.2
LDL cholesterol (mg/dL)	131±36[a]	134±27[a]	0.7	0.2	0.3
Leukocytes (µL^{-1})	6,895±1,792	10,459±3,102	0.0024	0.0103	0.0130
CRP (mg/dL)	0.62±0.54	1.42±1.00	0.2	0.06	0.06
GOT (U/L)	22±5[b]	25±10[a]	0.6	0.7	0.7
GPT (U/L)	23±9[b]	37±21[a]	0.1	0.3	0.3
γ-GT (U/L)	25±13[b]	50±60[a]	0.2	0.06	0.07
Fetuin-A (µg/mL)	335±213[a]	372±165	0.6	0.6	0.6
SHBG (nmol/L)	54.0±76.5[a]	27.6±9.19	0.3	0.3	0.3
PAI-1 (ng/mL)	90.4±28.9[a]	134.7±33.1	0.007	0.0024	0.0034
Leptin (ng/mL)	71.3±32.2[a]	95.7±97.4	0.6	1.0	1.0
Adiponectin (µg/mL)	9.17±2.61[a]	6.26±2.45	0.0391	0.07	0.08

Data represent number (N) or means ±SD. Prior to statistical analysis, data were log$_e$-transformed in order to approximate normal distribution and adjusted; p = unadjusted p-value; p1 = p-value after adjustment for gender and age; p2 = p-value after adjustment for gender, age, and BMI. # defined by criteria from International Diabetes Federation 2005 and American Heart Association 2005; [a] Available from only 9 subjects; [b] available from 8 subjects.

specific aspects. The aim of this study was, to carve out possible adipocyte-specific metabolic differences between MHO and MUHO, and to figure out novel adipocyte-related functional biomarkers leading to pathways discriminating MHO and MUHO. To accomplish this study, we applied targeted metabolomics.

Methods

Population

20 morbidly obese (BMI >40 kg/m^2) subjects of Western European Descendent undergoing bariatric (gastric sleeve) surgery were selected. Based on insulin sensitivity index, subjects were divided into an IR and an IS group. Participants were matched for gender, age, BMI and percentage of body fat (see also table 1). Overt diabetes as well as other severe diseases (besides morbid obesity) and/or medication affecting glucose tolerance were exclusion criteria. All included participants underwent physical examination. Informed written consent was given by all individuals; the study protocol has been approved by the ethics committee of the university Tübingen and was in accordance with the declaration of Helsinki.

Phenotyping

All participants underwent a 2 h 75 g OGTT, insulin sensitivity was calculated using the method of Matsuda and DeFronzo (10,000/square root of [fasting glucose x fasting insulin x mean glucose x mean insulin]) [17]. Routine laboratory tests were performed, partly by ELISAs (see table 1). In-depth-description is given in File S1.

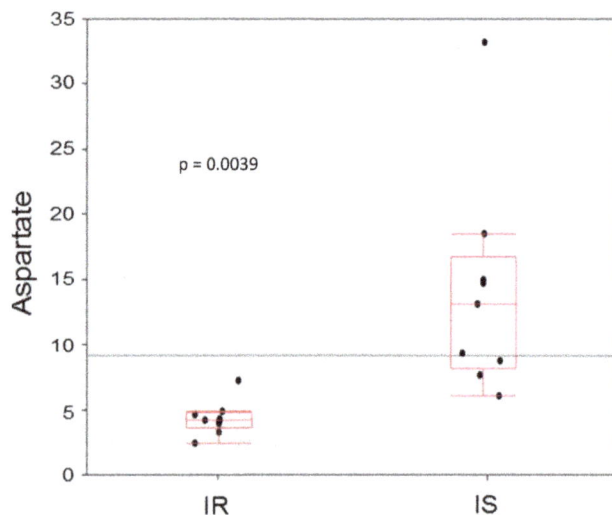

Figure 1. Aspartate. Intracellular levels in µM; IR vs. IS, n = 9; test: Wilcoxon. Horizontal line means grand mean.

Table 2. Intracellular differences between IR and IS.

Assay	Metabolite	Test	N (IR vs IS)	p-value	IR
EMI	Aspartate	Wil	8 vs 10	0.0097	L
	Hexose	HE	9 vs 10	0.0383	H
p180	Aspartate	Wil	8 vs. 9	0.0039	L
	Glutamine	HO	8 vs. 9	0.007	H
	Histidine	HE	9 vs. 9	0.0226	H
	Spermidine	Wil	8 vs. 9	0.0161	H
	lysoPC C18:0	HO	9 vs. 9	0.0321	H
	PC aa C32:3	HE	9 vs. 9	0.0394	H *
	PC aa C34:4	Wil	9 vs. 9	0.0218	H
	PC aa C36:4	Wil	9 vs. 9	0.0325	H
	PC aa C36:5	HO	9 vs. 9	0.0175	H
	SM C16:1	HE	9 vs. 9	0.0499	H

Metabolites with nominal inter-group difference (p<0.05); EMI: Energy Metabolite Intermediates; HE= heteroscedastic unpaired two-sided t-test, HO= homoscedastic unpaired two-sided t-test, Wil = Wilcoxon test, ME= median test; p-value: $p_{Bonferroni} \leq 0.0004$. H/L: metabolite-values in IR higher/lower vs. IS; PC: Phosphatidylcholine, aa/ae: acyl/ether side chain; SM: sphingolipids. * contrarily regulated in extracellular milieu.

Isolation and culture of human adipocytes

Human subcutaneous fat biopsies were obtained during gastric sleeve surgery after overnight fast prior to surgery. Human primary preadipocytes were isolated as previously described [18]. Then, preadipocytes were grown up and subsequently differentiated into mature adipocytes over a 20-day culture period. Exact concentration and medium contents are described in ESM. Adipocytes from all donors were used in second pass. Differentiation success was checked microscopically by NileRed/DAPI- and OilRedO-staining (see exemplarily Figure S1). Moreover, density of OilRed- staining per well was estimated using the publicly available JPEG-plugin colorcounter.

Sample Preparation

At day 20 of differentiation, sample collection was performed. For extracellular milieu, cell culture medium was collected exactly 48 h after the last medium exchange (6 wells were pooled to account for inter-well differences) and sterile filtered (0.2 µm; Corning, Wiesbaden, Germany). Where necessary, 0.001% butylated hydroxytoluene was added to prevent auto-oxidation of prostanoids. Thereafter, the samples were aliquotted and stored in a −80°C freezer until measurement. For cell lysates, the layer was washed twice with pre-warmed PBS; quenching and extraction was performed by cell scrapping in 80% methanol (pre-cooled to −20°C) and transferred to a tube, immediately cooled in liquid nitrogen. Prior to analysis, 3 wells were pooled and filled in a vial containing glass beads (VK-05; Peqlab, Erlangen, Germany). Homogenization took place in the Precellys24 (PeqLab) homogenizer at 4°C for three times over 30 seconds at 5500 rpm. After centrifugation, the supernatant was used for analysis.

Metabolomic analysis

Adipocytes from the MHO and MUHO were characterized with targeted metabolomics. The p180 kit of Biocrates Life Sciences AG (Innsbruck, Austria) allows a simultaneous quantification of 186 metabolites, including free carnitine, 40 acylcarnitines (Cx:y), 21 amino acids, 19 biogenic amines, hexoses, 90 glycerophospholipids (14 lysophosphatidylcholines (lysoPC) and 76 phosphatidylcholines (PC)), and 15 sphingolipids (SMx:y). The

abbreviations Cx:y are used to describe the total number of carbons and double bonds of all chains, respectively. The assay procedures of the AbsoluteIDQ™ p180 kit as well as the metabolite nomenclature have been described in detail previously [19,20]. Sample handling was performed by a Hamilton Microlab STAR™ robot (Hamilton Bonaduz AG, Bonaduz, Switzerland) and an Ultravap nitrogen evaporator (Porvair Sciences, Leatherhead, U.K.). Mass spectrometric (MS) analyses were done on a API 4000 LC/MS/MS System (AB Sciex Deutschland GmbH, Darmstadt, Germany) equipped with a 1200 Series HPLC (Agilent Technologies Deutschland GmbH, Böblingen, Germany) and a HTC PAL auto sampler (CTC Analytics, Zwingen, Switzerland) controlled by the software Analyst 1.5.1. Data evaluation for quantification of metabolite concentrations and quality assessment is performed with the MetIDQ software package, which is an integral part of the AbsoluteIDQ kit. Internal standards served as reference for the calculation of metabolite concentrations.

Further assays for free fatty acids, eicosanoids and oxidized fatty acids (prostaglandins), as well as energy metabolism intermediates were performed at Biocrates AG. Metabolites were measured by gas chromatography coupled with MS detection (for free fatty acids) or high performance liquid chromatography tandem MS with Multiple Reaction Monitoring (MRM) (for eicosanoids). For energy metabolites detection hydrophilic interaction liquid chromatography electrospray tandem MS method in highly selective negative MRM detection mode was used. Further details are given in File S1.

All values below detection limit (LOD) were set to zero, and metabolites with 'zero' or 'not applicable' in all individuals and/or with values 'not applicable' in more than 4 individuals of one group have been excluded. Regarding lysates, 129 metabolites remained. The multivariate analyses require complete datasets as well as same number of individuals for every single metabolite. Thus, the multivariate analyses of lysates only were performed with 82 metabolites, measured with p180 kit (table S1 in File S1). Concerning conditioned medium, 274 metabolites remained, and for multivariate analyses 121 metabolites (table S2 in File S1) were used.

Table 3. Differences between IR and IS in extracellular milieu.

Assay	Metabolite	Test	N (IR vs IS)	p-value	IR
FFA	C18:0 (stearic acid)	ME	9 vs. 10	0.0427	L
	C18:3 (linoleic acid)	HO	9 vs. 10	0.0488	H
	C20:4 (arachidonic acid)	HO	9 vs.10	0.0100	H
Eicosanoids	15-S-HETE	Wil	9 vs. 10	0.0014	H
	AA	Wil	9 vs. 10	0.0055	H
	DHA	**Wil**	**9 vs. 10**	**0.0033**	**H**
p180	Serotonin	HO	8 vs. 10	0.0166	H
	PC aa C32:0	HO	8 vs.10	0.0370	H
	PC aa C32:3	HO	8 vs. 10	<0.0032	L *
	PC aa C36:6	ME	8 vs. 10	0.0257	L
	PC ae C34:3	HO	8 vs. 10	0.0494	L
	PC ae C42:2	HO	8 vs. 10	0.0059	H
	SM C20:2	ME	8 vs. 10	0.0245	L
	SM C22:3	ME	8 vs. 10	0.0455	H

Metabolites with nominal inter-group difference (p<0.05); tests: HE = heteroscedastic unpaired two-sided t-test, HO = homoscedastic unpaired two-sided t-test, Wil = Wilcoxon test, ME = median test; corrected p-values: $p_{Bonferroni}$<0.0002. Asterisk (*) marks statistical significance after Bonferroni correction. PC: Phosphatidylcholine, aa/ae: acyl/ether side chain; SM: sphingolipids. **Bold**: also affected in plasma of our probands. * contrarily regulated intracellularly. H/L: metabolite-values in IR higher/lower vs. IS.

For analysis in blood, 500 µl of EDTA (ethylenediaminetetra-acetic acid) plasma were withdrawn from each participant after overnight-fasting and immediately frozen until measurement. The metabolomic analysis took place at Biocrates, Austria. Same analyses were performed as for the adipocytes.

Multiplex Assay (BioPlex Pro Human Cytokine 3-Plex-Assay, BioRad, Munich, Germany) was performed according to manufacturer's instructions to measure MCP-1, TNFα and IL-6. All metabolites and cytokines were normalized for the differentiation level of adipocytes, measured by percentage of OilRed staining per well (expressed as arbitrary units [AU]).

Statistics

For all statistical analyses JMP 10.0 (SAS Institute Inc., USA) was used. Regarding multivariate analysis, Principal Component Analysis (PCA) was performed to reduce the magnitude of data and to identify groups [21]. To verify the discriminative potential of the metabolite subsets, a linear discriminant analysis (IR vs. IS) was used (Figures S2 and S3).

For further statistical analysis, an unpaired, two-sided t-test was performed, if normal distribution was given; either a hetero- or homoscedastic test was applied, depending on the equality of variances. The equality of variances was determined with 5 different tests (O'Brien, Brown-Forsythe, Levene, Bartlett, and two-sided F-Test) and assumed, if all tests didn't reject the null hypothesis. Non-parametric tests were performed as indicated. Correction for multiple testing was done with the Bonferroni procedure $(p_{Bonferroni} = 1 - 0.95^{1/n})$. A p-value$\leq p_{Bonferroni}$ was considered to be statistically significant; intracellularly: p$\leq$0.0004, extracellularly: p$\leq$0.0002, ratios: p$\leq$0.0029, plasma: 0.0002.

Results

Cell donors'clinical characteristics

Anthropometric and laboratory characteristics of the participants are summarized in table 1. 20 individuals from southwest

Germany were matched for gender, age, BMI and percentage of body fat. Based on the selection process, there was a marked intergroup difference regarding the OGTT-derived whole-body insulin sensitivity. Although all participants were non-diabetic, a significant difference regarding HbA1c and $AUC_{Glucose}$ could be detected. As expected, MUHO had higher inflammation markers (e.g., serum leukocytes), but there was no difference in liver parameters. Adiponectin levels were reduced in IR subjects, but did not reach significance. In contrast, a clear difference was seen in plasminogen activator inhibitor (PAI)-1, with higher concentrations (almost 1.5-fold; p = 0.0034) in the IR group.

There were no differences in degree of differentiation between IR and IS adipocyte cultures (p = 0.3).

Intracellular differences between IR and IS in amino acids and PCs

To illustrate the plenty of data, a PCA was performed (Figure S4). Based on scree-plot (Figure S4A), the first three components were meaningful pertaining to PCA. As Eigen-values were decreasing rapidly, only the first two components with Eigen-values more than ten (Figure S4B) were taken into account for PCA (Figure S4C). Discriminant analysis showed good separation between the groups (Figure S2).

Appropriate t-tests or non-parametric tests, respectively, revealed 12 metabolites with nominal differences (p<0.05) between groups (table 2): notably, aspartate was found to be decreased to one third in IR cells (Figure 1; p = 0.0039), which was replicated in another kit (p = 0.0097). These results partly resisted additional adjustment for age (p = 0.03 and 0.07). Other amino acids were elevated in IR (table 2), namely glutamine (p = 0.0070), histidine (p = 0.0226) and spermidine (p = 0.0161). Hexose (~2.1-fold, p = 0.03) was higher in IR cells. Several PCs were affected, most species higher in IR adipocytes (table 2).

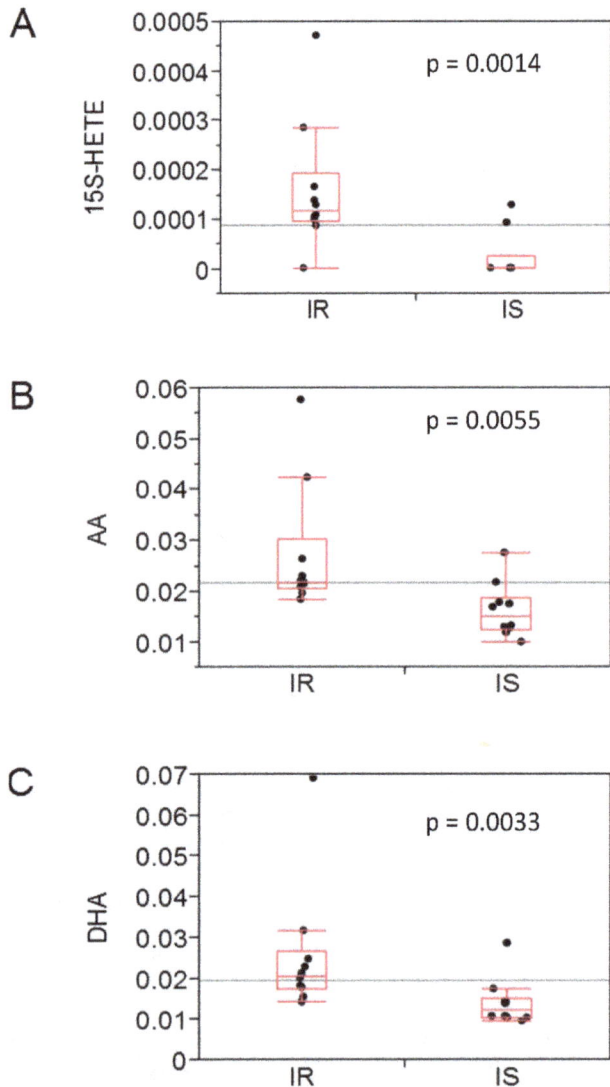

Figure 2. Arachidonic acid metabolism. Extracellular milieu; metabolite levels in µM; IR vs. IS; n = 10; (A) 15S-HETE: 15-hydroxy-eicosatetraenoic acid, median test; (B) AA: arachidonic acid, Wilcoxon; (C) DHA: docosahexaenoic acid (Wilcoxon). Horizontal line means grand mean.

Extracellular differences between IR and IS in fatty acids, eicosanoids, and PCs

Figure S5 shows the PCA of extracellular metabolites. Scree-plot (Figure S5A) and Eigen-values (Figure S5B) revealed the first two components being important performing the PCA (Figure S5C). These two components explain more than 35% of the variance of all 121 successfully measured metabolites (p180 kit). Also extracellularly, a good inter-group separation was confirmed by discriminant analysis (Figure S3).

Analyzed with the appropriate tests, there were 13 metabolites with nominal differences (table 3); among others, the saturated fatty acid C18:0 (stearic acid; 22-fold; p = 0.0427) was lower in extracellular milieu of MUHO.

Furthermore, 15(S)-HETE (15-hydroxy-eicosatetraenoic acid; 0 vs. 120 nM; p = 0.0014), arachidonic acid (AA; 1.5-fold; p = 0.0055) and docosahexaenoic acid (DHA, C22:6; 2-fold; p = 0.0033) emerged, all higher in IR (Figure 2), and all related

to AA metabolism (Figure 3A, orange pathway). AA was confirmed also by the free fatty acid kit (p = 0.01). After additional adjustment for age, p-values decreased to: 15(S)-HETE (p = 0.08), AA (p = 0.12; second kit p = 0.02), and DHA (p = 0.02). PCaa32:3 was reduced in IR (p = 0.0032), while elevated intracellularly (p = 0.0394).

Additionally, several ratios or sums of metabolites were investigated (see table S3 in File S1); thereof, two remained significant after correction for multiple testing ($p_{Bonferroni} \leq 0.0029$): citrulline/ornithine-ratio, displaying the ornithine carbamoylphosphate transferase activity (mean IRvs.IS: 0.08vs.0.06; p = 0.0002); and ornithine/arginine-ratio (arginase activity), (mean IRvs.IS: 0.10vs.0.13; p = 0.00005). Measurements of cytokines showed elevated levels of IL-6 (p = 0.0275) in IS. MCP-1 (p = 0.2) revealed no difference between the groups. TNFα was below limit of detection. Though, there was no correlation of IL-6 with the OGTT-derived insulin sensitivity index or adipose insulin resistance index neither ($r^2 = 0.1$; p = 0.2, 0.1, respectively).

Correlation of metabolites with adipose insulin resistance index

To strengthen our results, correlation analyses were made for the revealed metabolites (see Figure S6). Intracellularly, we saw significant correlation with adipose insulin resistance index for, e.g., aspartate (negatively correlated; p = 0.0157, p = 0.0016 second kit), and, among others, PCaa32:3 (positively correlated; p = 0.0354), that was found to be altered intra- as well as extracellularly.

Plasma metabolite differences between IR and IS

Plasma samples of the study participants were analyzed. 16 nominal significant metabolites are listed in table 4. Some fatty acids, as well as lysophosphatidylcholines and phosphatidylcholines were different between the groups. Divergent from the extracellular milieu, DHA was reduced in plasma of IR, so it may not derive abundantly from adipocytes to play a systemic role.

Discussion

Aim of this study was, to uncover new insights in adipocyte metabolism of MHO versus MUHO. For this purpose, and to find novel functional discriminating biomarkers in adipocytes, the metabolic differences between *in vitro* differentiated subcutaneous adipocytes of IR vs. IS morbidly obese individuals were analysed using a targeted metabolomics approach. With respect to the participants' serum parameters (table 1), some of the results were expected, i.e., the observed increase in levels of inflammation markers in IR subjects and a slightly elevated gamma-glutamyl-transferase level. Notably, there was no significant difference in fatty acids between the groups. The higher levels of PAI-I in the IR group was somewhat surprising, as plasma levels of this adipokine correlate very well with BMI [22,23]. However, elevation of PAI-1 per se is in line with several studies that linked PAI-1 not only to hypofibrinolysis, but also to inflammation and increased cardiovascular risk [24,25]. Our results indicate that it is independent of adipose tissue mass, as the groups were well matched for body adiposity. Certainly, this finding will need further replication in larger cohorts.

As expected, adiponectin levels were reduced in the IR subjects, but this difference did not reach statistical significance. This could be due to the strong association of adiponectin levels with adipocyte mass, which was equal in both groups. In addition, we did not find significant differences between the groups regarding liver markers (e.g. transaminases, fetuin-A, SHBG). This is in

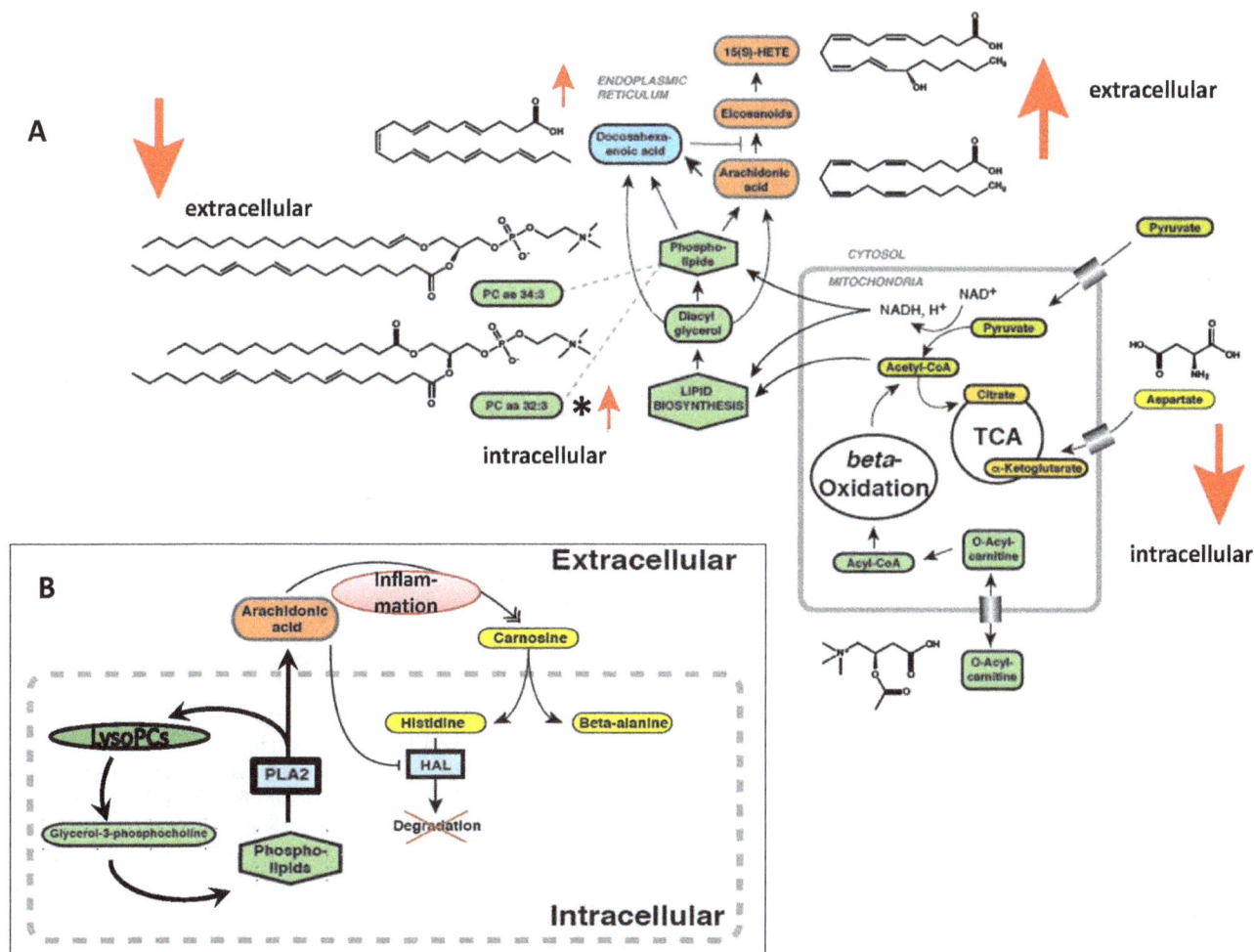

Figure 3. Overview on metabolite changes. Connecting processes like cofactors and intermediates are shown. Large arrows indicate change direction in the IR group. (A) Intracellular pathways; (B) Interactions between intracellular and extracellular metabolites; * Contrarily regulated intracellularly. HAL: histidine ammonia-lyase.

contrast to [16] and may be due to the limited sample size. To study the adipocyte-specific impact on MUHO, we used the cell culture system. This minimized the influence of other cell types, i.e., macrophages and other immune cells escorting adipose tissue.

Even though being an *in vitro* project with culture time of several weeks, *in vivo* phenotypes seem to be conserved, pointing to genetic/epigenetic termination. The analysis of fat cell metabolism of IR vs. IS subjects revealed prominent differences in glycerophospholipids and sphingomyelins (see Figure 3 for an overview on contributing metabolites). Extracellularly as well as in plasma, almost all PCs were reduced in MUHO, interestingly, in contrast to higher PCs (same species) in MUHO's intracellular milieu; this is possibly due to an increased endogenous PC synthesis and/or reduced PC release in IR adipocytes (see Figure 3A).

Furthermore, PCs, same like sphingomyelins, are components of cell membranes; a contribution of membrane fluidity and flexibility to metabolic diseases is known [26], i.e., accumulation of those with decreased saturation level resulted in improved cell membrane fluidity.

Extracellular reduction of an even-numbered saturated fatty acid in MUHO (stearic acid) might reflect the insulin resistance-induced decrease in lipogenesis. However, it may also be linked to an increased level of glycerophospholipids intracellularly, includ-

ing lysoPC C18:0 and PCaaC36, containing chains with different saturation level. The saturation variants in PCaaC36 suggest desaturation of stearic acid inside the cells and its incorporation into PCs. Desaturation can be catalyzed by SCD1 or FADS2 molecules, known to play a role in obesity [27] and inflammatory diseases [28].

As adipose tissue inflammation plays a major role in obesity-induced insulin resistance, the AA pathway, we found elevated extracellularly in IR, is very interesting. Albeit only nominally significant (Figure 2) for the single pathway member, multiple intermediates of the AA metabolism were elevated (Figure 3A, orange pathway): first, DHA, an ω-3 fatty acid, also called cervonic acid; as DHA is an inhibitor of prostaglandin synthase [29], this probably displays a counter-regulatory - albeit insufficient - mechanism of MUHO's adipocytes. Second, another altered PUFA was arachidonic acid (AA), a very important local inflammatory metabolite. The AA pathway is linked to several complications of the metabolic syndrome/diabetes, e.g. vascular disease, diabetic retinopathy and nephropathy [30], at least in cell culture systems or mammals. Of note, it's difficult to translate results from one species to another, as great species-specific differences in AA metabolism are known [30]. AA itself stimulates glucose uptake in 3T3-L1 adipocytes [31]. Also an adipogenic

Table 4. Differences between IR and IS in plasma.

Metabolite	p-value	IR
C16 (acylcarnitine)	0.0108	L
C18:1 (acylcarnitine)	0.0479	L
C 22:4 (adrenic acid)	0.0331	L
C 22:6 (cervonic acid [=DHA])	0.0449	L §
lysoPC C16:0	0.0122	L ‡
lysoPC C16:1	0.0150	L
lysoPC C18:1	0.0095	L
lysoPC C20:3	0.0281	L
lysoPC C20:4	0.0372	L
PC ae 36:4	0.0261	L
PC ae 36:5	0.0295	L -
PC ae 38:5	0.0194	L
PC ae 38:6	0.0248	L -
SM C26:0	0.0483	L
glutamic acid	0.0160	H
Hexosephosphate	0.0291	L

Metabolites with nominal difference (p<0.05) analyzed by t-tests. PC: Phosphatidylcholine, ae: acyl/ether side chain; SM: sphingolipids; n = 10 vs. 10; H/L: metabolite-values in IR higher/lower vs. IS; DHA = docosahexaenoic acid; ‡ also found by [12,13]; § contrarily found extracellularly.

effect of AA is discussed [32]. On the other hand, AA reduces basal glucose uptake in adipocytes and, furthermore, insulin-dependent AA-uptake is reduced in adipocytes of obese subjects [33]. This could be another explanation for elevated AA levels in IR and needs further clarification. Release of arachidonic acid (AA) can be catalyzed by phospholipase A2 (PLA2) or phospholipase C. Higher activities of some types of PLA2 are positively associated to diabetes [34]. Another intermediate of the arachidonate metabolism was concordantly affected (please see Figure 3A, orange pathway): 15S-HETE (15S-hydroxyeicosatetraenoic acid), one of the fatty acids derived from AA oxidation. The first step towards leukotriene synthesis is catalyzed by lipoxygenases (LOXs) producing HPETEs (hydroxyperoxyeicosatetraenoic acids). The intermediates are biologically active per se and/or can serve as precursors for lipid mediators [30]. LOXs are expressed in adipose tissue and promote adipogenesis, at least in mice and cell lines (3T3-L1) [35]. In humans, little is known about the 12-/15-LOXs. Interestingly, 15S-HETE is known to act as an agonist of PPAR (peroxisome proliferator-activated receptor) δ and PPARγ [36,37], two important regulators of lipid metabolism. 12-HETE, which was also higher in the IR group but did not reach nominal significance, was already shown to directly promote insulin resistance and inflammation in adipocytes [38]. The extracellularly elevated levels of pro-inflammatory molecules may stimulate intracellular accumulation of histidine (an anti-inflammatory molecule and an essential amino acid). This finding can be supported by [39], where anti-oxidative and anti-inflammatory protection of histidine and carnosine against diabetic deterioration were reported.

One biogenic amine found to differ between the groups was serotonin, elevated extracellularly in IR. Serotonin is a hormone and neurotransmitter with versatile effects: e.g., on brain, endothelial cells, smooth muscles, heart, gut and coagulation, etc., usually depending on the particular receptor. Until now, it

was not discovered to differ systemically in lean/obese or healthy/diabetic individuals; our finding could imply altered autocrine/paracrine effects in adipocytes of IR subjects. Very recently emerged that, at least in rats, there is a functional system of serotonin synthesis, reuptake and receptor activation in visceral adipose tissue [40].

The intracellularly reduced aspartate levels in IR individuals (Figure 1), could, via aspartate aminotransferase, reflect an altered citric acid cycle with relative depletion in IR subjects, what was already speculated at least in muscle cells [41,42]. Furthermore, also a reduced aspartate uptake from medium (concentration: 50 μM) by IR adipocytes has to be discussed. Ornithine carbamoylphosphate transferase (calculated by the ratio of citrulline to ornithine) was significantly elevated in IR subjects in our study, perhaps reflecting an increased urea cycle flux in IR adipocytes, supported by reduced intracellular aspartate, which also supplies the urea cycle. Besides, arginine metabolism is known to play a role in insulin-stimulated glycogen-synthesis [43].

To close the circle, our *in vitro* results were checked for systemic relevance *in vivo*. Plasma samples of corresponding probands revealed no congruency of several extracellular metabolites (tables 1, 2, and 3), indicating a local role of the described metabolites.

A comparison of our plasma metabolite results with a very recently published study by Floegel et al [44] looking for serum metabolites associating with incidence of type 2 diabetes, did not show analogies, perhaps indicating different pathomechanisms for MUHO as for diabetes per se. With reduced lysoPC C16:0 in IR a bridge is built to metabolically malign fatty liver [12], confirming the complex interaction between multiple organs regarding the pathogenesis of metabolic syndrome. Furthermore, lower lysoPC C20:4 levels in IR are in good agreement with recent studies [8,13], where serum metabolites in diabetic vs. non-diabetic participants were measured, and lysoPC C20:4 was negatively associated with diabetes.

The systemically reduced DHA in IR reflects the decrease of beneficial ω3-FAs in IR and enforces our hypothesis of local (adipocyte-specific) counterregulatory mechanisms.

Of course, there are several limitations of this study: due to study design, we are not able to differentiate between cause and consequence of IR and/or elevated blood glucose, but the goal of this study was to find hints for novel adipocyte-related pathways and functional biomarkers. These biomarkers for MUHO/MHO of course have to be validated in larger but appropriate cohorts. Furthermore, our groups are not matched for daily eating habits; FA composition of tissues is at least partially influenced by diet, but we believe that this effect is negligible in morbidly obese subjects, who usually consume high-caloric diet. There is upcoming evidence that there are important sex differences regarding metabolism, but our study unfortunately does not have the power to discriminate between genders. Insulin sensitivity of our probands was estimated by an OGTT-derived index, not measured by clamps. Lastly, the findings result from an in vitro situation. But the differences sustained despite a several weeks lasting culture period. Thus, our findings reflecting insulin sensitivity are probably due to epigenetic long-term alterations in the adipocytes.

To conclude, this study reveals novel insights into the adipocyte-specific impact on IR. Several differences in cell membrane components, amino acids and fatty acids emerged. Alteration of the arachidonic acid metabolism points to a – albeit insufficient – counterregulation with negative feedback mechanism of MUHO's adipocytes.

Supporting Information

Figure S1   In vitro differentiated adipocytes.

Figure S2   Discriminant Analysis of intracellular metabolites.

Figure S3   Discriminant Analysis of extracellular milieu.

Figure S4   Graphical inter-group description intracellularly.

Figure S5   Graphical inter-group description extracellularly.

Figure S6   Correlation of metabolites with AdipoIR index.

File S1   File includes Supplementary Research Design and Methods, Supplemental References, legends for Figures S1-S6, and Tables S1–S3.

Acknowledgments

We thank Carina Haas, Christina Lukas, and Mika Scheler for support in laboratory work in Tübingen and München; as well as Dr. Cornelia Prehn, Dr. Werner Römisch-Margl, Julia Scarpa, and Katharina Sckell for support in metabolomics measurements performed at the Helmholtz Centrum München, Genome Analysis Center, Metabolomics Core Facility.

Author Contributions

Conceived and designed the experiments: AB AH NS AF AK HUH MHA JA HS. Performed the experiments: AB AH. Analyzed the data: AB AH RL NS JA HS. Contributed reagents/materials/analysis tools: TM MZ AK NS AF HUH. Wrote the paper: AB. Read and edited the manuscript: AB AH TM MZ RL CW NS AF AK HUH MHA JA HS.

References

1. Stefan N, Haring HU (2013) The role of hepatokines in metabolism. Nature reviews Endocrinology 9: 144–152.
2. Ouchi N, Parker JL, Lugus JJ, Walsh K (2011) Adipokines in inflammation and metabolic disease. Nature reviews Immunology 11: 85–97.
3. Stefan N, Kantartzis K, Machann J, Schick F, Thamer C, et al. (2008) Identification and characterization of metabolically benign obesity in humans. Archives of internal medicine 168: 1609–1616.
4. McLaughlin T, Abbasi F, Lamendola C, Reaven G (2007) Heterogeneity in the prevalence of risk factors for cardiovascular disease and type 2 diabetes mellitus in obese individuals: effect of differences in insulin sensitivity. Archives of internal medicine 167: 642–648.
5. Grundy SM (2012) Pre-diabetes, metabolic syndrome, and cardiovascular risk. Journal of the American College of Cardiology 59: 635–643.
6. Ryden L, Standl E, Bartnik M, Van den Berghe G, Betteridge J, et al. (2007) Guidelines on diabetes, pre-diabetes, and cardiovascular diseases: executive summary. The Task Force on Diabetes and Cardiovascular Diseases of the European Society of Cardiology (ESC) and of the European Association for the Study of Diabetes (EASD). European heart journal 28: 88–136.
7. Oberbach A, Bluher M, Wirth H, Till H, Kovacs P, et al. (2011) Combined proteomic and metabolomic profiling of serum reveals association of the complement system with obesity and identifies novel markers of body fat mass changes. Journal of proteome research 10: 4769–4788.
8. Suhre K, Meisinger C, Doring A, Altmaier E, Belcredi P, et al. (2010) Metabolic footprint of diabetes: a multiplatform metabolomics study in an epidemiological setting. PLoS One 5: e13953.
9. Suhre K, Wallaschofski H, Raffler J, Friedrich N, Haring R, et al. (2011) A genome-wide association study of metabolic traits in human urine. Nat Genet 43: 565–569.
10. Wang TJ, Larson MG, Vasan RS, Cheng S, Rhee EP, et al. (2011) Metabolite profiles and the risk of developing diabetes. Nature medicine 17: 448–453.
11. Newgard CB, An J, Bain JR, Muehlbauer MJ, Stevens RD, et al. (2009) A branched-chain amino acid-related metabolic signature that differentiates obese and lean humans and contributes to insulin resistance. Cell metabolism 9: 311–326.
12. Lehmann R, Franken H, Dammeier S, Rosenbaum L, Kantartzis K, et al. (2013) Circulating lysophosphatidylcholines are markers of a metabolically benign nonalcoholic Fatty liver. Diabetes care 36: 2331–2338.
13. Zhao X, Fritsche J, Wang J, Chen J, Rittig K, et al. (2010) Metabonomic fingerprints of fasting plasma and spot urine reveal human pre-diabetic metabolic traits. Metabolomics 6: 362–374.
14. Lucio M, Fekete A, Weigert C, Wagele B, Zhao X, et al. (2010) Insulin sensitivity is reflected by characteristic metabolic fingerprints—a Fourier transform mass spectrometric non-targeted metabolomics approach. PLoS One 5: e13317.
15. Wang-Sattler R, Yu Z, Herder C, Messias AC, Floegel A, et al. (2012) Novel biomarkers for pre-diabetes identified by metabolomics. Mol Syst Biol 8: 615.
16. Kloting N, Fasshauer M, Dietrich A, Kovacs P, Schon MR, et al. (2010) Insulin-sensitive obesity. American journal of physiology Endocrinology and metabolism 299: E506–515.
17. Matsuda M, DeFronzo RA (1999) Insulin sensitivity indices obtained from oral glucose tolerance testing: comparison with the euglycemic insulin clamp. Diabetes care 22: 1462–1470.
18. Schling P, Mallow H, Trindl A, Loffler G (1999) Evidence for a local renin angiotensin system in primary cultured human preadipocytes. International journal of obesity and related metabolic disorders: journal of the International Association for the Study of Obesity 23: 336–341.
19. Römisch-Margl W PC, Bogumil R, Röhring C, Suhre K, Adamski J (2012) Procedure for tissue sample preparation and metabolite extraction for high-throughput targeted metabolomics. Metabolomics 8: 133–142. Doi:10.1007/s11306-011-0293-4
20. Zukunft S SM, Prehn C, Möller G, Adamski J (2013) Targeted Metabolomics of Dried Blood Spot Extracts. Chromatographia. Doi: 10.1007/s10337-013-2429-3.
21. Moller T (2012) Formation and paleoclimatic interpretation of a continuously laminated sapropel S5: a window to the climate variability during the Eemian interglacial in the Eastern Mediterranean http://nbn-resolving.de/urn:nbn:de:bsz:21-opus-63524.pp. 46.
22. Alessi MC, Bastelica D, Morange P, Berthet B, Leduc I, et al. (2000) Plasminogen activator inhibitor 1, transforming growth factor-beta1, and BMI are closely associated in human adipose tissue during morbid obesity. Diabetes 49: 1374–1380.
23. Nieuwdorp M, Stroes ES, Meijers JC, Buller H (2005) Hypercoagulability in the metabolic syndrome. Curr Opin Pharmacol 5: 155–159.
24. Van De Craen B, Declerck PJ, Gils A (2012) The Biochemistry, Physiology and Pathological roles of PAI-1 and the requirements for PAI-1 inhibition in vivo. Thrombosis research 130: 576–585.
25. Iwaki T, Urano T, Umemura K (2012) PAI-1, progress in understanding the clinical problem and its aetiology. Br J Haematol 157: 291–298.
26. Weijers RN (2012) Lipid composition of cell membranes and its relevance in type 2 diabetes mellitus. Curr Diabetes Rev 8: 390–400.
27. Stefan N, Peter A, Cegan A, Staiger H, Machann J, et al. (2008) Low hepatic stearoyl-CoA desaturase 1 activity is associated with fatty liver and insulin resistance in obese humans. Diabetologia 51: 648–656.
28. Obukowicz M, Welsch D, Salsgiver W, Martin-Berger C, Chinn K, et al. (1999) Novel, selective delta6 or delta5 fatty acid desaturase inhibitors as antiinflammatory agents in mice. Lipids 34 Suppl: S149.
29. Corey EJ, Shih C, Cashman JR (1983) Docosahexaenoic acid is a strong inhibitor of prostaglandin but not leukotriene biosynthesis. Proceedings of the National Academy of Sciences of the United States of America 80: 3581–3584.
30. Dobrian AD, Lieb DC, Cole BK, Taylor-Fishwick DA, Chakrabarti SK, et al. (2011) Functional and pathological roles of the 12- and 15-lipoxygenases. Prog Lipid Res 50: 115–131.
31. Nugent C, Prins JB, Whitehead JP, Wentworth JM, Chatterjee VK, et al. (2001) Arachidonic acid stimulates glucose uptake in 3T3-L1 adipocytes by increasing GLUT1 and GLUT4 levels at the plasma membrane. Evidence for involvement of lipoxygenase metabolites and peroxisome proliferator-activated receptor gamma. The Journal of biological chemistry 276: 9149–9157.
32. Massiera F, Saint-Marc P, Seydoux J, Murata T, Kobayashi T, et al. (2003) Arachidonic acid and prostacyclin signaling promote adipose tissue development: a human health concern? J Lipid Res 44: 271–279.
33. Malipa AC, Meintjes RA, Haag M (2008) Arachidonic acid and glucose uptake by freshly isolated human adipocytes. Cell biochemistry and function 26: 221–227.
34. Nelson TL, Biggs ML, Kizer JR, Cushman M, Hokanson JE, et al. (2012) Lipoprotein-associated phospholipase A2 (Lp-PLA2) and future risk of type 2

diabetes: results from the Cardiovascular Health Study. The Journal of clinical endocrinology and metabolism 97: 1695–1701.

35. Madsen L, Petersen RK, Sorensen MB, Jorgensen C, Hallenborg P, et al. (2003) Adipocyte differentiation of 3T3-L1 preadipocytes is dependent on lipoxygenase activity during the initial stages of the differentiation process. The Biochemical journal 375: 539–549.

36. Naruhn S, Meissner W, Adhikary T, Kaddatz K, Klein T, et al. (2010) 15-hydroxyeicosatetraenoic acid is a preferential peroxisome proliferator-activated receptor beta/delta agonist. Molecular pharmacology 77: 171–184.

37. Shappell SB, Gupta RA, Manning S, Whitehead R, Boeglin WE, et al. (2001) 15S-Hydroxyeicosatetraenoic acid activates peroxisome proliferator-activated receptor gamma and inhibits proliferation in PC3 prostate carcinoma cells. Cancer research 61: 497–503.

38. Cole BK, Morris MA, Grzesik WJ, Leone KA, Nadler JL (2012) Adipose tissue-specific deletion of 12/15-lipoxygenase protects mice from the consequences of a high-fat diet. Mediators Inflamm 2012: 851798.

39. Lee YT, Hsu CC, Lin MH, Liu KS, Yin MC (2005) Histidine and carnosine delay diabetic deterioration in mice and protect human low density lipoprotein against oxidation and glycation. European journal of pharmacology 513: 145–150.

40. Stunes AK, Reseland JE, Hauso O, Kidd M, Tommeras K, et al. (2011) Adipocytes express a functional system for serotonin synthesis, reuptake and receptor activation. Diabetes, obesity & metabolism 13: 551–558.

41. Gaster M, Nehlin JO, Minet AD (2012) Impaired TCA cycle flux in mitochondria in skeletal muscle from type 2 diabetic subjects: marker or maker of the diabetic phenotype? Archives of physiology and biochemistry 118: 156–189.

42. Schrauwen P, Hesselink MK (2008) Reduced tricarboxylic acid cycle flux in type 2 diabetes mellitus? Diabetologia 51: 1694–1697.

43. Egan JM, Henderson TE, Bernier M (1995) Arginine enhances glycogen synthesis in response to insulin in 3T3-L1 adipocytes. The American journal of physiology 269: E61–66.

44. Floegel A, Stefan N, Yu Z, Muhlenbruch K, Drogan D, et al. (2012) Identification of Serum Metabolites Associated With Risk of Type 2 Diabetes Using a Targeted Metabolomic Approach. Diabetes.

23

Ursolic Acid Increases Glucose Uptake through the PI3K Signaling Pathway in Adipocytes

Yonghan He[1,2,3], Wen Li[4], Ying Li[1], Shuocheng Zhang[2,5], Yanwen Wang[2,5]*, Changhao Sun[1]*

1 Department of Nutrition and Food Hygiene, Public Health College, Harbin Medical University, Harbin, Heilongjiang, People's Republic of China, 2 Aquatic and Crop Resource Development, Life Sciences Branch, National Research Council Canada, Charlottetown, Prince Edward Island, Canada, 3 State Key Laboratory of Genetic Resources and Evolution, Kunming Institute of Zoology, Chinese Academy of Sciences, Kunming, Yunnan, People's Republic of China, 4 Department of Endocrinology, Third People's Hospital of Yunnan Province, Kunming, Yunnan, People's Republic of China, 5 Department of Biomedical Sciences, University of Prince Edward Island, Charlottetown, Prince Edward Island, Canada

Abstract

Background: Ursolic acid (UA), a triterpenoid compound, is reported to have a glucose-lowering effect. However, the mechanisms are not fully understood. Adipose tissue is one of peripheral tissues that collectively control the circulating glucose levels.

Objective: The objective of the present study was to determine the effect and further the mechanism of action of UA in adipocytes.

Methods and Results: The 3T3-L1 preadipocytes were induced to differentiate and treated with different concentrations of UA. NBD-fluorescent glucose was used as the tracer to measure glucose uptake and Western blotting used to determine the expression and activity of proteins involved in glucose transport. It was found that 2.5, 5 and 10 μM of UA promoted glucose uptake in a dose-dependent manner (17%, 29% and 35%, respectively). 10 μM UA-induced glucose uptake with insulin stimulation was completely blocked by the phosphatidylinositol (PI) 3-kinase (PI3K) inhibitor wortmannin (1 μM), but not by SB203580 (10 μM), the inhibitor of mitogen-activated protein kinase (MAPK), or compound C (2.5 μM), the inhibitor of AMP-activated kinase (AMPK) inhibitor. Furthmore, the downstream protein activities of the PI3K pathway, phosphoinositide-dependent kinase (PDK) and phosphoinositide-dependent serine/threoninekinase (AKT) were increased by 10 μM of UA in the presence of insulin. Interestingly, the activity of AS160 and protein kinase C (PKC) and the expression of glucose transporter 4 (GLUT4) were stimulated by 10 μM of UA under either the basal or insulin-stimulated status. Moreover, the translocation of GLUT4 from cytoplasm to cell membrane was increased by UA but decreased when the PI3K inhibitor was applied.

Conclusions: Our results suggest that UA stimulates glucose uptake in 3T3-L1 adipocytes through the PI3K pathway, providing important information regarding the mechanism of action of UA for its anti-diabetic effect.

Editor: Chih-Hsin Tang, China Medical University, Taiwan

Funding: This research was supported by the Internal Research Project of the Third People's Hospital of Yunnan Province (YJ201202) and the National Natural Science Fund of China (81130049). The funders had no role in study design, data collection and analysis, decision to publish, or preparation of the manuscript.

Competing Interests: The authors have declared that no competing interests exist.

* Email: yanwen.wang@nrc.ca (YW); sun2002changhao@yahoo.com (CS)

Introduction

The prevalence of diabetes has dramatically increased and results in a considerably higher rate of mortality worldwide. Insulin resistance has been considered as a well-known metabolic disorder of diabetes, which is closely related with serious complications such as cardiovascular and kidney diseases [1]. Insulin is critical in glucose homeostasis and stimulates the transport of blood glucose into the cells for metabolism in the peripheral tissues (such as muscle, fat tissue and liver) by regulating the expression and translocation of glucose transporters [2,3]. When insulin resistance occurs, the insulin-mediated glucose uptake is impaired, leading to reduced glucose uptake into muscle,

adipose or liver cells and consequently the elevation of blood glucose concentration. Accordingly, agents with an ability of stimulating glucose uptake in these tissues are used to improve or treat insulin resistance and diabetes.

Although some effective therapeutic drugs have been developed and used for many years to treat diabetes, most of these drugs produce undesirable or severe side effects, such as induction of fat accumulation [4], inhibition of hepatic regeneration [5], and causing osteoporosis [6]. Therefore, there is a need to develop new anti-diabetic products, especially through an approach of stimulating glucose uptake and utilization in peripheral tissues without causing obvious side effects. In this regard, natural products have provided a new avenue and been considered having great potential.

Ursolic acid (UA) is a natural pentacyclic triterpenoid and present in many different plants, fruits and herbs. Accumulating evidence has shown that UA possesses multiple nutritional and pharmacological functions [7,8]. Recent studies have revealed that UA decreases weight gain and abdominal fat mass in mice fed a high-fat diet [9,10]. Further studies have demonstrated that UA reduces adiposity by enhancing lipolysis [11,12] and inhibiting adipogenesis [13]. It is well established that central obesity is closely related to insulin resistance and diabetes [14]. We hypothesized that UA might be beneficial to insulin resistant or diabetic patients partially through regulating fat and glucose metabolism. Indeed, emerging evidence demonstrates that UA is able to lower blood glucose and improve insulin resistance and diabetes [15–19]. Although several mechanisms have been reported, such as promoting the glucose uptake and utilization in muscle cells [20,21], increasing liver glycogen synthesis and deposition [22], and increasing pancreatic β-cell function [16], it is not clear whether and how UA modulates glucose uptake and metabolism in adipose tissue, which plays an important role in glucose homeostasis through taking up glucose when the circulating glucose level is elevated [23]. Accordingly, the present study was conducted to determine the effect of UA on glucose uptake and further on the protein expression and activity of the insulin signaling pathway. Here we report that UA promotes glucose uptake in adipocytes through the phosphatidylinositol (PI) 3-kinase (PI3K) pathway and enhancing glucose transporter 4 (GLUT4) translocation and expression.

Materials and Methods

Chemicals and reagents

Ursolic acid, cytochalasin B, insulin, 3-isobutyl-1-methylxan-thine (IBMX), dexamethasone, wortmannin, SB203580, com-pound C, protease inhibitor and bovine serum albumin (BSA) were purchased from Sigma (St. Louis, MO, USA). High glucose Dulbecco's modified Eagle's medium (DMEM) was from Media-tech, Inc. (Cellgro Mediatech, Inc. Manassas, VA). Fetal bovine serum (FBS) was bought from PAA Laboratories (Etobicoke, ON, Canada). Bovine calf serum (BCS) was purchased from Cayman Chemical Company (Ann Arbor, Michigan, USA). The BCA protein assay kit was obtained from Thermo Scientific (San Jose, CA, USA). RIPA lysis buffer was from Millpore (MA, USA). Protein loading buffer was from Bio-Rad (Montreal, QC, Canada). Antibodies against phospho-phosphoinositide-dependent kinase (pPDK), phosphoinositide-dependent kinase (PDK), phos-pho-protein kinase C (PKC), protein kinase C (PKC), phospho-AS160 (pAS160), AS160, GLUT4, glucose transporter 1 (GLUT1), phospho-phosphoinositide-dependent serine/threonine kinase (pAKT), phosphoinositide-dependent serine/threonine kinase (AKT) and clathrin were from Cell Signaling Technology, Inc. (Beverly, Massachusetts, USA). 2-NBD-glucose was purchased from Invitrogen Life Technologies (Carlsbad, CA, USA). BM chemiluminescence blotting substrate kit was from Roche Diag-nosis (Laval, QC, Canada).

Cell culture

3T3-L1 mouse embryo fibroblasts were obtained from Amer-ican Type Culture Collection (Rockville, MD) and cultured in DMEM containing 10% BCS until confluent, and were then maintained in the same medium for additional 2 d. The cells were then induced to differentiate according to the method reported previously [13,24].

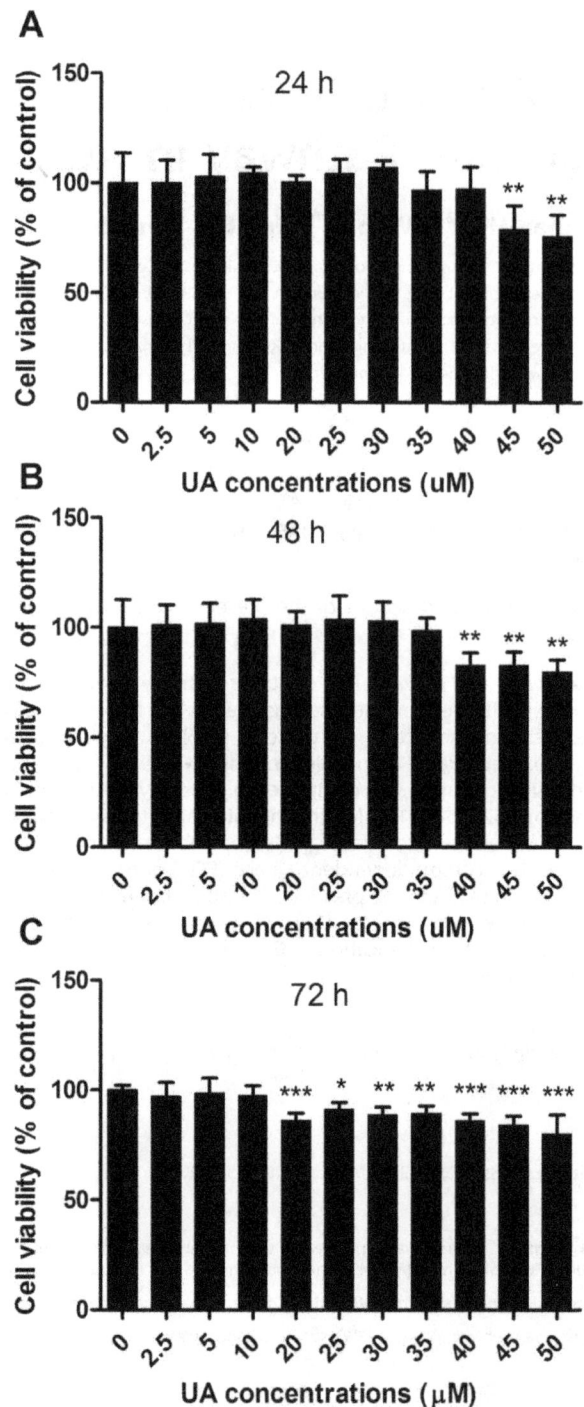

Figure 1. Effect of UA on the viability of 3T3-L1 adipocytes. Mature 3T3-L1 adipocytes were incubated with different concentrations of UA for 24, 48, or 72 h, respectively. The MTT reagents were added to the medium. After 4 h of incubation, the medium was aspirated and 150 μL DMSO was added to each well. The absorbance was measured at 570 nm. Data are expressed as means ± SD (n = 3). *P<0.05, **P< 0.001 and ***P<0.001 vs. the control of 0 μM UA.

Cell viability

After differentiation, 3T3-L1 adipocytes were cultured in the presence of 2.5 to 50 μM of UA for 24, 48 and 72 h, respectively. At each time point, the cells were treated with MTT assay reagents

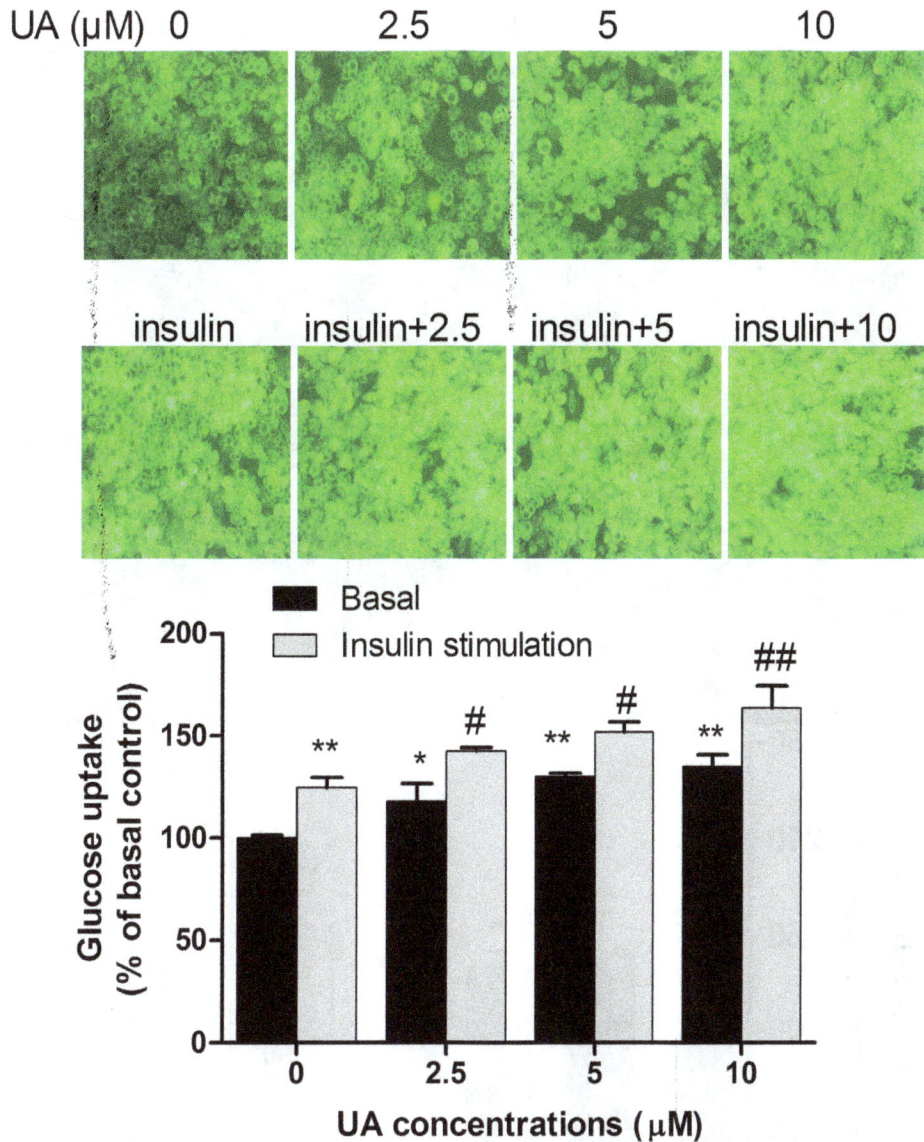

Figure 2. Effect of UA on glucose uptake in 3T3-L1 adipocyte. Mature 3T3-L1 adipocytes were incubated with 2.5 μM, 5 μM, or 10 μM of UA for 2 h and glucose uptake was measured in the presence or absence of 1 μg/mL insulin. The fluorescence intensity of NBD-glucosewas measured at 466/550 nm on a Varioskan Flash spectral scanning multimode plate reader. Data are expressed as means ± SD (n = 3). * P<0.05 and **P<0.01 vs. the control of 0 μM UA; #P<0.05 and ##P<0.01 vs. 1 μg/mL of insulin.

(1 mg/mL) for 4 h and the resulting formazan was solubilized in 150 μL dimethyl sulfoxide (DMSO) and further diluted 10 times with DMSO. The absorbance was read at 570 nm on a Varioskan Flash spectral scanning multimode plate reader (Thermo Fisher Scientific, Waltham, MA).

Measurement of glucose uptake

3T3-L1 preadipocytes were cultured in 96-well plates and induced to differentiate for 8 d. The cells were then starved overnight in DMEM with 0.1% BSA and further incubated in Krebs Ringer bicarbonate buffer (110 mM NaCl, 4.4 mM KCl, 1.45 mM KH_2PO_4, 1.2 mM $MgCl_2$, 2.3 mM $CaCl_2$, 4.8 mM $NaHCO_3$, 10 mM HEPES and 0.3% BSA) containing 100 μM NBD-glucose, 2.8 mM glucose and different concentrations of UA for 2 h at 37°C in the presence or absence of 1 μg/mL insulin. After 2 h incubation, the reaction was terminated by 20 μM of

cytochalasin B. The cells were washed twice with cold Krebs Ringer bicarbonate buffer (4°C), and then 100 uL cold PBS (4°C) were added to each well. The fluorescence intensity was immediately measured at 466/550 nm on a Varioskan Flash spectral scanning multimode plate reader (Thermo Fisher Scientific, Waltham, MA). For the inhibition experiments, the cells were pretreated with PI3K inhibitor wortmannin (1 μM), MAPK inhibitor SB203580 (10 μM), and AMPK inhibitor compound C (2.5 μM), respectively, for 30 min.

Western blotting

3T3-L1 preadipocytes were grown in 75 cm² flasks and differentiated. After treatment with different concentrations of UA, total protein was extracted using the method described previously [24]. For measuring the translocation of GLUT4, membrane proteins were separated using a membrane protein

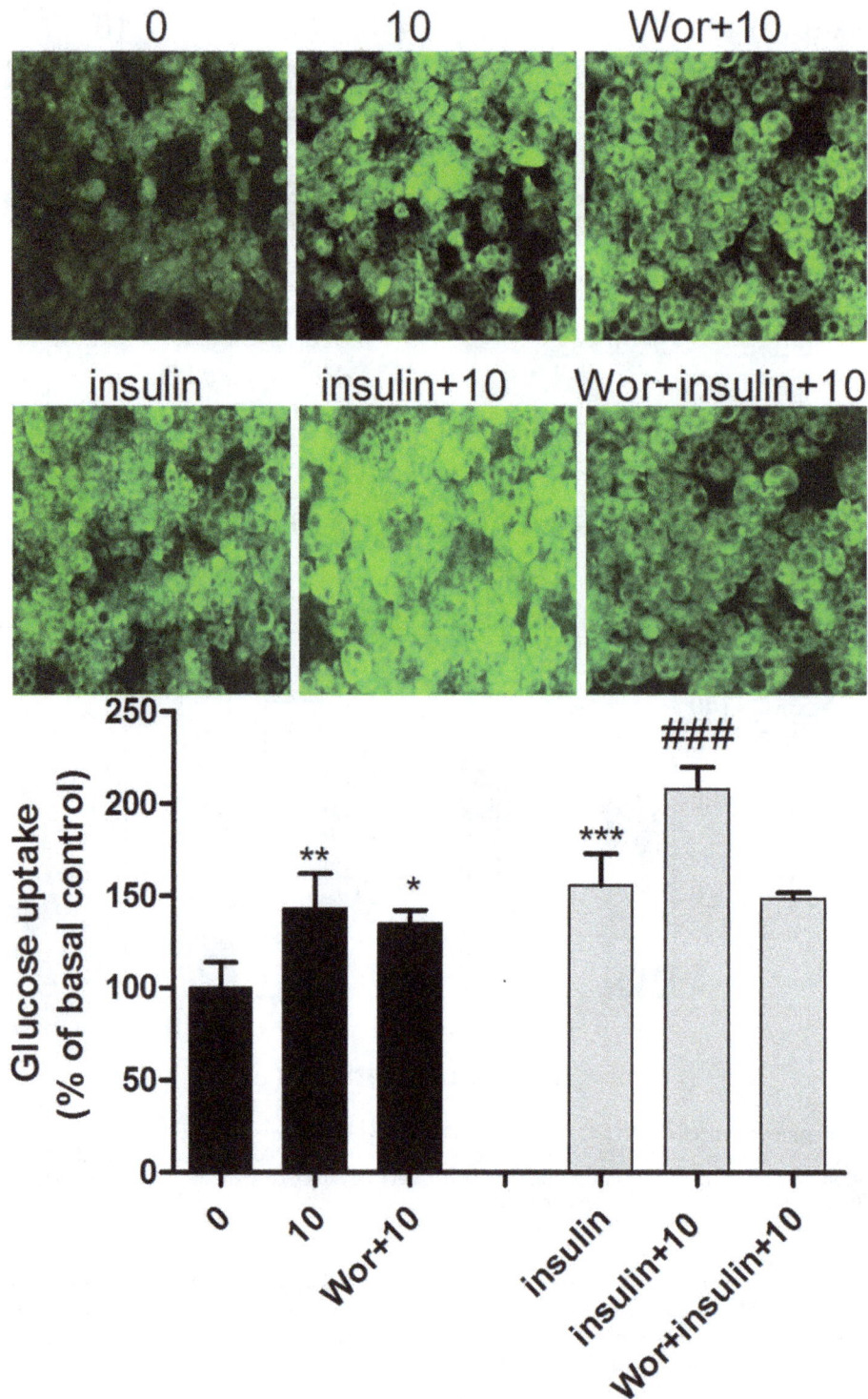

Figure 3. Effect of the PI3K inhibitor wortmannin on glucose uptake in 3T3-L1 adipocyte. Mature 3T3-L1 adipocytes were incubated with 10 μM of UA for 2 h, or pretreated with 1 μM of wortmannin for 30 min before incubation with 10 μM of UA and 1 μM of wortmannin for 2 h. Glucose uptake was measured in the presence or absence of 1 μg/mL insulin. The fluorescence intensity of NBD-glucose was measured at 466/550 nm on a Varioskan Flash spectral scanning multimode plate reader. Data are expressed as means ± SD (n = 3). *$P < 0.05$ and **$P < 0.01$ vs. the control of 0 μM UA; #$P < 0.05$, ##$P < 0.01$ and ###$P < 0.001$ vs. the insulin control of 1 μg/mL. Wor indicates 1 μM of wortmannin.

extraction kit (Abcam, Cambridge, MA) following the manufacturers' protocol. The protein of GLUT4 was determined using the Western blotting, with clathrin being used as the loading control.

Immunofluorescence assay

3T3-L1 preadipocytes were cultured in glass-bottomed dishes and differentiated in the induction medium. The differentiated adipocytes were starved in DMEM with 0.1% BSA for 3 h. After

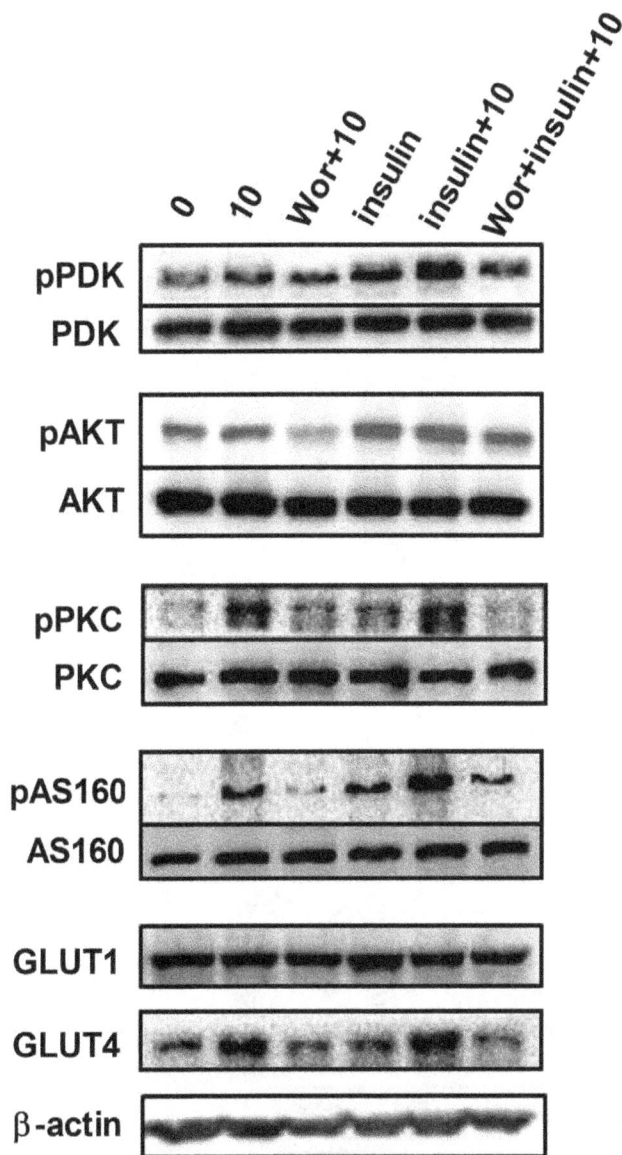

Figure 4. Effect of UA on the activity of PDK, AKT, PKC and AS160, and the expression of GLUT1 and GLUT4. Mature 3T3-L1 cells were treated with 10 μM of UA in the absence or presence of 1 μg/mL insulin for 24 h, or pretreated with 1 μM of wortmannin for 30 min before incubation 10 μM of UA and 1 μM of wortmannin for 24 h. The activity of PDK, AKT, PKC and AS160, and the expression of GLUT1 and GLUT4 were assessed by Western blotting. Data are expressed as means ± SD (n = 3). Wor indicates 1 μM of wortmannin.

pretreatment with wortmannin for 30 min, the cells were treated with 10 μM of UA for 2 h in the presence or absence of 1 μg/mL insulin. They were washed once with ice-cold PBS, fixed for 15 min in 4% paraformaldehyde, permeablized in 0.25% Triton X-100 for 5 min at 4°C, and washed 3 times using ice-cold PBS. After blocking in 10% normal donkey serum at room temperature for 1 h, the cells were washed and incubated at 4°C with anti-GLUT4 antibody overnight. After three washes of 10 min each with PBS, the FITC-conjugated secondary antibody was applied to the samples at room temperature for 1 h. After washing with PBS, images were immediately captured under a Nikon inverted microscope (ECLIPSE TE200).

Statistical analysis

The statistical analyses were performed using SPSS 13.0 statistical program (version 13.01S; Beijing Stats Data Mining Co. Ltd). The treatment effect was determined using one-way ANOVA and followed by a post-hoc Dunnett's or Bonferroni's multiple comparisons test, where a P value less than 0.05 was considered significant. Data are presented as means ± SD.

Results

Effect of UA on fat cell viability

The MTT assay results revealed that UA at concentrations up to 35 μM did not affect cell viability after 24 or 48 h of incubation (**Figure. 1A, B**), while 20 μM and above being toxic after 72 h of incubation in differentiated 3T3-L1 adipocytes (**Figure 1C**). The concentrations of 20 μM and higher were also toxic in 3T3-L1 preadipocytes [13]. Therefore, a maximal concentration of 10 μM was used in the subsequent experiments.

UA increases glucose uptake in 3T3-L1 adipocytes

To investigate the effect of UA on glucose uptake, differentiated 3T3-L1 adipocytes were cultured in DMEM supplemented with different concentrations of UA for 2 h in the presence or absence of 1 μg/mL of insulin. As shown in **Figure 2**, 2.5, 5, or 10 μM of UA significantly increased glucose uptake by 17%, 29% and 35%, respectively, which was supported by the increase of intracellular fluorescent intensity of NBD-glucose. Glucose uptake was stimulated by insulin at 1 μg/mL and further increased by UA in a dose-dependent manner (**Figure 2**).

UA stimulates glucose uptake through the PI3K pathway

To identify the pathway through which UA stimulated glucose uptake, the differentiated 3T3-L1 adipocytes were pretreated with the PI3K, MAPK and AMPK inhibitors, respectively, and then treated with 10 μM of UA in the presence or absence of 1 μg/mL insulin. PI3K inhibitor wortmannin at 1 μM completely blocked the glucose uptake stimulated by insulin, while showing weak effect at the basal level, i.e., in the absence of insulin (**Figure 3**). MAPK inhibitor SB203580 at 10 μM or AMPK inhibitor compound C at 2.5 μM did not have any effect on the UA-stimulated glucose uptake at either the basal or insulin-stimulated status (Fig. S1). These results suggest that the PI3K pathway was responsible for the UA-induced increase of glucose uptake, especially under the conditions of insulin stimulation.

UA stimulates glucose uptake through regulating protein activities in the PI3K pathway

To confirm the role of PI3K pathway in upregulating glucose uptake in adipocytes by UA, we further determined the expression or the activity of key proteins of this pathway in the presence or absence of insulin. The activity of PDK and AKT was increased when the cells were treated with 10 μM of UA and more obvious when 1 μg/mL of insulin was applied (**Figure 4**), which was however inhibited by the PI3K inhibitor wortmannin. This observation supported the notion that PI3K pathway was responsible for the enhancing effect of UA on glucose uptake, especially under insulin stimulation in differentiated 3T3-L1 adipocytes. AS160 was a downstream target protein of AKT, and the PKC was a parallel kinase to AKT, which both serve as the effectors facilitating GLUT4 translocation and subsequent glucose uptake [25]. In this study we also observed increases in the activity of AS160 and PKC by UA at 10 μM at either the basal or insulin-stimulated status.

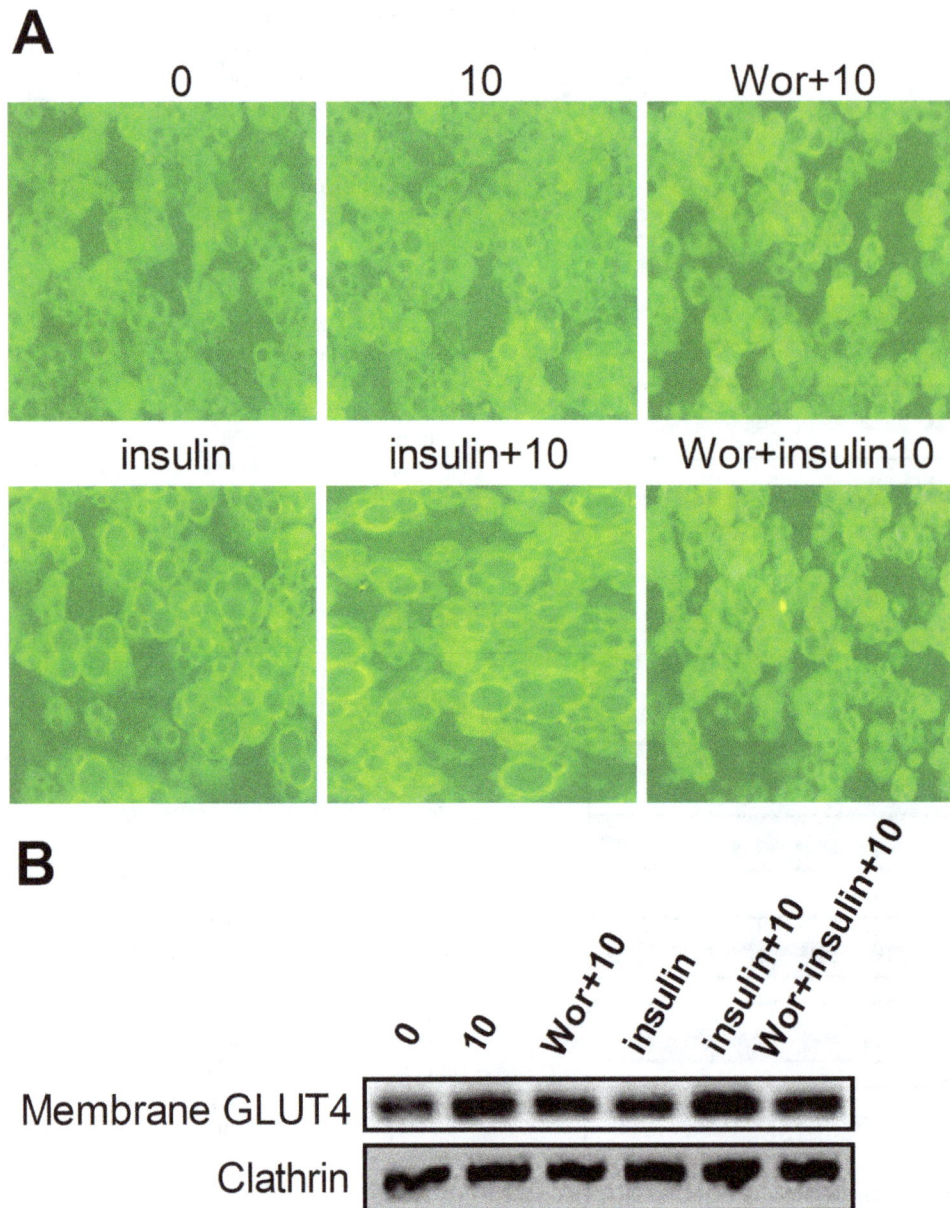

Figure 5. Effect of UA on GLUT4 expression and translocation in 3T3-L1 adipocyte. (A) Mature 3T3-L1 cells were treated with 10 µM of UA in the absence or presence of 1 µg/mL insulin for 24 h, or pretreated with 1 µM of wortmannin for 30 min before incubation with 10 µM of UA and 1 µM of wortmannin. The expression level of GLUT4 was determined by immunofluorescence. (B) Mature 3T3-L1 cells were treated with 10 µM of UA in the absence or presence of 1 µg/mL insulin for 24 h, or pretreated with 1 µM of wortmannin for 30 min and then with 10 µM of UA and 1 µM of wortmannin. Cell membrane was obtained and the expression of GLUT4 was determined with Western blotting (n = 3). Wor indicates 1 µM of wortmannin.

UA enhances GLUT4 expression and translocation

GLUT4 is the key molecule that transports glucose into cells and is critical for glucose uptake by adipose and muscle tissues and thus postprandial glucose clearance from the circulating system. We observed that after 24 h of incubation with 10 µM of UA not only increased the expression of total cellular protein of GLUT4 (**Figure 4**) but also increased its presence on the cell membrane at either the basal or insulin stimulated status (**Figure 5B**). This effect was attenuated by the pretreatment of cells with PI3K inhibitor wortmannin. The result of the immunoflurence assay provided additional support (**Figure 5A**). GLUT1 was reported to function in the process of glucose uptake under a basal status;

however, there were not any effects of UA on GLUT1 expression (**Figure 4**). Together, these results imply that the enhancement of GLUT4 expression and translocation was responsible for the observed increase of glucose uptake by UA in 3T3-L1 adipocytes.

Discussion

Ursolic acid is well known to possess a wide range of biological functions, including anti-inflammatory, anti-oxidative, anti-muta-genic, anti-carcinogenic, hepatoprotective, anti-microbial, anti-atherosclerotic, and anti-hyperlipidemic effects [7,8]. We have previously demonstrated that UA inhibits adipogenesis through the LKB1/AMPK pathway [13] and promotes lipolysis in adipocytes via the PPARγ signaling [13], and shows an anti-obesity effect *in vivo* [26]. Our recent study showed that UA improved insulin resistance, inflammation and oxidative stress in high-fat diet-induced rats [26]. Obesity is highly related to insulin resistance and T2DM through a mechanism of increased release of fatty acids, glycerol, hormones, pro-inflammatory cytokines and other risk factors from adipose tissue [14]. Adipose insulin resistance contributes to the total insulin resistance and liver complications caused by obesity [27–30]. Since UA possesses anti-obesity and anti-insulin resistance effects and has benefits to the adipose tissue fat metabolism, we wondered whether and how UA regulates glucose metabolism in adipocytes. In this study, we demonstrated that UA stimulated glucose uptake in adipocytes through upregulating the PI3K pathway and GLUT4 expression and translocation.

Several studies have demonstrated the hypoglycemic effect of UA [15–19]. The reported mechanisms include the inhibition of protein tyrosine phosphatase 1B (PTP1B) [21], increase of liver glycogen synthesis [22], enhancement of pancreatic β-cell function [16] and the activation of skeletal muscle AKT activity [20]. Glucose homeostasis is determined by glucose production and utilization in the insulin-sensitive organs and tissues, including muscle, liver and adipose tissue. Glucose uptake in adipose tissue plays a critical role in the body glucose control [23], which is demonstrated by the selective depletion of GLUT4 in adipose tissues of mice [31]. We observed that UA stimulated glucose uptake in adipocytes in a dose-dependent manner at either the basal or insulin-stimulated status. Wortmannin is a PI3K inhibitor, when it was added in the culture medium of 3T3-L1 adipocytes, the effect of UA on glucose uptake was almost completely abolished. PDK is the downstream target of the PI3K and functions as an activator of AKT [25]. UA activated the PDK and AKT in the presence of insulin and again this effect was attenuated by wortmannin. PKC is a parallel kinase to AKT [32] and AS160 is the substrate of AKT [25]. They are all involved the regulation of GLUT4 translocation. Interestingly, the UA alone or together with insulin increased the activities of PKC and AS160, both are important effectors in modulating glucose uptake [25]. These effects of UA were suppressed by the PI3K inhibitor. The findings suggest that the PI3K pathway is responsible for the UA-stimulated glucose uptake in adipocytes.

Although the results of the present study suggested that UA enhanced glucose uptake through the PI3K pathway, we could not rule out other pathways that may also contribute to the increased glucose uptake in adipose tissue. MAPK has been shown to modulate glucose uptake stimulated by insulin or other factors in adipocytes and muscle cells [33,34]. AMPK is reported to be a key regulator of glucose transport in 3T3-L1 adipocytes [35]. We demonstrated previously that UA inhibited adipogenesis in 3T3-L1 adipocytes through stimulating the AMPK activity [13], suggesting a possible role of AMPK in the UA-enhanced glucose uptake. To understand the role of these molecules in UA-regulated glucose uptake, we further investigated the effect of the kinase inhibitors on the UA-induced increase of glucose uptake in adipocytes. Surprisingly, AMPK inhibitor (compound C) or MAPK inhibitor (SB203580) did not block the stimulatory effect of UA on glucose uptake, indicating that the regulation of UA on glucose uptake in adipocytes was independent of the MAPK and AMPK pathways.

Glucose uptake in adipocytes is regulated by glucose transporters, GLUT1 and GLUT4 [36,37]. Of them, GLUT1 is essential for basal glucose transport in various tissues, whereas GLUT4 is selectively expressed in the insulin-responsive tissues, such as adipose and skeletal muscle cells. UA did not show any effect on GLUT1 expression but significantly upregulated GLUT4 levels in adipocytes. When blood glucose level is elevated, insulin is released into the blood stream and triggers insulin signaling. The GLUT4 moves from cytoplasm to the cell membrane where it transports glucose across the membrane into the cells. Thus, the total expression and translocation of GLUT4 is critical in glucose transport and uptake, and subsequently glucose disposal and clearance from the circulation. Both the protein expression and immonofluorescence assay results revealed that UA upregulated GLUT4 expression and translocation, in good agreement with the increased activity of AS160, which is a key regulator of GLUT4 trafficking in 3T3-L1 adipocytes [38,39]. This notion was further supported by the effect on PKC that regulates GLUT4 distribution in 3T3-L1 adipocytes [40]. We did not determine the effect of UA on the activity of insulin receptor and insulin receptor substrate, which are important proteins at the upstream of the PI3K pathway. However, UA has been reported to increase insulin receptor phosphorylation in the presence of insulin [18]. It should be pointed out that UA increases the phosphorylation and activity of AMPK and the expression of CPT1, thus inhibits fatty acid synthesis while enhancing fat oxidation [13]. As a result, UA stimulated glucose uptake but did not promote the synthesis and accumulation of fat in adipocytes.

In conclusion, UA increased glucose uptake in 3T3-L1 adipocytes by activating the PI3K pathway and GLUT4 translocation. The results provide additional information regarding the mechanism of action of UA for its anti-diabetic effect.

Supporting Information

Figure S1   Effect of the AMPK inhibitor compound C or the MAPK inhibitor SB203580 on glucose uptake in 3T3-L1 adipocyte. Mature 3T3-L1 adipocytes were incubated with 10 μM of UA for 2 h, or pretreated with 2.5 μM of coumpound C or pretreated with 10 μM of SB203580 for 30 min before incubation with 10 μM of UA in the presence of indicated concentrations of inhibitors for 2 h. Glucose uptake was measured in the presence or absence of 1 μg/mL insulin. The fluorescence intensity of NBD-glucose was measured at 466/550 nm on a Varioskan Flash spectral scanning multimode plate reader. Data are expressed as means ± SD (n = 3). *P<0.05 and **P<0.01 vs. the control of 0 μM UA; CC indicates 2.5 μM of coumpound C and SB indicates 10 μM of SB203580.

Acknowledgments

Thanks to Ben Perry and Tiantian Zhao for their technical support during the experiments.

Author Contributions

Conceived and designed the experiments: YWW CHS. Performed the experiments: YHH SCZ. Analyzed the data: YHH WL. Contributed reagents/materials/analysis tools: YL WL. Contributed to the writing of the manuscript: WL YHH YWW.

References

1. Grundy SM, Benjamin IJ, Burke GL, Chait A, Eckel RH, et al. (1999) Diabetes and cardiovascular disease: a statement for healthcare professionals from the American Heart Association. Circulation 100: 1134–1146.
2. Chang L, Chiang SH, Saltiel AR (2004) Insulin signaling and the regulation of glucose transport. Mol Med 10: 65–71.
3. Khan AH, Pessin JE (2002) Insulin regulation of glucose uptake: a complex interplay of intracellular signalling pathways. Diabetologia 45: 1475–1483.
4. de Souza CJ, Eckhardt M, Gagen K, Dong M, Chen W, et al. (2001) Effects of pioglitazone on adipose tissue remodeling within the setting of obesity and insulin resistance. Diabetes 50: 1863–1871.
5. Turmelle YP, Shikapwashya O, Tu S, Hruz PW, Yan Q, et al. (2006) Rosiglitazone inhibits mouse liver regeneration. FASEB J 20: 2609–2611.
6. Rzonca SO, Suva LJ, Gaddy D, Montague DC, Lecka-Czernik B (2004) Bone is a target for the antidiabetic compound rosiglitazone. Endocrinology 145: 401–406.
7. Ikeda Y, Murakami A, Ohigashi H (2008) Ursolic acid: an anti- and pro-inflammatory triterpenoid. Mol Nutr Food Res 52: 26–42.
8. Liu J (2005) Oleanolic acid and ursolic acid: research perspectives. J Ethnopharmacol 100: 92–94.
9. Jayaprakasam B, Olson LK, Schutzki RE, Tai MH, Nair MG (2006) Amelioration of obesity and glucose intolerance in high-fat-fed C57BL/6 mice by anthocyanins and ursolic acid in Cornelian cherry (Cornus mas). J Agric Food Chem 54: 243–248.
10. Rao VS, de Melo CL, Queiroz MG, Lemos TL, Menezes DB, et al. (2011) Ursolic acid, a pentacyclic triterpene from Sambucus australis, prevents abdominal adiposity in mice fed a high-fat diet. J Med Food 14: 1375–1382.
11. Kim J, Jang DS, Kim H, Kim JS (2009) Anti-lipase and lipolytic activities of ursolic acid isolated from the roots of Actinidia arguta. Arch Pharm Res 32: 983–987.
12. Li Y, Kang Z, Li S, Kong T, Liu X, et al. (2010) Ursolic acid stimulates lipolysis in primary-cultured rat adipocytes. Mol Nutr Food Res 54: 1609–1617.
13. He Y, Li Y, Zhao T, Wang Y, Sun C (2013) Ursolic acid inhibits adipogenesis in 3T3-L1 adipocytes through LKB1/AMPK pathway. PLoS One 8: e70135.
14. Kahn SE, Hull RL, Utzschneider KM (2006) Mechanisms linking obesity to insulin resistance and type 2 diabetes. Nature 444: 840–846.
15. Jang SM, Kim MJ, Choi MS, Kwon EY, Lee MK (2010) Inhibitory effects of ursolic acid on hepatic polyol pathway and glucose production in streptozotocin-induced diabetic mice. Metabolism 59: 512–519.
16. Jang SM, Yee ST, Choi J, Choi MS, Do GM, et al. (2009) Ursolic acid enhances the cellular immune system and pancreatic beta-cell function in streptozotocin-induced diabetic mice fed a high-fat diet. Int Immunopharmacol 9: 113–119.
17. Kazmi I, Rahman M, Afzal M, Gupta G, Saleem S, et al. (2012) Anti-diabetic potential of ursolic acid stearoyl glucoside: a new triterpenic gycosidic ester from Lantana camara. Fitoterapia 83: 142–146.
18. Kunkel SD, Suneja M, Ebert SM, Bongers KS, Fox DK, et al. (2011) mRNA expression signatures of human skeletal muscle atrophy identify a natural compound that increases muscle mass. Cell Metab 13: 627–638.
19. Lee J, Yee ST, Kim JJ, Choi MS, Kwon EY, et al. (2010) Ursolic acid ameliorates thymic atrophy and hyperglycemia in streptozotocin-nicotinamide-induced diabetic mice. Chem Biol Interact 188: 635–642.
20. Kunkel SD, Elmore CJ, Bongers KS, Ebert SM, Fox DK, et al. (2012) Ursolic acid increases skeletal muscle and brown fat and decreases diet-induced obesity, glucose intolerance and fatty liver disease. PLoS One 7: e39332.
21. Zhang W, Hong D, Zhou Y, Zhang Y, Shen Q, et al. (2006) Ursolic acid and its derivative inhibit protein tyrosine phosphatase 1B, enhancing insulin receptor phosphorylation and stimulating glucose uptake. Biochim Biophys Acta 1760: 1505–1512.
22. Azevedo MF, Camsari C, Sa CM, Lima CF, Fernandes-Ferreira M, et al. (2010) Ursolic acid and luteolin-7-glucoside improve lipid profiles and increase liver glycogen content through glycogen synthase kinase-3. Phytother Res 24 Suppl 2: S220–224.
23. Rosen ED, Spiegelman BM (2006) Adipocytes as regulators of energy balance and glucose homeostasis. Nature 444: 847–853.
24. He Y, Li Y, Zhang S, Perry B, Zhao T, et al. (2013) Radicicol, a heat shock protein 90 inhibitor, inhibits differentiation and adipogenesis in 3T3-L1 preadipocytes. Biochem Biophys Res Commun 436: 169–174.
25. Krook A, Wallberg-Henriksson H, Zierath JR (2004) Sending the signal: molecular mechanisms regulating glucose uptake. Med Sci Sports Exerc 36: 1212–1217.
26. Li S, Liao X, Meng F, Wang Y, Sun Z, et al. (2014) Therapeutic role of ursolic acid on ameliorating hepatic steatosis and improving metabolic disorders in high-fat diet-induced non-alcoholic fatty liver disease rats. PLoS One 9: e86724.
27. Donnelly KL, Smith CI, Schwarzenberg SJ, Jessurun J, Boldt MD, et al. (2005) Sources of fatty acids stored in liver and secreted via lipoproteins in patients with nonalcoholic fatty liver disease. J Clin Invest 115: 1343–1351.
28. Guerre-Millo M (2004) Adipose tissue and adipokines: for better or worse. Diabetes Metab 30: 13–19.
29. Haukeland JW, Damas JK, Konopski Z, Loberg EM, Haaland T, et al. (2006) Systemic inflammation in nonalcoholic fatty liver disease is characterized by elevated levels of CCL2. J Hepatol 44: 1167–1174.
30. Pagano C, Soardo G, Pilon C, Milocco C, Basan L, et al. (2006) Increased serum resistin in nonalcoholic fatty liver disease is related to liver disease severity and not to insulin resistance. J Clin Endocrinol Metab 91: 1081–1086.
31. Abel ED, Peroni O, Kim JK, Kim YB, Boss O, et al. (2001) Adipose-selective targeting of the GLUT4 gene impairs insulin action in muscle and liver. Nature 409: 729–733.
32. Bandyopadhyay G, Standaert ML, Zhao L, Yu B, Avignon A, et al. (1997) Activation of protein kinase C (alpha, beta, and zeta) by insulin in 3T3/L1 cells. Transfection studies suggest a role for PKC-zeta in glucose transport. J Biol Chem 272: 2551–2558.
33. Bazuine M, Ouwens DM, Gomes de Mesquita DS, Maassen JA (2003) Arsenite stimulated glucose transport in 3T3-L1 adipocytes involves both Glut4 translocation and p38 MAPK activity. Eur J Biochem 270: 3891–3903.
34. Somwar R, Kim DY, Sweeney G, Huang C, Niu W, et al. (2001) GLUT4 translocation precedes the stimulation of glucose uptake by insulin in muscle cells: potential activation of GLUT4 via p38 mitogen-activated protein kinase. Biochem J 359: 639–649.
35. Yamaguchi S, Katahira H, Ozawa S, Nakamichi Y, Tanaka T, et al. (2005) Activators of AMP-activated protein kinase enhance GLUT4 translocation and its glucose transport activity in 3T3-L1 adipocytes. Am J Physiol Endocrinol Metab 289: E643–649.
36. Scheepers A, Joost HG, Schurmann A (2004) The glucose transporter families SGLT and GLUT: molecular basis of normal and aberrant function. JPEN J Parenter Enteral Nutr 28: 364–371.
37. Shepherd PR, Kahn BB (1999) Glucose transporters and insulin action-implications for insulin resistance and diabetes mellitus. N Engl J Med 341: 248–257.
38. Eguez L, Lee A, Chavez JA, Miinea CP, Kane S, et al. (2005) Full intracellular retention of GLUT4 requires AS160 Rab GTPase activating protein. Cell Metab 2: 263–272.
39. Larance M, Ramm G, Stockli J, van Dam EM, Winata S, et al. (2005) Characterization of the role of the Rab GTPase-activating protein AS160 in insulin-regulated GLUT4 trafficking. J Biol Chem 280: 37803–37813.
40. Bosch RR, Bazuine M, Span PN, Willems PH, Olthaar AJ, et al. (2004) Regulation of GLUT1-mediated glucose uptake by PKClambda-PKCbeta(II) interactions in 3T3-L1 adipocytes. Biochem J 384: 349–355.

Permissions

List of Contributors

Olga Franck
Department of Internal Medicine, Division of Endocrinology, Diabetology, Vascular Disease, Nephrology and Clinical Chemistry, University of Tübingen, Tübingen, Germany

Stefan Z. Lutz, Anja Böhm, Hans-Ulrich Häring and Harald Staiger
Department of Internal Medicine, Division of Endocrinology, Diabetology, Vascular Disease, Nephrology and Clinical Chemistry, University of Tübingen, Tübingen, Germany
Institute for Diabetes Research and Metabolic Diseases of the Helmholtz Centre Munich at the University of Tübingen, Tübingen, Germany
German Centre for Diabetes Research (DZD), Tübingen, Germany

Andreas Fritsche
Department of Internal Medicine, Division of Endocrinology, Diabetology, Vascular Disease, Nephrology and Clinical Chemistry, University of Tübingen, Tübingen, Germany
Institute for Diabetes Research and Metabolic Diseases of the Helmholtz Centre Munich at the University of Tübingen, Tübingen, Germany
German Centre for Diabetes Research (DZD), Tübingen, Germany
Department of Internal Medicine, Division of Nutritional and Preventive Medicine, University of Tübingen, Tübingen, Germany

Fausto Machicao
Institute for Diabetes Research and Metabolic Diseases of the Helmholtz Centre Munich at the University of Tübingen, Tübingen, Germany
German Centre for Diabetes Research (DZD), Tübingen, Germany

Jürgen Machann and Fritz Schick
Institute for Diabetes Research and Metabolic Diseases of the Helmholtz Centre Munich at the University of Tübingen, Tübingen, Germany
German Centre for Diabetes Research (DZD), Tübingen, Germany
Department of Diagnostic and Interventional Radiology, Section on Experimental Radiology, Eberhard Karls University Tübingen, Tübingen, Germany

Jia-Ling Lee, Yow-Rong Liao, Yao-Ming Wu, Ming-Chih Ho and Hong-Shiee Lai
Department of Surgery, National Taiwan University Hospital and National Taiwan University College of Medicine, Taipei, Taiwan

Tzu-Min Hung and Yen-Chun Liu
Department of Surgery, National Taiwan University Hospital and National Taiwan University College of Medicine, Taipei, Taiwan
Department of Medical Research, E-DA Hospital, Kaohsiung, Taiwan

Cheng-Maw Ho
Department of Surgery, National Taiwan University Hospital and National Taiwan University College of Medicine, Taipei, Taiwan
Graduate Institute of Clinical Medicine, College of Medicine, National Taiwan University, Taipei, Taiwan

Po-Huang Lee
Department of Surgery, National Taiwan University Hospital and National Taiwan University College of Medicine, Taipei, Taiwan
Department of Surgery, E-DA Hospital, Kaohsiung, Taiwan

Chien-Hung Chen
Department of Internal Medicine, National Taiwan University Hospital and National Taiwan University College of Medicine, Taipei, Taiwan

Serenella Salinari
Department of Computer and System Science, University of Rome "Sapienza", Rome, Italy

Cyrille Debard, Christine Durand and Hubert Vidal
Lyon 1 University, CarMeN Laboratory, INSERM U1060, Oullins, France

Alessandro Bertuzzi
Institute of Systems Analysis and Computer Science, National Research Council, Rome, Italy

Paul Zimmet
Baker IDI Heart and Diabetes Institute, Melbourne, Victoria, Australia

Geltrude Mingrone
Department of Internal Medicine, Catholic University, School of Medicine, Rome, Italy

Qiuwei Wang, Ruiping Huang, Bin Yu, Fang Cao, Huiyan Wang, Ming Zhang, Xinhong Wang, Bin Zhang and Hong Zhou and Ziqiang Zhu
Changzhou Women and Children Health Hospital Affiliated to Nanjing Medical University, Changzhou, Jiangsu Province, China

Norbert Stefan, Cora Weigert and Harald Staiger
Department of Internal Medicine, Division of Endocrinology, Diabetology, Angiology, Nephrology and Clinical Chemistry, Eberhard Karls University Tübingen, Tübingen, Germany
Institute for Diabetes Research and Metabolic Diseases of the Helmholtz Centre Munich at the University of Tübingen, Tübingen, Germany
German Centre for Diabetes Research (DZD), Neuherberg, Germany

Hans- Ulrich Häring
Department of Internal Medicine, Division of Endocrinology, Diabetology, Angiology, Nephrology and Clinical Chemistry, Eberhard Karls University Tübingen, Tübingen, Germany
Institute for Diabetes Research and Metabolic Diseases of the Helmholtz Centre Munich at the University of Tübingen, Tübingen, Germany
German Centre for Diabetes Research (DZD), Neuherberg, Germany
Institute of Experimental Genetics, Helmholtz Centre Munich, German Research Centre for Environmental Health, Neuherberg, Germany

Andreas Fritsche
Department of Internal Medicine, Division of Endocrinology, Diabetology, Angiology, Nephrology and Clinical Chemistry, Eberhard Karls University Tübingen, Tübingen, Germany
Institute for Diabetes Research and Metabolic Diseases of the Helmholtz Centre Munich at the University of Tübingen, Tübingen, Germany
German Centre for Diabetes Research (DZD), Neuherberg, Germany
Department of Internal Medicine, Division of Nutritional and Preventive Medicine, Eberhard Karls University Tübingen, Tübingen, Germany

Anja Böhm
Department of Internal Medicine, Division of Endocrinology, Diabetology, Angiology, Nephrology and Clinical Chemistry, Eberhard Karls University Tübingen, Tübingen, Germany
German Centre for Diabetes Research (DZD), Neuherberg, Germany
Institute of Experimental Genetics, Helmholtz Centre Munich, German Research Centre for Environmental Health, Neuherberg, Germany

Fausto Machicao
Institute for Diabetes Research and Metabolic Diseases of the Helmholtz Centre Munich at the University of Tübingen, Tübingen, Germany
German Centre for Diabetes Research (DZD), Neuherberg, Germany

Jürgen Machann and Fritz Schick
Institute for Diabetes Research and Metabolic Diseases of the Helmholtz Centre Munich at the University of Tübingen, Tübingen, Germany
German Centre for Diabetes Research (DZD), Neuherberg, Germany
Department of Diagnostic and Interventional Radiology, Section on Experimental Radiology, Eberhard Karls University Tübingen, Tübingen, Germany

Mika Scheler and Lucia Berti
German Centre for Diabetes Research (DZD), Neuherberg, Germany
Institute of Experimental Genetics, Helmholtz Centre Munich, German Research Centre for Environmental Health, Neuherberg, Germany

Martin Hrabĕ de Angelis
German Centre for Diabetes Research (DZD), Neuherberg, Germany
Institute of Experimental Genetics, Helmholtz Centre Munich, German Research Centre for Environmental Health, Neuherberg, Germany
Chair for Experimental Genetics, Technical University Munich, Freising, Germany

Anna Krook
Department of Physiology and Pharmacology, Karolinska Institute, Stockholm, Sweden

Ki-Chul Sung and Bum-Soo Kim
Division of Cardiology, Department of Medicine, Kangbuk Samsung Hospital, Sungkyunkwan University School of Medicine, Seoul, Republic of Korea

Jin-Ho Choi, Hyeon-Cheol Gwon and Seung-Hyuk Choi
Division of Cardiology, Cardiac and Vascular Center, Department of Medicine, Samsung Medical Center, Sungkyunkwan University School of Medicine, Seoul, Republic of Korea

Hyon Joo Kwag
Department of Radiology, Kangbuk Samsung Hospital Sungkyunkwan, University School of Medicine, Seoul, Republic of Korea

Sun H. Kim
Division of Endocrinology, Department of Medicine, Stanford University School of Medicine, Stanford, California, United States of America

Ji Hye Huh, Byung-Wan Lee, Eun Seok Kang, Bong Soo Cha and Hyun Chul Lee
Division of Endocrinology and Metabolism, Department of Internal Medicine, Yonsei University College of Medicine, Seoul, Korea

Kwang Joon Kim
Severance Executive Healthcare Clinic, Severance Hospital, Seoul, Korea,

Dong Wook Kim
Division of Medical Statistics, Yonsei University College of Medicine, Seoul, Korea

Md. Rafiqul Islam, John Attia, Mark McEvoy, Patrick McElduff, Roseanne Peel, Khanrin P. Vashum and Abul Hasnat Milton
Centre for Clinical Epidemiology and Biostatistics (CCEB), School of Medicine and Public Health, The University of Newcastle, New Lambton Heights, New South Wales, Australia

Ariful Basher
Department of Medicine, Mymensingh Medical College, Ministry of Health and Family Welfare, Government of Bangladesh, Mymensingh, Bangladesh

Iqbal Arslan and Waliur Rahman
Department of Biochemistry, Bangobondhu Sheikh Mujib Medical University (BSMMU), Dhaka, Bangladesh

Ayesha Akhter
Department of Obstetrics and Gynaecology, Tairunnessa Memorial Medical College, Gazipur, Dhaka, Bangladesh

Shahnaz Akter
Department of Paediatrics, Institute of Child and Mother Health (ICMH), Dhaka, Bangladesh

Henry Jansen, Anneke Hijmans and Cees J. Tack
Department of Medicine, Radboud University Medical Centre, Nijmegen, The Netherlands

Peter van Essen and Janna A. van Diepen
Department of Medicine, Radboud University Medical Centre, Nijmegen, The Netherlands
Institute for Genomic and Metabolic Disease, Radboud University Medical Centre, Nijmegen, The Netherlands

Dov B. Ballak
Department of Medicine, Radboud University Medical Centre, Nijmegen, The Netherlands
Institute for Genomic and Metabolic Disease, Radboud University Medical Centre, Nijmegen, The Netherlands
Nijmegen Institute for Infection Inflammation and Immunity, Radboud University Medical Centre, Nijmegen, The Netherlands

Rinke Stienstra
Department of Medicine, Radboud University Medical Centre, Nijmegen, The Netherlands
Institute for Genomic and Metabolic Disease, Radboud University Medical Centre, Nijmegen, The Netherlands
Department of Human Nutrition, Wageningen University and Research Centre, Wageningen, The Netherlands

Mihai G. Netea and Leo A. B. Joosten
Department of Medicine, Radboud University Medical Centre, Nijmegen, The Netherlands
Nijmegen Institute for Infection Inflammation and Immunity, Radboud University Medical Centre, Nijmegen, The Netherlands

Tetsuya Matsuguchi
Department of Oral Biochemistry, Field of Developmental Medicine, Kagoshima University, Graduate School of Medical and Dental Sciences, Sakuragaoka, Kagoshima, Japan

Helmut Sparrer
Novartis Pharma AG, Basel, Switzerland

Farrell Cahill, Mariam Shahidi, Jennifer Shea, Danny Wadden, Wayne Gulliver, Sudesh Vasdev and Guang Sun
Division of Medicine, Faculty of Medicine, Memorial University of Newfoundland, St. John's, Canada,

Edward Randell
Discipline of Laboratory Medicine, Faculty of Medicine, Memorial University of Newfoundland, St. John's, Canada

Kristína Simon Klenovics
Department of Clinical and Experimental Pharmacotherapy, Medical Faculty, Slovak Medical University, Bratislava, Slovakia
Institute of Physiology, Medical Faculty, Comenius University, Bratislava, Slovakia

Katarína Šebeková
Department of Clinical and Experimental Pharmacotherapy, Medical Faculty, Slovak Medical University, Bratislava, Slovakia
Institute of Molecular BioMedicine, Medical Faculty, Comenius University, Bratislava, Slovakia

Peter Celec
Institute of Molecular BioMedicine, Medical Faculty, Comenius University, Bratislava, Slovakia

Peter Boor
Institute of Molecular BioMedicine, Medical Faculty, Comenius University, Bratislava, Slovakia
Division of Nephrology and Institute of Pathology, RWTH University of Aachen, Aachen, Germany

Veronika Somoza
German Research Center for Food Chemistry, Garching, Germany
Department of Nutritional and Physiological Chemistry, University of Vienna, Vienna, Austria

Vincenzo Fogliano
Department of Food Science, University of Naples Federico II, Naples, Italy

Petronella E. Deetman, Stephan J. L. Bakker, Arjan J. Kwakernaak, Gerjan Navis and Robin P. F. Dullaart
Department of Internal Medicine, University of Groningen, University Medical Center Groningen, The Netherlands

Qing-Qing Yin, Ding-Zhen Luo, Si-Qing Dong and Meng-Han Sun
Department of Senile Neurology, Provincial Hospital Affiliated to Shandong University, Jinan, Shandong, P. R. China

Xue-Ping Liu
Department of Senile Neurology, Provincial Hospital Affiliated to Shandong University, Jinan, Shandong, P. R. China
Department of Anti-Ageing, Provincial Hospital Affiliated to Shandong University, Jinan, Shandong, P. R. China

Jin-Jing Pei
Department of KI-Alzheimer Disease Research Center, Karolinska Institutet, Stockholm, Sweden,

Song Xu and Zhi- Jian Sun
Department of Anti-Ageing, Provincial Hospital Affiliated to Shandong University, Jinan, Shandong, P. R. China

Li You
Department of Central Lab, Provincial Hospital Affiliated to Shandong University, Jinan, Shandong, P. R. China

Dalong Zhu, Yan Bi and Donghui Yang
Department of Endocrinology, Nanjing Drum Tower Hospital, Nanjing University School of Medicine, Nanjing, China

Ran Meng
Department of Endocrinology, Nanjing Drum Tower Hospital, Nanjing University School of Medicine, Nanjing, China
Department of Medical Genetics, Nanjing University School of Medicine, Nanjing, China
Jiangsu Key Laboratory of Molecular Medicine, Nanjing University, Nanjing, China

Yaping Wang
Department of Medical Genetics, Nanjing University School of Medicine, Nanjing, China
Jiangsu Key Laboratory of Molecular Medicine, Nanjing University, Nanjing, China

John A. Corbin, Vinay Bhaskar, Daniel H. Bedinger, Angela Lau, Kristen Michelson, Lisa M. Gross, Hua F. Kuan, Catarina Tran, Llewelyn Lao, Masahisa Handa, Susan R. Watson, Ajay J. Narasimha, Shirley Zhu, Raphael Levy, Lynn Webster, Sujeewa D. Wijesuriya, Naichi Liu, Xiaorong Wu, David Chemla-Vogel, Steve R. Lee, Steve Wong, Diane Wilcock and Mark L. White
Department of Preclinical Research, XOMA Corporation, Berkeley, California, United States of America

Ira D. Goldfine and Betty A. Maddux
Department of Medicine, University of California San Francisco, San Francisco, California, United States of America

Baojun Yuan, Yue Dai and Gaolin Wu
Department of Nutrition and Food Hygiene, Jiangsu Provincial Center for Disease Control and Prevention, Nanjing, China

Hui Zuo
Department of Nutrition and Food Hygiene, Jiangsu Provincial Center for Disease Control and Prevention, Nanjing, China
Department of Community Medicine, Institute of Health and Society, Faculty of Medicine, University of Oslo, Oslo, Norway

Akhtar Hussain
Department of Community Medicine, Institute of Health and Society, Faculty of Medicine, University of Oslo, Oslo, Norway

Zumin Shi
Discipline of Medicine, University of Adelaide, Adelaide, Australia

Jacqueline L. Beaudry, Emily C. Dunford, Trevor Teich, Dessi Zaharieva and Michael C. Riddell
School of Kinesiology and Health Science, Faculty of Health, Muscle Health Research Center and Physical Activity and Chronic Disease Unit, York University, Toronto, Ontario, Canada

Hazel Hunt and Joseph K. Belanoff
Corcept Therapeutics, Menlo Park, California, United States of America

Leonardo B. Leiria, José M. Dora, Simone M. Wajner, Aline A. F. Estivalet, Daisy Crispim and Ana Luiza Maia
Thyroid Section, Endocrine Division, Hospital de Clínicas de Porto Alegre, Universidade Federal do Rio Grande do Sul, Porto Alegre, RS, Brazil

Mathias Rask-Andersen, Gaëtan Philippot, Robert Fredriksson and Helgi B. Schiöth
Department of Neuroscience, Functional Pharmacology, Uppsala University, BMC, Uppsala, Sweden

George Moschonis, George Dedoussis and YannisManios
Department of Nutrition and Dietetics, Harokopio University, Athens, Greece

Claude Marcus
Department for Clinical Science, Intervention and Technology, Karolinska Institutet, Division of Pediatrics, National Childhood Obesity Centre, Stockholm, Sweden

Klaus Straßburger, Roshan Livingstone, Kathrin Keßel and Jong-Hee Hwang
Institute for Clinical Diabetology, German Diabetes Center at Heinrich-Heine University, Düsseldorf, Germany

Sabine Kahl and Bettina Nowotny
Institute for Clinical Diabetology, German Diabetes Center at Heinrich-Heine University, Düsseldorf, Germany
Department of Endocrinology and Diabetology, Heinrich-Heine University Düsseldorf, Düsseldorf, Germany

Michael Roden
Institute for Clinical Diabetology, German Diabetes Center at Heinrich-Heine University, Düsseldorf, Germany
Department of Endocrinology and Diabetology, Heinrich-Heine University Düsseldorf, Düsseldorf, Germany
German Center for Diabetes Research, Partner Düsseldorf, Germany

Birgit Klüppelholz and Guido Giani
Institute for Biometrics and Epidemiology, German Diabetes Center at Heinrich-Heine University, Düsseldorf, Germany

Barbara Hoffmann
IUF – Leibniz Research Institute for Environmental Medicine, Düsseldorf, Germany

Giovanni Pacini
National Research Council, Institute of Biomedical Engineering, Metabolic Unit, Padova, Italy

Amalia Gastaldelli
National Research Council, Institute of Clinical Physiology, Pisa, Italy

Bo-Mi Song
Department of Public Health, Graduate School of Yonsei University, Seoul, Korea

Dong Phil Choi
Department of Public Health, Graduate School of Yonsei University, Seoul, Korea
Cardiovascular and Metabolic Diseases Etiology Research Center, Yonsei University College of Medicine, Seoul, Korea

Sun Min Oh, Ju-Mi Lee, Hye Min Cho and Won Joon Lee
Department of Preventive Medicine, Yonsei University College of Medicine, Seoul, Korea

Hyeon Chang Kim
Department of Preventive Medicine, Yonsei University College of Medicine, Seoul, Korea
Cardiovascular and Metabolic Diseases Etiology Research Center, Yonsei University College of Medicine, Seoul, Korea

Yumie Rhee
Department of Internal Medicine, Yonsei University College of Medicine, Seoul, Korea

Anna Halama
Helmholtz Zentrum München, German Research Center for Environmental Health, Institute of Experimental Genetics, Genome Analysis Center, Neuherberg, Germany

Anja Böhm, Cora Weigert, Hans-Ulrich Häring and Harald Staiger
Helmholtz Zentrum München, German Research Center for Environmental Health, Institute of Experimental Genetics, Genome Analysis Center, Neuherberg, Germany
Department of Internal Medicine IV, Division of Endocrinology, Diabetology, Angiology, Nephrology, and Clinical Chemistry, University Hospital, Eberhard Karls University, Tübingen, Germany
German Center for Diabetes Research, Neuherberg, Germany
Institute for Diabetes Research and Metabolic Diseases of the HelmholtzCenter München at the Eberhard Karls University of Tübingen, Tübingen, Germany

Martin Hrabě de Angelis and Jerzy Adamski
Helmholtz Zentrum München, German Research Center for Environmental Health, Institute of Experimental Genetics, Genome Analysis Center, Neuherberg, Germany
German Center for Diabetes Research, Neuherberg, Germany
Chair of Experimental Genetics, Technical University München, Freising-Weihenstephan, Germany

Rainer Lehmann, Andreas Fritsche and Norbert Stefan
Department of Internal Medicine IV, Division of Endocrinology, Diabetology, Angiology, Nephrology, and Clinical Chemistry, University Hospital, Eberhard Karls University, Tübingen, Germany
German Center for Diabetes Research, Neuherberg, Germany
Institute for Diabetes Research and Metabolic Diseasues of the HelmholtzCenter München at the Eberhard Karls University of Tübingen, Tübingen, Germany

Tobias Meile, Marty Zdichavsky and Alfred Königsrainer
Department of General, Visceral and Transplant Surgery, University Hospital, Eberhard Karls University, Tübingen, Germany

Ying Li and Changhao Sun
Department of Nutrition and Food Hygiene, Public Health College, Harbin Medical University, Harbin, Heilongjiang, People's Republic of China

Yonghan He
Department of Nutrition and Food Hygiene, Public Health College, Harbin Medical University, Harbin, Heilongjiang, People's Republic of China
Aquatic and Crop Resource Development, Life Sciences Branch, National Research Council Canada, Charlottetown, Prince Edward Island, Canada
State Key Laboratory of Genetic Resources and Evolution, Kunming Institute of Zoology, Chinese Academy of Sciences, Kunming, Yunnan, People's Republic of China

Shuocheng Zhang and Yanwen Wang
Aquatic and Crop Resource Development, Life Sciences Branch, National Research Council Canada, Charlottetown, Prince Edward Island, Canada
Department of Biomedical Sciences, University of Prince Edward Island, Charlottetown, Prince Edward Island, Canada

Wen Li
Department of Endocrinology, Third People's Hospital of Yunnan Province, Kunming, Yunnan, People's Republic of China

Index

www.ingramcontent.com/pod-product-compliance
Lightning Source LLC
Chambersburg PA
CBHW080647200326

41458CB00013B/4759